Law, Ethics, and Policy in Healthcare Administration

Joel Teitelbaum and George Pozgar

JONES & BARTLETT
LEARNING

World Headquarters
Jones & Bartlett Learning
5 Wall Street
Burlington, MA 01803
978-443-5000
info@jblearning.com
www.jblearning.com

Jones & Bartlett Learning books and products are available through most bookstores and online booksellers. To contact Jones & Bartlett Learning directly, call 800-832-0034, fax 978-443-8000, or visit our website, www.jblearning.com.

This book is produced through PUBLISH – a custom publishing service offered by Jones & Bartlett Learning. For more information on PUBLISH, contact us at 800-832-0034 or visit our website at www.jblearning.com.

Disclaimer

This publication is sold with the understanding that the publisher is not engaged in rendering medical, legal, accounting, or other professional services. If medical, legal, accounting, or other professional service advice is required, the service of a competent professional should be sought. The authors, editor, and publisher have designed this publication to provide accurate information with regard to the subject matter covered. However, they are not responsible for errors, omissions, or for any outcomes related to the use of the contents of this publication and make no guarantee and assume no responsibility or liability for the use of the products and procedures described, or the correctness, sufficiency, or completeness of stated information, opinions, or recommendations. Treatments and side effects described in this publication are not applicable to all people; required dosages and experienced side effects will vary among individuals. Drugs and medical devices discussed herein are controlled by the Food and Drug Administration (FDA) and may have limited availability for use only in research studies or clinical trials. Research, clinical practice, and government regulations often change accepted standards. When consideration is being given to the use of any drug in the clinical setting, the health care provider or reader is responsible for determining FDA status of the drug, reading the package insert, and reviewing prescribing information for the most current recommendations on dose, precautions, and contraindications and for determining the appropriate usage for the product. This is especially important in the case of drugs that are new or seldom used. Any references in this publication to procedures to be employed when rendering emergency care to the sick and injured are provided solely as a general guide; other or additional safety measures might be required under particular circumstances. This publication is not intended as a statement of the standards of care required in any particular situation; circumstances and the physical conditions of patients can vary widely from one emergency to another. This publication is not intended in any way to advise emergency personnel concerning their legal authority to perform the activities or procedures discussed. Such local determination should be made only with the aid of legal counsel. Some images in this publication feature models; these models do not necessarily endorse, represent, or participate in the activities represented in the images.

Cover Image: © Photos.com

6048
Printed in the United States of America
16 15 14 13 12   10 9 8 7 6 5 4 3 2 1

Contents

INTRODUCTION TO ETHICS

I expect to pass through this world but once. Any good therefore that I can do, or any kindness I can show to any creature, let me do it now. Let me not defer it, for I shall not pass this way again.

–STEPHEN GRELLET

LEARNING OBJECTIVES

Upon completion of this chapter, the reader will be able to:

- Explain what ethics is, its importance, and its application to ethical dilemmas.
- Describe the concepts of morality, codes of conduct, and moral judgments.
- Understand relevant ethical theories and principles.
- Describe virtue ethics and values and how they more clearly describe one's moral character.

- Understand how religious ethics can affect one's moral character.
- Explain the concept of situational ethics and how changes in circumstances can alter one's behavior.
- Understand the importance of reasoning in the decision-making process.

INTRODUCTION

Good can triumph over evil.

—AUTHOR UNKNOWN

This chapter provides the reader with an overview of ethics, moral principles, virtues, and values. The intent here is not to burden the reader with the philosophical arguments surrounding ethical theories, morals, and principles; however, as with the study of any new subject, "words are the tools of thought." The reader who thoroughly absorbs and applies the content of the theories and principles of ethics discussed herein will have the tools necessary to empathize with and guide patients through the conflicts they will face when making difficult care decisions. Therefore, some new vocabulary is a necessary tool, as a building block for the reader to establish a foundation for applying the abstract theories and principles of ethics in order to make practical use of them.

Theories, principles, virtues, and values are a necessary beginning point for the study of ethics. Words are merely labels for ideas and best used for helping the reader to wire his or her mind to think through difficult dilemmas more easily. The directions on a map are of little value until we make the journey. So it is with ethics; we must begin to make the journey inward with a lot of hard mind work so that we can more easily make the right decisions when faced with ethical dilemmas. The learning process for ethics becomes a more enjoyable and rewarding journey as we grasp the ideas, build upon them, and practice all the good we learn by helping all the people we can as long as we can.

ETHICS

How we perceive right and wrong is influenced by what we feed on.

—AUTHOR UNKNOWN

Ethics is the branch of philosophy that seeks to understand the nature, purposes, justification, and founding principles of moral rules and the systems they comprise. Ethics and morals are derivatives from the Greek and Latin terms (roots) for custom. The etymology of the words "ethics" and "morality" are derived from the roots "ethos" and "mos," which both convey a meaning describing customs or habits. This etymology supports the claims of anthropologist Ruth Benedict that all values are rooted in customs and habits of a culture because the words moral and ethics themselves were essentially created to describe these topics.[1]

Ethics deals with values relating to human conduct. It focuses on the rightness and wrongness of actions, as well as the goodness and badness of motives and ends. Ethics encompasses the decision-making process of determining ultimate actions—what should I do and is it the right thing to do. It involves how individuals decide to live with one another within accepted boundaries and how they live in harmony with the environment as well as one another. Ethics is concerned with human conduct as it ought to be, as opposed to what it actually is.

Microethics involves an individual's view of what is right and wrong based on one's personal life teachings, tradition, and experiences. *Macroethics* involves a more global view of right and wrong. Although no person lives in a vacuum, solving ethical dilemmas involves consideration of ethical issues from both a micro and macro perspective.

Man's duty is to improve himself; to cultivate his mind; and, when he finds himself going astray, to bring the moral law to bear upon himself.

—IMMANUEL KANT

The term *ethics* is used in three distinct but related ways, signifying (1) *philosophical ethics*, which involves inquiry about ways of life and rules of conduct; (2) a *general pattern or way of life*, such as religious ethics (e.g., Judeo-Christian ethics); and (3) a *set of rules* of conduct or "moral code" (e.g., professional codes for ethical behavior).

The scope of health care ethics encompasses numerous issues, including the right to choose or refuse treatment and the right to limit the suffering one will endure. Incredible advances in technology and the resulting capability to extend life beyond what would be considered a reasonable quality of life have complicated the process of health care decision making. The scope of health care ethics is not limited to philosophical issues but embraces economic, medical, political, social, and legal dilemmas.

Bioethics addresses such difficult issues as the nature of life, the nature of death, what sort of life is worth living, what constitutes murder, how we should treat people who are especially vulnerable, and the responsibilities that we have to other human beings. It is about making better decisions when faced with diverse and complex circumstances.

WHY STUDY ETHICS?

We study ethics to help us make sound judgments, good decisions, and right choices; if not right choices, then better choices. To those in the health care industry, it is about anticipating and recognizing health care dilemmas and making good judgments and decisions based on universal values that work in unison with the laws of the land and our constitution. Where the law remains silent, we rely on the ability of caregivers to make sound judgments, guided by the Wisdom of Solomon to do good. Doing the right thing by applying the universal morals and values described in this text (e.g., the 10 Commandments) will help shield and protect all from harm.

MORALITY

The three hardest tasks in the world are neither physical feats nor intellectual achievements, but moral acts: to return love for hate, to include the excluded, and to say, "I was wrong."

—SYDNEY J. HARRIS

The following news clippings portray how a deficiency in the morality of society can lead to a betrayal of humanity. Lawlessness and heartless actions run rampant in a land void of courage and compassion. The reader who thoroughly absorbs, understands, and practices the virtues and values discussed in the pages that follow will spring forth hope in what often seems a desperate and hopeless world.

Vietnam—Terror of War

Fire rained down on civilians. Women and children ran screaming. Ut snapped pictures. A little girl ran toward him, arms outstretched, eyes shut in pain, clothes burned off by Napalm. She said, "Too hot, please help me!"

1973 Spot News, Newseum, *Washington, DC*

Ethiopian Famine (1985 Feature)

People searched everywhere for food. Some 30,000 tons of it, from the United States, had been held up by an Ethiopian government determined to starve the countryside into submission. And starve the people it did—half a million Ethiopians, many of them children so hungry their bodies actually consumed themselves.

I'll never forget the sounds of kids dying of starvation.

Newseum, *Washington, DC*

Waiting Game for Sudanese Child . . .

Carter's winning photo shows a heartbreaking scene of a starving child collapsed on the ground, struggling to get to a food center during a famine in the Sudan in 1993. In the background, a vulture stalks the emaciated child.

Carter was part of a group of four fearless photojournalists known as the "Bang Bang Club" who traveled throughout South Africa capturing the atrocities committed during apartheid.

Haunted by the horrific images from Sudan, Carter committed suicide in 1994 soon after receiving the award.

A Pulitzer-Winning Photographer's Suicide, National Public Radio, (NPR), *March 2, 2006*

Trek of tears describes many horrible historic events, from broken treaties with American Indians to an African Journey of horror, where people would flee together as a village to escape the barbaric slaughter of men, women, and children as the remainder of the world stood cowardly by watching the death and starvation of hundreds of thousands of people. Human atrocities committed by humans. Is it not time to stand up and be counted on to do what is right and leave all excuses behind for our complacency toward the genocide that continues throughout the world?

–GP

There are those who have been brainwashed into believing, in the name of religion, that if they blow themselves up in public places, killing innocent people, that they will be rewarded in the afterlife. This is not religion and it is not culture; it is evil people brainwashing young minds to do evil things.

–GP

Aim above morality. Be not simply good; be good for something.

–HENRY DAVID THOREAU

Morality describes a class of rules held by society to govern the conduct of its individual members. It implies the quality of being in accord with standards of right and good conduct. Morality is a code of conduct. It is a guide to behavior that all rational persons should put forward for governing their behavior. Morality requires us to reach a decision as to the rightness or wrongness of an action. *Morals* are ideas about what is right and what is wrong; for example, killing is wrong, whereas helping the poor is right, and causing pain is wrong, whereas easing pain is right. Morals are deeply ingrained in culture and religion and are often part of its identity. Morals should not be confused with religious or cultural habits or customs, such as wearing a religious garment (e.g., veil, turban). That which is considered morally right can vary from nation to nation, culture to culture, and religion to religion. In other words, there is no universal morality that is recognized by all people in all cultures at all times.

CODE OF CONDUCT

A *code of conduct* generally prescribes standards of conduct, states principles expressing responsibilities, and defines the rules expressing duties of professionals to whom they apply. Most members of a profession subscribe to certain "values" and moral standards written into a formal document called a code of ethics. Codes of conduct often require interpretation by caregivers as they apply to the specific circumstances surrounding each dilemma.

Michael D. Bayles, a famous author and teacher, describes the differences between standards, principles, and rules:

- *Standards* (e.g., honesty, respect for others, conscientiousness) are used to guide human conduct by stating desirable traits to be exhibited and undesirable ones (dishonesty, deceitfulness, self-interest) to be avoided.
- *Principles* describe responsibilities that do not specify what the required conduct should be. Professionals need to make a judgment about what is desirable in a particular situation based on accepted principles.
- *Rules* specify specific conduct; they do not allow for individual professional judgment.

MORAL JUDGMENTS

Moral judgments are those judgments concerned with what an individual or group believes to be the right or proper behavior in a given situation. Making a moral judgment is being able to choose an option from among choices. It involves assessing another person's moral character based on how he or she conforms to the moral convictions established by the individual and/or group. A lack of conformity can result in moral disapproval and possibly ridicule of one's character.

MORALITY LEGISLATED

When it is important that disagreements be settled, morality is often legislated. Law is distinguished from morality by having explicit rules and penalties, as well as officials who interpret the laws and apply penalties when laws are broken. There is often considerable overlap in the conduct governed by morality and that governed by law. Laws are created to set boundaries for societal behavior. They are enforced to ensure that the expected behavior happens.

MORAL DILEMMAS

Moral dilemmas in the health care setting often arise when values, rights, duties, and loyalties conflict. Caregivers often find that there appears to be no right or wrong answer when faced with the daunting task of deciding which decision path to follow. The best answer when attempting to resolve an ethical dilemma includes the known wishes of the patient and other pertinent information, such as a living will, that might be available when the patient is considered incompetent to make his or her own choices. The right answer is often elusive when the patient is in a coma and there are no known documents as to a patient's wishes and there are no living relatives. However, an understanding of the concepts presented here will help the caregiver in resolving complex ethical dilemmas.

ETHICAL THEORIES

Ethics, too, are nothing but reverence for life. This is what gives me the fundamental principle of morality, namely, that good consists in maintaining, promoting, and enhancing life, and that destroying, injuring, and limiting life are evil.

—ALBERT SCHWEITZER

Ethics seeks to understand and to determine how human actions can be judged as right or wrong. Ethical judgments can be made based on our own experiences or based upon the nature of or principles of reason.

Ethical theories and principles introduce order into the way people think about life. They are the foundations of ethical analysis and provide guidance in the decision-making process. Various theories present varying viewpoints that assist caregivers in making difficult decisions when faced with ethical dilemmas that affect the lives of others. The more commonly discussed ethical theories are presented here.

Metaethics is the study of the origin and meaning of ethical concepts. Metaethics seeks to understand ethical terms and theories and their application. "Metaethics explores as well the connection between values, reasons for action, and human motivation, asking how it is that moral standards might provide us with reasons to do or refrain from doing as it demands,

6

and it addresses many of the issues commonly bound up with the nature of freedom and its significance (or not) for moral responsibility."[2]

NORMATIVE ETHICS

Normative ethics is prescriptive in that it attempts to determine what moral standards should be followed so that human behavior and conduct may be morally right. Normative ethics is primarily concerned with establishing standards or norms for conduct and is commonly associated with investigating how one ought to act. It involves the critical study of major moral precepts, such as what things are right, what things are good, and what things are genuine. One of the central questions of modern normative ethics is whether human actions are to be judged right or wrong solely according to their consequences.

The determination of a universal moral principle for all humanity is a formidable task and most likely not feasible due to the diversity of people and their cultures. However, there is a need to have a commonly held consensus as to right and wrong to avoid chaos. Thus, there are generally accepted moral standards around which laws are drafted.

Normative Ethics and Assisted Suicide

Oregon's Death with Dignity Act of 1997 allows terminally ill state residents to end their lives through the voluntary self-administration of a lethal dose of medications prescribed by a physician.[3] Although this act was voted upon by the Oregon state legislature and agreed upon by referendum, there are those who disagree with the law from a religious or moral standpoint. The Oregon act is controversial at best and has placed morality and the law in conflict. In the middle of the continuing controversy is the terminally ill patient who must make the ultimate decision of life versus death. It could be argued that it is morally wrong to take one's own life regardless of the law or it can be argued that ending one's life is a morally permissible right because the law provides the opportunity for terminally ill patients to make end-of-life decisions that include the right to self-administer a lethal dose of medications.

As there is a diversity of cultures, there is diversity of opinions as to the rightness and wrongness of the Oregon act. From a microethics point of view as it relates to the Oregon law, each individual must decide what is the right thing to do.

Normative ethics prescribes how people should act and descriptive ethics describes how people act. Both theories have application in the Oregon act. The controversial nature of physician-assisted suicide in the various states is but one of many health care dilemmas caregivers will experience during their careers (e.g., abortion, euthanasia).

DESCRIPTIVE ETHICS

Descriptive ethics, also known as comparative ethics, is the study of what people believe to be right and wrong and why they believe it. Descriptive ethics describes how people act, whereas normative ethics prescribes how people ought to act.

APPLIED ETHICS

Applied ethics is "the philosophical search (within western philosophy) for right and wrong within controversial scenarios."[4] *Applied ethics* is the application of normative theories to practical moral problems, such as abortion, euthanasia, and assisted suicide.

CONSEQUENTIAL ETHICS

The end excuses any evil.

—Sophocles, *Electra* (c. 409 B.C.)

The *consequential theory* of ethics emphasizes that the morally right action is whatever action leads to the maximum balance of good over evil. From a contemporary standpoint, theories that judge actions by their consequences have been referred to as consequential ethics. Consequential ethical theories revolve around the premise that the rightness or wrongness of an action depends on the consequences or effects of an action. The theory of consequential ethics is based on the view that the value of an action derives solely from the value of its consequences. The consequentialist considers the morally right act or failure to act is one that will produce a good outcome. The goal of a consequentialist is to achieve the greatest good for the greatest number. It involves asking such questions as:

- What will be the effects of each course of action?
- Who will benefit?
- What action will cause the least harm?
- What action will lead to the greatest good?

These questions should be applied when answering the questions in the following *reality check*.

No Good Deed Goes Unpunished

Matt was assigned to survey "Community Medical Center" (CMC) in Minnesota with a team of three surveyors and one observer. He related to me his experience of surveying the children's dental clinic.

Following his tour of CMC's dental clinic, Matt reviewed with the clinic's staff the dental program, which served the city's underserved children. He also reviewed the care rendered several patients based on common and complex diagnoses, as well as the clinic's performance improvement activities. During the survey Dr. Seiden, the clinic director asked, "Are surveyors trained about the importance of dental care in disease prevention? As you know, dentistry is often a stepchild when it comes to allocation of scarce resources. Departments like surgery and radiology often receive the lion's share of funds." Matt responded by describing a film sponsored by the American Dental Association that was shown when he was in training to become a surveyor. The film presented a man whose dental care had been sorely neglected throughout his life and not been addressed prior to replacement of a heart valve. The patient developed a systemic infection following surgery, which led to deterioration of the heart valve and the patient's ultimate death. The film described the lessons learned and opportunities for performance improvement that included the need for a dental evaluation by a dentist prior to valve replacement. Dr. Seiden was pleased to learn that the importance of dentistry is included in surveyor training.

Following Matt's survey of the dental clinic, the staff relayed to him their concern that the clinic was going to be closed for lack of funds. Cheryl, the clinic manager, explained, "I sometimes feel the importance of the dental clinic to the underserved population is not well-understood." A bit emotional, Cheryl said, "Matt, have you surveyed other dental clinics?" Matt replied, "Yes, several well-funded clinics that come to mind were in Philadelphia and New York." Cheryl then asked, "Matt, do you have any ideas as to how we can save our clinic from closing?" Matt replied, "I have some time before lunch and I can share a few ideas with you." Cheryl replied, "The staff will be eager to listen." The staff proceeded to place several chairs in a semicircle and brainstormed with Matt a variety of ideas for saving the clinic. The staff discussed several fund-raising activities including a car wash by children to bring awareness to Any Town's dental clinic." Matt looked at his watch and said, "I need to get back to my survey team, but I want to leave you with one other thought to ponder that could be applicable to any department in the hospital. I was surveying a veteran's hospital physical therapy department and noticed on their bulletin board the staff's dream plan for renovation of their department. I asked the physical therapy staff about the plan. They related how their vision of a new physical therapy department had been sketched out and placed on their bulletin board. Several weeks later, a veteran who had been sitting in the waiting area became curious about their dream. After studying the board during his visits for therapy, he walked to the reception desk on his last visit and asked about their vision for physical therapy. They explained it was a $200,000 dream. Gary looked at the staff at the reception desk and said, "It is no longer a dream. I don't have much, but what I do have is enough to make your dream come true." And, so he did. Matt continued, "You see, if people know your dreams, something as small as a bulletin board can make all the difference." Dr. Seiden smiled and said, "I see where this is going, community awareness as to the need to fund the clinic. It's really not merely about a car wash, it's about a concept of how the hospital can save not only the dental clinic but other programs earmarked for closing." Matt smiled, as the staff regained hope. Dr. Seiden, seeing that Matt had little time for lunch, stood up, extended his hand and said, "Matt, you gave us hope when we believed there was none. Thank you so much. I will be sure to discuss this with administration."

Matt presented his observations the following morning to the organization's leadership, which included his round table discussion with the staff. He was however cut short in his presentation by the surveyor team leader, Brad, who later reported to Victor, Matt's manager, that Matt should not be discussing how to save a dental clinic by opening a car wash. Matt received a reprimand from Victor and was removed at the end of day 4 of a 5-day survey without explanation.

Anonymous

Discussion

1. Discuss Matt's approach to addressing the staff's concerns for saving the children's dental clinic.
2. If Matt's round table session led to saving the clinic, was Matt's reprimand worth the risk if he could have foreseen the resulting reprimand?
3. The goal of a consequentialist is to achieve the greatest good for the greatest number. Discuss how this applies in this *reality check*.

Happiness often sneaks in a door you did not think was open.

−Author Unknown

The utilitarian theory of ethics involves the concept that the moral worth of an action is determined solely by its contribution to overall usefulness. It describes doing the greatest good for the most people. It is thus a form of consequential ethics, meaning that the moral worth of an action is determined by its outcome, and, thus, the ends justify the means. The utilitarian commonly holds that the proper course of an action is one that maximizes utility, commonly defined as maximizing happiness and reducing suffering, as noted in the following *reality check*.

Maximizing Happiness and Reducing Suffering

Daniel was the last of five interviews for the CEO's position at Anytown Medical Center. During the interview, a member of the finance committee asked, "Daniel, how would maximize an allocation of $100,000 to spend as you wished for improving patient care, aside from capital budget and construction projects?" Bishop Paul, the board chairman added, "Daniel, think about the question. I will give you five minutes to form an answer." Daniel responded, "Bishop Paul, I am ready now to answer your question." The trustees looked somewhat surprised, as Bishop Paul with a smile quickly responded, "You may proceed with your answer." Daniel replied, "An old Chinese proverb came to mind as quickly as the question was asked: 'Give a man a fish and you feed him for a day. Teach a man to fish and you feed him for a lifetime.' You are interviewing me as CEO of your hospital. I see my job as assuring you that employees are thoroughly trained to care for the patients the hospital serves. I will maximize the value of each and every dollar by determining the staff skill sets that are lacking and retrain staff in the areas deficiencies are noted." Bishop Paul looked around the long oval table at the trustees, "This has been a long day and a grueling interview process for Daniel. Are there any other questions you would like to ask him." There was silence, as the trustees nodded their heads no. Bishop Paul looked at Daniel and thanked him for his interest in becoming the hospital's next CEO.

As Daniel began to leave the boardroom, Bishop Paul smiled and turned his swivel chair around as Daniel was walking towards the exit and asked, "Daniel, could you not leave the building just yet. If you could, just wait outside the room and have a seat in the doctors' lounge area." After about 20 minutes, a trustee went into the lounge where Daniel was sitting and asked him to return to the boardroom. As he entered the room, Bishop Paul stood up and looked at Daniel straight in his eyes and said, "Daniel, you were the last to be interviewed because you were on the 'short list' of candidates selected to be interviewed. Speaking for the board, your response to the last question was merely icing on the cake confirming our interest in you joining our staff. Both the Board of Trustees and members of the Medical Executive Committee unanimously have recommended you as our CEO, with which I unconditionally concur! Welcome to Anytown hospital." The trustees stood and clapped their hands. The bishop turned to the trustees and said, "Wow, that's a first."

Anonymous

Discussion

1. Discuss how Daniel's response to the trustee's question of how he would spend the $100,000 fits the utilitarian theory of ethics.
2. Did Daniel, metaphorically speaking, succeed in maximizing happiness in the eyes of the board? Discuss your answer.

DEONTOLOGICAL ETHICS

Act in such a way that you always treat humanity, whether in your own person or in the person of any other, never simply as a means, but always at the same time as an end.

–IMMANUEL KANT

Deontological ethics is commonly attributed to the German philosopher Immanuel Kant (1724–1804). Kant believed that although doing the right thing is good, it might not always lead to or increase the good and right thing sought after. It focuses on one's duties to others and others' rights. It includes telling the truth and keeping your promises. Deontology ethics is often referred to as duty-based ethics. It involves ethical analysis according to a moral code or rules, religious or secular. *Deon* is derived from the Greek word meaning "duty." Kant's theory differs from consequentialism in that consequences are not the determinant of what is right; therefore, doing the right thing may not always lead to an increase in what is good.

> Duty-based approaches are heavy on obligation, in the sense that a person who follows this ethical paradigm believes that the highest virtue comes from doing what you are supposed to do—either because you have to, e.g., following the law, or because you agreed to, e.g., following an employer's policies. It matters little whether the act leads to good consequences; what matters is "doing your duty."[5]

The following *reality check* illustrates how duty-based ethics focuses on the act and not the consequences of an act.

Duty Compromises Patient Care

At 33 years of age, I was the youngest administrator in New York State and was about to learn that adhering to company policy sometimes conflicts with the needs of the patient. In this case it was a 38-year-old employee who had been diagnosed with cancer. I remember the day well, even though it was more than 30 years ago. My secretary alerted me that Carol, a practical nurse and employee, had been admitted to the 3-North medical-surgical unit, where she worked. Without delay, I left my office and went to the nursing unit and inquired as to what room Carol was in. Beth, the unit's nurse manager, overheard my question. She walked up to me and asked, "Daniel, could I please talk to you for a moment before you visit with Carol?" I looked at her and nodded my head yes and without thought we both walked to her office. She closed the door and said, "As you know, we are self-insured and the health insurance program we have does not cover Carol's chemotherapy treatments. She cannot bear the cost. Is there anything you can do to help her?" I replied that I would make an inquiry with our human resources director to see what could be done.

Beth asked, "Would you mind if I went with you to Carol's room for a few minutes." Daniel compassionately replied, "Of course you can."

They walked to Carol's room. Her husband and children had just left. Beth stayed for a few minutes while Daniel remained behind chatting with Carol for a few moments and said he would be back to talk with her more.

Daniel went to speak with Christine, the human resources director for his hospital. There were two other hospitals in the multihospital system. He explained Carol's financial situation and her lack of funds for chemotherapy treatment. Christine replied, "Daniel, this is corporate policy that is applicable to all three hospitals with which we must comply." Following much discussion, Daniel said, "Christine, Carol is an employee and I realize there are conflicting duties here. One is to follow corporate policy or choose to do, as I see it, what is right for Carol. If you prefer, I can request an exception to the rule. To me, right trumps duty." Christine looked at Daniel and said, "Daniel, I will see what I can do. I have a good relationship with the corporate vice president for human resources. If anyone can make an exception, he can make it happen. I know you would do the same for me and any other employee."

Anonymous

Discussion

1. Discuss the potential long-term effect of granting an exception for Carol.
2. Do you believe that duty should be trumped by good? Discuss your answer.
3. Would you describe Daniel as consequentialist because he favors evaluating the outcome of an act rather than the act itself? Discuss your answer.
4. Discuss how deontological ethics in this case is in conflict with consequential thinking.

NONCONSEQUENTIAL ETHICS

The *nonconsequential ethical theory* denies that the consequences of an action are the only criteria for determining the morality of an action. In this theory, the rightness or wrongness of an action is based on properties intrinsic to the action, not on its consequences. In other words, the nonconsequentialist believes right or wrong depends on the intention not the outcome.

Bad Outcome, Good Intentions

Chelsea was preparing to drape Mr. Smith's leg in OR 6 for surgery, when she was approached by Nicole, the nurse manager, asked, "Chelsea, please come to OR 3. We have an emergency there and urgently need your skills to assist the surgeon." Chelsea turned to Daniel, the surgical technician, and asked him to continue prepping Mr. Smith's leg for surgery. Daniel prepped the leg prior to the surgeon entering the room. The surgeon entered the room a few minutes later and asked, "Where is Chelsea?" Daniel replied, "She was called away for an emergency in OR 3. Karen will be in shortly to assist us."

Following surgery, Mr. Smith was transferred to the recovery room. While he was in the recovery room a nurse was looking at the patient's medical record as to the notes regarding the patient's procedure during surgery. She noticed that surgery was conducted on the wrong leg.

Although there was heated discussion between the surgeon and nursing staff, each member of the staff had good intentions but the outcome was not so good. Nonconsequentialists believe that right or wrong depends on the intention. They generally focus more on deeds and whether those deeds are good or bad. In this case the intentions were good but the outcome was bad. It should be noted that nonconsequentialists do not always ignore the consequences. They accept the fact that sometimes good intentions can lead to bad outcomes. In summary nonconsequentialists focus more on character as to whether someone is a good person or not. Nonconsequentialists believe that right or wrong depends on the intention. Generally, the consequentialist will focus more on outcomes as to whether or not they are good or bad.

Discussion

1. Describe how the nonconsequential theory of ethics applies in this case.
2. What questions might the consequentialist raise after reviewing the facts of this case?

ETHICAL RELATIVISM

The theory of *ethical relativism* holds that morality is relative to the norms of the culture in which an individual lives. In other words, right or wrong depends on the moral norms of the society in which it is practiced. A particular action by an individual may be morally right in one society or culture and wrong in another. What is acceptable in one society may not be considered as such in another. Slavery may be considered an acceptable practice in one society and unacceptable and unconscionable in another. The administration of blood may be acceptable as to one's religious beliefs and not acceptable to another within the same society. The legal rights of patients vary from state to state, as is well borne out, for example, by Oregon's Death with Dignity Act. Caregivers must be aware of cultural, religious, and legal issues that can affect the boundaries of what is acceptable and what is unacceptable practice, especially when delivering health care to persons with beliefs different from their own. As the various cultures of the world merge together in communities, the education and training of caregivers become more complex. The caregiver must not only grasp the clinical skills of his or her profession but also have a basic understanding of what is right and what is wrong from both a legal and ethical point of view. Although decision making is not always perfect, the knowledge gained from this text will aid the reader in making better decisions.

PRINCIPLES OF ETHICS

You cannot by tying an opinion to a man's tongue, make him the representative of that opinion; and at the close of any battle for principles, his name will be found neither among the dead, nor the wounded, but the missing.

—E.P. WHIPPLE (1819–1886)

An army of principles can penetrate where an army of soldiers cannot.

—Thomas Jefferson

Ethical principles are universal rules of conduct, derived from ethical theories that provide a practical basis for identifying what kinds of actions, intentions, and motives are valued. Ethical principles assist caregivers in making choices based on moral principles that have been identified as standards considered worthwhile in addressing health care–related ethical dilemmas. As noted by the principles discussed in the following sections, caregivers, in the study of ethics, will find that difficult decisions often involve choices between conflicting ethical principles.

AUTONOMY

No right is held more sacred, or is more carefully guarded, by the common law, than the right of every individual to the possession and control of his own person, free from all restraint or interference of others, unless by clear and unquestioned authority of law.

—Union Pacific Ry. Co. v. Botsford [141 U.S. 250, 251 (1891)]

The principle of *autonomy* involves recognizing the right of a person to make one's own decisions. "Auto" comes from a Greek word meaning "self" or the "individual." In this context, it means recognizing an individual's right to make his or her own decisions about what is best for him or herself. Autonomy is not an absolute principle. The autonomous actions of one person must not infringe upon the rights of another. The eminent Justice Benjamin Cardozo, in *Schloendorff v. Society of New York Hospital*, stated:

> Every human being of adult years and sound mind has a right to determine what shall be done with his own body and a surgeon who performs an operation without his patient's consent commits an assault, for which he is liable in damages, except in cases of emergency where the patient is unconscious and where it is necessary to operate before consent can be obtained.[6]

Each person has a right to make his or her own decisions about health care. A patient has the right to refuse to receive health care even if it is beneficial to saving his or her life. Patients can refuse treatment, refuse to take medications, and refuse invasive procedures regardless of the benefits that may be derived from them. They have a right to have their decisions adhered to by family members who may disagree simply because they are unable to let go. Although patients have a right to make their own choices, they also have a concomitant right to know the risks, benefits, and alternatives to recommended procedures.

Autonomous decision making can be affected by one's disabilities, mental status, maturity, or incapacity to make decisions. Although the principle of autonomy may be inapplicable in certain cases, one's autonomous wishes may be carried out through an advance directive and/or an appointed health care agent in the event of one's inability to make decisions.

What happens when the right to autonomy conflicts with other moral principles, such as beneficence and justice? Conflict can arise, for example, when a patient refuses a blood transfusion considered necessary to save his or her life whereas the caregiver's principal obligation is to do no harm. What is the right thing to do when the spouse decides to have the physician withhold from his wife her true diagnosis?

Spouse's Grief Leads to Withholding the Truth

Annie, a 27-year-old woman with one child, began experiencing severe pain in her abdomen while visiting her family in May. After describing the excruciating pain to her husband Daniel, he scheduled Annie for an appointment with Dr. Sokol, a gastroenterologist, who ordered a series of tests. While conducting a barium scan, a radiologist at Community Hospital noted a small bowel obstruction. Dr. Sokol recommended surgery to which both Annie and Daniel agreed.

After the surgery, on July 7, Dr. Brown, the operating surgeon, paged Daniel over the hospital intercom as he walked down a corridor on the ground floor. Daniel, hearing the page, picked up a house phone and dialed zero for an operator. The operator inquired, "May I help you?" "Yes," Daniel replied. "I was just paged." The operator replied, "Oh, yes. Dr. Brown would like to talk to you. I will connect you with him. Hang on. Don't hang up." (Daniel's heart began to pound.) Dr. Brown asked, "Is this you, Daniel?" Daniel replied, "Yes, it is." Dr. Brown replied, "Well, surgery is over. Your wife is recovering nicely in the recovery room." Daniel was relieved but for a moment. "That's good." Daniel sensed Dr. Brown had more to say. Dr. Brown continued, "I am sorry to say that she has carcinoma of the colon." Daniel replied, "Did you get it all?" Dr. Brown reluctantly replied, "I am sorry, but the cancer has spread to her lymph nodes and surrounding organs." Daniel, with the tears in his eyes, asked, "Can I see her?" Dr. Brown replied, "She is in the recovery room." Before hanging up, Daniel told Dr. Brown, "Please do not tell Annie that she has cancer. I want her to always have hope." Dr. Brown agreed, "Don't worry, I won't tell her. You can tell her that she had a narrowing of the colon."

Daniel hung up the phone and proceeded to the recovery room. After entering the recovery room, he spotted his wife. His heart sank. Tubes seemed to be running out of every part of her body. He walked to her bedside. His immediate concern was to see her wake up and have the tubes pulled out so that he could take her home.

Later, in a hospital room, Annie asked Daniel, "What did the doctor find?" Daniel replied, "He found a narrowing of the colon." "Am I going to be okay?" "Yes, but it will take a while to recover." "Oh, that's good. I was so worried," said Annie. "You go home and get some rest." Daniel said, "I'll be back later," as Annie fell back to sleep.

Daniel left the hospital and went to see his friends, Jerry and Helen, who had invited him for dinner. As Daniel pulled up to Jerry and Helen's home, he got out of his car and just stood there, looking up a long stairway leading to Jerry and Helen's home. They were standing there looking down at Daniel. It was early evening. The sun was setting. A warm breeze was blowing, and Helen's eyes were watering. Those few moments seemed like a lifetime. Daniel discovered a new emotion, as he stood there speechless. He knew then that he was losing a part of himself. Things would never be the same.

Annie had one more surgery 2 months later in a futile attempt to extend her life. In November 2002, Annie was admitted to the hospital for the last time. Annie was so ill that even during her last moments she was unaware that she was dying. Dr. Brown entered the room and asked Daniel, "Can I see you for a few moments?" "Yes," Daniel replied. He followed Dr. Brown into the hallway. "Daniel, I can keep Annie alive for a few more days, or we can let her go." Daniel, not responding, went back into the room. He was now alone with Annie. Shortly thereafter, a nurse walked into the room and gave Annie an injection. Daniel asked, "What did you give her?" The nurse replied, "Something to make her more comfortable." Annie had been asleep; she awoke, looked at Daniel, and said, "Could you please cancel my appointment to be sworn in as a citizen? I will have to reschedule. I don't think I will be well enough to go." Daniel replied, "Okay, try to get some rest." Annie closed her eyes, never to open them again.

Discussion

1. Do you agree with Daniel's decision not to tell Annie about the seriousness of her illness? Explain your answer.
2. Should the physician have spoken to Annie as to the seriousness of her illness regardless of Daniel's desire to give Annie hope and not a death sentence? Explain your answer.
3. Describe the ethical dilemmas in this case (e.g., how Annie's rights were violated).
4. Place yourself in Annie's shoes, the physician's shoes, and Daniel's shoes, and then discuss how the lives of each may have been different if the physician had informed Annie as to the seriousness of her illness.

This true life case raises numerous questions, often resulting in conflicts among ethics, the law, patient rights, and family wishes. From a professional ethics point of view, the American Medical Association provides in its *Principles of Medical Ethics* that:

> IV. A physician shall respect the rights of patients, colleagues, and other health professionals, and shall safeguard patient confidences and privacy within the constraints of the law.[7]

Legally, pursuant to the Patient Self-Determination Act of 1990, patients have a right to make their own health care decisions, to accept or refuse medical treatment, and to execute an advance health care directive. Practically speaking, as discussion of this case illustrates, one shoe does not fit all. Both legal and ethical edicts have often served to raise an unending stream of questions that involve both the law and ethics. Although discussed later, a case here has been made for the need of a well-balanced ethics committee to help caregivers, patients, and family come to a consensus in the decision-making process.

Life or Death: The Right to Choose

A Jehovah's Witness executed a release requesting that no blood or its derivatives be administered during hospitalization. The Connecticut Superior Court determined that the hospital had no common law right or obligation to thrust unwanted medical care on the patient because she had been sufficiently informed of the consequences of the refusal to accept blood transfusions. She had competently and clearly declined that care. The hospital's interests were sufficiently protected by her informed choice, and neither it nor the trial court in this case was entitled to override that choice.

BENEFICENCE

Beneficence describes the principle of doing good, demonstrating kindness, showing compassion, and helping others. In the health care setting, caregivers demonstrate beneficence by providing benefits and balancing benefits against risks. Beneficence requires one to do good. Doing good requires knowledge of the beliefs, culture, values, and preferences of the patient—what one person may believe to be good for a patient may in reality be harmful. For example, a caregiver may decide to tell a patient frankly, "There is nothing else that I can do for you." This could be injurious to the patient if the patient really wants encouragement and information about care options from the caregiver. Compassion here requires the caregiver to tell the patient, "I am not aware of new treatments for your illness; however, I have some ideas about how I can help treat your symptoms and make you more comfortable. In addition, I will keep you informed as to any significant research that may be helpful in treating your disease processes."

Paternalism

Paternalism is a form of beneficence. People sometimes believe that they know what is best for another and make decisions that they believe are in that person's best interest. It may involve, for example, withholding information, believing that the person would be better off that way. Paternalism can occur due to one's age, cognitive ability, and level of dependency.

CPR and Paternalism in Nursing Homes

Some nursing homes have implemented facilitywide no CPR policies, as noted in the following Centers for Medicare and Medicaid Services Memorandum. Nursing home patients have a right to make their own care decisions. To eliminate that option in the nursing home sitting by having a policy of no resuscitation measures is a paternalistic approach to patient care and is a clear violation of patient rights and autonomous decision making. Such policies are unconditionally morally and legally wrong.

Memorandum Summary

- **Initiation of CPR**—Prior to the arrival of emergency medical services (EMS), nursing homes must provide basic life support, including initiation of CPR, to a resident who experiences cardiac arrest (cessation of respirations and/or pulse) in accordance with that resident's advance directives or in the absence of advance directives or a Do Not Resuscitate (DNR) order. CPR-certified staff must be available at all times.
- **Facility CPR Policy**—Some nursing homes have implemented facilitywide no CPR policies. Facilities must not establish and implement facilitywide no CPR policies.
- **Surveyor Implications**—Surveyors should ascertain that facility policies related to emergency response require staff to initiate CPR as appropriate and that records do not reflect instances where CPR was not initiated by staff even though the resident requested CPR or had not formulated advance directives.[8]

Physicians and Paternalism

Medical paternalism involves making decisions for patients who are capable of making their own choices. Physicians often find themselves in situations where they can influence a patient's health care decision simply by selectively telling the patient what he or she prefers based on personal beliefs. This directly violates patient autonomy. The problem of paternalism involves a conflict between the principles of autonomy and beneficence, each of which may be viewed and weighed differently, for example, by the physician and patient, physician and family member, or even the patient and a family member.

Employment-Related Paternalism

Employment-related paternalism at its best is a shared and cooperative style of management in which the employer recognizes and considers employee rights when making decisions in the workplace. Paternalism at its worst occurs when the employer's style of management becomes more authoritarian, sometimes arbitrary, and unpredictable, as noted in the *reality check* presented next. In this scenario the employer has complete discretion in making workplace decisions and the individual employee's freedom is subordinate to the employer's authority. Here the employer requires strict obedience to follow orders without question. The employer in this case lacks respect and consideration for the employee.

Paternalism and Breach of Confidentiality

Nina traveled with her husband, Dan, to a work assignment in Michigan. While visiting with her brother in Michigan, Nina believed that her potassium was low, which was a frequent occurrence with her for many years. Nina's brother suggested she could have her blood tested at a local blood drawing station. Dan later learned Nina's potassium was low.

Later that morning, while at work, Joan, Dan's colleague, called Bill, Dan's supervisor, to discuss Nina's health. Bill, however, had overslept and had not yet arrived at work. Joan decided to speak to the supervisor on call. After that conversation, Joan, being led by three staff members from the organization, tracked Dan down on several occasions that morning. On the first occasion, at approximately 10:15 A.M., Dan was surveying the organization's family practice center when Joan arrived. She rudely called Dan aside, excusing the organization's staff from the immediate area. Joan said, with surprise, "Dan, you are working?" Dan, even more surprised at the question, "Yes, I have been working." Joan replied, "Well, anyway, the corporate office wants to speak to you." Dan said he would call during lunch hour. Joan, somewhat agitated, walked away.

Joan again tracked Dan down with an entourage of the organization's staff at 11:30 A.M. She located Dan while he was in the organization's transfusion center. Again she rudely entered the conference room where Dan was discussing the care being rendered to a cancer patient. She once again asked in a stern tone of voice, "Could everyone please leave the room. I need to talk to Dan." The organization's staff left the room and the nurse said, "I finally reached Bill and he wants you to call him." Dan inquired, "Is he pulling me off this assignment?" The nurse replied, "Yes, he is. I spoke to Bill, and he has decided that out of concern for Nina you should be removed from this particular assignment. He wants you to call him." Dan replied, "I don't understand why you did this, calling Bill and continuously interrupting my work and sharing with others confidential information about my wife. I will wrap up with the staff my review of this patient and call Bill." As Joan left the conference room Dan said, "I trusted you and you shared confidential information about my wife?" Joan, realizing that she had no right to share the information, quickly walked away.

Dan called Bill during his lunch break. During that call Bill said, "I am going to remove you from your assignment because I think your wife's health needs should be addressed, and this could be disruptive to the survey." Dan replied, "The only disruption has been the nurse tracking me down with staff from the organization and not conducting her work activities." Bill said, "My decision stands. You can opt to take vacation time for the remainder of the week."

Discussion

1. Discuss what examples of paternalism you have gleaned from this case.
2. Do you think Dan was treated fairly? Discuss your answer.
3. Discuss the issues of trust, confidentiality, and fairness as they relate to this case.

At present, our federal employment discrimination laws fail to provide uniform and consistent legal protection when an employer engages in applicant-specific paternalism—the practice of excluding an applicant merely to protect that person from job-related safety and/ or health risks uniquely attributable to his or her federally protected characteristic(s). Under Title VII of the Civil Rights Act of 1964, the courts and the Equal Employment Opportunity Commission (EEOC) reject such paternalism, demanding that the applicant alone decide whether to pursue (and accept) a job that poses risks related to his or her sex, race, color, religion, or national origin.[9]

CAN A PHYSICIAN "CHANGE HIS OR HER MIND"?

Walls had a condition that caused his left eye to be out of alignment with his right eye. Walls discussed with Shreck, his physician, the possibility of surgery on his left eye to bring both eyes into alignment. Walls and Shreck agreed that the best approach to treating Walls was to attempt surgery on the left eye. Before surgery, Walls signed an authorization and consent form that included the following language:

- I hereby authorize Dr. Shreck . . . to perform the following procedure and/or alternative procedure necessary to treat my condition . . . of the left eye.
- I understand the reason for the procedure is to straighten my left eye to keep it from going to the left.
- It has been explained to me that conditions may arise during this procedure whereby a different procedure or an additional procedure may need to be performed, and I authorize my physician and his assistants to do what they feel is needed and necessary.

During surgery, Shreck encountered excessive scar tissue on the muscles of Walls's left eye and elected to adjust the muscles of the right eye instead. When Walls awoke from the anesthesia, he expressed anger at the fact that both of his eyes were bandaged. The next day,

Walls went to Shreck's office for a follow-up visit and adjustment of his sutures. Walls asked Shreck why he had operated on the right eye, and Shreck responded that "he reserved the right to change his mind" during surgery.

Walls filed a lawsuit. The trial court concluded that Walls had failed to establish that Shreck had violated any standard of care. It sustained Shreck's motion for directed verdict, and Walls appealed. The court stated that the consent form that had been signed indicated that there can be extenuating circumstances when the surgeon exceeds the scope of what was discussed presurgery. Walls claimed that it was his impression that Shreck was talking about surgeries in general.

Roussel, an ophthalmologist, had testified on behalf of Walls. Roussel stated that it was customary to discuss with patients the potential risks of a surgery, benefits, and the alternatives to surgery. Roussel testified that medical ethics requires informed consent.

Shreck claimed that he had obtained the patient's informed consent not from the form but from what he discussed with the patient in his office. The court found that the form itself does not give or deny permission for anything. Rather, it is evidence of the discussions that occurred and during which informed consent was obtained. Shreck therefore asserted that he obtained informed consent to operate on both eyes based on his office discussions with Walls.

Ordinarily, in a medical malpractice case, the plaintiff must prove the physician's negligence by expert testimony. One of the exceptions to the requirement of expert testimony is the situation whereby the evidence and the circumstances are such that the recognition of the alleged negligence may be presumed to be within the comprehension of laypersons. This exception is referred to as the "common knowledge exception."

The evidence showed that Shreck did not discuss with Walls that surgery might be required on both eyes during the same operation. There was evidence that Walls specifically told Shreck he did not want surgery performed on the right eye.

Expert testimony was not required to establish that Walls did not give express or implied consent for Shreck to operate on his right eye. Absent an emergency, it is common knowledge that a reasonably prudent health care provider would not operate on part of a patient's body if the patient told the health care provider not to do so.

On appeal, the trial court was found to have erred in directing a verdict in favor of Shreck. The evidence presented established that the standard of care in similar communities requires health care providers to obtain informed consent before performing surgery. In this case, the applicable standard of care required Shreck to obtain Walls's express or implied consent to perform surgery on his right eye.

[*Walls v. Shreck*, 658 N.W.2d 686 (2003)]

Ethical and Legal Issues

1. Discuss the conflicting ethical principles in this case.
2. Did the physician's actions in this case involve medical paternalism? Explain your answer.

NONMALEFICENCE

Nonmaleficence is an ethical principle that requires caregivers to avoid causing patients harm. It derives from the ancient maxim *primum non nocere*, translated from the Latin, "first, do no harm." Physicians today still swear by the code of Hippocrates, pledging to do no harm. Medical ethics require health care providers to "first, do no harm." A New Jersey court in *In re Conroy*,[10] found that "the physician's primary obligation is . . . First do no harm." Telling the truth, for example, can sometimes cause harm. If there is no cure for a patient's disease, you may have a dilemma. Do I tell the patient and possibly cause serious psychological harm, or do I give the patient what I consider to be false hopes? Is there a middle ground? If so, what is it? To avoid causing harm, alternatives may need to be considered in solving the ethical dilemma.

The caregiver, realizing that he or she cannot help a particular patient, attempts to avoid harming the patient. This is done as a caution against taking a serious risk with the patient or doing something that has no immediate or long-term benefits.

Law and Ethics Intersect

Peninsula Child Psychiatrist William Ayres Sentenced to Eight Years for Molesting Patients

REDWOOD CITY—As one victim after another testified, calling William Ayres a monster and a serial child-abuser who robbed them of their innocence, the once-renowned child psychiatrist sat stoically Monday as a judge sentenced him to eight years in prison for molesting his former patients.

• • •

Ayres used his work with boys having trouble at school, at home or with the law as a setting to abuse them, the victims said. His position of authority allowed him to deflect suspicions about his sexual interest in boys and keep parents from believing their sons' complaints, victims said.

Joshua Melvin, San Jose Mercury News, *August 27, 2013*[11]

The patients described in the news clipping were harmed because the physician who was trained to do good did wrong by taking advantage of the patients' weaknesses. The beneficent person does good and not harm (nonmaleficence). The law in the news clipping is clear. If a person with intent and action causes harm to the patient, that person will be punished.

One of the many lessons in the next *reality check* teaches the reader that one may have good intent but that intent can lead to a perceived wrong and thus be damaging to one's good character and possibly his or her career path.

Patient Questions Physical Exam

Dear Sir:

I was a patient on your short-term acute-care psychiatric unit. It was a voluntary admission as is with all patients on that unit. Dr. X was my psychiatrist. Although he was very good as a psychiatrist, I was somewhat disturbed in the way he conducted my physical examination. He had come to my room on the day of my admission and said that he needed to perform a physical exam. He had already conducted a thorough history of my physical ailments and thoroughly reviewed my family history as far back as I could remember.

We were in the room alone when he entered. He had a gown in his hand and asked me to put it on. He then walked out of the room and said he would be back in a few minutes, as soon as I was gowned. When he returned he began his physical examination. Early on in the exam he asked when I had my last breast examination. I told him that I was 28 and never had one. He said, "Well, I better do one." I thought it was a bit odd that he conducted the exam without a female nurse present. I became more concerned when he touched my breasts in what I considered a sensual manner. It was uncanny. It seemed to be a bit more than what I would've expected during a breast examination. He seemed to be caressing my breasts, as opposed to examining them. I don't know if this is a routine procedure, but I was very uncomfortable in the situation. I think it would be better if you considered having a female nurse present when conducting female examinations in a patient room on a psychiatric unit or on any other unit for that matter.

Thanks for listening to my concerns.

Anonymous

Administrator

I called Dr. X into my office and discussed the patient's concerns with him. He said this is what physicians are trained to do. "We are trained to conduct both history and physical examinations." He had brought with him a letter from one of his professional associations that stated psychiatrists are permitted to perform physical examinations on their patients. I asked him why he did not have someone in the room with him when he examined the patient. He stated, "I generally do but I was extremely busy and the staff was swamped with other patients. It was just a hectic day."

Discussion

1. Discuss how you would respond to the patient.
2. Describe how you would resolve this issue with the physician; assuming this was the first complaint that you had received regarding his care.
3. Explain what policy decisions you would implement.
4. Knowing that the physician is in a position of trust with his patient, discuss what action the physician should take to prevent complaints of this nature from recurring.

The intersection of "law" and "ethics" is clear. Deviation from either can lead to unsatisfactory outcomes for both physicians and patients. Although a caregiver may be trained to conduct a physical examination, the question may not be "can I do it" but "should I do it."

Nonmaleficence and Ending Life

The principle of nonmaleficence is defeated when a physician is placed in the position of ending life by removing respirators, giving lethal injections, or writing prescriptions for lethal doses of medication. Helping patients die violates the physician's duty to save lives. In the final analysis, there needs to be a distinction between killing patients and letting them die. It is clear that killing a patient is never justified.

JUSTICE

Justice is the obligation to be fair in the distribution of benefits and risks. Justice demands that persons in similar circumstances be treated similarly. A person is treated justly when he or she receives what is due, is deserved, or can legitimately be claimed. Justice involves how people are treated when their interests compete with one another.

Distributive justice is a principle requiring that all persons be treated equally and fairly. No one person, for example, should get a disproportional share of society's resources or benefits. There are many ethical issues involved in the rationing of health care. This is often a result of limited or scarce resources, limited access as a result of geographic remoteness, or a patient's inability to pay for services combined with many physicians who are unwilling to accept patients who are perceived as "no-pays" with high risks for legal suits.

Senator Edward M. Kennedy, speaking on health care at the John F. Kennedy Presidential Library in Boston, Massachusetts on April 28, 2002, stated:

> It will be no surprise to this audience that I believe securing quality, affordable health insurance for every American is a matter of simple justice. Health care is not just another commodity. Good health is not a gift to be rationed based on ability to pay. The time is long overdue for America to join the rest of the industrialized world in recognizing this fundamental need.

Later, speaking at the Democratic National Convention on August 25, 2008, Kennedy said:

> And this is the cause of my life—new hope that we will break the old gridlock and guarantee that every American—North, South, East, West, young, old—will have decent, quality health care as a fundamental right and not a privilege.

Although Kennedy did not live to see the day his dream would come true, President Barack Obama signed into law the final piece of his administration's historic health care bill on March 23, 2010.

The costs of health care have bankrupted many, and research dollars have proven to be inadequate, yet many members of Congress elected to address the needs of the country have elected to continue their bipartisan bickering while they "enjoy" the lowest acceptance ratings in the nation's history. They have, however, ensured that their health care needs are met with the best of care in the best facilities with the best doctors. They have taken care of themselves. Their pensions are intact, whereas many Americans have to face such dilemmas as which medications they will take and which they cannot afford. Many often have to decide between food and medications. Is this justice or theft of the nation's resources by the few incompetents who have been elected to protect the American people? Unfortunately, these problems continue to this day as Congress continues to wrangle over national health insurance.

Justice and Government Spending

He Won His Battle With Cancer. Thus, Why Are Millions of Americans Still Losing Theirs?

For an increasing number of cancer activists, researchers and patients, there is too much death and too much waiting for new drugs and therapies. They want a greater sense of urgency, a new approach that emphasizes translational research over basic research—turning knowledge into therapies and getting them to patients pronto. The problem is, that's not the way our sclerotic research paradigm—principally administered by the National Institutes of Health and the National Cancer Institute (NIH/NIC)—is set up. "The fact that we jump up and down when cancer deaths go from 562,000 to 561,000, that's ridiculous. That's not enough," says Lance Armstrong, the cyclist and cancer survivor turned activist, through his Lance Armstrong Foundation (LAF).

Time, *September 15, 2008*

Scarce resources are challenging to the principles of justice. Justice involves equality; nevertheless, equal access to health care, for example, across the United States does not exist. How should government allocate a trillion dollars? Consider the following questions:

* Should the money be distributed equally among families?
* Should the money be distributed equally among all citizens?
* Should the money be invested and saved for a rainy day?
* Should the money be used to improve educational programs, build libraries, build state-of-the-art hospitals, or fund afterschool programs for disadvantaged youths?
* Should the money include both savings for that rainy day and funding for the programs described previously?
* What would be the greater good for all?
* Should health care be rationed based on one's ability to pay?
* Should those individuals found to be ethically corrupt be condemned to poverty and stand in the same food lines as the poorest of Americans?

States Have Double Standards

It is no secret that states have had double standards over the years, one for health care organizations and one for physicians and investors, who often duplicated the financially more lucrative hospital services, while referring Medicaid patients and no-pays to hospital programs for care. As administrator of one hospital, allow me to give you a few examples.

1. A radiology group was able to purchase their own Computed Tomography (CT) scanner, while I had to jump through hoops to be able to purchase one.
2. A group of surgeons and private investors established a surgery center in direct competition with my hospital without scrutiny. At the same time, I was required to justify the hospital's proposed surgery center. The hospital was required to complete lengthy questionnaires and gather supporting documentation to justify construction and operation of an outpatient surgery center.
3. The hospital had to justify opening an outpatient rehabilitation program within the hospital in order to provide a continuum of care for patients needing physical therapy services. While I was busy justifying the need for an outpatient rehabilitation program, orthopedic surgeons were busy setting up their own outpatient programs to compete with the hospital.

I remember walking to my car one day after work and one of my orthopedic surgeons caught up to me and said, "You know Dan, I have made enough money in the 3 years that I have been on your staff to buy your hospital."

Discussion

1. Discuss the issues of justice as they apply to this scenario.
2. Discuss the issues of fairness and how physician competition with hospitals can affect the quality of patient care.

Injustice for the Insured

Even if you're insured, getting ill could bankrupt you. Hospitals are garnishing wages, putting liens on homes and having patients who can't pay arrested. It's enough to make you sick. Think You're Covered? Think Again.

−SARA AUSTIN, *SELF*, OCTOBER 2004

Hospitals are receiving between $4 million and $60 million annually in charity funds in New York City alone, according to Elizabeth Benjamin, director of the health law unit of the Legal Aid Society of New York City; however, even the insured face injustice. In 2003, almost 1 million Americans declared bankruptcy because of medical issues, accounting for nearly half of all of the bankruptcies in the country. When an insured patient gets ill and exhausts his or her insurance benefits, should the hospital be able to:

- Withhold the money from the patient's wages?
- Place a lien on the patient's home?
- Arrest the patient?
- Block the patient from applying for the hundreds of millions of dollars in government funds designated to help pay for care for those who need it?

Age and Justice

New Kidney Transplant Rules Would Favor Younger Patients

The nation's organ transplant network is considering giving younger, healthier people preference over older, sicker patients for the best kidneys.

Some also complain that the new system would unfairly penalize middle-aged and elderly patients at a time when the overall population is getting older.

If adopted, the approach could have implications for other decisions about how to allocate scarce resources, such as expensive cancer drugs and ventilators during hurricanes and other emergencies. . . .

Rob Stein, The Washington Post, *February 24, 2011*

- Should an 89-year-old patient get a heart transplant, rather than a 10-year-old girl, just because he or she is higher on the waiting list?
- Should a 39-year-old single patient, rather than a 10-year-old boy, get a heart transplant because he or she is higher on the waiting list?
- Should a 29-year-old mother of three get a heart transplant, rather than a 10-year-old girl, because she is higher on the waiting list?
- Should a 29-year-old pregnant mother with two children, rather than a 10-year-old boy, get a heart transplant because she is higher on the waiting list?

Justice and Emergency Care

When two patients arrive in the emergency department in critical condition, consider who should receive treatment first. Should the caregiver base his or her decision on the:

- First patient who walks through the door?
- Age of the patients?
- Likelihood of survival?
- Ability of the patient to pay for services rendered?
- Condition of the patient?

Patients are to be treated justly, fairly, and equally. What happens, however, when resources are scarce and only one patient can be treated at a time? What happens if caregivers decide that age should be the determining factor as to who is treated first? One patient is saved, and another dies. What happens if the patient saved is terminal and has an advance directive in his wallet requesting no heroic measures to save his life? What are the legal issues intertwined with the ethical issues in this case?

The principle of distributive justice raises numerous issues, including how limited resources should be allocated. For example, when there is a reduction in staff in health care organizations, managers are generally asked to eliminate "nonessential" personnel. In the health care industry, this translates to those individuals not directly involved in patient care (e.g., maintenance and housekeeping employees). Is this fair? Is this just? Is this the right thing to do?

In Search of Economic Justice

Avery Comarow, in his article "Under the Knife in Bangalore" (*U.S. News and World Report*, May 12, 2008), wrote that the high cost of U.S. hospital care is motivating patients to travel to places like India and Thailand for major procedures. There would be no need for uninsured patients to go abroad if the prices they were quoted in the United States were more in line with what insurers and Medicare pay. The uninsured often pay full price for medical procedures in the United States. For example, a self-pay patient will pay between $70,000 and $133,000 for coronary bypass surgery, whereas Medicare will pay between $18,609 and $23,589. Commercial insurance plans often get up to a 60% discount off the list cost of medical procedures. In India, the same surgery will cost the patient $7,000, and in Thailand, it will be $22,000.

To avoid bankruptcy and loss of assets, maybe their homes, Americans risk the unknowns of going abroad for health care.

Boomer Bubble "Bioeconomics"

As baby boomers become Medicare eligible, there is likely to be a huge strain on the federal budget. Is this dramatically increased cost justified, beneficial, and necessary to the country as a whole?

The revenue from working, taxpaying baby boomers over the past 4 decades has fueled unprecedented prosperity. That revenue has made many entitlements possible, but it is going to diminish drastically as boomers retire and become recipients instead of contributors to the revenue base. Advances in medical technology have increased longevity dramatically, and boomers therefore are likely to be on the receiving end of entitlements for a long time. Medical advances, however, also can increase productivity as well as longevity. Boomers with a lifetime of work experience can be a valuable resource if they are kept healthy enough to remain gainfully employed at some level. Maintenance of a skilled American workforce is essential for future prosperity and economic stability. Boomers are a substantial resource of experienced skilled workers. It is a political necessity that they are encouraged to stay productive. The government's subsidizing health care through Medicare and other programs is therefore an investment that can facilitate this worthwhile goal. Additional incentives may even be appropriate. Even on an ethical basis, boomers that fueled our economy for so long deserve to be taken care of in their later years. Hopefully, many of them will be healthy enough and willing enough to continue being productive beyond the usual retirement age. Thus, from a political perspective, the healthful, moral, and ethical choice may also turn out to be the profitable choice for our society.

Physician

VIRTUE ETHICS AND VALUES

Virtue ethics focuses on the inherent character of a person rather than on the specific actions he or she performs. A *virtue* is a positive trait of moral excellence. Virtues are those characteristics that differentiate good people from bad people. Virtues such as courage, honesty, and justice are abstract moral principles. A morally virtuous person is one who does the good and right thing by habit, not merely based on a set of rules of conduct. The character of a virtuous person is naturally good, as exhibited by his or her unswerving good behavior and actions.

Resilience of the Health Caregiver Spirit

I've been in leadership roles for two sister hospitals in southeast Louisiana, with each experiencing the devastation of hurricane damage twice in the past 3 years. The first experience was temporarily suspending normal operations in New Orleans, and recently, history repeated itself at the sister hospital in Houma, Louisiana.

In both instances, I was stunned at the determination and strength of health care teams to rebuild. Both hospitals needed to resort to MASH-type tent hospitals to allow rebuilding of the hospitals. Health care for the communities was not interrupted. Back-to-basics care ensued, but not without close attention to needed regulatory compliance standards. The regulatory agencies were called and involved from the get-go, and the caregiver teams and support service staff flourished with enthusiasm to survive and care for the patients in need. Was this because of the nonprofit nature of our state-sponsored hospitals? I don't think so. The human spirit takes over when it comes to patient care, no matter what.

I am happy to say that both New Orleans and Houma are back on track, with care being provided in top-quality hospitals. This is only due to the diligence of all, including facilities management, housekeeping, and multiple direct and indirect caregiver departments. What is the ethical issue here? There is no issue. Support for the art of care-giving will never be disappointed—at least not in southeast Louisiana. I stand in awe of what I have seen and look forward to growing with this team of devoted professionals.

Nurse

Values are standards of conduct. They are used for judging the goodness or badness of some action. A *moral value* is the relative worth placed on some virtuous behavior.

Values are rooted in customs and habits of a culture because the words moral and ethics themselves were essentially created to describe these topics.[12]

Values are the standards by which we measure the goodness in our lives. *Intrinsic value* is something that has value in and of itself (e.g., happiness). *Instrumental value* is something that helps to give value to something else (e.g., money is valuable for what it can buy).

Values may change as needs change. If one's basic needs for food, water, clothing, and housing have not been met, one's values may change such that a friendship, for example, might be sacrificed if one's basic needs can be better met as a result of the sacrifice. As mom nears the end of her life, a financially well-off family member may want to take more aggressive measures to keep mom alive despite the financial drain on her estate. Another family member, who is struggling financially, may more readily see the futility of expensive medical care and find it easier to let go. Values give purpose to each life. They make up one's moral character.

All people make value judgments and make choices among alternatives. Values are the motivating power of a person's actions and necessary to survival, both psychologically and physically.

The relationship between abstract virtues (principles) and values (practice) is often difficult to grasp. The virtuous person is one who does good, and his or her character is known through the values he or she practices consistently by habit.

We begin our discussion here with an overview of those virtues commonly accepted as having value when addressing difficult health care dilemmas. The reader should not get overly caught up in the philosophical morass of how virtues and values differ but should be aware that virtues and values have been used interchangeably. This text is not about memorizing words; it is about applying what we learn for the good of all whose lives we touch.

Whether we call compassion a virtue or a value or both, the importance for our purposes in this text is to understand what compassion is and how it is applied in the health care setting.

PILLARS OF MORAL STRENGTH

I am part of all I have met.

—ALFRED TENNYSON

There is a deluge of ethical issues in every aspect of human existence. Although cultural differences, politics, and religion influence who we are, it is all of life experiences that affect who we have become. If we have courage to do right, those who have influenced our lives were most likely courageous. If we are compassionate, it is most likely because we have been influenced by the compassionate.

The *Pillars of Moral Strength* illustrated in **Figure 1** describes a virtuous person. What is it that sets each person apart? In the final analysis, it is one's virtues and values that build moral character. Look beyond the words and ask, "Do I know their meanings?" "Do I apply their concepts?" "Do I know their value?" "Are they part of me?"

FIGURE 1 Pillars of Moral Strength

COURAGE AS A VIRTUE

Courage is the greatest of all virtues, because if you haven't courage, you may not have an opportunity to use any of the others.

–SAMUEL JOHNSON

Courage is the mental or moral strength to persevere and withstand danger. Courage can be characterized as the ladder upon which all the other virtues mount. Courage is the strength of character necessary to continue in the face of fears and the challenges in life. It involves balancing fear, self-confidence, and values. Without courage, we are unable to take the risks necessary to achieve the things most valued. A courageous person has good judgment and a clear sense of his or her strengths, correctly evaluates danger, and perseveres until a decision is made and the right goal that is being sought has been achieved.

My Journey–How Lucky Am I?

No words can be scripted to say what I have been through, so I will just speak from my heart and off the cuff. From the day the Dr. said to me, "Denise, you have a rare cancer and we are sorry there is nothing we can do. I did not waver in my faith in God. He was in me, he was thru me and he was around me. I just asked the Dr., "What Do I Do?" And yet, although he said a whole bunch of words, I wasn't focused so much on what was being said. It's like a calmness was over me, not much worry, just a feeling of I will never be ALONE on this new journey I'm about to experience. I felt calm. Not until I looked at my loved ones FACES did I realize, oh my, this can be bad. But again, a feeling came over me that I will not face this ALONE. God has plans for me and I will surrender in his grace and as time past [sic], I realized how lucky and blessed I am, for most people who may feel that death may be close by, I didn't feel that way. What I felt was WOW!! Everyone gets to show me their love in the NOW and not in the later when I am no longer HERE. How lucky am I.

—Denise

Courage, in differing degrees, helps to define one's character (the essence of one's being) and offers the strength to stand up for what is good and right. It crosses over and unites and affects all other values. Courage must not be exercised to an extreme, causing a person to become so foolish that his or her actions are later regretted.

When the passion to destroy another human being becomes such an obsession that one is willing to sacrifice the lives of others, that person has become a bully and a coward and not a person of courage. History is filled with men and women who have hidden their fears by inciting others to do evil. Such people are not the models of character that we wish to instill thoughts of in the minds of our children.

WISDOM AS A VIRTUE

True wisdom comes to each of us when we realize how little we understand about life, ourselves, and the world around us.

—SOCRATES

We can learn from history how past generations thought and acted, how they responded to the demands of their time and how they solved their problems. We can learn by analogy, not by example, for our circumstances will always be different than theirs were. The main thing history can teach us is that human actions have consequences and that certain choices, once made, cannot be undone. They foreclose the possibility of making other choices and thus they determine future events.

—GERDA LERNER (PIONEER OF WOMEN'S HISTORY)

Wisdom is the judicious application of knowledge. Wisdom begins first by learning from the failures and successes of those who have preceded us. Marcus Tullius Cicero (106–43 BC), a Roman philosopher and politician, is reported to have said, "The function of wisdom is to discriminate between good and evil." In the health care setting, when the patient's wishes and end-of-life preferences are unknown, wisdom with good judgment without bias or prejudice springs forth more easily.

TEMPERANCE AS A VIRTUE

Being forced to work, and forced to do your best, will breed in you temperance and self-control, diligence and strength of will, cheerfulness and content, and a hundred virtues which the idle will never know.

—CHARLES KINGSLEY

Temperance involves self-control and restraint. It embraces moderation in thoughts and actions. Temperance is evidenced by orderliness and moderation in everything one says and does. It involves the ability to control one's actions so as not to go to extremes. The question arises, without the ability to control oneself from substance abuse, for example, how can a person possibly live the life of a virtuous person. The old adage, "the proof is in the pudding" lies in one's actions. A virtuous person stands out from the crowd by actions and deeds.

COMMITMENT

Unless commitment is made; there are only promises and hopes; but no plans.

—PETER F. DRUCKER

I know the price of success: dedication, hard work, and an unremitting devotion to the things you want to see happen.

—FRANK LLOYD WRIGHT

Commitment is the act of binding oneself intellectually or emotionally to a course of action (e.g., pursue a career, adhere to a religious belief) or person (e.g., marriage, family, patient care). It is an agreement or pledge to do something. It can be ongoing, such as in a marriage, or a pledge to do something in the future, such as an engagement as a commitment to marry a particular person.

COMPASSION

Compassion is the basis of morality.

—ARTHUR SCHOPENHAUER

The Fear Factor and Patient Satisfaction

Nurses tend to score highly on measures of empathy, care, and compassion . . . Here is some specific advice about what hospitals can do to help nurses improve at calming their patients' fears.

- Encourage nurses to be sensitive to the level of fear their patients experience when they're admitted to the hospital. Empathy and communication are key . . .
- Set nurses up for success through training and support. In many instances, it is easy to deal with safety concerns by providing detailed protocols, policies, and procedures . . .

Rick Blizzard, D.B.A., Gallup, *August 6, 2013*[13]

Hospital Video Shows No One Helped Dying Woman

A shocking video shows a woman dying on the floor in the psych ward at Kings County Hospital, while people around her, including a security guard, did nothing to help. After an hour, another mental patient finally got the attention of the indifferent hospital workers, according to the tape obtained by the *New York Daily News*.

Worse still, the surveillance tape suggests hospital staff may have falsified medical charts to cover the utter lack of treatment provided to Esmin Green before she died.

John Marzulli, Daily News, *June 30, 2008*

Compassion is the deep awareness of and sympathy for another's suffering. The ability to show compassion is a true mark of moral character. There are those who argue that compassion will blur one's judgment. Caregivers need to show the same compassion for others, as they would expect for themselves or their loved ones.

Elderly Patient Hit by Motorcycle Dies in Japan After Being Rejected by 14 Hospitals

After getting struck by a motorcycle, an elderly Japanese man with head injuries waited in an ambulance as paramedics phoned 14 hospitals, each refusing to treat him.

He died 90 minutes later at the facility that finally relented—one of thousands of victims repeatedly turned away in recent years by understaffed and overcrowded hospitals in Japan.

Maria Yamaguchi, Associated Press, *February 5, 2009*

Compassion is a moral value expected of all caregivers. Those who lack compassion have a weakness in their moral character. In 1996, Dr. Linda Peeno, featured in Michael Moore's 2007 film *Sicko*, testified before Congress (Important issue facing House-Senate conference on health care reform, House of Representatives—March 28, 2000—Page: H1465) to discuss her prior work for Humana, where she worked as a claims reviewer for several health maintenance organizations (HMOs). Dr. Peeno showed compassion as she testified before the Committee on Commerce on May 30, 1996. Here is her story in part:

> I wish to begin by making a public confession. In the spring of 1987, I caused the death of a man. Although this was known to many people, I have not been taken before any court of law or called to account for this in any professional or public forum. In fact, just the opposite occurred. I was rewarded for this. It brought me an improved reputation in my job and contributed to my advancement afterwards. Not only did I demonstrate that I could do what was asked, expected of me, I exemplified the good company employee. I saved a half a million dollars.

Since that day, I have lived with this act and many others eating into my heart and soul. The primary ethical norm is do no harm. I did worse, I caused death. Instead of using a clumsy bloody weapon, I used the simplest, cleanest of tools: my words. This man died because I denied him a necessary operation to save his heart. I felt little pain or remorse at the time. The man's faceless distance soothed my conscience. Like a skilled soldier, I was trained for the moment. When any moral qualms arose, I was to remember, "I am not denying care; I am only denying payment."

Duty-based ethics required Dr. Peeno to follow the rules of her job. In so doing, a life was lost. Although Dr. Peeno eventually came forward with her story, the irony here lies in the fact that Dr. Peeno lacked the courage, integrity, and compassion to report her story sooner. The lack of compassion for others plagues the health care industry in a variety of settings.

Teaching Doctors to Care

At Harvard and other medical schools across the country, educators are beginning to realize that empathy is as valuable to a doctor as any clinical skill . . . doctors who try to understand their patients may be the best antidote for the widespread dissatisfaction with today's health care system.

Nathan Thornburgh, Time magazine, *March 29, 2006*

Detachment

Detachment, or lack of concern for the patient's needs, often translates into mistakes that result in patient injuries. Those who have excessive emotional involvement in a patient's care may be best suited to work in those settings where patients are most likely to recover and have good outcomes (e.g., maternity units). As with all things in life, there needs to be a comfortable balance between compassion and detachment.

Never apologize for showing feeling. When you do so, you apologize for the truth.

–Benjamin Disraeli

Policy Ruled—Compassion Missing

Mr. Jones was trying to get home from a long trip to see his ailing wife. Mrs. Jones had been ill for several years, suffering a great deal of pain. His flight was to leave at 7:00 PM. Upon arrival at the airport in New York at 4:30 pm, he inquired at the ticket counter, "Is there an earlier flight that I can take to Washington?" The counter agent responded, "There is plenty of room on the 5:00 pm flight, but you will have pay a $200 change fee." The passenger inquired, "Could you please waive the change fee? I need to get home to my ailing wife." The ticket agent responded, "Sorry, your ticket does not allow me to make the change. You can, however, try at the gate."

The passenger made a second attempt at the gate to get on an earlier flight, but the manager at the gate was unwilling to authorize the change, saying, "I don't make the rules."

Mr. Jones decided to give it one more try. He called the airline's customer service center. The customer service agent responded to Mr. Jones's plea: "We cannot overrule the agent at the gate. Sorry, you just got the wrong supervisor. He is going by the book."

Anonymous

Discussion

1. Should rules be broken for a higher good? Discuss your answer.
2. Do the rules seem to be consistently or inconsistently applied in this *reality check*? Discuss your answer.

CONSCIENTIOUS

The most infectiously joyous men and women are those who forget themselves in thinking about and serving others.

–ROBERT J. MCCRACKEN

A *conscientious* person is one who has moral integrity and a strict regard for doing what is considered the right thing to do. An individual acts conscientiously if he or she is motivated to do what is right, believing it is the right thing to do. Conscience is a form of self-reflection on and judgment about whether one's actions are right or wrong, good or bad. It is an internal sanction that comes into play through critical reflection. This sanction often appears as a bad conscience in the form of painful feelings of remorse, guilt, shame, disunity, or disharmony as the individual recognizes that his or her acts were wrong.

Kill the Messenger

Frank, working as a hospital inspector, found a number of things wrong in his recent building inspection. At first glance the building looked clean and polished—Frank was amazed by how the floors sparkled in the old building. But then, as Frank always does, he asked to look behind a corridor door. Behind the door, Frank found a small storage closet with medical records strewn on the floor and others stored in cardboard boxes. The records had been soaked by water and floor wax that had seeped under the door when the corridors where cleaned. Entries on the records were blurred, making them difficult to read, and the records appeared to have black mold growing on them.

Behind another door was a medical equipment repair room. Dust balls floated on the floor as the door was opened. There was food on the floor, and a can of soda had been spilled and allowed to dry. Equipment parts were also scattered on the floor.

The staff complained about Frank's findings. Before he left, the staff corrected the issues he had noted and asked, "Frank, could you remove these comments from your report.

We cleaned the room and it is spotless. In addition, we stored the records in the medical records department." Frank replied, "I could not in good conscience remove my findings. Yes, the room may be clean but what about the information that had been recorded on the medical records that is not readable. Further, our process for inspecting your facility is a sampling process. I did not look behind every door and I am not sure what we would find if we did. I would suggest, as we discussed earlier, that a written plan of action be prepared and implemented to address the issues I identified. More important, your action plan should be implemented facilitywide. For example, no boxes should be stored on the floors, including medical supplies, as well as medical records."

Anonymous

Discussion

1. Should Frank have overlooked his findings, as the staff pressed him not to report them? Discuss your answer.
2. Assuming you were Frank, would you have deleted the findings from your report? Explain your answer.

DISCERNMENT

Get to know two things about a man—how he earns his money and how he spends it—and you have the clue to his character, for you have a searchlight that shows up the innermost recesses of his soul. You know all you need to know about his standards, his motives, his driving desires, and his real religion.

–ROBERT J. MCCRACKEN

Discernment is the ability to make a good decision without personal biases, fears, and undue influences from others. A person who has discernment has the wisdom to decide the best course of action when there are many possible actions to choose from.

9/11 Value Judgment

James had been scheduled to fly Monday evening, September 10, 2001, from Ronald Reagan Washington National Airport to New York LaGuardia Airport, and then rent a car and drive to Greenwich, Connecticut, where he was assigned to inspect a hospital. As luck would have it, there was one flight cancellation after another. After the last flight to LaGuardia was canceled, he went to the ticket counter and scheduled the first flight out Tuesday morning, September 11, 2001, at 6:00 AM.

The following morning James flew into LaGuardia, picked up his car, and drove to Connecticut to work with an assigned team led by Dr. Matthews. Not long after he arrived at the hospital, the first plane hit the World Trade Center. Shortly after the second plane crashed into the World Trade Center, the corporate office called and asked if the hospital wanted to reschedule the survey. The hospital opted to continue the survey.

On Thursday, the last day of the survey, a hospital staff member approached Dr. Matthews and asked if he and his survey team would like to attend a short memorial service in the lobby at noon for the victims and workers of 9/11. Without hesitation, Dr. Matthews replied, "No, we really have to finish our reports."

Anonymous

Discussion

1. Did the team leader make an appropriate decision? Discuss your answer.
2. Describe the various virtues and values that come into play in this case.
3. Discuss how you would have addressed the hospital's request to attend the memorial service.
4. Realizing that hindsight is 20/20, could you defend the decision not to attend the ceremony? Explain your answer.

FAIRNESS

Do all the good you can, By all the means you can, In all the ways you can, In all the places you can, At all the times you can, To all the people you can, As long as you ever can.

–JOHN WESLEY

In ethics, *fairness* requires each person to be objective, unbiased, dispassionate, impartial, and consistent with the principles of ethics. Fairness is the ability to make judgments free from discrimination, dishonesty, or one's own bias. It is the ability to be objective without prejudice or bias. We often tolerate mediocrity. We sometimes forget to thank those who just do their jobs, and we often praise the extraordinary, sometimes despite questionable faults. To be fair, it is important to see the good in all and to reward that good.

Questions of fairness in the Affordable Care Act have led to lawsuits in a number of the nation's top hospitals including the Mayo Clinic in Minnesota and Cedars-Sinai in Los Angeles because they are cut out of most insurance plans sold on the exchange.

Health Costs Cut by Limiting Choice

"Exchanges exclude, doctors, hospitals; in backlash, some providers file lawsuits"

The result, some argue, is a two-tiered system of health care: Many of the people who buy health plans on the exchanges have fewer hospitals and doctors to choose from than those with coverage through their employers.

• • •

Insurers "looked at the people expected to go on the exchanges and thought: 'these are people coming out of the ranks of the uninsured. They don't care about the Mayo Clinic or the Cleveland Clinic. They will go to community providers,'" explained Robert Laszewski, a consultant to the health-care industry.

Sandhya Somashekhar and Ariana Eunjung Cha, The Washington Post, *August 21, 2013*

Although care is generally cheaper at community-based hospitals than academic medical centers, the quality of that care often comes into question, as noted in the following *reality check*.

Community Hospital v. Respected Medical Center

My closest friend Nick was admitted to a small community hospital for what was described as a minor surgical procedure. During surgery, the surgeon unknowingly nicked the large bowel, which went unknown for several days. Nick, as a result, developed a methicillin-resistant staphylococcus aureus (MRSA) infection. Further surgeries were conducted, complicating an already botched surgery. One evening a nurse called his family aside and said, although I am jeopardizing my job, "I would get Nick out of here if I was you." The family decided to move Nick to a major teaching medical center several hours away from his hometown. Following an extended stay at the medical center and discharged home under hospice care, I visited Nick at his home. He looked intensely straight at me with deep sadness and said, "they took my life from me." He told another friend, "My life is over."

Anonymous

So where are we as it relates to fairness in the delivery of health care? Is it true that people coming out of the ranks of the uninsured don't care about the Mayo Clinic, Cleveland Clinic, the Lahey Hospital and Medical Center, or the Massachusetts General Hospital, to name but a few? Or do they care but just don't know the quality differences from one hospital to the next. Or is it a question of accessibility in remote areas of the country. Do we need hospital selection exchanges more then we need insurance exchanges? If one has money or connections is he or she more likely to get a higher quality of medical care than a poorer patient? Who determines what routine care is? Is routine care based on each patient's needs and comorbidities? Should those who have a financial interest in where a patient is treated be excluded from the decision-making process? Cheaper is not always better and providing care very well may not be enough. Although fairness in the delivery of health is a laudable value, it is most likely unachievable. The disparity as to who holds the nation's wealth continues to widen, as noted in the news clippings that follow. With so much wealth in the hands of the few, fairness in the delivery of high-quality health care for all is unlikely. However, the human race must continue to strive to meet the needs of all.

Of the 1%, by the 1%, for the 1%

Americans have been watching protests against oppressive regimes that concentrate massive wealth in the hands of an elite few. Yet in our own democracy, 1 percent of the people take nearly a quarter of the nation's income—an inequality even the wealthy will come to regret.

Joseph E. Stiglitz, Vanity Fair, *May 2011*

World's Richest 1% Own 40% of All Wealth, UN Report Discovers

The richest 1% of adults in the world own 40% of the planet's wealth, according to the largest study yet of wealth distribution. The report also finds that those in financial services and the internet sectors predominate among the super rich.

Europe, the US and some Asia Pacific nations account for most of the extremely wealthy. More than a third live in the US. Japan accounts for 27% of the total, the UK for 6% and France for 5%.

James Randerson, The Guardian, *December 2006*

FIDELITY

Nothing is more noble, nothing more venerable, than fidelity. Faithfulness and truth are the most sacred excellences and endowments of the human mind.

—CICERO

Fidelity is the virtue of faithfulness, being true to our commitments and obligations to others. A component of fidelity, veracity, implies that we will be truthful and honest in all our endeavors. It involves being faithful and loyal to obligations, duties, or observances. The opposite of fidelity is infidelity, meaning unfaithfulness.

FREEDOM

You can only protect your liberties in this world by protecting the other man's freedom. You can only be free if I am free.

—DOROTHY THOMPSON

Freedom is the quality of being free to make choices for oneself within the boundaries of law. Freedoms enjoyed by citizens of the United States include the freedom of speech, freedom of religion, freedom from want, and freedom from physical aggression.

HONESTY/TRUSTWORTHINESS/TRUTH TELLING

A lie can travel halfway around the world while the truth is still putting on its shoes.
—MARK TWAIN (AMERICAN HUMORIST, WRITER, AND LECTURER, 1835–1910)

Honesty and trust involve confidence that a person will act with the right motives. It is the assured reliance on the character, ability, strength, or truth of someone or something. To tell the truth, to have integrity, and to be honest are most honorable virtues. *Veracity* is devotion to and conformity with what is truthful. It involves an obligation to be truthful.

Truth telling involves providing enough information so that a patient can make an informed decision about his or her health care. Intentionally misleading a patient to believe something that the caregiver knows to be untrue may give the patient false hopes. There is

FIGURE 2 Freedom Speaks (© Keith Bell/Shutterstock, Inc.)

always apprehension when one must share bad news; the temptation is to play down the truth for fear of being the bearer of bad news. To lessen the pain and the hurt is only human, but in the end, truth must win over fear.

Speaking the truth in times of universal deceit is a revolutionary act.

—GEORGE ORWELL

36,000 Feet over Texas

A few weeks before Frank was to travel to Dodge City, Texas, for a work assignment, he received a call from Dr. Layblame: "Hi Frank. This is Dr. Layblame. Can you be ready for an early afternoon departure from Dodge City on Friday?" Frank replied, "Well you know we have been instructed not to leave early, and the last flight leaves at 4:30 P.M. Anyway, I don't mind flying out Saturday morning." Dr. Layblame replied, "Well, it's only an hour early. If you write most of your report the night before and during lunch on Friday, we should be able to finish up work by 2:30 P.M. The airport is small and close to the hospital. Besides, my team has to drive to Louisiana and we would like to get there so we can go out to dinner and enjoy evening. I am the tour leader, so it should not be a problem." Frank said OK and scheduled a 4:30 P.M. return flight.

While Frank was in a flight to Washington, DC following his work assignment, Ronald, Frank's supervisor was dictating a voicemail message to him. When Frank returned home at about 10:30 that evening, he retrieved his voicemail messages. Ronald had left Frank a message at 4:30 P.M. earlier that day asking Frank, "Call me as soon as you get this message. I will be in my office until about 5:30 P.M. If you miss me, you can reach me over the weekend. My cell phone number is xxx/xxx-xxxx."

Frank called Ronald that evening and the next morning; however, Ronald never answered, nor did he return his call. Frank called Ronald Monday morning. As luck would have it, Ronald was out of the office for the day. Frank called Ronald again on Tuesday morning and Ronald answered. Frank asked, "Ronald, you called?" He replied, "Yes, I did. How were you able to get to the airport on Friday and catch a 4:30 P.M. flight without leaving your job early? I had your flight schedule and you left the survey early. You could not possibly have traveled to the airport in time to catch your flight without leaving early."

Frank replied, "I did not schedule the exit time from the survey. The physician team leader determined the time of the exit. He said that he was conducting a system tour and would like to get the exit briefing started as soon as possible. He asked for everybody to be ready to exit by having draft reports ready the night before." Ronald replied, "Dr. Layblame told me the team had to exit early because you scheduled an early flight."

Frank asked, "Just one question, Ronald. Why would you leave a message for me at 4:30 P.M. to call you by 5:30 P.M. when you knew I was 36,000 feet high in the sky? And why didn't you call the team leader at the beginning of the assignment and not after it was completed? Since you know flight schedules, why would you wait until the assignment was completed to raise this issue? Sounds a bit peculiar, don't you think? Sort of like observing a protocol not being followed in the OR and then chastising the OR team after the surgery is completed for not following protocol. This is a serious business we are in. You need to ask yourself why you would allow an event to occur if you believed it to be wrong."

Discussion

1. Discuss the ethical issues involved in this case.
2. Discuss what you would do if you found yourself in Frank's situation.
3. What should Frank have said if his manager said, "You should have reported Dr. Layblame"?
4. How would you describe Ronald's management style?

Declining Trust in the Health Care System

The declining trust in the nation's ability to deliver high-quality health care is evidenced by a system caught up in the quagmire of managed care companies, which have in some instances inappropriately devised ways to deny health care benefits to their constituency. In addition, the continuing reporting of numerous medical errors serves only to escalate distrust in the nation's political leadership and the providers of health care.

Physicians find themselves vulnerable to lawsuits, often because of misdiagnosis. As a result, patients are passed from specialist to specialist in an effort to leave no stone unturned. Fearful to step outside the boundaries of their own specialties, physicians escalate the problem by ineffectively communicating with the primary care physician responsible for managing the patient's overall health care needs. This can also be problematic if no one physician has taken overall responsibility to coordinate and manage a patient's care.

Cancer Doctor Allegedly Prescribed $35 Million Worth of Totally Unnecessary Chemotherapy

A Michigan oncologist has been charged with giving $35 million in needless chemotherapy to patients—some of whom didn't even have cancer, The Today Show reported.

Popular physician Farid Fata, who had more than 1,000 patients, allegedly misdiagnosed people with cancer just so he could bill Medicare.

He's also accused of giving chemo to "end-of-life" patients who wouldn't benefit and had to endure the treatment's nasty side effects during their final days.

Christina Sterbenz, Business Insider, *August 15, 2013*

Politics and Distrust

Lies or the appearance of lies are not what the writers of our Constitution intended for our country—it's not the America we salute every Fourth of July, it's not the America we learned about in school, and it is not the America represented in the flag that rises above our land.

—ANONYMOUS

Truthfulness is just one measure of one's moral character. Unfortunately, politicians do not always set good examples for the people they serve. The following news clipping is an example of how political decisions can lead to distrust in government.

Cheney's Staff Cut Testimony on Warming

In a letter to Sen. Barbara Boxer (D-Calif.), former EPA deputy associate administrator Jason K. Burnett said an official from Cheney's office ordered last October that six pages be edited out of the testimony of Julie L. Gerberding, director of the Centers for Disease Control and Prevention. Gerberding had planned to say that the "CDC considers climate change a serious public health concern."

Juliet Eilperin, The Washington Post, *July 9, 2008*

Discussion

1. Discuss how headlines such as this affect your opinion of politicians.
2. Assuming a cover-up, discuss how the principles of beneficence and nonmaleficence apply.
3. At the end of our days, the most basic principles of life—trust and survival—are on trial. What is your verdict, if indeed there was a cover-up?

Nearly all men can stand adversity, but if you want to test a man's character, give him power.

–ABRAHAM LINCOLN

Wrong-Operation Doctor

Hospitals find it hard to protect patients from wrong-site surgery

Last year a jury returned a $20 million negligence verdict against Arkansas Children's Hospital for surgery on the wrong side of the brain of a 15-year-old boy who was left psychotic and severely brain damaged. Testimony showed that the error was not disclosed to his parents for more than a year. The hospital issued a statement saying it deeply regretted the error and had "redoubled our efforts to prevent" a recurrence.

"Healthcare has far too little accountability for results . . . . All the pressures are on the side of production; that's how you get paid," said Peter Pronovost, a prominent safety expert and medical director of the Johns Hopkins Center for Innovation in Quality Patient Care, who added that increased pressure to turn over operating rooms quickly has trumped patient safety, increasing the chance of error.

Sandra G. Boodman, Kaiser Health News, The Washington Post, *June 20, 2011*

Discussion

1. Discuss the issues of integrity in this case.
2. Should criminal charges be a consideration in this case, if accurately reported? Discuss your answer.

Integrity involves a steadfast adherence to a strict moral or ethical code and a commitment not to compromise this code. A person with integrity has a staunch belief in and faithfulness to, for example, his or her religious beliefs. Patients and professionals alike often make health care decisions based on their integrity and their strict moral beliefs. For example, Jehovah's Witnesses generally refuse blood transfusions because it is contrary to their religious beliefs, even if such refusal may result in death. A provider of health care may refuse to participate in an abortion because it is against the provider's moral beliefs. A person without personal integrity lacks sincerity and moral conviction and may fail to act on professed moral beliefs.

Behind the Smiles

Jeff well remembers what happened after Bill left the hospital boardroom. He, however, remembers more clearly how Bill, a consultant, was treated while he was in the room after presenting his organizational improvement report to the hospital's leadership. Bill was treated with kindness and assurances as to how well he took an educational approach to his audit findings with the staff and how employees appreciated his suggestions for improvement.

Prior to exiting the conference room, Bill asked whether there were any questions about his report. No questions, just smiles, accolades, and goodbyes. Jeff thought to himself, wow, it is good to see good people take suggestions and be so willing to make the changes that Bill suggested.

Oops, hold on, it turns out Bill wasn't as wonderful as the leadership described. The organization's leadership was now disgruntled about Bill's report. Bill was gone and now vilified. Jeff, a consultant not scheduled to finish his assignment for another 2 weeks, asked, "Why didn't you ask questions while Bill was here?" Carol, the finance director replied, "I spent 2 weeks with Bill. He just made up his mind. There was just no changing his mind." Jim said, "Are you saying that you disagree with Bill's report?" Carol, replied, "Yes, I do disagree with it." Jeff continued, "But you did not state that while he was here. You told him you liked his suggestions and that you were already in the process of implementing them." Carol replied, "That's true, but since we made the suggested changes while he was here, he did not have to include them in his written report." Bill replied, "It speaks well of leadership that you have done so; however, it is the hospital board that asked for the audit. We must report what we found." Carol, disgruntled, remained silent. Jim thought to himself, integrity includes being honest and truthful and surely not criticizing a person after leaving the conference room.

Anonymous

Discussion

1. Should Bill have left his findings off the report? Explain your answer.
2. Discuss why Bill's integrity in reporting the deficiencies he found and reported were important to both ABC consulting and the hospital board, which had contracted with ABC to conduct the audit.

Employee Satisfaction Survey

The human resources department manager was reporting on an employee satisfaction survey at a leadership roundtable session with the organization's employees. To maintain employee confidentiality, a third-party consulting firm had conducted the survey. Approximately 49% of employees had responded to the survey, compared with 47% 3 years earlier. The HR manager commented that it is was the first satisfaction survey conducted in 3 years and that the results were excellent, with a 4.2% rise in overall employee satisfaction. Management was all smiles as they sat listening to the report. The HR manager had actually briefed the organization's leadership prior to the roundtable session. Following the report, she asked if there were any questions. The silence was deadly—no one responded. Finally, one employee, Richard, placed his hands on the table to stand up, but he felt a nudge on his right shoulder from Phil, a physician friend. Phil whispered, "Richard, are you sure you want to ask any questions? There is nothing to gain here." Richard, looking down with a smile, said, "I agree, but I can't help myself." Richard then stood up and asked the HR manager, "Do you know what the employee turnover rate has been during the past 3 years?" She responded, "Well, ugh, yes, it was about 30%." Richard replied, "So, then, does this report reflect that we have had a 30% turnover?" The manager replied, "Good point, I will have to get back to you on that."When he returned to his seat, Phil said, "Do you really think you will ever hear back an answer to your question?" Richard smiled and replied, "Not really." Richard was right; she never did get back to him.

Discussion

1. Discuss why employees are often reluctant to ask questions when their questions are solicited by leadership.
2. Knowing that the HR manager never followed up with Richard, should he have followed up with the manager as to the validity of the survey data? Explain your answer.

Medical Integrity and Patient Autonomy

The integrity of the medical profession is not threatened by allowing competent patients to decide for themselves whether a particular medical treatment is in their best interests. Patient autonomy sets the foundation of one's right to bodily integrity, including the right to accept or refuse treatment. Those rights are superior to the institutional considerations of hospitals and their medical staffs. A state's interest in maintaining the ethical integrity of a profession does not outweigh, for example, a patient's right to refuse blood transfusions.

KINDNESS

When you carry out acts of kindness, you get a wonderful feeling inside. It is as though something inside your body responds and says, yes, this is how I ought to feel.

—HAROLD KUSHNER

Kindness involves the quality of being considerate and sympathetic to another's needs. Some people are takers, and others are givers. If you go through life giving without the anticipation of receiving, you will be a kinder and happier person.

Kindness Is Not Always Returned

The widely known saying "actions speak louder than words" is well demonstrated in this *reality check*. Joe was a health care consultant. He had collected thousands of documents of helpful information to share with health care organizations with which he had worked. His thinking was this: Why should hospitals have to reinvent the wheel? If organizations are willing to share with others, why not disseminate such information for the benefit of other hospitals? His hopes were that larger trade organizations would eventually collect the information and freely share with their constituents. After all, the goal was better care for all wherever they lived. Joe would provide copies of his CD to fellow consultants and encourage them to share the information with others. One day upon arriving at work he noticed that one of the consultants to whom he had given a copy of the CD had four or five newspaper clippings about hospitals spread out on a conference room table. Joe thought they looked interesting and asked, "Could I have a copy of your clippings?" The consultant said, "No, these are proprietary information."

On another occasion, after sharing his CD with an organization, he asked, "Would you be willing to share your '12 Step Addiction Program' with other health care organizations?" A representative from the organization said, "We will share it with you but not others." Joe kindly said, "That's okay. I can accept only what you are willing to share with others."

Anonymous

Discussion

1. Should Joe have asked for his CD back from the consultant and organization? Discuss your answer.
2. Discuss why an organization might not be willing to share program information.

RESPECT

Respect for ourselves guides our morals; respect for others guides our manners.

–LAURENCE STERNE

Respect is an attitude of admiration or esteem. Kant was the first major Western philosopher to put respect for persons, including oneself as a person, at the center of moral theory. He believed that persons are ends in themselves with an absolute dignity, which must always be respected. In contemporary thinking, respect has become a core ideal extending moral respect to things other than persons, including all things in nature.

Caregivers who demonstrate respect for one another and their patients will be more effective in helping them cope with the anxiety of their illness. Respect helps to develop trust between the patient and caregiver and improve healing processes. If caregivers respect the family of a patient, cooperation and understanding will be the positive result, encouraging a team effort to improve patient care.

HOPEFULNESS

Hope is the last thing that dies in man; and though it be exceedingly deceitful, yet it is of this good use to us, that while we are traveling through life, it conducts us in an easier and more pleasant way to our journey's end.

–FRANCOIS DE LA ROCHEFOUCAULD

Brooke Greenberg: 20-Year-Old "Toddler's" Legacy of Hope and Love

The baffling case of Brooke Greenberg, a 20-year-old who never developed beyond the toddler stage, may provide clues to help scientists unlock the secrets of longevity and fight age-related disorders, such as Alzheimer's, Parkinson's, and heart disease. Brooke, who passed away last Thursday, had the body and cognitive function of a 1-year-old. She didn't grow after the age of 5—and basically, she stopped aging entirely.

Brooke may have been the only person in the world suffering from a mysterious genetic disease that her doctors called Syndrome X. "Finding out that her DNA makeup is completely different than anyone else brought to our attention that we could help," her father, Howard Greenberg, told Yahoo Shine in a previous interview. "So eventually, at the end of the rainbow, there will be something that comes out of all this. I believe everyone is here for a reason."

Sarah B. Weir, Healthy Living, *October 29, 2013*[14]

Hopefulness in the patient care setting involves looking forward to something with the confidence of success. Caregivers have a responsibility to balance truthfulness while promoting hope. The caregiver must be sensitive to each patient's needs and provide hope. As noted by Brooke's father, we can pass on hope and love to others.

TOLERANCE

There is a criterion by which you can judge whether the thoughts you are thinking and the things you are doing are right for you. The criterion is: Have they brought you inner peace? If they have not, there is something wrong with them—so keep seeking! If what you do has brought you inner peace, stay with what you believe is right.

—PEACE PILGRIM

Tolerance can be viewed in two ways, positive or negative. *Positive tolerance* implies that a person accepts differences in others and that one does not expect others to believe, think, speak, or act as he or she does. Tolerant people are generally free of prejudice and discrimination. Recognizing this fact, Thomas Jefferson incorporated theories of tolerance into the U.S. Constitution. *Negative tolerance* implies that one will reluctantly put up with another's beliefs. In other words, he or she merely tolerates the views of others.

Although tolerance can be viewed as a virtue, however, not all tolerance is virtuous nor is all intolerance necessarily wrong. An exaggerated tolerance may amount to a vice, whereas intolerance may sometimes be a virtue. For example, tolerating everything regardless of its repugnance (e.g., persecution for religious beliefs) is no virtue, and having intolerance for that which should not be tolerated and is evil is no vice (e.g., mass executions).

If we do not hang together, we will all hang separately.

—BENJAMIN FRANKLIN (1706–1790)

Cooperation is the process of working with others. In the health care setting, caregivers must work together to improve patient outcomes. The health care worker today works in an environment where change is the norm. Those unwilling to accept change and work in unity will eventually be working alone. Change is the only constant in today's workplace and society in general. Technological change is occurring at a pace faster than the human mind can absorb, thus requiring teamwork between individuals with a wide variety of skills sets. Congress, as noted in the following news clipping, is an example of how little can be accomplished when its members are dysfunctional and unwilling to cooperate and work together towards common goals.

Congress Gets Stuck Again—Over FAA

Parties Blame Each Other in Funding Dispute and Partial Shutdown

A dispute over funding for the Federal Aviation Administration has left an estimated 74,000 people out of work for a dozen days and tossed Congress into the throes of yet another interparty battle.

Now, with lawmakers leaving town or already on recess, there seems to be little hope of a resolution on the horizon.

Ashley Halsey III, The Washington Post, *August 4, 2011*

Failure to cooperate has a rippling effect in any setting. The failure of Congress to cooperate and resolve funding issues for the Federal Aviation Administration (FAA) before taking its summer recess in 2011 left 74,000 people out of work, costing the nation nearly a billion dollars for the month of August. Failure of the few to cooperate and act responsibly not only affected employees placed on a leave of absence but also placed a financial hardship on their families, not to mention the effect it has had on the communities where they live. In addition, passenger safety on airline flights was placed in jeopardy. If hospitals operated in this manner, there would be even more recorded bad outcomes. Teamwork is effective only as long as each member of the team cooperates and fulfills the duties assigned. High-quality patient care is more likely to be better in those organizations where respect and cooperation abounds.

Tying together the Patient Protection and Portable Care Act, commonly referred to as Obamacare, as a prerequisite to approving the national budget has merely resulted in name-calling by government officials, which has stirred bitterness between citizens of varying beliefs. Pundits and politicians alike fill the airways with contemptuous remarks that stoke the flames of division. The need to win one's point of view has selfishly become the norm and more important than the nation itself. Pride and self-appointed power brokers are the hallmarks of those responsible for crisis after crisis. Change comes when the players learn to cooperate for the common good.

Forgiveness is a virtue of the brave.

−INDIRA GANDHI

Forbearing one another, and forgiving one another, if any man have a quarrel against any:
even as Christ forgave you, so also do ye.

−COLOSSIANS 3:13 KJV

Forgiveness is a virtue and a value. It is the willingness to pardon someone who has wronged you in some way. It is also a form of mercy. Forgiveness is to forgive and let lose the bonds of blame. It is a form of cleansing souls of both those who forgive and those who accept the forgiveness offered.

The following *reality check* is an excerpt of a Facebook discussion between two friends involving courage and forgiveness by two very special people.

Courage and Forgiveness

7:38 am

Scotty: Did you see this link http://www.josieking.org/page.cfm?pageID=10 on the internet?

7:38 am

Diane: Reading it now

[Josie was 18 months old.... In January of 2001 Josie was admitted . . . after suffering first and second degree burns from climbing into a hot bath. She healed well and within weeks was scheduled for release. Two days before she was to return home she died of severe dehydration and misused narcotics ...

Josie spent 10 days in the PICU. I [Josie's mother] was by her side every day and night. I paid attention to every minute detail of the doctors' and nurses' care, and I was quick to ask questions. I bonded with them and was in constant awe of the medical attention she received . . . . She was sent down to the intermediate care floor with expectations of being sent home in a few days. Her three older siblings prepared for her welcome home celebration . . .

The following week her central line had been taken out. I began noticing that every time she saw a drink she would scream for it, and I thought this was strange. I was told not to let her drink. While a nurse and I gave her a bath, she sucked furiously on a washcloth. As I put her to bed, I noticed that her eyes were rolling back in her head. Although I asked the nurse to call the doctor, she reassured me that oftentimes children did this and her vitals were fine. I told her Josie had never done this and perhaps another nurse could look at her. After yet another reassurance from another nurse that everything was fine, I was told that it was okay for me to sleep at home. I called to check in two times during the night and returned to the hospital at 5:30 am. I took one look at Josie and demanded that a doctor come at once. She was not fine. Josie's medical team arrived and administered two shots of Narcan. I asked if she could have something to drink. The request was approved, and Josie gulped down nearly a liter of juice. Verbal orders were issued for there to be no narcotics given. As I sat with Josie, I noticed that the nurse on morning duty was acting very strangely. She seemed nervous, overly demonstrative and in a hurry. Uneasy, I asked the other nurses about her and they said she had been a nurse for a long time. Still worried, I expressed my concern to one of the doctors, and he agreed that she was acting a bit odd. Meanwhile, Josie started perking up. She was more alert and had kept all liquids down. I was still scared and asked her doctors to please stay close by. At 1:00 the nurse walked over with a syringe of methadone. Alarmed, I told her that there had been an order for no narcotics. She said the orders had been changed and administered the drug.

Josie's heart stopped as I was rubbing her feet. Her eyes were fixed, and I screamed for help. I stood helpless as a crowd of doctors and nurses came running into her room. I was ushered into a small room with a chaplain.

The next time I saw Josie she had been moved back up to the PICU. Doctors and nurses were standing around her bed. No one seemed to want to look at me. She was hooked up to many machines, and her leg was black and blue. I looked into their faces, and said to them, You did this to her now YOU must fix her. I was told to pray. Two days later Jack, Relly and Eva were brought to the hospital to kiss their beloved Josie goodbye. Josie was taken off of life support. She died in our arms on a snowy night in what's considered to be one of the best hospitals in the world. Our lives were shattered and changed forever.

Josie died from severe dehydration and misused narcotics. Careless human errors. On top of our overwhelming sorrow and intense grief we were consumed by anger. They say anger can do one of two things to you. It can cause you to rot away or it can propel you forward. There were days when all I wanted was to destroy the hospital and then put an end to my own pain. My three remaining children were my only reason for getting out of bed and functioning. One day I will tell them how they saved my life. My husband Tony and I decided that we had to let the anger move us forward. We would do something good that would help prevent this from ever happening to a child again.

7:43 am

Diane: I've experience first hand human error in the hospital. I was told by my Dr. it could have been critical and I would have died.

7:45 am

Diane: The nurses don't like him and he told me to write a letter to file a complaint, but the thing is, the nursing staff was so good to me before and after that incident. Evidently when it was happening he yelled at the staff without me knowing. I had no clue what had happened till days later the nurse involved apologized to me profusely.

7:46 am

Diane: But I was so ill I didn't give it much thought you ever heard of tpn? Its a sugar mixture via iv cuz i couldn't eat. Supposedly it was supposed to be infused in me I think over a 12 hr period?

7:47 am

Diane: But the nurse put it for 4 hrs. I could have gone into diabetic shock. I do remember trying to wake up but I couldn't open my eyes and I heard a lot of movement in my room with the nurses. I yelled out. I can't open my eyes and I'm dretched in sweat. I had no idea wat was happening. I was then put on insulin.

7:50 am

Scotty: I must say you are an amazing young lady.

Anonymous Patient

Discussion

1. This young lady forgave the nurse and suggested that when the nurse was setting the timing for the TPN, she may have distracted the nurse, and she blamed herself for the wrong setting. Discuss how courage and forgiveness were displayed in this case.
2. Discuss the similarities in values that Josie's mother and the young lady on the Internet have in common.
3. Discuss your thoughts as to how human errors can be prevented; including what roles patients, families, caregivers, hospitals, and regulatory agencies should play in preventing similar errors.

RELIGIOUS ETHICS

The Great Physician: Dear Lord, You are the great physician. I turn to you in my sickness, asking you for help. I place myself under Your loving care, praying that I may know Your healing grace and wholeness. Help me to find love in this strange world and to feel your presence by my bed both day and night. Give my doctors and nurses wisdom, that they may understand my illness. Steady and guide them with your strong hand. Reach out Your hand to me and touch my life with Your peace. Amen.

—University of Pennsylvania Health System

FIGURE 3 Religious Influence on Ethics (© Pack-Shot/Shutterstock, Inc.)

Religious ethics serve a moral purpose by providing codes of conduct for appropriate behavior through revelations from a divine source. These codes of conduct are enforced through fear of pain and suffering in the next life and/or reward in the next life for adhering to religious codes and beliefs. The prospect of divine justice helps us to tolerate the injustices in this life, where goodness is no guarantee of peace, happiness, wellness, or prosperity.

Many Think God's Intervention Can Revive the Dying

When it comes to saving lives, God trumps doctors for many Americans. An eye-opening survey reveals widespread belief that divine intervention can revive dying patients. And, researchers said, doctors "need to be prepared to deal with families who are waiting for a miracle."

Lindsey Tanner, USA Today, *August 18, 2008*

Religion should be a component of the education, policy development, and consultative functions of ethics committees. There is a need to know, for example, how to respond to Jehovah's Witnesses who refuse blood transfusions. Some hospitals provide staff with materials that describe various religious beliefs and how those beliefs might affect the patient's course of care while in the hospital.

Religion is often used as a reason to justify what otherwise could be considered unjustifiable behavior. Political leaders often use religion to legitimize and consolidate their power. Leaders in democratic societies speak of the necessity to respect the right to "freedom of religion."

Political leaders often use religion to further their political aspirations. They have often used religion to justify their actions. Religious persecution has plagued humanity from the beginning of time.

Syrian Rebels Combat al-Qaeda Force

The ISIS extremists "have not the support of the people because they treated them badly. They were cutting off people's heads all of the time to scare them in the name of religion," said Col. Qassim Saadeddine, spokesman for the Revolutionary Front.

Liz Sly, The Washington Post, *January 6, 2013*

The world today, with the aid of the news media, is able to see firsthand the results of what can happen to innocent people in the name of religion. The atrocities of evil people strapping bombs to the mentally deficient with the purpose of blowing themselves up in public places, killing and maiming men, women, and children, are but a few of the numerous atrocities of what has occurred throughout the ages.

Spirituality implies that there is purpose and meaning to life; spirituality generally refers to faith in a higher being. For a patient, injury and sickness are frightening experiences. This fear is often heightened when the patient is admitted to a hospital or nursing facility. Health care organizations can help reduce patient fears by making available to them appropriate emotional and spiritual support and coping resources. It is a well-proven fact that patients who are able to draw on their spirituality and religious beliefs tend to have a more comfortable and often improved healing experience. To assist both patients and caregivers in addressing spiritual needs, patients should be provided with information as to how their spiritual needs can be addressed.

Surgeon Uses Ministry in Medical Practice

DALLAS–At 83, Carl Smith found himself facing quadruple bypass surgery and the real possibility that he might not survive.

Within hours on this spring morning, Dr. Daniel Pool would temporarily bring Smith's heart to a stop in an attempt to circumvent its blocked passages.

And to help his patient confront the uncertainty, Pool did something unusual in his profession: He prayed with him.

The power of healing: Medicine and religion have had their day, and they haven't always been able to coexist. But as today's medical treatment becomes more holistic, doctors are increasingly taking spirituality into account.

Marc Ramirez, Altoona Mirror, *August 9, 2013*

Discussion

1. Discuss the pressure, if any, placed on the patient in responding to the suggestion of prayer prior to surgery.
2. Describe how you, as the surgeon, would address a patient's religious or spiritual needs if the risks of a complex surgical procedure appear to be threatening.

Difficult questions regarding a patient's spiritual needs and how to meet those needs are best addressed on admission by first collecting information about the patient's religious or spiritual preferences. Caregivers often find it difficult to discuss spiritual issues for fear of offending a patient who may have beliefs different from their own. If caregivers know from admission records a patient's religious beliefs, the caregiver can share with the patient those religious and spiritual resources available in the hospital and community.

A variety of religions are described next for the purpose of understanding some of the basic tenets of these religions. They are presented here to note the importance of better understanding why patients differ in decision-making processes and how religion affects their beliefs and to encourage further study of how each religion affects the decision-making process. Hospitals should maintain a directory of the various religions that includes contacts for referral and consultation purposes.

JUDAISM

Jewish Law refers to the unchangeable 613 mitzvot (commandments) that God gave to the Jews. Halakhah (Jewish Law) comes from three sources: (1) the Torah (the first five books of the Bible); (2) laws instituted by the rabbis; and (3) longstanding customs. The Jewish People is another name for the Children of Israel, referring to the Jews as a nation in the classical sense, meaning a group of people with a shared history and a sense of a group identity rather than a specific place or political persuasion.[15]

Judaism is a monotheistic religion based on principles and ethics embodied in the Hebrew Bible (Old Testament). The notion of right and wrong is not so much an object of philosophical inquiry as an acceptance of divine revelation. Moses, for example, received a list of 10 laws directly from God. These laws were known as the 10 Commandments. Some of the 10 Commandments are related to the basic principles of justice that have been adhered to by society since they were first proclaimed and published. For some societies, the 10 Commandments were a turning point, where essential commands such as "thou shalt not kill" or "thou shalt not commit adultery" were accepted as law. The 10 Commandments (King James Version of the Bible) are as follows:

1. Thou shalt have no other gods before me.
2. Thou shalt not make unto thee any graven image, or any likeness of anything that is in heaven above, or that is in the earth beneath, or that is in the water under the earth. Thou shalt not bow down thyself to them, nor serve them.
3. Thou shalt not take the name of the Lord thy God in vain.
4. Remember the Sabbath day, to keep it holy.
5. Honor thy father and thy mother: that thy days may be long upon the land which the Lord thy God giveth thee.
6. Thou shalt not kill.
7. Thou shalt not commit adultery.
8. Thou shalt not steal.
9. Thou shalt not bear false witness against thy neighbor.
10. Thou shalt not covet thy neighbor's house, thou shalt not covet thy neighbor's wife, nor his manservant, nor his maidservant, nor his ox, nor his ass, nor anything that is thy neighbor's.

When caring for the dying, family members will normally want to be present and prayers spoken. If a rabbi is requested, the patient's own rabbi should be contacted first.

HINDUISM

Hinduism is a polytheistic religion with many gods and goddesses. Hindus believe that God is everything and is infinite. The earliest known Hindu Scriptures were recorded around 1200 BC. Hindus believe in reincarnation and that one's present condition is a reflection of one's virtuous behavior or lack thereof in a previous lifetime.

When caring for the dying, relatives may wish to perform rituals at this time. In death, jewelry, sacred threads, or other religious objects should not be removed from the body. Washing the body is part of the funeral rites and should be carried out by the relatives.[16]

BUDDHISM

Buddhism is a religion and philosophy encompassing a variety of traditions, beliefs, and practices, based largely on teachings attributed to Prince Siddhartha Gautama (563–483 BC), son of King Suddhodana and Queen Mayadevi, who lived in the present-day border area between India and Nepal. He had gone on a spiritual quest and eventually became enlightened at the age of 35, and from then on, he took the name Buddha. Simply defined, Buddhism is a religion to some and a philosophy to others that encourages one "to do good, avoid evil, and purify the mind."

When caring for the dying, Buddhists like to be informed about their health status in order to prepare themselves spiritually. A side room with privacy is preferred.[17]

Falun Gong

Falun Gong, also referred to as *Falun Dafa*, is a traditional Chinese spiritual discipline belonging to the Buddhist school of thought. It consists of moral teachings, a meditation, and four exercises that resemble tai chi and are known in Chinese culture as *qigong*. Falun Gong does not involve physical places of worship, formal hierarchies, rituals, or membership and is taught without charge. The three principles practiced by the followers are truthfulness, compassion, and forbearance/tolerance toward others. The followers of Falun Gong claim a following in 100 countries.

Zen

Zen evolved from Buddhism in Tibet. It emphasizes dharma practice (from the master to the disciple) and experiential wisdom based on learning through the reflection on doing, going beyond scriptural readings. In Zen, Buddhism learning comes through a form of seated meditation known as *zazen*, where practitioners perform meditation to calm the body and the mind and experience insight into the nature of existence and thereby gain enlightenment.

TAOISM

Taoists believe that ultimate reality is unknowable and unperceivable. The founder of Taoism is believed to be Lao Tzu (6 BC). Taoist doctrine includes the belief that the proper way of living involves being in tune with nature. Everything is ultimately interblended and interacts.

CHRISTIANITY

Christianity is based on the Bible's New Testament teachings. Christians accept both the Old and New Testament as being the word of God. The New Testament describes Jesus as being God, taking the form of man. He was born of the Virgin Mary, sacrificed his life by suffering crucifixion, and after being raised from the dead on the third day, he ascended into Heaven from which he will return to raise the dead, at which time the spiritual body will be united with the physical body. His death, burial, and resurrection provide a way of salvation through belief in Him for the forgiveness of sin. God is believed to be manifest in three persons: the Father, Son, and Holy Spirit.

The primary and final authority for Christian ethics is found in the life, teachings, ministry, death, and resurrection of Jesus Christ. He clarified the ethical demands of a God-centered life by applying the obedient love that was required of Peter. The 10 Commandments are accepted and practiced by both Christians and Jews.

Christians, when determining what is the right thing to do, often refer to the Golden Rule, which teaches us to "do unto others as you would have them do unto you," a common principle in many moral codes and religions.

There have been and continue to be numerous interpretations of the meaning of the scriptures and their different passages by Christians over the centuries. This has resulted in a plethora of churches with varying beliefs. As noted later, such beliefs can affect a patient's wishes for health care. However, the heart of Christian beliefs is found in the book of John:

For God so loved the world, that he gave his only begotten Son, that whoever believeth in him should not perish, but have everlasting life.

– King James Version, John 3:16

The Apostle Paul proclaimed that salvation cannot be gained through good works but through faith in Jesus Christ as savior. He recognized the importance of faith in Christ over good works in the pursuit of salvation.

That if thou shalt confess with thy mouth the Lord Jesus, and shalt believe in thine heart that God hath raised him from the dead, thou shalt be saved.

– King James Version, Romans 10:9

The Apostle Paul, however, did not dismiss the importance of good works. Works are the fruit of one's faith. In other words, good works follows faith.

Anointing of the Sick

When caring for the dying, services of the in-house chaplain and/or one's religious minister should be offered the patient. A Catholic priest should be offered when last rites need to be administered to those of the Catholic faith.

Islam

The Islamic religion believes there is one God: Allah. Muhammad (570–632 AD) is considered to be a prophet/messenger of God. He is believed to have received revelations from God. These revelations were recorded in the Qur'an, the Muslim Holy Book. Muslims accept Moses and Jesus as prophets of God. The Qur'an is believed to supersede that of the Torah and the Bible. Muslims believe that there is no need for God's grace and that their own actions can merit God's mercy and goodness. Humans are believed to have a moral responsibility to submit to God's will and to follow Islam as demonstrated in the Qur'an. The five pillars of the practice of Islam are believing the creed, performing five prayers daily, giving alms, fasting during Ramadan, and making a pilgrimage to Mecca at least once in a lifetime.

When caring for the dying, patients may want to die facing Mecca (toward the southeast) and be with relatives. In death, many Muslims follow strict rules in respect of the body after death.

Religious beliefs and codes of conduct sometimes conflict with the ethical duty of caregivers to save lives. For example, Jehovah's Witnesses, believe that it is a sin to accept a blood transfusion because the Bible states that we must "abstain from blood" (Acts 15:29). Current Jehovah's Witness doctrine, in part, states that blood must not be transfused. In order to respect this belief, bloodless surgery is available in a number of hospitals to patients who find it against their religious beliefs to receive a blood transfusion.

Every attempt should be made to resolve blood transfusion issues prior to any elective surgery. The transfusion of blood to an emergent unconscious patient may be necessary to save the patient's life. Because some Jehovah's Witnesses would accept blood in such situations, most courts would most likely find such a transfusion acceptable. When transfusion of a minor becomes necessary and parental consent is refused, it may be necessary to seek a court order to allow for such transfusions. Because time is of the essence in many cases, it is important for hospitals to work out such issues in advance with legislative bodies and the judicial system in order to provide legal protection for caregivers who find it necessary to transfuse blood in order to save a life. In those instances in which the patient has a right to refuse a blood transfusion, the hospital should seek a formal signed release from the patient.

SECULAR ETHICS

Unlike religious ethics, *secular ethics* is based on codes developed by societies that have relied on customs to formulate their codes. The Code of Hammurabi, for example, carved on a black Babylonian column 8 feet high, now located in the Louvre in Paris, depicts a mythical sun god presenting a code of laws to Hammurabi, a great military leader and ruler of Babylon (1795–1750 BC). Hammurabi's code of laws is an early example of a ruler proclaiming to his people an entire body of laws. The following excerpts are from the Code of Hammurabi.

Code of Hammurabi

5

If a judge try a case, reach a decision, and present his judgment in writing; if later error shall appear in his decision, and it be through his own fault, then he shall pay twelve times the fine set by him in the case, and he shall be publicly removed from the judge's bench, and never again shall he sit there to render judgment.

194

If a man give his child to a nurse and the child die in her hands, but the nurse unbeknown to the father and mother nurse another child, then they shall convict her of having nursed another child without the knowledge of the father and mother and her breasts shall be cut off.

215

If a physician make a large incision with an operating knife and cure it, or if he open a tumor (over the eye) with an operating knife, and saves the eye, he shall receive ten shekels in money.

217

If he be the slave of some one, his owner shall give the physician two shekels.

218

If a physician make a large incision with the operating knife, and kill him, or open a tumor with the operating knife, and cut out the eye, his hands shall be cut off.

219

If a physician make a large incision in the slave of a freed man, and kill him, he shall replace the slave with another slave.

221

If a physician heal the broken bone or diseased soft part of a man, the patient shall pay the physician five shekels in money.

ATHEISM

Atheism is the rejection of belief in any god, generally because atheists believe there is no scientific evidence that can prove God exists. They argue that there is no objective moral standard for right and wrong and that ethics and morality are the products of culture and politics, subject to individual convictions.

Those of various religious faiths, however, believe there is overwhelming evidence that there is reason to believe that God does exist and that the evidence through historical documents, archeological finds, and the vastness of space and time clearly supports and confirms the existence of God. Christians often refer to the Old Testament and cite the book of Isaiah:

It is He that sitteth upon the circle of the earth . . .

—Isaiah 40:22 (King James Version)

Christians argue when citing this verse that Isaiah could not possibly know that the earth is the shape of a circle. He presents no magical formula or scientific argument in his writings as to why the earth is round. Furthermore, Isaiah does not belabor the fact that the earth is round. The argument continues in the book of Job:

He stretcheth out the north over the empty place, and hangeth the earth upon nothing.

—Job 26:7 (King James Version)

The obvious question then arises, how did Job know, 3,000 years before it became a scientific, verifiable fact, the earth hangs upon nothing?

SITUATIONAL ETHICS

Be careful how you judge others. . . . As Scottish author J.M. Barrie said, "Never ascribe to an opponent motives meaner than your own." We tend to judge others based on their behavior, and ours based on our intent. In almost all situations, we would do well to recognize the possibility— even probability—of good intent in others . . . sometimes despite their observable behavior.

—Stephen M. R. Covey, *The Speed of Trust* (Free Press)

Situational ethics is concerned with the outcome or consequences of an action in which the ends can justify the means. It refers to those times when a person's beliefs and values can change as circumstances change. Why do good people behave differently in similar situations? Why do good people sometimes do bad things? The answer is fairly simple: One's moral character can sometimes change as circumstances change; thus the term situational ethics. A person, therefore, may contradict what he believes is the right thing to do and do what he morally considers wrong. For example, a decision not to use extraordinary means to sustain the life of an unknown 84-year-old may result in a different decision if the 84-year-old is one's mother.

The news clipping that follows illustrates how far society can regress when there are no common rules, values, or boundaries to guide us.

Viet Cong Execution

"And out of nowhere came this guy who we didn't know." Gen. Nguyen Ngoc Loan, chief of South Viet Nam's national police, walked up and shot the prisoner in the head. His reason: The prisoner, a Viet Cong lieutenant, had just murdered a South Vietnamese colonel, his wife, and their six children.

The peace movement adopted the photo as a symbol of the war's brutality. But Adams, who stayed in touch with Loan, said the photo wrongly stereotyped the man. "If you're this general and you caught this guy after he killed some of your people . . . how do you know you wouldn't have pulled that trigger yourself? You have to put yourself in that situation. . . . It's a war."

1969 Spot News, Newseum, *Washington, DC*

Have we lost our way? Have we lost our sense as to what is right and what is wrong? We say we have become a melting pot with some common themes but uncommon beliefs. In religion, there are those who sometimes seek a place of worship not always because one seeks what is right but because unconsciously it supports an individual's beliefs of what is right and wrong. Sometimes one's ever-changing choice of lifestyle contradicts earlier beliefs and can often result in a change in place of worship.

The values held ever so strongly in one situation may conflict with the same values given a different fact pattern. To better understand the concept of situational ethics, consider the desire to live and the extreme measures one will take in order to do so, remembering that ethical decision making is the process of determining the right thing to do when faced with moral dilemmas.

Consider the account of the plane crash on October 13, 1972, high in the Andes Mountains. The survivors of the crash, until the day they were rescued, were faced with difficult decisions in order to survive. Of the original 40 passengers and 5 crewmembers, 16 emerged alive 72 days later to tell the story of the difficult ethical dilemmas and survival decisions they had to make.

Those who wished to survive had to eat the flesh of those who did not. They realized that to survive, they would have to deviate from their beliefs that teach it is morally wrong to eat the flesh of another human being. Given a different fact pattern, where there would have been an abundance of food at the site of the plane crash, the survivors would have found it reprehensible to eat human flesh. This is a gruesome story indeed, but it illustrates how there are no effective hard and fast rules or guidelines to govern ethical behavior when faced with life or death decisions. The reader here should consider here how one's beliefs, decisions, and or actions can change as circumstances change. Such is the case in the patient care setting where individual differences emerge based on needs, beliefs, and values.

ABSENCE OF A MORAL COMPASS

© marekuliasz/Shutterstock

The world is a dangerous place. Not because of the people who are evil; but because of the people who don't do anything about it.

—ALBERT EINSTEIN

The nation's health care system is off course as noted by the absence of a moral compass. Trust in the health care system continues to decline when those who are entrusted with providing health care prescribe unnecessary procedures (e.g., cardiac catheterizations, hysterectomies, tonsillectomies), molest our children, secretly record photographic pictures of patients while they are receiving physical examinations, numerous fraudulent billing scams costing the nation billions of dollars annually, tampering with chemotherapy agents by diluting them (unbeknown by patients who trust they are being treated by caregivers with integrity), unwarranted high-risk life-saving treatment delays for our veterans and falsification of records, and the list of unethical behavior continues to grow, seemingly unabated. The failure of government and those in leadership roles have failed to reset the nation's moral compass. The present path to better health care for all continues on an unacceptable course of corruption and is increasingly becoming a disturbing public concern.

Political corruption, antisocial behavior, declining civility, and rampant unethical conduct have heightened discussions over the nation's moral decline and decaying value systems in the delivery of health care. The numerous instances of questionable political decisions; numbers-cooking executives with exorbitant salaries, including health care executives working for both profit and nonprofit organizations, have all contributed to the nation's moral decline.

The continuing trend of consumer awareness of declining value systems mandates that the readers of this book understand ethics and the law and how they intertwine. Applying the generally accepted ethical principles (e.g., do good and not harm) and the moral values (e.g., respect, trust, integrity, compassion) described in this chapter will help sit a better course for those who are guided by a moral compass. It is the responsibility of every person to participate in resetting the moral compass, in our nation and in the world at large.

SUMMARY THOUGHTS

Be careful of your thoughts, for your thoughts inspire your words. Be careful of your words, for your words precede your actions. Be careful of your actions, for your actions become your habits. Be careful of your habits, for your habits build your character. Be careful of your character, for your character decides your destiny.

—Chinese Proverb

Although you cannot control the amount of time you have in this lifetime, you can control your behavior by adopting the virtues and values that will define who you are and what you will become and how you will be remembered or forgotten.

Become who you want to be and behave how you want to be remembered. The formula is easy and well described previously in what has been claimed to be a Chinese proverb. Read it. Reread it. Write it. Memorize it. Display it in your home, at work, and in your car, and most of all, practice it, always remembering that it all begins with thoughts.

Control your thoughts, and do not let them control you. As to words, they are the tools of thought. They can be sharper than any double-edged sword and hurt, or they can do good and heal.

It is never too late to change your thoughts, as long as you have air to breathe. Your legacy may be short, but it can be powerful. Remember the Gettysburg address. In the final analysis:

People are often unreasonable, illogical and self-centered; forgive them anyway. If you are kind, people may accuse you of selfish, ulterior motives; be kind anyway. If you are successful, you will win some false friends and some true enemies; succeed anyway. What you spend years building, someone may destroy overnight; build anyway. The good you do today, people will often forget tomorrow; do good anyway. Give the world the best you have, and it may never be enough; give the world the best you have anyway. You see, in the final analysis, it is between you and God; It was never between you and them anyway.

—Author Unknown

1. *Ethics* is the branch of philosophy that seeks to understand the nature, purposes, justification, and founding principles of moral rules and the systems they compose.
   - *Microethics* involves an individual's view of what is right and wrong based on his or her life experiences.
   - *Macroethics* involves a more generalized view of right and wrong.
2. *Bioethics* addresses such difficult issues as the nature of life, the nature of death, what sort of life is worth living, what constitutes murder, how we should treat people who are especially vulnerable, and the responsibilities we have to other human beings.
3. We study ethics to aid us in making sound judgments, good decisions, and right choices.
4. Ethics signifies a general pattern or way of life, such as religious ethics; a set of rules of conduct or "moral code," which involves professional ethics; or philosophical ethics, which involves inquiry about ways of life and rules of conduct.
5. *Morality* is a code of conduct. It is a guide to behavior that all rational persons would put forward for governing the behavior of all moral agents.
6. There is no "universal morality." Whatever guide to behavior that an individual regards as overriding and wants to be universally adopted is considered that individual's morality.
7. *Moral judgments* are those judgments concerned with what an individual or group believes to be the right or proper behavior in a given situation.
8. Morality is often legislated when differences cannot be resolved because of conflicting moral codes with varying opinions as to what is right and what is wrong (e.g., abortion). Laws are created to set boundaries for societal behavior, and they are enforced to ensure that the expected behavior is followed.
9. *Ethical theories* and principles introduce order into the way people think about life. *Metaethics* seeks to understand ethical terms and theories and their application. The following are ethical theories:
   - *Normative ethics* is the attempt to determine what moral standards should be followed so that human behavior and conduct may be morally right.
   - *Descriptive ethics*, also known as comparative ethics, deals with what people believe to be right and wrong.
   - *Applied ethics* is the application of normative theories to practical moral problems. It is the attempt to explain and justify specific moral problems such as abortion, euthanasia, and assisted suicide.
   - The *consequential theory* emphasizes that the morally right action is whatever action leads to the maximum balance of good over evil. The consequential theory is based on the view that the value of an action derives solely from the value of its consequences.
   - *Utilitarian ethics* involves the concept that the moral worth of an action is determined solely by its contribution to overall utility, that is, its contribution to happiness or pleasure as summed among all persons.

- *Deontological ethics* focuses on one's duties to others. It includes telling the truth and keeping your promises. Deontology is an ethical analysis according to a moral code or rules.
- The *nonconsequential ethical theory* denies that the consequences of an action or rule are the only criteria for determining the morality of an action or rule.
- *Ethical relativism* is the theory that holds that morality is relative to the norms of one's culture.

10. Common principles of ethics include:
- *Autonomy* involves recognizing the right of a person to make his or her own decisions.
- *Beneficence* describes the principle of doing good, demonstrating kindness, showing compassion, and helping others.
  - *Paternalism* is a form of beneficence. It may involve withholding information from a person because of the belief that doing so is in the best interest of that person.
  - *Medical paternalism* involves making choices for (or forcing choices on) patients who are capable of choosing for themselves. It directly violates patient autonomy.
- *Nonmaleficence* is an ethical principle that requires caregivers to avoid causing harm to patients.
- *Justice* is the obligation to be fair in the distribution of benefits and risks.
  - *Distributive justice* is a principle that requires treatment of all persons equally and fairly.

11. *Virtue ethics and values*
- *Virtue* is normally defined as some sort of moral excellence or beneficial quality. In traditional ethics, virtues are characteristics that differentiate good people from bad people.
- *Virtue ethics* focuses on the inherent character of a person rather than on the specific actions he or she performs.
- *Value* is something that has worth. Values are used for judging the goodness or badness of some action.
  - *Ethical values* imply standards of worth.
  - *Intrinsic value* is something that has value in and of itself.
  - *Instrumental value* is something that helps to give value to something else (e.g., money is valuable for what it can buy).
  - Values may change as needs change.

12. *Religious ethics* serves a moral purpose by providing codes of conduct for appropriate behavior through revelations from a divine source.

13. *Secular ethics* is based on codes developed by societies that have relied on customs to formulate their codes.

14. *Situational ethics* describes how a particular situation may influence how one's reaction and values may change in order to cope with changing circumstances.

15. The acceptance, understanding, and application of the ethical and moral concepts learned in this chapter will provide a *Moral Compass* to guide the reader through life's journey.

TERMINOLOGY

applied ethics
autonomy
beneficence
bioethics
code of ethics
commitment
compassion
conscientiousness
consequential theory
cooperation
courage
deontological ethics
descriptive ethics
detachment
distributive justice
discernment
employment-related
   paternalism
ethical principles

ethical relativism
ethical theories
ethics
fairness
fidelity
freedom
honesty
hopefulness
instrumental value
integrity
intrinsic value
justice
kindness
macroethics
medical paternalism
metaethics
microethics
moral dilemmas
moral judgments

morality
moral values
nonconsequential ethics
nonmaleficence
normative ethics
paternalism
religious ethics
respect
secular ethics
situational ethics
spirituality
tolerance
truth telling
values
veracity
virtue ethics
virtues

REVIEW QUESTIONS

1. What is ethics?

2. Why should one study ethics?

3. What is morality?

4. Describe the ethical theories presented in this chapter.

5. What is ethical relativism? What is the relevance of this concept to individuals of various cultures living in the same society?

6. Describe the various ethical principles reviewed and how they might be helpful in resolving health care ethical dilemmas.

7. Describe virtue ethics and values. How do virtues and values differ?

8. Discuss why "courage" could be considered as the greatest of all virtues.

9. Discuss how religion can affect one's character.

10. Describe the principle of justice and how it can affect the decision-making process.

11. Explain how you would allocate scarce resources in the provision of health care?

12. What is "situational ethics"? Why do people behave differently in different situations?

NOTES

1. http://www.bukisa.com/articles/15091_the-root-of-ethics-and-morality.
2. Ayer, A. J., 1946. "A Critique of Ethics," in *Language, Truth and Logic*, London: Gollanz, pp. 102–114.
3. http://public.health.oregon.gov/ProviderPartnerResources/EvaluationResearch/DeathwithDignityAct/Pages/index.aspx.
4. http://www.ethicsmorals.com/ethicsapplied.html.
5. http://smallbusiness.chron.com/workplace-example-duty-based-ethics-11972.html
6. 105 N.E. 92, 93 (N.Y. 1914).
7. http://www.ama-assn.org/ama/pub/physician-resources/medical-ethics/code-medical-ethics/principles-medical-ethics.page
8. http://www.healthlawyers.org/Members/PracticeGroups/PALS/emailalerts/Documents/131111_Surveyand-CertLetter.pdf.
9. Craig Robert Senn, Fixing Inconsistent Paternalism Under Federal Employment Discrimination Law 58 UCLA L. Rev. 947. http://uclalawreview.org/?p=1679.
10. 464 A.2d 303, 314 (N.J. Super. Ct. App. Div. 1983).
11. http://www.mercurynews.com/san-mateo-county-times/ci_23948856/peninsula-child-psychiatrist-william-ayres-sentenced-eight-years?source=rss&cid=dlvr.it.
12. http://www.bukisa.com/articles/15091_the-root-of-ethics-and-morality.
13. http://www.gallup.com/poll/7288/Fear-Factor-Patient-Satisfaction.aspx.
14. http://shine.yahoo.com/healthy-living/brooke-greenberg-20-old-8220-toddler-8217-8221-185100345.html.
15. Tracey R. Rich, "Halakhah: Jewish Law," http://www.jewfaq.org/halakhah.htm (accessed October 13, 2010).
16. *Id.*
17. *Id.*

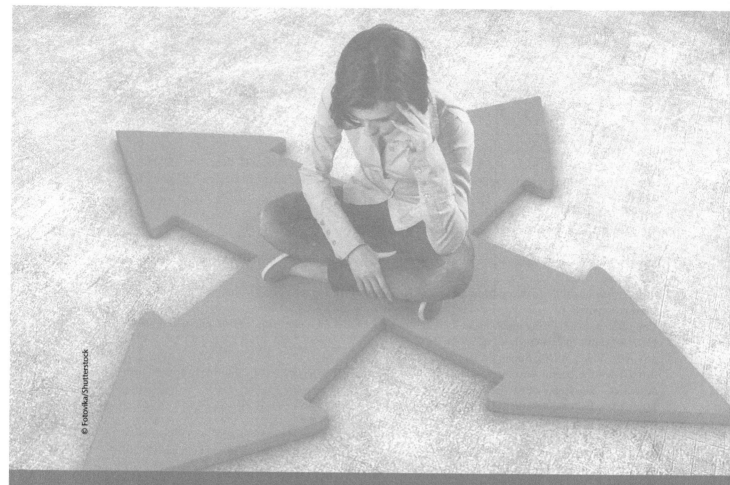

CONTEMPORARY ETHICAL DILEMMAS

No right is held more sacred, or is more carefully guarded, by the common law, than the right of every individual to the possession and control of his own person, free from all restraint or interference of others, unless by clear and unquestioned authority of law.

—UNION PAC. RY. CO. V. BOTSFORD[1]

LEARNING OBJECTIVES

Upon completion of this chapter, the reader will be able to:

- Describe various historical events that have had an impact on the resolution of ethical dilemmas.
- Describe common ethical dilemmas and the various ethical issues that have in many instances divided many segments of the population. Topics include abortion; sterilization; artificial insemination; surrogacy; organ donations; research, experimentation, and clinical trials; human genetics, stem cell research; and, AIDS.

INTRODUCTION

An *ethical dilemma* arises in situations where a choice must be made between unpleasant alternatives. It can occur whenever a choice involves giving up something good and suffering something bad, no matter what course of action is taken. Ethical dilemmas often require care-givers to make decisions that may break some ethical norm or contradict some ethical value. For example, should I choose life knowing that an unborn child will be born with severe disabilities, or should I choose abortion and thus prevent pain for both parent and child? Should I adhere to my spouse's wishes not to be placed on a respirator, or should I choose life over death, disregarding her wishes and right to self-determination? Should I encourage my daughter—the victim of a gang rape—to have an abortion or should I choose life and "do no harm" to the unborn child? Such dilemmas give rise to conflicting answers.

There is a wide range of ethical and legal issues impacting the health care system. This chapter focuses on some of the more common ethical and legal dilemmas facing the providers of health care. In reviewing this chapter, the reader should apply court decisions and the ethical theories, principles, and values previously discussed.

NOTEWORTHY HISTORICAL EVENTS

I was created at the end of the Renaissance, watched pirates rule the oceans as Ivan the Terrible ruled Russia, and witnessed the arrest of Galileo for believing the earth revolved around the sun.

–I AM HISTORY

The historical events presented in this section describe some of the many milestones that have had a significant impact on health care ethics.

58,000–68,000 BC

Neanderthal Burial Sites

Evidence of belief in an afterlife was found in Neanderthal burial sites, where various implements and supplies were buried with the deceased.

> According to anthropologist F. Clark Howell the flexed position of the body, and discoveries of other sites where stone slabs were placed over the Neanderthal graves, along with food and tools, suggests that Neanderthal man believed in life after death. Their concept of the afterlife must not have been that much different than the life they experienced on earth; they provided the dead with food, tools, and other every-day items, much like the Egyptians did for their journey to the next life.[2]

1932–1972

Tuskegee Study of Syphilis

The Tuskegee Study of Syphilis, involving African American men, was designed to analyze the natural progression of untreated syphilis. The study was conducted from 1932 through the early 1970s. The participants were not told during the study that there was a cure for syphilis (e.g., penicillin). They believed that they were receiving adequate care and unknowingly suffered unnecessarily. The Tuskegee syphilis study used disadvantaged, rural black men to investigate the untreated course of a disease, one that is by no means confined to that population. We know now that the selection of research subjects must be closely monitored to ensure that specific classes of individuals (e.g., terminally ill patients, welfare patients, racial and ethnic minorities, or persons confined to institutions) are not selected for research studies because of their easy availability, compromised position, or manipulability. Rather, they must be selected for reasons directly related to the research being conducted.

1933–1945

The Holocaust

The Holocaust was one of the most violent events in human history. Over 6 million Jews were murdered as well as millions of people from other cultural groups, including Slavs, homosexuals, and Gypsies.

Doctors have always been thought of as the saviors of mankind, the healers, and caretakers of our utter existence. Even ancient civilizations revered the medicine men as having special power to protect life. The trust of a physician is sacred. This is why the practice of medicine by the doctors of the Third Reich is egregious, outrageous, and shocking. The Nazi doctors violated the trust placed in them by humanity. The most painful truth is for the most part the doctors escaped their crimes against Humanity and lived a life, unlike their victims.[3]

1946

Military Tribunal for War Crimes

In 1946, the Military Tribunal for War Crimes began criminal proceedings against 23 German physicians and administrators for war crimes and crimes against humanity. As a direct result of these proceedings, the Nuremberg Code was established, which made it clear that the voluntary and informed consent of human subjects is essential to research and that benefits of research must outweigh risks to human subjects involved.[4]

1949

WMA International Code of Medical Ethics

The World Medical Association International Code of Medical Ethics was adopted in October 1949 after it was learned that the Nazis conducted numerous inhumane experiments on prisoners in concentration camps. Prisoners were exposed to cholera, diphtheria, malaria, mustard gas, yellow fever, and typhus and forced to participate in other horrendous experiments, ultimately claiming thousands of lives. This exploitation of unwilling prisoners as research subjects was condemned as a particularly flagrant injustice. The code was amended at the 57th WMA General Assembly, Pilanesberg, South Africa, October 2006.[5]

1954

Guidelines on Human Experimentation

The National Institutes of Health published guidelines on human experimentation following the first kidney transplant[6] conducted in 1954. The transplantation of human organs has generated numerous ethical issues (e.g., the harvesting and selling of organs, who should have first access to freely donated human organs, how death is defined).

1960s

Cardiopulmonary Resuscitation Raises Ethical Dilemmas

Cardiopulmonary resuscitation was developed, leading to numerous ongoing ethical dilemmas because it involves the prolonging of life beyond what would reasonably be expected. Should limited resources, for example, be spent on those who have been determined to be in a comatose vegetative state without hope of recovery? Or, should limited resources be spent on preventative medicine, aimed at improving the quality of life?

1964

WHO Guidelines for Conducting Biomedical Research

The World Medical Association[7] established guidelines for medical doctors conducting biomedical research involving human subjects. The Declaration of Helsinki is the basis for advanced clinical practices today.[8]

1968

Harvard Ad Hoc Committee on Brain Death

The Harvard Ad Hoc Committee on Brain Death published the following criteria to aid in determining a permanently nonfunctioning brain, a condition it referred to as "irreversible coma," now known as brain death:

1. Patient shows total unawareness to external stimuli and unresponsiveness to painful stimuli.
2. No movements or breathing: All spontaneous muscular movement, spontaneous respiration, and response to stimuli are absent.
3. No reflexes: Fixed, dilated pupils; no eye movement even when hit or turned, or when ice water is placed in the ear; no response to noxious stimuli; no tendon reflexes.

In addition to these criteria, the report recommended adding the presence of a flat electroencephalogram.[9]

1970

Patient as a Person

The Patient as a Person by Paul Ramsey discusses the question of *paternalism*. As physicians are faced with many options for saving lives, transplanting organs, and furthering research, they also must wrestle with new and troubling choices, for example, who should receive scarce resources (e.g.., organ transplants), how to determine when life ends, and what limits should be placed on care for the dying.

1971

Kennedy Institute of Ethics

The Joseph P. and Rose F. Kennedy Institute of Ethics was established at Georgetown University in 1971 by a generous grant from the Joseph P. Kennedy, Jr., Foundation. Today it is the world's oldest and most comprehensive academic bioethics center. The institute and its library serve as an unequaled resource for those who research and study ethics, as well as those who debate and make public policy. The Kennedy Institute is home to scholars who engage in research, teaching, and public service on issues that include protection of research subjects, reproductive and feminist bioethics, end-of-life care, health care justice, intellectual disability, cloning, gene therapy, eugenics, and other major bioethical issues. Institute scholars figure prominently among the pioneers of the discipline. They are extending the boundaries of the field to incorporate emerging issues of racial and gender equality, international justice and peace, and other policies affecting the world's most vulnerable populations.[10]

1972

Informed Consent

Informed consent in the *Canterbury v. Spence*[11] case set the *reasonable man standard*, requiring informed consent for treatment. Patients must be informed of the risks, benefits, and alternatives associated with recommended treatments. The court found that Dr. Spence negligently failed to disclose a risk of serious disability inherent in the operation and that the Washington Hospital Center provided negligent postoperative care.[12]

1973

Women's Right to Abortion

The *Roe v. Wade*[13] abortion case gave strength to a woman's right to privacy in the context of matters relating to her own body, including how a pregnancy would end.

1974

National Research Act (NRA) of 1974

Because of publicity from the Tuskegee Syphilis Study, the National Research Act (NRA) of 1974 was passed. The NRA created the National Commission for the Protection of Human Subjects of Biomedical and Behavioral Research. One of the commission's charges was to identify the basic ethical principles that should underlie the conduct of biomedical and behavioral research involving human subjects and to develop guidelines to ensure that such research is conducted in accordance with those principles.[14]

The commission was directed to consider the following:[15]

1. The boundaries between biomedical and behavioral research and the accepted and routine practice of medicine
2. The role of assessment of risk-benefit criteria in determining the appropriateness of research involving human subjects
3. Appropriate guidelines for the selection of human subjects for participation in such research
4. The nature and definition of informed consent in various research settings

1976

Substitute Judgment—Karen Ann Quinlan

The New Jersey Supreme Court in the *Matter of Karen Ann Quinlan*[16] rendered a unanimous decision providing for the appointment of Joseph Quinlan as personal guardian of his daughter, Karen Ann Quinlan. The record was remanded to the trial court to implement without further testimonial hearing:

> To appoint Joseph Quinlan as guardian of the person of Karen Quinlan with full power to make decisions with regard to the identity of her treating physicians.
>
> We repeat for the sake of emphasis and clarity that upon the concurrence of the guardian and family of Karen, should the responsible attending physicians conclude that there is no reasonable possibility of Karen's ever emerging from her present comatose condition to a cognitive, sapient state and that the life-support apparatus now being administered to Karen should be discontinued, they shall consult with the hospital "Ethics Committee" or like body of the institution in which Karen is then hospitalized. If that consultative body agrees that there is no reasonable possibility of Karen's ever emerging from her present comatose condition to a cognitive, sapient state, the present life-support system may be withdrawn and said action shall be without any civil or criminal liability therefor, on the part of any participant, whether guardian, physician, hospital or others.
>
> By the above ruling we do not intend to be understood as implying that a proceeding for judicial declaratory relief is necessarily required for the implementation of comparable decisions in the field of medical practice.

First Living Will Legislation Enacted

In California, the first living will legislation was enacted, permitting a person to sign a declaration stating that if there is no hope of recovery, no heroic measures need to be taken to prolong life. This provision is now available in every state.

1978

Commission for the Study of Ethical Problems

The President's Commission for the Study of Ethical Problems in Medicine includes studies regarding the ethical and legal issues of informed consent for research participants;

the matter of defining death, including the advisability of developing a uniform definition of death; the voluntary testing, counseling, and information and education programs with respect to genetic diseases and conditions, taking into account the essential equality of all human beings, born and unborn; the differences in the availability of health services, as determined by the income or residence of the persons receiving the services; current procedures and mechanisms designed to safeguard the privacy of human subjects of behavioral and biomedical research, to ensure the confidentiality of individually identifiable patient records and to ensure appropriate access of patients to information; and such other matters relating to medicine or biomedical or behavioral research as the president may designate for study by the commission.[17]

1980

Hemlock Society

The Hemlock Society was an organization formed to advocate for physician-assisted dying for the terminally ill, mentally competent patient suffering with incurable illnesses.

Controversial in death as in life, the Hemlock Society USA as a name died suddenly on June 13, 2003, in a boardroom in Denver, Colorado. It was 23 years old. Public relations experts and political strategists—leaning heavily on focus groups—were on hand to usher in the death knell. Months of agonizing debate had preceded the decision because no one could think of a better name![18]

1983

First Durable Power of Attorney Legislation

California enacted the first durable power of attorney legislation permitting an advance directive to be made describing the kind of health care that one would desire when facing death by designating an agent to act on the patient's behalf. Currently the California Health Care Directive form in part reads:

You have the right to give instructions about your own health care. You also have the right to name someone else to make health care decisions for you. This form lets you do either or both of these things. It also lets you express your wishes regarding donation of organs and the designation of your primary physician. If you use this form, you may complete or modify all or any part of it. You are free to use a different form. [CALIFORNIA PROBATE CODE SECTION 4700-4701][19]

Compassion and Choices

The Hemlock Society evolved into "End-of-Life Choices, which in 2005 merged with Compassion in Dying to form Compassion & Choices."[20]

Compassion & Choices is the leading nonprofit organization committed to helping everyone have the best death possible. We offer free counseling, planning resources, referrals and guidance, and across the nation we work to protect and expand options at the end of life.

For over thirty years we have reduced people's suffering and given them some control in their final days—even when injury or illness takes their voice. We are experts in what it takes to die well.[21]

1990

Patient Self-Determination Act

The Patient Self-Determination Act of 1990[22] was enacted to ensure that patients are informed of their rights to execute advance directives and accept or refuse medical care. The act was intended to reinforce a person's constitutional right to make his or her own health care decisions. The act requires that federally funded health care organizations explain to patients their right to complete an advance directive.

Nancy Cruzan Feeding Tube Removed

The Supreme Court ruled that the parents of Nancy Cruzan, a 32-year old woman who had been unconscious since a 1983 car accident, could have her feeding tube removed.[23] The court determined the Missouri Department of Health was permitted to require clear and convincing evidence of the wishes of a patient regarding provision of artificial nutrition and hydration.[24] Thus affirming the right of Americans to refuse unwanted medical treatment and their right to appoint a healthcare proxy.

Kevorkian Illegally Assists Terminally Ill Patients in Suicide

Dr. Jack Kevorkian assisted terminally ill patients in suicide outside the boundaries of law. He used a suicide machine to assist Janet Adkins, a 54-year-old woman with Alzheimer's disease, in ending her life at her request.

Timothy Quill and Prescription for Death

Timothy Quill, a primary care physician, published an article describing how he had prescribed a lethal dose of sedatives to end the life of a young woman whose suffering from leukemia had become unbearable.

Final Exit and Freedom of Speech

Derek Humphry's popular text, *Final Exit: The Practicalities of Self-Deliverance and Assisted Suicide for the Dying,* was published. Although there were calls for it to be banned, it was not possible under the First Amendment to the U.S. Constitution.

Congress shall make no law respecting an establishment of religion, or prohibiting the free exercise thereof; or abridging the freedom of speech, or of the press; or the right of the people peaceably to assemble, and to petition the Government for a redress of grievances.[25]

1993

Patient's Wishes Honored

In the case of *DeGrella v. Elston,* the Kentucky Supreme Court ruled on an incompetent's right to die. The decision determined that a patient's wishes will be honored if the attending physician, the hospital, or nursing home ethics committee where a patient resides and the legal guardian or next of kin all agree upon and document the patient's wishes and the patient's condition. If no one disputes their decision, no court order is required to proceed to carry out the patient's wishes. Future criminal sanctions or civil liability turn not on the existence or absence of a court order, but on the facts of the case. No liability attaches to a decision to refuse or withdraw treatment if the necessary facts are established and carefully documented by the parties involved. In contrast, the court cannot absolve the parties from liability where the facts do not exist to support the action taken.[26]

1994

Oregon—Physician Assisted Suicide Legal

Oregon's Death with Dignity Act, involving physician-assisted suicide, became a legal medical option for terminally ill patients in Oregon. The Oregon Death with Dignity Act allows terminally ill Oregon residents to obtain from their physicians and use prescriptions for self-administered, lethal medications.

Michigan—Physician Assisted Suicide Illegal

The Supreme Court of Michigan ruled on December 13, 1994, that assisted suicide is illegal in the state of Michigan. The ruling overturned several lower court decisions. The court determined that there is no constitutional right to aid in carrying out a suicide in Michigan. Jack Kevorkian, a physician, assisted terminally ill patients in suicide outside the boundaries of the law. He claims to have assisted 130 patients.

1996

Health Insurance Portability and Accountability Act

The Health Insurance Portability and Accountability Act (Public Law 104191) was enacted to protect the privacy, confidentiality, and security of patient information.

Dolly the Sheep Cloned

Ian Wilmut Keith Campbell and colleagues at the Roslin Institute, University of Edinburgh and the biotechnology company PPL Therapeutics near Edinburgh in Scotland successfully cloned Dolly, the Sheep.

> Several clones had been produced in the lab before Dolly, including frogs, mice, and cows, which had all been cloned from the DNA from embryos. Dolly was remarkable in being the first mammal to be cloned from an adult cell. This was a major scientific achievement as it demonstrated that the DNA from adult cells, despite having specialised as one particular type of cell, can be used to create an entire organism.[27]

Fourteenth Amendment and Terminally Ill

The Second and Ninth U.S. Circuit Courts of Appeals ruled that there is a constitutional right under the Fourteenth Amendment for a terminally ill person to receive help from a physician when dying.

1997

Physician-Assisted Suicide

Physician-assisted suicide, through referendum, became a legal medical option within narrowly prescribed circumstances for terminally ill Oregon residents.

Kevorkian Charged with Murder

Kevorkian was charged with murder in five cases of physician-assisted suicide and was acquitted.

Supreme Court—States May Enact Assisted Suicide Laws

The Supreme Court ruled that it is up to the individual states to enact laws regarding medically assisted death.

1998

Oregon Voters Reaffirm Death with Dignity Act

Oregon voters reaffirm their support for the Death with Dignity Act by a 60% majority.

Kevorkian Administers Lethal Injection

Kevorkian administered a lethal injection to Thomas Youk, a 52-year-old man with Lou Gehrig's disease, on national television.

Ballot Physician-Assisted Suicide Defeated

Michigan voters defeated a ballot measure that would legalize physician-assisted suicide.

1999

Kevorkian Convicted of Second-Degree Murder

Kevorkian was convicted of second-degree murder for Youk's death and sentenced 10 to 20 years in prison.

Patients Receive Lethal Doses of Medication

Twenty-three terminally ill patients were reported as having received lethal doses of medication since passage of Oregon's Death with Dignity Act.

2000

Seven Myths About End-of-Life Care

Legal myths about end-of-life care may prevent doctors and patients and families from providing adequate comfort measures to dying patients, according to an article published in the November 15 issue of the *Journal of the American Medical Association* (AMA).[28]

2001

President's Council on Bioethics

President George W. Bush created the President's Council on Bioethics. The council was charged with advising the president on bioethical issues that may emerge as a consequence of advances in biomedical science and technology.

Assisted Suicide Act Challenged

U.S. Attorney General John Ashcroft abrogated former Attorney General Janet Reno's mandate allowing physician-assisted suicide. Instead, he decided that physician-assisted suicide was a violation of the federal Controlled Substance Act. In *State of Oregon v. Ashcroft*, CV01-1647 (D-Oregon), the judge allowed Oregon's law to remain in effect.

Oregon—Assisted Suicide Cases

Since 1991, the total number of physician-assisted suicide cases totaled 129. On April 17, U.S. District Court Judge Robert Jones upheld Oregon's Death with Dignity Act.

2002

Attorney General Appeals District Court's Ruling

Attorney General John Ashcroft filed an appeal, asking the Ninth U.S. Circuit Court of Appeals to lift the District Court's ruling.

2003

Human Genome System Fully Sequenced

The human genome system became fully sequenced, allowing molecular genetics and medical research to accelerate at an unprecedented rate. The ethical implications of human genome research are as immense as the undertaking of the totality of the research that was conducted to map the human genome system (e.g., cloning of humans).[29]

Oregon—Assisted Suicide Cases

Forty-two residents of the State of Oregon ingested medications under provisions of the Death with Dignity Act.

2004

Death with Dignity Act Upheld

The U.S. Circuit Court of Appeals upheld Oregon's Death with Dignity Act, blocking the attempt by the U.S. Justice Department, under Attorney General Ashcroft, to use the federal Controlled Substances Act to prevent doctors in the state from prescribing drugs to assist the suicide of their patients. The Ashcroft directive interfered with Oregon's authority to regulate medical care within its borders and therefore altered the usual constitutional balance between state and the federal governments.[30]

2005

The United Nations Educational, Scientific, and Cultural Organization released the second edition to the 2005 *Human Cloning, Ethical Issues* publication.[31]

2006

U.S. Supreme Court Upholds Death with Dignity Act

On January 17, 2006, the U.S. Supreme Court voted six to three to uphold an Oregon physician-assisted suicide law in the case *Gonzales v. Oregon*,[32] ruling that former Attorney General John Ashcroft overstepped his authority in seeking to punish doctors who prescribed drugs to help terminally ill patients end their lives. In the decision, the Supreme Court said that the Oregon law supersedes federal authority to regulate physicians and that the Bush administration improperly attempted to use the Controlled Substances Act to prosecute Oregon physicians who assist in patient suicides.

Supreme Court Blocks Bush's Attempt to Punish Doctors

The Supreme Court blocks the Bush administration's attempt to punish doctors who help terminally ill patients die, protecting Oregon's one-of-a-kind assisted-suicide law.[33]

Morning-after Pill

The Food and Drug Administration approved the morning-after pill to prevent contraception for use without a prescription. This decision has added another dimension to the ongoing controversy between right-to-life and pro-choice advocates. Opponents claim that it is just another way to end human life.

2009

Right to Know End-of-Life Options

On January 1, the Terminal Patients' Right to Know End-of-Life Options Act, AB 2747, goes into effect in California.

2010

California—Living Donor Registry

Legislation was introduced in California that would make it the first state in the country to build a living donor registry. Under Senate Bill 1395, people could declare their wishes regarding organ donation by checking a box when obtaining or renewing their driver's license.

2013

Information and Referral Service for Kidney Donors

California launched a state-authorized information and referral service to inspire and inform people to be altruistic living kidney donors. Through its website, www.LivingDonationCalifornia.org, the free service provides information about living kidney donation and refers potentially eligible individuals for evaluation at a transplant center.[34]

NEWS

Vermont Set to Become Third U.S. State to Allow Assisted Suicide

Vermont is poised to become the third U.S. state to allow doctor-assisted suicide, after its legislature passed a bill allowing physicians to prescribe lethal drugs to terminally ill patients.

The bill passed late on Monday, and the governor has pledged to sign it into law.

Oregon and Washington state have legalized doctor-assisted suicide in voter referendums.

Scott Malone, Reuters, May 14, 2013

ABORTION

We shall have to fight the politician, who remembers only that the unborn have no votes and that since posterity has done nothing for us we need do nothing for posterity.

–WILLIAM RALPH INGE (1860–1954)[35]

An *abortion* is the termination of pregnancy by removal or expulsion from the uterus of a fetus or embryo before it is viable. The question of viability has been strongly debated between pro-life (the right to life) and pro-choice (the right to choose) advocates. An abortion can be a spontaneous abortion, often referred to as a miscarriage, or it can be an elective abortion, meaning purposely induced, which continues to be a hotly debated controversial issue nationwide. The controversy in its simplest form involves the question of the rights of the fetus to be born and the rights of the mother to make decisions regarding her body.

A consensus as to when life begins has not been reached. There has been no final determination as to the proper interplay among a mother's liberty, the interests of an unborn child, and the state's interests in protecting life. In abortion cases, the law presupposes a theory of ethics and morality, which in turn presupposes deeply personal ideas about being and existence. Answers to such questions as when life begins define ethical beliefs, and these ethical beliefs should determine how we govern ourselves. Abortion in this context is less a question about constitutional law and more about who we are as a people. This is a decision the Supreme Court cannot make. Taking these issues out of the public discourse threatens to foment hostility, stifle the search for answers, distance people from the Constitution, and undermine the credibility of that document.[36]

With more than 1 million abortions performed annually in the United States, it is certain that the conflict between pro-choice and pro-life advocates will continue to pervade America's landscape. The issues are numerous and emotions run high. Common ethical dilemmas include:

- When does life begin?
- Who decides?
- Who protects the unborn fetus?
- What are the rights of the child or woman who has been raped?
- What are the rights of the spouse?
- What are the rights of the father of an unwed child or woman?
- What are the rights of society and the state to interfere with another's rights?
- Should the principles of autonomy and right to self-determination prevail?
- Should an abortion be considered murder?
- Can the use of contraception be considered a form of killing by preventing a birth that might have otherwise occurred?
- What are the religious implications of a woman who is Catholic, for example, who chooses to undergo an abortion?
- Is it morally acceptable to save the life of the mother by aborting the fetus?
- Is an abortion for mere convenience morally wrong?
- What role should education play in the woman's decision to undergo an abortion?
- What alternatives should the woman be educated about (e.g., the choice of adoption) before undergoing an abortion?
- At what age should the decision to abort be that of the mother?
- Should the feelings of guilt that may accompany an abortion and how those feelings may haunt the mother through the years be explained?
- Should the feelings that might occur after giving birth be explained to the victim of a rape (e.g., anger and resentment)?
- When does control over one's body begin, and when does it end?

These are but a few of the many questions that need to be addressed in the pursuit of doing the right thing. As the following pages point out, for each new issue decided in the courts, numerous new issues arise, all of which seem to involve both legal and moral questions as to what is acceptable behavior. In addition to having substantial ethical, moral, and religious implications, abortion has proven to be a major political issue and will continue as such in the future. As the following court decisions illustrate, new laws will be enacted by the various states and challenged, often winding their way up to the Supreme Court for decision.

The *Roe v. Wade* 1973 landmark case gave strength to a woman's right to privacy in the context of matters relating to her own body, including how a pregnancy would end.[37] The U.S. Supreme Court has also recognized the interest of the states in protecting potential life and has attempted to spell out the extent to which the states may regulate and even prohibit abortions. The Supreme Court in this case found the Texas penal abortion law unconstitutional, stating, "State criminal abortion statutes . . . that except from criminality only a lifesaving procedure on behalf of the mother, without regard to the stage of her pregnancy and other interests involved, is violating the Due Process Clause of the Fourteenth Amendment."[38] The court then went on to delineate what regulatory measures a state lawfully may enact during the three stages of pregnancy.

First Trimester

During the first trimester of pregnancy, the decision to undergo an abortion procedure is between the woman and her physician. A state may require that abortions be performed by a licensed physician pursuant to law; however, a woman's right to an abortion is not unqualified because the decision to perform the procedure must be left to the medical judgment of her attending physician. "For the stage prior to approximately the end of the first trimester, the abortion decision and its effectuation must be left to the medical judgment of the pregnant woman's attending physician."[39]

Second Trimester

In *Roe v. Wade*, the Supreme Court stated, "For the stage subsequent to approximately the end of the first trimester, the State, in promoting its interest in the health of the mother, may, if it chooses, regulate the abortion procedure in ways that are reasonably related to maternal health."[40] Thus, during approximately the fourth to sixth months of pregnancy, the state may regulate the medical conditions under which the procedure is performed. The constitutional test of any legislation concerning abortion during this period would be its relevance to the objective of protecting maternal health.

Third Trimester

The Supreme Court reasoned that by the time the final stage of pregnancy has been reached the state has acquired a compelling interest in the product of conception, which would override the woman's right to privacy and justify stringent regulation even to the extent of prohibiting abortions. In the *Roe v. Wade* case, the court formulated its ruling as to the last trimester in the following words: "For the stage subsequent to viability, the State in promoting its interest in the potentiality of human life, may, if it chooses, regulate, and even proscribe, abortion except where it is necessary, in appropriate medical judgment, for the preservation of the life or health of the mother."[41]

Thus, during the final stage of pregnancy, a state may prohibit all abortions except those deemed necessary to protect maternal life or health. The state's legislative powers over the performance of abortions increase as the pregnancy progresses toward term.

Abortion Committee Review

In a 1973 companion decision, the U.S. Supreme Court ruled in *Doe v. Bolton,*[42] that Georgia's abortion statute requiring residency requirements for women seeking an abortion and calling for the procedure to be performed in a hospital accredited by the Joint Commission is constitutionally invalid. Further, the court found there was no constitutionally justifiable rationale for a statutory requirement necessitating advance approval by the abortion committee of the hospital's medical staff prior to abortion. The court ruled that "interposition of the hospital abortion committee is unduly restrictive of the patient's rights and needs that . . . have already been medically delineated and substantiated by her personal physician. To ask more serves neither the hospital nor the State."[43] Insofar as statutory consultation requirements are concerned, the court reasoned that the acquiescence of two copractitioners has no rational connection with a patient's needs and, further, unduly infringes on the physician's right to practice.

Abortion Counseling

The U.S. Supreme Court in 1983 in *City of Akron v. Akron Center for Reproductive Health*[44] decided that the different states cannot (1) mandate what information physicians give abortion patients or (2) require that abortions for women more than 3 months pregnant be performed in a hospital. With respect to a requirement that the attending physician must inform the woman of specified information concerning her proposed abortion, it was found unreasonable for a state to insist that only a physician is competent to provide information and counseling relative to informed consent. A state may not adopt regulations to influence a woman's informed choice between abortion and childbirth.

With regard to a second-trimester hospital requirement, this could significantly limit a woman's ability to obtain an abortion. This is especially so in view of the evidence that a second-trimester abortion may cost more than twice as much in a hospital as in a clinic.

Undue Burden Rule

In *Planned Parenthood v. Casey,*[45] the U.S. Supreme Court ruling, as enunciated in *Roe v. Wade,* reaffirmed:

* The constitutional right of women to have an abortion before viability of the fetus, as first enunciated in *Roe v. Wade*
* The state's power to restrict abortions after fetal viability, so long as the law contains exceptions for pregnancies that endanger a woman's life or health
* The principle that the state has legitimate interests from the outset of the pregnancy in protecting the health of the woman and the life of the fetus

The U.S. Supreme Court rejected the trimester approach in *Roe v. Wade,* which limited the regulations states could issue on abortion depending on the development stage of the fetus. In place of the trimester approach, the court will evaluate the permissibility of state abortion rules based on whether they unduly burden a woman's ability to obtain an abortion. A rule is an *"undue burden"* if its purpose or effect is to place a substantial obstacle in the path of a woman seeking an abortion before the fetus attains viability. The Supreme Court ruled that it is "not an undue burden" to require that a woman be informed of the nature of the abortion procedure and the risks involved, be offered information on the fetus and alternatives to abortion, and be given informed consent before the abortion procedure. In addition, it is not an undue burden to require parental consent for a minor seeking an abortion, providing for a judicial bypass option if a minor does not wish to or cannot obtain parental consent, and requiring a 24-hour waiting period before any abortion can be performed.

FUNDING

Some states have placed an indirect restriction on abortion through the elimination of funding. Under the Hyde Amendment, the U.S. Congress, through appropriations legislation, has limited the types of medically necessary abortions for which federal funds may be spent under the Medicaid program. Although the Hyde Amendment does not prohibit states from funding nontherapeutic abortions, this action by the federal government opened the door to state statutory provisions limiting the funding of abortions.

Denial of Financial Assistance for Elective Abortions

In *Beal v. Doe*[46] in 1977, the Pennsylvania Medicaid plan was challenged based on denial of financial assistance for nontherapeutic abortions. The U.S. Supreme Court held that Title XIX of the Social Security Act (the Medicaid program) does not require the funding of nontherapeutic abortions as a condition of state participation in the program. The state has a strong interest in encouraging normal childbirth, and nothing in Title XIX suggests that it is unreasonable for the state to further that interest. The court ruled that it is not inconsistent with the Medicaid portion of the Social Security Act to refuse to fund unnecessary (although perhaps desirable) medical services.

In *Maher v. Roe*[47] in 1977, the U.S. Supreme Court considered the Connecticut statute that denied Medicaid benefits for first-trimester abortions that were not medically necessary. The court rejected the argument that the state's subsidy of medical expenses incident to pregnancy and childbirth created an obligation on the part of the state to subsidize the expenses incident to nontherapeutic abortions. The Supreme Court voted six to three that states may refuse to spend public funds to provide nontherapeutic abortions for women.

Funding Not Required for Therapeutic Abortions

The U.S. Supreme Court in 1980 in *Harris v. McRae*,[48] upheld in a five-to-four vote the Hyde Amendment, which restricts the use of federal funds for Medicaid abortions. Under this case, the different states are not compelled to fund Medicaid recipients' medically necessary abortions for which federal reimbursement is unavailable but may choose to do so.

Funding Bans Unconstitutional in California

The California Supreme Court in 1981 held that funding bans were unconstitutional; the court asked rhetorically:

> If the state cannot directly prohibit a woman's right to obtain an abortion, may the state by discriminatory financing indirectly nullify that constitutional right? Can the state tell an indigent person that the state will provide him with welfare benefits only

upon the condition that he join a designated political party or subscribe to a particular newspaper that is favored by the government? Can the state tell a poor woman that it will pay for her needed medical care but only if she gives up her constitutional right to choose whether or not to have a child?[49]

Funding Discrimination Prohibited in Arizona

The Arizona Supreme Court, in 2002 in *Simat Corp. v. Arizona Health Care Cost Containment Sys.*,[50] found that the state's constitution does not permit the state and the Arizona Health Care Cost Containment System (AHCCCS) to refuse to fund medically necessary abortion procedures for pregnant women suffering from serious illness while funding such procedures for victims of rape or incest or when the abortion was necessary to save the woman's life (A.R.S. § 35-196.02. AHCCCS). After the state has chosen to fund abortions for one group of indigent, pregnant women for whom abortions are medically necessary to save their lives, the state may not deny the same option to another group of women for whom the procedure is also medically necessary to save their health. An example is cancer, for which chemotherapy or radiation therapy ordinarily cannot be provided if the patient is pregnant, making an abortion necessary before proceeding with the recognized medical treatment. Other therapy regimens that must at times be suspended during pregnancy include those for heart disease, diabetes, kidney disease, liver disease, chronic renal failure, inflammatory bowel disease, and lupus. In many of the women suffering from these diseases, suspension of recognized therapy during pregnancy will have serious and permanent adverse effects on their health and lessen their life span. In such a situation, the state is not simply influencing a woman's choice but is actually conferring the privilege of treatment on one class and withholding it from another.

A woman's right to choose preservation and protection of her health and, therefore, in many cases, her life is at least as compelling as the state's interest in promoting childbirth. The court's protection of the fetus and promotion of childbirth cannot be considered so compelling as to outweigh a woman's fundamental right to choose and the state's obligation to be evenhanded in the design and application of its health care policies. The majority of states that have examined similar Medicaid funding restrictions have determined that their state statutes or constitutions offer broader protection of individual rights than does the U.S. Constitution, and they have found that medically necessary abortions should be funded if the state also funds medically necessary expenses related to childbirth. The case was remanded to the trial court for further proceedings consistent with this opinion.

Refusal to Fund Abortion Counseling Not Unconstitutional

Federal regulations that prohibit abortion counseling and referral by family planning clinics that receive funds under Title X of the Public Health Service Act were found not to violate the constitutional rights of pregnant women or Title X grantees in a five-to-four decision by the Supreme Court in *Rust v. Sullivan*.[51] Proponents of abortion counseling argued (1) that the regulations impermissibly burden a woman's privacy right to abortion and (2) that by prohibiting the delivery of abortion information, even as to where such information could be obtained, the regulations deny a woman her constitutionally protected right to choose under the First Amendment. The question arises: How can a woman make an informed choice between two options when she cannot obtain information as to one of them? The plaintiff had argued that the government may not condition receipt of a benefit on the relinquishment of constitutional rights. In *Sullivan*, however, the Supreme Court found that there was no violation of a woman's or provider's First Amendment rights to freedom of speech. The court extended the doctrine that government need not subsidize the exercise of the fundamental rights to free speech.

SPOUSAL CONSENT

Husband's Interest Insufficient

Provisions of the Florida Therapeutic Abortion Act, which required a married woman to obtain the husband's consent before abortion, were found to be unconstitutional in *Poe v. Gerstein*.[52] The state's interest was found not to be sufficiently compelling to limit a woman's right to abortion. The husband's interest in the baby was held to be insufficient to force his wife to face the mental and physical risks of pregnancy and childbirth.

Husband's Required Consent Unconstitutional

In *Doe v. Zimmerman* (1975),[53] the court declared unconstitutional the provisions of the Pennsylvania Abortion Control Act, which required that the written consent of the husband of a married woman be secured before performing an abortion. The court found that these provisions impermissibly permitted the husband to withhold his consent either because of his interest in the potential life of the fetus or for capricious reasons. The natural father of an unborn fetus in *Doe v. Smith* (1988)[54] was not entitled to an injunction to prevent the mother from submitting to an abortion. Although the father's interest in the fetus was legitimate, it did not outweigh the mother's constitutionally protected right to an abortion, particularly in light of evidence that the mother and father had never married.

In the 1992 decision of *Planned Parenthood v. Casey*, the Supreme Court ruled that spousal consent would be an undue burden on the woman.

PARENTAL CONSENT

Competent Persons Under 18

The U.S. Supreme Court ruled in 1973 in *Danforth v. Planned Parenthood*[55] that it is unconstitutional to require all women younger than the age of 18 years to obtain parental consent in writing prior to obtaining an abortion. The court, however, failed to provide any definitive guidelines as to when and how parental consent may be required if the minor is too immature to comprehend fully the nature of the procedure.

The U.S. Supreme Court in 1979 in *Bellotti v. Baird*[56] ruled eight to one that a Massachusetts statute requiring parental consent before an abortion could be performed on an unmarried woman younger than the age of 18 years was unconstitutional. Justice John P. Stevens, joined by Justices William J. Brennan, Jr., Thurgood Marshall, and Harry Blackmun, concluded that the Massachusetts statute was unconstitutional because under that statute as written and construed by the Massachusetts Supreme Judicial Court, no minor, no matter how mature and capable of informed decision making, could receive an abortion without the consent of either both parents or a superior court judge, thus making the minor's abortion subject in every instance to an absolute third-party veto.

Incompetent Persons

Abortion was found to be proper by a family court in *In re Doe* (1987)[57] for a profoundly retarded woman. She had become pregnant during her residence in a group home as a result of a sexual attack by an unknown person. The record had supported a finding that if the woman had been able to do so she would have requested the abortion. The court properly chose welfare agencies and the woman's guardian ad litem (a guardian appointed to prosecute or defend a suit on behalf of a party incapacitated by infancy, mental incompetence, etc.) as the surrogate decision makers.

Parental Notification Permitted

The U.S. Supreme Court in 1981 in *H. L. v. Matheson*,[58] by a six-to-three vote, upheld a Utah statute that required a physician to "notify, if possible" the parents or guardian of a minor on whom an abortion is to be performed. In this case, the physician advised the patient that an abortion would be in her best medical interest but, because of the statute, refused to perform the abortion without notifying her parents. The Supreme Court ruled that although a state may not constitutionally legislate a blanket, unreviewable power of parents to veto their daughter's abortion, a statute setting out a mere requirement of parental notice when possible does not violate the constitutional rights of an immature, dependent minor.

Emancipated Minor

The trial court in 1987 *In re Anonymous*[59] was found to have abused its discretion when it refused a minor's request for waiver of parental consent to obtain an abortion. The record indicated that the minor lived alone, was within 1 month of her 18th birthday, lived by herself most of the time, and was employed full time.

Parental Notification Not Required

The issue in 2000 in *Planned Parenthood v. Owens*[60] was whether the Colorado Parental Notification Act (Colorado Revised Statute §§ 12-37.5-101, et seq. [1998]), which requires a physician to notify the parents of a minor prior to performing an abortion upon her, violates the minor's rights protected by the U.S. Constitution. The act, a citizen-initiated measure, was approved at Colorado's general election. The act generally prohibits physicians from performing abortions on an unemancipated minor until at least 48 hours after written notice has been delivered to the minor's parent, guardian, or foster parent.

The U.S. District Court decided that the act violated the rights of minor women protected by the Fourteenth Amendment. The Supreme Court, for more than a quarter of a century, has required that any abortion regulation except from its reach an abortion medically necessary for the preservation of the mother's health. The act fails to provide such a health exception.

INFORMED CONSENT

The Fifth U.S. Circuit Court of Appeals determined that a Texas law requiring a pregnant mother to undergo an ultrasound prior abortion is constitutional. Although a pregnant woman cannot be compelled to view the ultrasound image, the physician is required to describe what the image shows. The pregnant woman, however, has a concomitant right to refuse to listen to any detailed explanation. Chapter 171 of the Texas Health and Safety Code requires the following as prerequisites for a woman's informed and voluntary consent to an abortion:

(1) the physician who is to perform the abortion, or a certified sonographer agent thereof, must perform a sonogram on the pregnant woman;

(2) the physician must display the sonogram images "in a quality consistent with current medical practice" such that the pregnant woman may view them;

(3) the physician must provide, "in a manner understandable to a layperson," a verbal explanation of the results of the sonogram images, including a variety of detailed descriptions of the fetus or embryo; and

(4) the physician or certified sonographer agent must "make . . . audible the heart auscultation for the pregnant woman to hear, if present, in a quality consistent with current medical practice and provide . . . , in a manner understandable to a layperson, a simultaneous verbal explanation of the heart auscultation," H.B. 15, Sec. 2 (amending TEX. HEALTH & SAFETY CODE ANN. Ann. § 171.012).

STATES MAY PROTECT FETUS

The U.S. Supreme Court in 1979 in *Colautti v. Franklin*[61] voted six to three that states can seek to protect a fetus that a physician has determined could survive outside the womb. Determination of whether a particular fetus is viable is, and must be, a matter for judgment of the responsible attending physician. State abortion regulations that impinge on this determination, if they are to be constitutional, must allow the attending physician the room that he or she needs to make the best medical judgment.

ABORTION RIGHTS NARROWED

Webster v. Reproductive Health Services[62] began the U.S. Supreme Court's narrowing of abortion rights by upholding a Missouri statute providing that no public facilities or employees should be used to perform abortions and physicians should conduct viability tests before performing abortions.

PARTIAL BIRTH ABORTION

The Supreme Court in 1998 in *Women's Medical Professional Corp. v. Voinovich*[63] involved an Ohio statute that banned the use of the intact dilation and extraction (D&X) procedure in the performance of any previability or postviability abortion. The Sixth Circuit Court of Appeals held that the statute banning any use of the D&X procedure was unconstitutionally vague. It is likely that a properly drafted statute will eventually be judged constitutionally sound.

Partial Birth Abortion Ban Struck Down

On June 28, 2002, the U.S. Supreme Court struck down a Nebraska ban on "partial-birth abortion," finding it an unconstitutional violation of *Roe v. Wade*. The court found these types of bans to be extreme descriptive attempts to outlaw abortion—even early in pregnancy—that jeopardizes women's health [192 F.3d 1142 (8th Cir. 1999), 120 S. Ct. 2597 (2000)].

Partial Birth Abortion Ban Made Law

President Bush, on November 6, 2003, signed the first federal restrictions banning late-term partial-birth abortions. (The *partial birth abortion,* also referred to as the D&X procedure, is a late-term abortion involving partial delivery of the baby before its being aborted.) Both houses of Congress passed the ban. The ban permits no exceptions when a woman's health is at risk or the fetus has life-threatening disabilities. A U.S. District Court in Nebraska issued a restraining order on the ban.

Partial-Birth Abortion Ban Unconstitutional

The Partial-Birth Abortion Ban Act, 18 U.S.C. Section 1531, in *National Abortion Fed'n v. Gonzages,*[64] was found to be unconstitutional because it lacked any exception to preserve the health of the mother, where such exception was constitutionally required. Also, the act was unconstitutional because it imposed an undue burden on a woman's right to choose previability abortion and was constitutionally vague.

STATE ABORTION STATUTES

The effect of the Supreme Court's 1973 decisions in *Roe* and *Doe* was to invalidate all or part of almost every state abortion statute then in force. The responses of state legislatures to these decisions were varied, but it is clear that many state laws had been enacted to restrict the performance of abortions as much as possible. Although *Planned Parenthood v. Casey* was expected to clear up some issues, it is evident that the states have been given more power to regulate the performance of abortions.

24-Hour Waiting Period Not Burdensome

In 1992, the U.S. Supreme Court in *Planned Parenthood of Southeastern Pennsylvania v. Casey*[65] determined that in asserting an interest in protecting fetal life, a state may place some restrictions on previability abortions, so long as those restrictions do not impose an "undue burden" on the woman's right to an abortion. The court determined that the 24-hour waiting period, the informed consent requirement, and the medical emergency definitions did not unduly burden the right to an abortion and were therefore constitutional.

The 1993 Utah Abortion Act Revision, Senate Bill 60, provides for informed consent by requiring that certain information be given to the pregnant woman at least 24 hours before performing an abortion. The law allows for exceptions to this requirement in the event of a medical emergency. The Utah Women's Clinic, in *Utah Women's Clinic, Inc. v. Leavitt,*[66] filed a 106-page complaint challenging the constitutionality of the new Utah law. It was determined that the 24-hour waiting period did not impose an undue burden on the right to an abortion. On appeal, a U.S. District Court held that the Utah abortion statute's 24-hour waiting period and informed consent requirements do not render the statute unconstitutionally vague.

The abortion issue is obviously one that invokes strong feelings on both sides. Individuals are free to urge support for their cause through debate, advocacy, and participation in the political process. The subject also might be addressed in the courts so long as there are valid legal issues in dispute. Where, however, a case presents no legitimate legal arguments, the courthouse is not the proper forum. Litigation, or the threat of litigation, should not be used as economic blackmail to strengthen one's hand in the political battle.[67]

The morality of abortion involves philosophy, ethics, and theology. It is a subject wherein reasonable people adhere to vastly divergent convictions and principles. The obligation of society is to define the liberties of all and not to mandate one's own moral code.[68]

Two or more ethical principles in conflict with one another are considered "ethical dilemmas," such as in the case of abortion. Further complication of ethical dilemmas occurs when laws and regulations affect the decision-making process and, further, when the courts enter the melting pot by interpreting laws and regulations while recognizing the rights of individuals as provided under the Constitution.

Pro-life advocates argue on constitutional, ethical, and religious grounds that the unborn child has a right to life and that right must be protected. Pro-choice advocates argue that a woman has a right to choose preservation and protection of her health, and therefore, in many cases, her life is at least as compelling as the state's interest in promoting childbirth. Two viewpoints, as different as day and night, opposite opinions surrounded by highly charged emotional and religious beliefs as to what is right and what is wrong.

Dr. Gosnell, a Philadelphia physician, was found guilty of murder in some instances by severing the spinal cord of a fetus during late-term abortions. As illustrated in the following news headlines, there is a stream of court cases that continue to stoke the flames of the abortion controversy.

Philadelphia Abortion Doctor Guilty of Murder in Late-Term Procedures

While abortion rights groups argued that Dr. Gosnell operated far outside the legalities and norms of women's health care, abortion opponents seized on the case to raise questions about the ethics of late-term abortions. Put simply, they asked why a procedure done to a living baby outside the womb is murder, but destroying a fetus of similar gestation before delivery can be legal.

John Hurdle and Trip Gabriel, The New York Times, *May 13, 2013*

Pa. Abortion Provider Convicted of Murder

. . . "Some abortionists may have cleaner sheets than Gosnell, and better sterilized equipment and better trained accomplices, but what they do—what Gosnell did—kill babies and hurt women is the same," Rep. Christopher H Smith (R-NJ) said in a statement.

Meanwhile, abortion-rights groups insisted that Gosnell's crimes are an anomaly and that the abysmal conditions inside his clinic persisted only because numerous regulators ignored red flags for years.

Brady Dennis, The Washington Post, *May 14, 2013*

To make the right choices in the resolution of ethical dilemmas, it is often necessary to value one ethical principle more than another. The difficulty in the abortion dilemma arises because beliefs, religion, culture, education, and life experiences can differ from person to person. Good people cannot be considered bad people merely because their beliefs differ from another's beliefs. Values differ, and, therefore, determinations of morality may differ. It is certain that the controversies and ethical dilemmas surrounding abortion will continue for many years to come.

Common ground must be the beginning point for resolving this emotionally charged dilemma.

Moral Persuasion on Abortion

If you wish to persuade someone to adopt your viewpoint on any issue, it is usually counter-productive to begin by insulting that person. The reason is simple: Your target is likely to want to defend himself or herself from the insult, and consequently will not be in a position to hear your argument.

Joseph B. Kadane, Huffington Post, *September 27, 2013*[69]

STERILIZATION

Sterilization is the termination of the ability to produce offspring. Sterilization often is accomplished by either a *vasectomy* for men or a tubal ligation for women. A vasectomy is a surgical procedure in which the vas deferens is severed and tied to prevent the flow of the seminal fluid into the urinary canal. A *tubal ligation* is a surgical procedure in which the fallopian tubes are cut and tied, preventing passage of the ovum from the ovary to the uterus. Sterilizations are often pursued for such reasons as:

- Birth control
- Economic necessity
- Therapeutic necessity (e.g., prevent harm to a woman's health)
- Genetic concerns (e.g., prevent birth defects)

ELECTIVE STERILIZATION

Voluntary or *elective sterilizations* on competent individuals present few legal problems, so long as proper consent has been obtained from the patient and the procedure is performed properly. Civil liability for performing a sterilization of convenience may be imposed if the procedure is performed in a negligent manner. Like abortion, voluntary sterilization is the subject of a variety of debates concerning its moral and ethical propriety.

THERAPEUTIC STERILIZATION

If the life or health of a woman may be jeopardized by pregnancy, the danger may be avoided by terminating: (1) her ability to conceive or (2) her husband's ability to impregnate. Such an operation is a *therapeutic sterilization*—one performed to preserve life or health. The medical necessity for sterilization renders the procedure therapeutic. Sometimes a diseased reproductive organ has to be removed to preserve the life or health of the individual. The operation results in sterility, although this was not the primary reason for the procedure. Such an operation technically should not be classified as sterilization because it is incidental to the medical purpose.

EUGENIC STERILIZATION

The term *eugenic sterilization* refers to the involuntary sterilization of certain categories of persons described in statutes, without the need for consent by, or on behalf of, those subject to the procedures. Persons classified as mentally deficient, feebleminded, and, in some instances, epileptic are included within the scope of the statutes. Several states also have included certain sexual deviants and persons classified as habitual criminals. Such statutes ordinarily are designed to prevent the transmission of hereditary defects to succeeding generations, but several statutes also have recognized the purpose of preventing procreation by individuals who would not be able to care for their offspring.

Although there have been judicial decisions to the contrary, the United States Supreme Court in *Buck v. Bell*[70] specifically upheld the validity of such eugenic sterilization statutes, provided that certain procedural safeguards are observed. Several states have laws authorizing eugenic sterilization. The decision in *Wade v. Bethesda Hospital*[71] strongly suggests that in the absence of statutory authority the state cannot order sterilization for eugenic purposes. Eugenic sterilization statutes provide the following: a grant of authority to public officials supervising state institutions for the mentally ill or prisons and to certain public health officials to conduct sterilizations; a requirement of personal notice to the person subject to sterilization and, if that person is unable to comprehend what is involved, notice to the person's legal representative, guardian, or nearest relative; a hearing by the board designated in the particular statute to determine the propriety of the prospective sterilization; at the hearing, evidence that may be presented, and the patient, who must be present or represented by counsel or the nearest relative or guardian; and an opportunity to appeal the board's ruling to a court.

The procedural safeguards of notice, hearing, and the right to appeal must be present in sterilization statutes to fulfill the minimum constitutional requirements of due process. An Arkansas statute was found to be unconstitutional in that it did not provide for notice to the incompetent patient and opportunity to be heard or for the patient's entitlement to legal counsel.[72]

NEGLIGENT STERILIZATION

The improper performance of sterilization can result in lawsuits based on such theories as *wrongful birth*, *wrongful life*, and *wrongful conception*. Wrongful life suits are generally unsuccessful, primarily because of the court's unwillingness, for public policy reasons, to permit financial recovery for the "injury" of being born into the world.

Some success, however, has been achieved in litigation by the patient (and his or her spouse) who allegedly was sterilized and subsequently proved fertile. Damages have been awarded for the cost of the unsuccessful procedure; pain and suffering as a result of the pregnancy; the medical expense of the pregnancy; and the loss of comfort, companionship services, and consortium of the spouse. Again, as a matter of public policy, the courts have indicated that the joys and benefits of having the child outweigh the cost incurred in the rearing process.

There have been many cases in recent years involving actions for wrongful birth, wrongful life, and wrongful conception. Litigation originated with the California case in which a court found that a genetic testing laboratory could be held liable for damages from incorrectly reporting genetic tests, leading to the birth of a child with defects.[73] Injury caused by birth had not been previously actionable by law. The court of appeals held that medical laboratories engaged in genetic testing owe a duty to parents and their unborn child to use ordinary care in administering available tests for the purpose of providing information concerning potential genetic defects in the unborn. Damages in this case were awarded on the basis of the child's shortened life span.

Wrongful Birth

In a wrongful birth action, the plaintiffs claim that but for a breach of duty by the defendant(s) (e.g., improper sterilization), the child would not have been born. A wrongful birth claim can be brought by the parent(s) of a child born with genetic defects against a physician who or a laboratory that negligently fails to inform them, in a timely fashion, of an increased possibility that the mother will give birth to such a child, therefore precluding an informed decision as to whether to have the child.

NEGLIGENT STERILIZATION

Chaffee performed a partial salpingectomy on Seslar. The purpose of the procedure was to sterilize Seslar, who had already borne four children, so that she could not become pregnant again. After undergoing the surgery, however, Seslar conceived and delivered a healthy baby. Seslar sued Chaffee.

The Court of Appeals held that damages for the alleged negligent sterilization procedure could not include the costs of raising a normal healthy child. Although raising an unplanned child is costly, all human life is presumptively invaluable. A child, regardless of the circumstances of birth, does not constitute harm to the parents so as to permit recovery for the costs associated with raising and educating the child. As with a majority of jurisdictions, the court held that the value of a child's life to the parents outweighs the associated pecuniary burdens as a matter of law. Recoverable damages may include pregnancy and childbearing expenses but not the ordinary costs of raising and educating a normal, healthy child conceived after an allegedly negligent sterilization procedure.[74]

Ethical and Legal Issues

1. Do you agree with the court's decision?
2. Under what circumstances would you not agree with the court's decision?
3. Describe the ethical issues in this case.

In a New Jersey case, *Canesi ex rel. Canesi v. Wilson*,[75] the New Jersey Supreme Court reviewed the dismissal of an action for wrongful birth on the claim of the parents that had the mother been informed of the risk that a drug, Provera, which she had been taking before she learned that she was pregnant, might cause the fetus to be born with congenital anomalies, such as limb reduction, she would have decided to abort the fetus. It was alleged that the physicians failed to disclose the risks associated with the drug. The physicians argued that the informed consent doctrine requires that the plaintiffs establish that the drug in fact caused the birth anomalies. The court rejected the argument and distinguished the wrongful birth action from one based on informed consent:[76]

> In sum, the informed consent and wrongful birth causes of action are similar in that both require the physician to disclose those medically accepted risks that a reasonably prudent patient in the plaintiff's position would deem material to her decision. What is or is not a medically acceptable risk is informed by what the physician knows or ought to know of the patient's history and condition. These causes of action, however, have important differences. They encompass different compensable harms and measures of damages. In both causes of action, the plaintiff must prove not only that a reasonably prudent patient in her position, if apprised of all material risks, would have elected a different course of treatment or care. In an informed consent case, the plaintiff must additionally meet a two-pronged test for proximate causation: She must prove that the undisclosed risk actually materialized and that it was medically caused by the treatment. In a wrongful birth case, on the other hand, a plaintiff need not prove that the doctor's negligence was the medical cause of her child's birth defect. Rather, the test of proximate causation is satisfied by showing that an undisclosed fetal risk was material to a woman in her position; the risk materialized was reasonably foreseeable and not remote in relation to the doctor's negligence; and had plaintiff known of that risk, she would have terminated her pregnancy. The emotional distress and economic loss resulting from this lost opportunity to decide for herself whether or not to terminate the pregnancy constitute plaintiff's damages.

With the increasing consolidation of hospital services and physician practices, a case could be made for finding a hospital liable for the physician's failure to obtain informed consent where the hospital actually owns or controls the physician's practice or where both the hospital and the physician's practice are owned or controlled by another corporation that sets policy for both the hospital and the physician's practice.

Wrongful Life

Wrongful life claims are initiated by the parent(s) or child based on harm suffered as a result of being born. The plaintiffs generally contend that the physician or laboratory negligently failed to inform the child's parents of the risk of bearing a genetically defective infant and hence prevented the parents' right to choose to avoid the birth.[77] Because there is no recognized legal right not to be born, wrongful life cases are generally not successful.

> [L]egal recognition that a disabled life is an injury would harm the interests of those most directly concerned, the handicapped. Disabled persons face obvious physical difficulties in conducting their lives. They also face subtle yet equally devastating

handicaps in the attitudes and behavior of society, the law, and their own families and friends. Furthermore, society often views disabled persons as burdensome misfits. Recent legislation concerning employment, education, and building access reflects a slow change in these attitudes. This change evidences a growing public awareness that the handicapped can be valuable and productive members of society. To characterize the life of a disabled person as an injury would denigrate both this new awareness and the handicapped themselves.[78]

A cause of action for wrongful life was not cognizable under Kansas law in *Bruggeman v. Schimke.*[79] Human life is valuable, precious, and worthy of protection. Not to be born rather than to be alive with deformities cannot be recognized. The Kansas Supreme Court held that there was no recognized cause for wrongful life.

In *Kassama v. Magat,*[80] Kassama alleged that Dr. Magat failed to advise her of the results of an alpha-fetoprotein blood test that indicated a heightened possibility that her child, Ibrion, might be afflicted with Down syndrome. Had she received that information, Kassama contends, she would have undergone amniocentesis, which would have confirmed that prospect. Kassama claims that if that had occurred she would have chosen to terminate the pregnancy through an abortion.

The Supreme Court of Maryland decided that for purposes of tort law, an impaired life was not worse than nonlife, and, for that reason, life itself was not and could not be considered an injury. There was no evidence that Ibrion was not deeply loved and cared for by her parents or that she did not return that love. Studies have shown that people afflicted with Down syndrome can lead productive and meaningful lives. They can be educated and employed, form friendships, and get along in society. Allowing a recovery of extraordinary life expenses on some theory of fairness—that the physician or his or her insurance company should pay not because the physician was negligent causing the injury or impairment but because the child was born—ignores that fundamental issue.

Wrongful birth is based on the premise that being born and having to live with the affliction are disadvantages and thus cognizable injuries. The injury sued upon was the fact that Ibrion was born; she bears the disability and will bear the expenses only because, due to the alleged negligence of Magat, her mother was unable to terminate the pregnancy and avert her birth. The issue here is whether Maryland law is prepared to recognize that kind of injury—the injury of life itself.

The child has not suffered any damage cognizable at law by being brought into existence. One of the most deeply held beliefs of our society is that life, whether experienced with or without a major physical handicap, is more precious than nonlife. No one is perfect, and each person suffers from some ailments or defects (whether major or minor) that make impossible participation in all of the activities life has to offer. Our lives are not thereby rendered less precious than those of others whose defects are less pervasive or less severe. Despite their handicaps, Down syndrome children are able to love and be loved and to experience happiness and pleasure—emotions that are truly the essence of life and that are far more valuable than the suffering that may be endured.

The right to life and the principle that all are equal under the law are basic to our constitutional order. To presume to decide that a child's life is not worth living would be to forsake these ideals. To characterize the life of a disabled person as an injury would denigrate the handicapped themselves. Measuring the value of an impaired life as compared with nonexistence is a task that is beyond mortals.

Unless a judgment can be made on the basis of reason rather than the emotion of any given case, that nonlife is preferable to impaired life—that the child–plaintiff would, in fact, have been better off had he or she never been born—there can be no injury, and if there can be no injury, whether damages can or cannot be calculated becomes irrelevant.

The crucial question, a value judgment about life itself, is too deeply immersed in each person's own individual philosophy or theology to be subject to a reasoned and consistent community response in the form of a jury verdict.

Wrongful Conception

Wrongful conception refers to a claim for damages sustained by the parents of an unexpected child based on an allegation that conception of the child resulted from negligent sterilization procedures or a defective contraceptive device.[81] Damages sought for a negligently performed sterilization might include:

* Pain and suffering associated with pregnancy and birth
* Expenses of delivery
* Lost wages
* Father's loss of consortium
* Damages for emotional or psychological pain
* Suffering resulting from the presence of an additional family member in the household
* The cost and pain and suffering of a subsequent sterilization
* Damages suffered by a child born with genetic defects

The most controversial item of damages claimed is that of raising a normal healthy child to adulthood. The mother in *Hartke v. McKelway*[82] had undergone sterilization for therapeutic reasons to avoid endangering her health from pregnancy. The woman became pregnant as a result of a failed sterilization. She delivered a healthy child without injury to herself. It was determined that "the jury could not rationally have found that the birth of this child was an injury to this plaintiff. Awarding child-rearing expense would only give Hartke a windfall."[83]

The cost of raising a healthy newborn child to adulthood was recoverable by the parents of the child conceived as a result of an unsuccessful sterilization by a physician employee at Lovelace Medical Center. The physician in *Lovelace Medical Center v. Mendez*[84] found and ligated only one of the patient's two fallopian tubes and then failed to inform the patient of the unsuccessful operation. The court held that:[85]

> the Mendezes' interest in the financial security of their family was a legally protected interest which was invaded by Lovelace's negligent failure properly to perform Maria's sterilization operation (if proved at trial), and that this invasion was an injury entitling them to recover damages in the form of the reasonable expenses to raise Joseph to maturity.

Some states bar damage claims for emotional distress and the costs associated with the raising of healthy children but will permit recovery for damages related to negligent sterilizations. In *Butler v. Rolling Hill Hospital*,[86] the Pennsylvania Superior Court held that the patient stated a cause of action for the negligent performance of a laparoscopic tubal ligation. The patient was not, however, entitled to compensation for the costs of raising a normal, healthy child. "In light of this Commonwealth's public policy, which recognizes the paramount importance of the family to society, we conclude that the benefits of joy, companionship, and affection which a normal, healthy child can provide must be deemed as a matter of law to outweigh the costs of raising that child."[87]

As the Court of Common Pleas of Lycoming County, Pennsylvania, in *Shaheen v. Knight,* stated:[88]

> Many people would be willing to support this child were they given the right of custody and adoption, but according to plaintiff's statement, plaintiff does not want such. He wants to have the child and wants the doctor to support it. In our opinion, to allow such damages would be against public policy.

ARTIFICIAL INSEMINATION

Artificial insemination is the process by which sperm is placed into the reproductive tract of a female, for the purpose of impregnating the female by using means other than sexual intercourse. There are two sources of the sperm for impregnation of a female: (1) homologous artificial insemination involves the use of the husband's semen to impregnate the female; and heterologous artificial insemination (HAI) involves the use of semen from a donor other than a woman's husband. The absence of answers to many questions concerning HAI may discourage couples from seeking to use the procedure and physicians from performing it. Some of the questions concern the procedure itself; others concern the status of the offspring, the effect of the procedure on the marital relationship, and the risk of multiple births that can be financially challenging. Further worrying is the potential for legal actions for multiple births and even lead to the loss of a physician's license to practice medicine such as occurred when the Medical Board of California revoked Dr. Michael Kamrava medical license. Dr. Kamrava had transplanted multiple embryos that resulted in the birth of octuplets. The Medical Board determined that Dr. Kamrava had acted beyond the reasonable judgment of a physician by implanting a number of embryos that exceeded existing guidelines. "The Board subsequently found Kamrava guilty of gross negligence, repeated negligent acts, and inadequate medical records in the first case. In the additional two cases, Kamrava was found guilty of gross negligence and repeated negligent acts in one case and guilty of repeated negligent acts in the other case."[89]

CONSENT

The Oklahoma HAI statute specifies that husband and wife must consent to the procedure.[90] It is clear that the wife's consent must be obtained; without it, the touching involved in the artificial insemination would constitute a battery. Besides the wife's consent, it is important to obtain the husband's consent to ensure against liability accruing if a court adopted the view that without the consent of the husband, HAI was a wrong to the husband's interest, for which he could sustain a suit for damages.

The Oklahoma statute also deals with establishing proof of consent. It requires the consent to be in writing, and it must be executed and acknowledged by the physician performing the procedure and by the local judge who has jurisdiction over the adoption of children, as well as by the husband and wife.

In states without specific statutory requirements, medical personnel should attempt to avoid such potential liability by establishing the practice of obtaining the written consent of the couple requesting the HAI procedure.

CONFIDENTIALITY

Another problem that directly concerns medical personnel involved in heterologous artificial insemination birth is preserving confidentiality. This problem is met in the Oklahoma HAI statute, which requires that the original copy of the consent be filed pursuant to the rules for filing adoption papers and is not to be made a matter of public record.[91]

SURROGACY

Surrogacy is a method of reproduction whereby a woman agrees to give birth to a child she will not raise but hand over to a contracted party, who is often unable to conceive a natural child of her or his own. A surrogate "may be the child's genetic mother (the more traditional form of surrogacy), or she may as a gestational carrier, carry the pregnancy to delivery after having been implanted with an embryo. In some cases surrogacy is the only available option for parents who wish to have a child that is biologically related to them."[92]

Surrogacy raises a variety of ethical and legal issues that should be considered before searching for a surrogate mother. For example, is it ethical to enter a contract with a woman by offering her money in exchange for bearing a child and then transferring all parental rights and physical custody of the child to the "commissioning couple"? Although the long-term effects of surrogacy contracts are not known, the adverse psychological impact could be detrimental to the child who learns that he or she is the offspring of someone who gave birth only to obtain money. Would the child want to search for his or her gestational mother? Should records be kept, and should the child have access to the records? After the child is taken, the surrogate mother may be negatively affected as her feeling of isolation is felt along with the reality of the sale of her body.

Although there are arguments offered for and against surrogacy contracts, there are many parents who have experienced the joy of raising happy, psychologically well-balanced, and career-successful surrogate children. Those who have done their research and understand the issues live as happy together as those in any other family relationship.

ORGAN DONATIONS

Becoming a Donor

Organ and tissue donation and transplantation provide a second chance at life for thousands of people each year. You have the opportunity to be one of the individuals who make these miracles happen.

By deciding to be a donor, you give the gift of hope ... hope for the thousands of individuals awaiting organ transplants and hope for the millions of individuals whose lives could be enhanced through tissue transplants. [organdonor.gov.]

U.S. Department of Health and Human Services[93]

Federal regulations require that hospitals have and implement written protocols regarding their organ procurement responsibilities. The regulations impose specific notification duties, as well as other requirements concerning informing families of potential donors. It encourages discretion and sensitivity in dealing with the families and in educating hospital staff on a variety of issues involved with donation matters in order to facilitate timely donation and transplantation.

Organ transplantations are performed to treat patients with end-stage organ disease who face organ failure. Developments in medical science have enabled physicians to take tissue from persons immediately after death for use in replacing or rehabilitating diseased or damaged organs or other parts of living persons. Interest in organ transplantation increased in 1954 when the Herrick twins became the first successful kidney transplant.[94] The success rates of organ transplants have improved because of advances in the patient selection process, improved clinical and operative management and skills, and immunosuppressant drugs that aid in decreasing the incidence of tissue rejection (e.g., cyclosporin A, which acts to suppress the production of antibodies that attack transplanted tissue); nevertheless, this progress has created the problem of obtaining a sufficient supply of replacement body parts. There is a corresponding cry for more organs as the success rate in organ transplantation increases. Because of the fear of people buying and selling organs, the National Organ Procurement Act was enacted in 1984, making it illegal to buy or sell organs. Throughout the country, there are tissue banks and other facilities that store and preserve organs and tissue that can be used for transplantation and other therapeutic services.

The ever-increasing success of organ transplants and the demand for organ tissue require the close scrutiny of each case, to make sure that established procedures have been followed in the care and disposal of all body parts. Section 1138, Title XI, of the Omnibus Budget Reconciliation Act of 1986 requires hospitals to establish organ procurement protocols or face a loss of Medicare and Medicaid funding. Physicians, nurses, and other paramedical personnel assigned this responsibility often are confronted with several legal issues. Liability can be limited by complying with applicable regulations. Organs and tissues to be stored and preserved for future use must be removed almost immediately after death; therefore, it is imperative that an agreement or arrangement for obtaining organs and tissue from a body be completed before death, or very soon after death, to enable physicians to remove and store the tissue promptly.

There is a shortage of cadavers needed for medical education and transplantation. Mark Zuckerburg, chairman and chief executive officer of Facebook, aware of the severe shortage, launched an organ donation campaign in 2012.

Facebook Launches Organ Donation Campaign

May 1 (Reuters)—Facebook on Tuesday launched an organ donation tool aimed at encouraging the 900 million users of the social networking site to help combat a shortage of organs needed for life-saving transplants.

"What we hope will happen is that by just having a simple tool, we think that people can really help spread awareness of organ donation and that they want to participate in this to their friends, and we think that can be a big part in helping to solve the crisis," chief executive Mark Zuckerberg said on ABC-TV's "Good Morning America" program on Tuesday.

Nicola Leske, Jill Serjeant, Patricia Reaney, Chicago Tribune, May 1, 2012

Some people may wish to make arrangements for the use of their bodies after death for such purposes. A surviving spouse may, however, object to such disposition. In such cases, the interest of the surviving spouse or other family member could supersede that of the deceased.

WHO LIVES? WHO DIES? WHO DECIDES?

Who lives? Who dies? Who decides? These are but a few of the ethical questions that arise when deciding to whom an organ shall be given. The answers are not easy. The decision makers, even with guidelines to follow, often become the judge and jury and often find that the answers to who lives and dies are not always easy decisions. If there were unlimited sources of organs, there would be no supply-and-demand issues. Because supply is limited, numerous ethical principles come into play. In the case of a 70-year-old patient with multiple life-threatening health problems, the patient may not be considered a suitable candidate for a transplant, whereas a 15-year-old patient with few health issues would be considered a more appropriate candidate.

UNIFORM ANATOMICAL GIFT ACT

The American Bar Association endorsed a *Uniform Anatomical Gift Act* drafted by the Commission on Uniform State Laws. This statute has been enacted by all 50 states and has many detailed provisions that apply to the wide variety of issues raised in connection with the making, acceptance, and use of anatomical gifts. The act allows a person to make a decision to donate organs at the time of death and allows potential donors to carry an anatomical donor card. State statutes regarding donation usually permit the donor to execute the gift during his or her lifetime.

The right to privacy of the donor and his or her family must be respected. Information should not be publicized regarding transplant procedures as well as the names the donor or donee without consent.

States have enacted legislation to facilitate donation of bodies and body parts for medical uses. Virtually all of the states have based their enactments on the Uniform Anatomical Gift Act, but it should be recognized that in some states there are deviations from this act or additional laws dealing with donation.

Individuals who are of sound mind and 18 years of age or older are permitted to dispose of their own bodies or body parts by will or other written instrument for medical or dental education, research, advancement of medical or dental science, therapy, or transplantation. Among those eligible to receive such donations are any licensed, accredited, or approved hospitals; accredited medical or dental schools; surgeons or physicians; tissue banks; or specified individuals who need the donation for therapy or transplantation. The statute provides that when only a part of the body is donated, custody of the remaining parts of the body shall be transferred to the next of kin promptly after removal of the donated part.

A donation by will becomes effective immediately on the death of the testator, without probate, and the gift is valid and effective to the extent that it has been acted on in good faith. This is true even if the will is not probated or is declared invalid for testimonial purposes.

FAILURE TO OBTAIN CONSENT

Although failure to obtain consent for removal of body tissue can give rise to a lawsuit, not all such claims are successful. In *Nicoletta v. Rochester Eye & Human Parts Bank*,[95] emotional injuries resulted from the removal of the eyes of Nicoletta's son for donation after a fatal motorcycle accident. The hospital was immune from liability under the provisions of the Uniform Anatomical Gift Act because the hospital had neither actual nor constructive knowledge that the woman who had authorized the donation was not the decedent's wife. The hospital was entitled to the immunity afforded by the "good faith" provisions of Section 4306(3) of the act, under which its agents had made reasonable inquiry as to the status of the purported wife, who had resided with the decedent for 10 years and was the mother of their two children. The hospital had no reason to believe that any irregularity existed. The father, who was present at the time his son was brought to the emergency department, failed to object to any organ donation and failed to challenge the authority of the purported wife to sign the emergency department authorization. There are several methods by which a donation may be revoked. If the document has been delivered to a named donee, it may be revoked by:

- A written revocation signed by the donor and delivered to the donee
- An oral revocation witnessed by two persons and communicated to the donee
- A statement to the attending physician during a terminal illness that has been communicated to the donee
- A written statement that has been signed and is on the donor's person or in the donor's immediate effects

If the written instrument of donation has not been delivered to the donee, it may be revoked by destruction, cancellation, or mutilation of the instrument. If the donation is made by a will, it may be revoked in the manner provided for revocation or amendment of wills. Any person acting in good-faith reliance on the terms of an instrument of donation will not be subject to civil or criminal liability unless there is actual notice of the revocation of the donation.

RESEARCH, EXPERIMENTATION, AND CLINICAL TRIALS

Medical progress and improved patient care are dependent on advances in medicine made through research. Research studies are designed to answer specific questions, including a drug or device's safety and effectiveness. Ethical considerations, to name but a few, that should be addressed when conducting research on human subjects include honesty, integrity, autonomy; self-determination; the Hippocratic maxim of do no harm; the application of justice; and, how to fairly conduct blind trials. The basic principle of research is honesty, which must be ensured through institutional protocols. Honesty and integrity must govern all stages of research.

The science of medicine, which by its very nature studies the human body, is prevented from making progress through direct experimentation. A necessary part of research is to conduct laboratory tests on animals and observe their effects prior to testing them on humans. Advances in research occurs by observation and study of how a normal healthy body functions and when the body malfunctions, studying the cause of those changes that occur and finding a way to slow and possibly reverse the progression of a disease.

Federal regulations control federal grants that apply to experiments involving new drugs, new medical devices, or new medical procedures. Generally, a combination of federal and state guidelines and regulations ensures proper supervision and control over experimentation that involves human subjects. For example, federal regulations require hospital-based researchers to obtain the approval of an *institutional review board.*

OFFICE OF RESEARCH INTEGRITY

The Office of Research Integrity (ORI) oversees and directs Public Health Service (PHS) research integrity activities on behalf of the Secretary of Health and Human Services with the exception of the research integrity activities of the Food and Drug Administration. The ORI carries out its responsibility by developing policies, procedures, and regulations related to the detection, investigation, and prevention of research misconduct and the responsible conduct of research. The ORI is responsible for implementing activities and programs to teach the responsible conduct of research, promote research integrity, prevent research misconduct, and improve the handling of allegations of research misconduct. The ORI administers programs for: maintaining institutional assurances, responding to allegations of retaliation against whistleblowers, approving intramural and extramural policies and procedures, and responding to Freedom of Information Act and Privacy Act requests.

FOOD AND DRUG ADMINISTRATION

The Food and Drug Administration (FDA) regulates the conduct of clinical trials. A variety of regulations that describe good clinical practices for studies with both human and nonhuman animal subjects are listed next. More detail on these and other research-related regulations can be found at the FDA website.[96]

- Electronic Records
- Protection of Human Subjects
- Informed Consent Elements
- Financial Disclosure by Investigators
- Institutional Review Boards
- Investigational Drug New Application
- Investigational Device Exemptions
- Good Laboratory Practice for Nonclinical Laboratory Studies
- Expanded Access to Investigational Drugs for Treatment

The FDA—after much criticism over the years because of the red tape involved in the approval of new drugs—issued new rules to speed up the approval process. The rules permit the use of experimental drugs outside a controlled clinical trial if the drugs are used to treat a life-threatening condition. In *Abigail Alliance for Better Access to Developmental Drugs v. Eschenbach,* [33] the U.S. Court of Appeals for the District of Columbia ruled that terminally ill patients have a "fundamental right" protected by the U.S. Constitution to access to experimental drugs that have not yet been fully approved by the FDA. The appeals court ruled that once the FDA has determined, after Phase I trials, that a potentially lifesaving new drug is sufficiently safe for expanded human trials, terminally ill patients have a constitutional right to seek treatment with the drug if no other FDA-approved drugs are available. The court said that if the FDA wishes to prevent such patients from gaining access to investigational drugs that have completed Phase I trials, it bears the burden of demonstrating that its restrictions are "narrowly tailored" to serve a compelling governmental interest.

Patients participating in research studies should fully understand the implications of their participation. Health care organizations involved in research studies should have appropriate protocols in place that protect the rights of patients. Consent forms should describe both the risks and benefits involved in the research activity.

INSTITUTIONAL REVIEW BOARD

Health care organizations conducting medical research must have a mechanism in place for approving and overseeing the use of investigational protocols. This is accomplished through the establishment of an institutional review board (IRB). An IRB is a committee designated by organizations (e.g., hospitals) conducting clinical trials to provide initial approval and periodic monitoring of biomedical research studies. The primary responsibilities of an IRB include:

- Protecting the rights and welfare of human subjects
- Ensuring protocols are presented by the sponsor(s)
- Ensuring sponsor(s) of a protocol discloses
  - Areas of concern that might give the impression of a conflict of interest in the outcome of the clinical research
  - Financial interests that might occur should the clinical trials prove to be successful or give the impression of success, including stock options and cash payouts
  - Reviewing, monitoring, and approving clinical protocols for investigations of drugs and medical devices involving human subjects
  - Ensuring that the rights, including the privacy and confidentiality, of each individual are protected
  - Ensuring that all research is conducted within appropriate state and federal guidelines (e.g., FDA guidelines)

INFORMED CONSENT

My husband . . . participated in a clinical trial involving both an autologous (self) and allogeneic (donor) transplant for a hopeful cure of the disease. We both understood the risks involved and the no-promise guarantee, as such is the nature of a clinical trial. The ultimate responsibility for whatever the outcome rested with us, as we were the ones who voluntarily entered into the program. Three years later, we have just learned of the disease's progression, but we continue to look forward, remain optimistic, and support those who dedicate their lives for the betterment of those afflicted with these cursed cancers.

The reality is that someday, probably sooner than later, my husband will lose the battle with this tenacious enemy, but we are still thankful for the compassionate and learned members of the Fred Hutchinson Cancer Research Center who helped and are still helping us to navigate a most challenging road.[97]

Mary Ellen Stokes and Bill Stokes, "Relentless Assault on a Research Hospital," *Wall Street Journal, March 15, 2004*

Health care organizations involved in research studies should have appropriate protocols in place that protect the rights of patients. Patients participating in research studies should fully understand the implications of their participation. Physicians have a clear duty to warn patients as to the risks, benefits, and alternatives of an experimental procedure. Written consent should be obtained from each patient who participates in a clinical trial. The consent form must not contain any coercive or exculpatory language through which the patient is forced to waive his or her legal rights, including the release of the investigator, sponsor, or organization from liability for negligent conduct.

Organizations conducting clinical trials on human subjects, at the very least, must:

- Fully disclose to the patient the inherent risks, benefits, and treatment alternatives to the proposed research protocol(s)
- Determine the competency of the patient to consent
- Obtain written consent from the patient
- Educate the staff as to the potential side effects, implementation of, and ongoing monitoring of protocols
- Require financial disclosure issues associated with the protocols
  - Promote awareness of ethical issues
  - Promote education in regard to ethical decision making
  - Increase nurse participation in ethical decision making
  - Have ongoing monitoring of approved protocols

The Centers for Medicare and Medicaid Services accreditation survey process for nursing facilities includes a review of the rights of nursing facility residents participating in experimental research. Surveyors will review the records of residents identified as participating in a clinical research study. They will determine whether informed consent forms have been executed properly. The form will be reviewed to determine whether all known risks have been identified. Appropriate questions may be directed to both the staff and residents or the residents' guardians.

Possible questions to ask staff include:[98]

- Is the facility participating in any experimental research?
- If yes, what residents are involved? (Interview a sample of these residents.)[99]
- Residents or guardians may be asked questions, such as:
  - Are you participating in the study?
  - Was this explained to you well enough so that you understand what the study is about and any risks that might be involved?

Experimental Subject's Bill of Rights

The following is a bill of rights developed by the Veterans Administration system for patients involved in research studies. Human subjects have the following rights. These rights include, but are not limited to, the subject's right to:[100]

- Be informed of the nature and purpose of the experiment
- Be given an explanation of the procedures to be followed in the medical experiment and any drug or device to be used
- Be given a description of any attendant discomforts and risks reasonably to be expected
- Be given an explanation of any benefits to the subject reasonably to be expected, if applicable
- Be given a disclosure of any appropriate alternatives, drugs, or devices that might be advantageous to the subject, their relative risks, and benefits
- Be informed of the avenues of medical treatment, if any, available to the subject after the experiment if complications should arise
- Be given an opportunity to ask questions concerning the experiment or the procedures involved
- Be instructed that consent to participate in the medical experiment may be withdrawn at any time and the subject may discontinue participation without prejudice
- Be given a copy of the signed and dated consent form
- Be given the opportunity to decide to consent or not to consent to a medical experiment without the intervention of any element of force, fraud, deceit, duress, coercion, or undue influence on the subject's decision

Case: Medical Research and Duty to Warn

About 5,000 patients at Michael Reese Hospital and Medical Center, located in Chicago, Illinois, were treated with X-ray therapy for some benign conditions of the head and neck from 1930 to 1960. Among them was Joel Blaz, now a citizen of Florida, who received this treatment for infected tonsils and adenoids while a child in Illinois from 1947 through 1948. He has suffered various tumors, which he now attributes to this treatment. Blaz was diagnosed with a neural tumor in 1987.

In 1974, Michael Reese set up the Thyroid Follow-Up Project to gather data and conduct research among the people who had been subjected to the X-ray therapy. In 1975, the program notified Blaz by mail that he was at increased risk of developing thyroid tumors because of the treatment. In 1976, someone associated with the program gave him similar information by phone and invited him to return to Michael Reese for evaluation and treatment at his own expense, which he declined to do.

Dr. Arthur Schneider was placed in charge of the program in 1977. In 1979, Schneider and Michael Reese submitted a research proposal to the National Institutes of Health stating that a study based on the program showed "strong evidence" of a connection between X-ray treatments of the sort administered to Blaz and various sorts of tumors: thyroid, neural, and others. In 1981, Blaz received but did not complete or return a questionnaire attached to a letter from Schneider in connection with the program. The letter stated that the purpose of the questionnaire was to "investigate the long-term health implications" of childhood radiation treatments and to "determine the possible associated risks." It did not say anything about "strong evidence" of a connection between the treatments and any tumors.

In 1996, after developing neural tumors, Blaz sued Michael Reese's successor, Galen Hospital in Illinois, and Dr. Schneider, alleging, among other things, that they failed to notify and warn him of their findings that he might be at greater risk of neural tumors in a way that might have permitted their earlier detection and removal or other treatment. There is a clear duty to warn the subject of previously administered radiation treatments when there is a strong connection between those treatments and certain kinds of tumors. The harm alleged, neural and other tumors would here be reasonably foreseeable as a likely consequence of a failure to warn and was in fact foreseen by Schneider. A reasonable physician, indeed any reasonable person, could foresee that if someone were warned of "strong evidence" of a connection between treatments to which he had been subjected and tumors, he would probably seek diagnosis or treatment and perhaps avoid these tumors, and if he were not warned he probably would not seek diagnosis or treatment, increasing the likelihood that he would suffer from such tumors. Other things being equal, therefore, a reasonable physician would warn the subject of the treatments.[101]

Ethical and Legal Issues

1. Discuss the ethical and legal principles violated in this case.
2. What preventative measures should be taken to prevent recurrence of cases such as this?

PATIENT RESPONSIBILITIES

Patients in National Institutes of Health (NIH) clinical trials have responsibilities, as well as rights. The following describes the responsibilities of NIH patients.

In the spirit of working together toward a common goal, our patients (and their parents, guardians, and surrogates) have responsibilities as partners in medical research and as patients at the Clinical Center.

You have the responsibility:

1. To provide, to the best of your knowledge, complete information about your current medical condition and past medical history, including current illness, prior hospitalizations, current medications, allergies, and all other health-related matters;
2. To discuss your protocol (study or treatment plan) with the research staff before indicating agreement to take part in it by signing a consent;
3. To inform the medical staff about your wishes regarding treatment plans. You may provide for a duly authorized family member or spokesperson to make medical decisions on your behalf in the event that you become unable to communicate;
4. To comply with your protocol, to cooperate with hospital staff, to ask questions if directions or procedures are not clear, and to participate in your health care decisions. You may withdraw from the study for any reason, but it is desirable to discuss your concerns with the attending physician before taking that action.

Parents of pediatric patients have the responsibility to indicate if and how they want to be involved in their child's plan of care;

5. To refrain from taking any medications, drugs, or alcoholic beverages while participating in the protocol, except those approved by an NIH physician;

6. To adhere to the no-smoking policy of the NIH;

7. To report on time for scheduled procedures and to keep all clinic appointments. If unable to do so, you have the responsibility of notifying the protocol physician and canceling and rescheduling the appointment;

8. To report promptly to the medical or nursing staff any unexpected problems or changes in your medical condition;

9. To inform the appropriate staff or the patient representative of any concerns or problems with the care and treatment that you feel are not being adequately addressed;

10. To respect the property of the U.S. government, fellow patients, and others; to follow NIH rules and regulations affecting patient care and treatment; to respect the rights of other patients and hospital staff. This includes the responsibility of respecting the privacy of other patients and treating information concerning them as confidential;

11. To pay all medical or laboratory expenses incurred outside the Clinical Center, except when you have received written authorization on the appropriate NIH form to have such expenses billed to the NIH;

12. To obtain medical care and medications from your own health care provider for all conditions unrelated to the protocol in which you are participating, except while being treated as an inpatient at the Clinical Center;

13. To provide your own transportation to and from the Clinical Center and to pay living expenses except when all or part of these expenses are covered by the protocol or authorized by the responsible NIH physician; to advise accompanying escorts or others who travel to and remain in the Bethesda area that they must pay for their travel and living expenses except when designated by NIH as a guardian for you when your expenses are covered;

14. To provide complete information, so that contacts and communications to schedule visits and monitor health status can be maintained. This information should include (1) your current address and phone number; (2) the names, addresses, and phone numbers of next of kin or persons to be notified in the event of an emergency; and (3) the names, addresses, and phone numbers of physicians responsible for your ongoing care, including your family physician and the physician(s) who referred you to the NIH;

15. To return to the care of your own health-care provider when participation in the protocol is completed or stopped and your medical condition permits.[102]

If you have questions about your rights, you may contact the Clinical Center Patient Representative.

PATENTS DELAY RESEARCH

The legal system—caught up in the rights of patent holders—has resulted in delayed cures. What happens to the rights of those who would have benefited from the cures? The rights of the few, those who could be viewed as seeing money as the ultimate good, hold hostage the rights of many. That is, until they need the cure. The legal system is so ruled by rules that it cannot get out of its own harmful way.

NEWS

Where Are the Cures? How Patent Gridlock Is Blocking the Development of Lifesaving Drugs

A curious thing happened on the way to the biotech revolution. While investment in biotech research and development has increased over the last three decades, new drugs that improve human health have not been forthcoming at the same rate.

What explains this drug discovery gap? Patent gridlock plays a large role. Since a 1980 Supreme Court decision allowing patents on living organisms, 40,000 DNA-related patents have been granted. Now picture a drug developer walking into an auditorium filled with dozens of owners of the biotech patents needed to create a potential lifesaving cure. Unless the drug maker can strike a deal with every person in the room, the new drug won't be developed.

Peter Ringrose, former chief science officer at Bristol-Myers Squibb, told the *New York Times* that the company would not investigate some 50 proteins that could be cancer-causing, because patent holders would either decline to cooperate or demand big royalties.

Michael Heller, Forbes, *August 11, 2008*

Discussion

- Discuss the ethical principles (e.g., beneficence [doing good] and nonmaleficence [avoiding causing harm]) and issues of morality of a legal system that delays research because of the legal rights of patent holders.
- Discuss what steps could be taken to right the wrongs of patents that delay and often discourage research.

HUMAN GENETICS

The most promising frontier of the future of medical practice is in the area of human genetics, which describes the study of inheritance as it occurs in human beings. It includes such areas as stem cell research, clinical genetics (e.g., genetic disease markers), and molecular genetics. Inevitably there will be ethical issues that will become manifest in these new areas. We have already had a preview of this in the controversy regarding the use of fetal stem cells versus adult stem cells for research and therapy.

The ethics of modern science is a challenging and evolving area, but it is nothing new. In ancient China, for instance, physician Sun Simiao (580–682 AD) had a difficult medical ethical dilemma. In his book *Qianjinfang (Prescriptions Worth a Thousand Pieces of Gold)*, he is credited with formulating the first ethical basis for the practice of medicine in China. The ethical conundrum he faced was the clash between Confucian and Buddhist ethics. The relatively new religion of Buddhism had taboos against using any animal-derived product for the treatment of disease, as this violated the principle of respect for all life. The more ancient Confucian idea of compassion and kindness could be interpreted to overrule this, however.

Sun Simiao dealt with this conflict by prohibiting a "standard physician" from using any medication derived from an animal source. He then included many prescriptions in his book that did have animal-sourced remedies. In other words, he seems to have artfully navigated an ethical gray zone between the two philosophies but with a less than clear distinction between right and wrong. Now in modern times we are still faced with continuing and evolving issues of ethics in the practice of medicine.[103]

GENETIC MARKERS

Genetic markers are genes or DNA sequences with a known location on a chromosome that can be used to identify specific cells and diseases, as well as individuals and species. They are often used to study the relationship between an inherited disease and its genetic cause in order to determine an individual's predisposition/proclivity to a specific disease. Genetic markers show observable information in DNA sequence variation, which may arise as a result of mutation of a specific gene. There are companies that will evaluate a person's DNA for these markers and provide a person with a report of his or her potential health risks. Health insurers, life insurers, employers, and others could potentially use this information to determine one's insurance premiums and even one's job future and so forth. There is going to be ethical issues that will arise. For instance, suppose a woman has a family history of breast cancer and has a genetic marker for it, but she is young (e.g., 30 years old) and free of any evidence of cancer. If a physician recommends prophylactic mastectomy or if the patient wants a prophylactic mastectomy, should this be covered by insurance? Should this same logic be extended to other body organs?

GENETIC INFORMATION NONDISCRIMINATION ACT OF 2008 (HR493)

On May 21, 2008, President George W. Bush signed into law the Genetic Information Nondiscrimination Act (GINA), which resulted largely from the efforts of Senator Ted Kennedy. The law prohibits discrimination on the basis of genetic information with respect to the availability of health insurance and employment. The GINA prohibits group health plans and insurers from denying coverage to a healthy individual or charging that person higher premiums based solely on a genetic predisposition to developing a specific disease (e.g., cancer or heart disease) at some future time. The GINA also prohibits employers from using an individual's genetic information when making hiring, firing, job placement, or promotion decisions.

The relatively recent mapping of the human genome and the likelihood of increasing clinical application of advances in genetic disease markers make this an issue of potential increasing importance in the practice of medicine. Most states also have legislation that addresses this issue. Unfortunately, there remains, no federal legislation that protects the individual from discrimination in the availability of life insurance, disability insurance coverage, or long-term care insurance. Because of this loophole, patients and their doctors need to consider the potential downside of ordering prognostic genetic tests.[104]

STEM CELL RESEARCH

Stem cell research involves the use of embryonic stem cells to create organs and various body tissues. It continues to be a highly controversial issue generally involving religious beliefs and fears as to how far scientists might go in their attempt to create, for example, another human being. Researchers must be free to unlock the secrets that stem cells hold and learn from them with the hope to develop effective therapies.

Some opponents of stem cell research argue that this practice is a slippery slope to reproductive cloning and fundamentally devalues the worth of a human being. Contrarily, some medical researchers in the field argue that it is necessary to pursue embryonic stem cell research because the resultant technologies could have significant medical potential and that excess embryos created for in vitro fertilization could be donated with consent and used for the research. This, in turn, conflicts with opponents in the pro-life movement, who advocate for the protection of human embryos. The ensuing debate has prompted authorities around the world to seek regulatory frameworks and highlighted the fact that embryonic stem cell research represents a social and ethical challenge that includes concern for the natural order of the ecosystem and, ultimately, the survival of the human race.

ACQUIRED IMMUNE DEFICIENCY SYNDROME

WHO Issues New HIV Recommendations Calling for Earlier Treatment

GENEVA—New HIV treatment guidelines by WHO recommend offering antiretroviral therapy (ART) earlier. Recent evidence indicates that earlier ART will help people with HIV to live longer, healthier lives, and substantially reduce the risk of transmitting HIV to others. The move could avert an additional 3 million deaths and prevent 3.5 million more new HIV infections between now and 2025.

News Release, World Health Organization, *June 30, 2013*

The epidemic of *acquired immune deficiency syndrome (AIDS)* is considered to be the deadliest epidemic in human history. The first case appeared in the literature in 1981.[105] It has been estimated that more than 35 million people have died of AIDS.

> **Global situation and trends:** Since the beginning of the epidemic, almost 70 million people have been infected with the HIV virus and about 35 million people have died of AIDS. Globally, 34.0 million (31.4–35.9 million) people were living with HIV at the end of 2011. An estimated 0.8% of adults aged 15–49 years worldwide are living with HIV, although the burden of the epidemic continues to vary considerably between countries and regions. Sub-Saharan Africa remains most severely affected, with nearly 1 in every 20 adults (4.9%) living with HIV and accounting for 69% of the people living with HIV worldwide.[106]

AIDS, generally, is accepted as a syndrome—a collection of specific, life-threatening, opportunistic infections and manifestations that are the result of an underlying immune deficiency. AIDS is caused by the human immunodeficiency virus (HIV) and is the most severe form of HIV, a highly contagious blood-borne virus. It is a fatal disease that destroys the body's capacity to ward off bacteria and viruses that ordinarily would be fought off by a properly functioning immune system. Although there is no effective long-term treatment of the disease, indications are that proper management of the disease can improve the quality of life and delay progression of the disease. Internationally, AIDS is posing serious social, ethical, economic, and health problems.

SPREAD OF AIDS

AIDS is spread by direct contact with infected blood or body fluids, such as vaginal secretions, semen, and breast milk. Currently, there is no evidence that the virus can be transmitted through food, water, or casual body contact. HIV does not survive well outside the body. Although there is currently no cure for AIDS, early diagnosis and treatment with new medications can help HIV-infected persons remain healthy for longer periods. High-risk groups include those who have had unprotected sexual encounters, intravenous drug users, and those who require transfusions of blood and blood products, such as hemophiliacs.

Blood Transfusions

The administration of blood is considered to be a medical procedure. It results from the exercise of professional medical judgment that is composed of two parts: (1) diagnosis, deciding the need for blood, and (2) therapy, the actual administration of blood.

Lawsuits often arise as a result of a person with AIDS claiming that he or she contracted the disease as a result of a transfusion of contaminated blood or blood products. In blood transfusion cases, the standards most commonly identified as having been violated concern blood testing and donor screening. An injured party generally must prove that a standard of care existed, that the defendant's conduct fell below the standard, and that this conduct was the proximate cause of the plaintiff's injury.

The most common occurrences that lead to lawsuits in the administration of blood involve:

- Transfusion of mismatched blood
- Improper screening and transfusion of contaminated blood
- Unnecessary administration of blood
- Improper handling procedures (e.g., inadequate refrigeration and storage procedures)

The risk of HIV infection and AIDS through a blood transfusion has been reduced significantly through health history screening and blood donations testing. Since May 1985, all blood donated in the United States has been tested for HIV antibodies. Blood units that do test positive for HIV are removed from the blood transfusion pool.

ADMINISTRATION OF THE WRONG BLOOD

The patient-plaintiff in *Bordelon v. St. Francis Cabrini Hospital* (1994)[107] was admitted to the hospital to undergo a hysterectomy. Before surgery, she provided the hospital with her own blood in case it was needed during surgery. During surgery, the patient did indeed need blood but was administered donor blood other than her own. The patient filed a lawsuit claiming that the hospital's failure to provide her with her own blood resulted in her suffering mental distress.

The court of appeals held that the plaintiff stated a cause of action for mental distress. It is well established in law that a claim for negligent infliction of emotional distress unaccompanied by physical injury is a viable claim of action. It is indisputable that HIV can be transmitted through blood transfusions even when the standard procedure for screening for the virus is in place. The plaintiff's fear was easily associated with receiving someone else's blood and therefore a conceivable consequence of the defendant's negligent act. The hospital had a "duty" to administer the plaintiff's own blood. The hospital breached that duty by administering the wrong blood.

Ethical and Legal Issues

1. Do you agree with the court's decision? Explain your answer.
2. In cases such as this, do you believe that financial awards are effective in preventing future incidents? Explain your answer.

Health Care Workers

NEWS

HIV test urged for 7,000 Oklahoma dental patients

Health officials are urging 7,000 patients of an Oklahoma dentist to be tested for potential exposure to HIV, hepatitis B and hepatitis C.

• • •

Harrington, an oral surgeon who has been licensed since the 1970s, surrendered his credentials March 20 and discontinued his practice after investigators discovered alleged health and safety violations. Authorities say he is cooperating.

Katharine Lackey and Michael Winter, USA Today, *March 28, 2013*[108]

Although transmission of HIV from an infected dentist, physician, or other caregiver to his or her patient during invasive procedures is not a common occurrence, there is a foreseeable risk. Because of the potentially deadly consequence of such transmission, physicians should not engage in any activity that creates a risk of transmission.

The ever-increasing likelihood that health care workers will come into contact with persons carrying the AIDS virus demands that health care workers comply with approved safety procedures. This is especially important for those who come into contact with blood and body fluids of HIV-infected persons.

An AIDS-infected surgeon in New Jersey was unable to recover on a discrimination claim when the hospital restricted his surgical privileges. In *Estate of Behringer v. Medical Center at Princeton* (1991),[109] the New Jersey Superior Court held that the hospital acted properly in initially suspending a surgeon's surgical privileges, thereafter imposing a requirement of informed consent and ultimately barring the surgeon from performing surgery. The court held that in the context of informed consent, the risk of a surgical accident involving an AIDS-positive surgeon and implications thereof would be a legitimate concern to a surgical patient that would warrant disclosure of the risk. "The 'risk of harm' to the patient includes not only the actual transmission of HIV from the surgeon to patient but the risk of a surgical accident (e.g.., a scalpel cut or needle stick), which may subject the patient to post-surgery HIV testing."[110]

CONFIDENTIALITY

Guidelines drafted by the Centers for Disease Control and Prevention call on health care workers who perform "exposure-prone" procedures to undergo tests voluntarily to determine whether they are infected. The guidelines also recommend that patients be informed. Both health care workers and patients claim that mandatory HIV testing violates their Fourth Amendment right to privacy. The dilemma is how to balance these rights against the rights of the public in general to be protected from a deadly disease.

State laws have been developed that protect the confidentiality of HIV related information. Some states have developed informational brochures and consent, release, and partner notification forms. The unauthorized disclosure of confidential HIV-related information can subject an individual to civil and/or criminal penalties. Information regarding a patient's diagnosis as being HIV positive must be kept confidential and should be shared with other health care professionals only on a need-to-know basis. Each person has a right to privacy as to his or her personal affairs. The plaintiff surgeon in *Estate of Behringer v. Medical Center at Princeton* (1991)[111] was entitled to recover damages from the hospital and its laboratory director for the unauthorized disclosure of his condition during his stay at the hospital. The hospital and the director had breached their duty to maintain confidentiality of the surgeon's medical records by allowing placement of the patient's test results in his medical chart without limiting access to the chart, which they knew was available to the entire hospital community. "The medical center breached its duty of confidentiality to the plaintiff, as a patient, when it failed to take reasonable precautions regarding the plaintiff's medical records to prevent the patient's AIDS diagnosis from becoming a matter of public knowledge."[112]

The hospital in *Tarrant County Hospital District v. Hughes* (1987)[113] was found to have properly disclosed the names and addresses of blood donors in a wrongful death action alleging that a patient contracted AIDS from a blood transfusion administered in the hospital. The physician–patient privilege expressed in the Texas Rules of Evidence did not apply to preclude such disclosure because the record did not reflect that any such relationship had been established. The disclosure was not an impermissible violation of the donors' right of privacy. The societal interest in maintaining an effective blood donor program did not override the plaintiff's right to receive such information. The order prohibited disclosure of the donors' names to third parties.

In *Doe v. University of Cincinnati* (1988),[114] a patient who was infected with HIV-contaminated blood during surgery brought an action against a hospital and a blood bank. The trial court granted the patient's request to discover the identity of the blood donor, and the defendants appealed. The court of appeals held that the potential injury to a donor in revealing his identity outweighed the plaintiff's modest interest in learning of the donor's identity. A blood donor has a constitutional right to privacy not to be identified as a donor of blood that contains HIV. At the time of the plaintiff's blood transfusion in July 1984, no test had been developed to determine the existence of AIDS antibodies. By May 27, 1986, all donors donating blood through the defendant blood bank were tested for the presence of HIV antibodies. Patients who had received blood from donors who tested positive were to be notified through their physicians. In this case, the plaintiff's family was notified because of the plaintiff's age and other disability.

HIV-related regulations must continue to address the rights and responsibilities of both patients and health care workers. Although this will always be a delicate balancing act, it must be handled with privacy, safety, and compassion in mind.

 ## DISCLOSURE OF PHYSICIAN'S HIV STATUS

The physician, Doe, was a resident in obstetrics and gynecology at a medical center. In 1991, he cut his hand with a scalpel while he was assisting another physician. Because of the uncertainty that blood had been transferred from Doe's hand wound to the patient through an open surgical incision, he agreed to have a blood test for HIV. His blood tested positive for HIV, and he withdrew himself from participation in further surgical procedures. The medical center and Harrisburg Hospital, where Doe also participated in surgery, identified those patients who could be at risk. The medical center identified 279 patients, and Harrisburg identified 168 patients, who fell into this category. Because hospital records did not identify those surgeries in which physicians may have accidentally cut themselves, the hospitals filed petitions in the Court of Common Pleas, alleging that there was, under the Confidentiality of HIV-Related Information Act [35 P.S. § 7608(a)(2)], a "compelling need" to disclose information regarding Doe's condition to those patients who conceivably could have been exposed to HIV. Doe argued that there was no compelling need to disclose the information and that he was entitled to confidentiality under the act.

The Pennsylvania Supreme Court held that a compelling need existed for at least a partial disclosure of the physician's HIV status.

The medical experts who testified agreed that there was some risk of exposure and that some form of notice should be given to the patients at risk. Even the expert witness presented by Doe agreed that there was at least some conceivable risk of exposure and that giving a very limited form of notice would not be unreasonable. Failure to notify the patients at risk could result in the spread of the disease to other noninfected individuals through sexual contact and through exposure to other body fluids. Doe's name was not revealed to the patients, only the fact that a resident physician who had participated in their care had tested HIV positive. "No principle is more deeply embedded in the law than that expressed in the maxim Salus populi suprema lex . . . (The welfare of the people is the supreme law), and a more compelling and consistent application of that principle than the one presented would be quite difficult to conceive."[115]

Ethical and Legal Issues

1. Do you agree that there was a need for a partial disclosure of the physician's HIV status?
2. If "the welfare of the people is the supreme law," did the court fall short of its responsibility by not allowing disclosure of the physician's name? Discuss your answer.

The Pennsylvania Superior Court in *Stenger v. Lehigh Valley Hospital Center*[116] upheld the Court of Common Pleas' order denying the petition of The Morning Call, Inc., which challenged a court order closing judicial proceedings to the press and public in a civil action against a hospital and physicians. A patient and her family had all contracted AIDS after the patient received a blood transfusion. The access of the media to pretrial discovery proceedings in a civil action is subject to reasonable control by the court in which the action is pending. The protective order limiting public access to pretrial discovery material did not violate the newspaper's First Amendment rights. The discovery documents were not judicial records to which the newspaper had a common-law right of access. Good cause existed for nondisclosure of information about the intimate personal details of the plaintiffs' lives, disclosure of which would cause undue humiliation.

HIV AUTONOMY AND CONFIDENTIALITY

Jones, a divorcee with two children, was sentenced to 10 years in prison for repeated robberies of three banks. He was in prison for 8 years. His wife, Nora, disappeared shortly after he was sentenced. Five of his close inmate friends at Sing Prison had tested positive for the HIV virus and had since passed away. Prison officials wanted to test Jones for the HIV virus. He objected and sought legal counsel. Local school officials were informed of the deaths of Mr. Jones's friends and his refusal to be tested for the HIV virus. Strangely, the community at large became aware of Jones's situation and the fact that his children were attending school with their children. The parents insisted that the Jones kids be removed from school or else they would remove their children from class. Meanwhile, Nora showed up at a local navy recruiting station posing as a single woman with no children. She admitted to being bisexual several years earlier but claimed that she was now straight. The navy learned of this situation and required her to undergo HIV testing. She objected and sought legal counsel.

Ethical and Legal Issues

1. What are Mr. Jones's rights?
2. What are the rights of other prisoners?
3. Is there a legitimate need for a physician to disclose otherwise confidential testing data to the spouse and other intimate sexual partners of an HIV-infected patient?

THE RIGHT TO TREATMENT

A variety of health care organizations have included in their ethics statements that HIV-infected patients have a right not to be discriminated against in the provision of treatment. The Ethics Committee of the American Academy of Dermatology, for example, states "it is unethical for a physician to discriminate against a class or category of patients and to refuse the management of a patient because of medical risk, real or imagined."[117] Patients with HIV infection, therefore, should receive the same compassionate and competent care provided to other patients.

Basketball Camp's Exclusion of HIV-Positive Boy Ruled Discrimination

An HIV-positive 10-year-old boy was discriminated against when he was denied admission to a New York basketball camp, a federal judge has ruled. Judge Donald C. Pogue granted a motion for declaratory relief, finding the camp had violated the Americans with Disabilities Act. "The court agrees that defendants were obligated to protect other campers from a very serious, life-threatening viral infection," Pogue said. "But this obligation does not excuse defendants' actions when based on unsubstantiated fears."

Mark Hamblet, New York Law Journal, *January 22, 2010*

DISCRIMINATION IN THE COMMUNITY

The plaintiff Adam Doe claimed that the defendants, Deer Mountain Day Camp, Inc. (DMDC) and Deer Mountain Basketball Academy (DMBA), discriminated against him by denying him admission to a basketball camp on the basis of his disability, an HIV infection, in violation of the Americans with Disabilities Act (ADA), 42 U.S.C. §§ 12101-213 (2000) (ADA) and the New York State Human Rights Law (NYHRL), N.Y. Exec. Law §§ 290301 (2004) (NYHRL).

Adam had contracted HIV at birth due to a perinatal infection. He took antiretroviral medications to treat his condition, and his syndrome has been undetectable for years. On the advice of Dr. Neu, Adam's HIV specialist, Adam and his mother had kept and continued to keep Adam's HIVseropositivity confidential. Adam liked to play basketball, and in 2004, his HIV clinic recommended that he attend a basketball camp.

Mrs. Doe had been notified that the camp was unable to make reasonable accommodations for Adam and, as a consequence, they could not allow him to attend DMBA. According to Mrs. Doe, she was told that Adam could potentially transmit HIV through blood in his urine or in his stool. Mrs. Doe denied that Adam had problems with bloody stool or urine. Mrs. Doe, however, was told that DMBA could not accept Adam. She later received a refund of Adam's admission fees.

The plaintiff brings this action for violations of Title III of the ADA and the NYHRL, arguing that the defendants unlawfully discriminated against him on the basis of his disability, e.g., his HIV-seropositivity, by excluding him from participation in the basketball camp. To redress his injuries, including emotional and psychological harm, Adam requested declaratory, compensatory, and injunctive relief, as well as attorney's fees and costs.

Both parties made motions for summary judgment. The defendants failed to present any evidence of the objective reasonableness of their determination that the plaintiff's condition posed a threat to other campers.

In their cross motions for summary judgment, the parties placed before the court the issues of whether HIV-seropositivity qualifies as a "disability" and whether defendants' denial of admission constitutes discrimination "on the basis of" that disability. The plaintiff's motion argued that the defendants conclusively qualify as "public accommodations," thus prohibiting them from engaging in such discrimination.

The United States District Court, S.D. of New York, granted the plaintiff's motion for Summary Judgment of ADA and NYHRL declaratory relief, as to DMDC's discrimination "on the basis of" Adam's disability, and denied the defendants' motion for summary judgment in its entirety.[118]

Ethical and Legal Issues

1. Since Adam's HIV syndrome has been undetectable for years, discuss why you agree or disagree with the basketball camp's decision to revoke Adam's registration.
2. Do you agree with the court's ruling? Discuss your answer.

AIDS EDUCATION

The ever-increasing likelihood that health care workers will come into contact with persons carrying HIV demands continuing development of and compliance with approved safety procedures. This is especially important for those who come into contact with blood and body fluids of HIV-infected persons. The Centers for Disease Control and Prevention (CDC) expanded its infection control guidelines and has urged hospitals to adopt universal precautions to protect their workers from exposure to patients' blood and other body fluids. Hospitals are following universal precautions in the handling of body fluids, which is the accepted standard for employee protection.

A wide variety of AIDS-related educational materials are available on the market. One of the most important sources of AIDS information is the CDC. The process of staff education in preparing to care for patients with AIDS is extremely important and must include a training program on prevention and transmission in the work setting. Educational requirements specified by the Occupational Safety and Health Administration (OSHA) for health care employees include epidemiology, modes of transmission, preventive practices, and universal precautions. See the following websites for some helpful information: www.aids.gov. and http://www.caps.ucsf.edu/.

CHAPTER REVIEW

1. Ethical dilemmas arises whenever a choice has to be made in which something good has to be given up or something bad has to be suffered no matter what is chosen.
2. Noteworthy historical events (see text at the beginning of the chapter).
3. *Abortion* is the premature termination of a pregnancy, either spontaneous or induced.
   - The morality of abortion is not a legal or constitutional issue; it is a matter of philosophy, ethics, and theology. It is a subject where reasonable people can and do adhere to vastly divergent convictions and principles.
   - *Partial birth abortion* is a late-term abortion that involves partial delivery of the baby prior to its being aborted.
4. *Sterilization* is defined as the termination of the ability to produce offspring.
   - *Therapeutic sterilization* is performed to preserve life or health.

- *Eugenic sterilization* refers to the involuntary sterilization of certain categories of persons described in statutes, without the need for consent by, or on behalf of, those subject to the procedures.
- *Wrongful birth* actions claim that, but for breach of duty by the defendant, a child would not have been born.
- *Wrongful life* suits—those in which a parent or child claims to have suffered harm as a result of being born—are generally unsuccessful.
- *Wrongful conception*/pregnancy actions claim that damages were sustained by the parents of an unexpected child based on the allegation that the child's conception was the result of negligent sterilization procedures or a defective contraceptive device.

5. *Artificial insemination* most often takes the form of the injection of seminal fluid into a woman to induce pregnancy.
   - *Homologous artificial insemination* is when the husband's semen is used in the procedure.
   - *Heterologous artificial insemination* is when the semen is from a donor other than the husband.

6. Surrogacy refers to a method of reproduction whereby a woman agrees to become pregnant for the purpose of gestating and giving birth to a child she will not raise but hand over to a contracted party.

7. Organ donations: Federal regulations require that hospitals have and implement written protocols regarding the organization's organ procurement responsibilities.
   - Organ transplantation is the result of the need for treating patients with end-stage organ disease facing organ failure.
   - Uniform Anatomical Gift Act has many provisions that apply to the wide variety of issues raised in connection with the making, acceptance, and use of anatomical gifts.
     - Act allows a person to make a decision to donate organs at the time of death.
     - Allows potential donors to carry an anatomical donor card.

8. Research, experimentation, and clinical trials.
   - Ethical principles that are relevant to the ethics of research involving human subjects include respect for person, beneficence, and justice. These principles cannot always be applied to resolve ethical problems beyond dispute. The objective in applying ethical principles is to provide an analytical framework that will guide the resolution of ethical problems arising from research involving human subjects.

9. Human genetics describes the study of inheritance as it occurs in human beings.
   - The Genetic Information Nondiscrimination Act (GINA) prohibits discrimination on the basis of genetic information with respect to the availability of health insurance and employment.

10. Stem cell research is being conducted to create tissues and organs that can be matched to patients for transplant.
    - Genetic markers are genes or DNA sequences that have a known location on chromosomes and can be associated with particular genes or traits.

11. *Acquired immune deficiency syndrome* is a fatal disease that destroys the body's ability to fight bacteria and viruses.
    - Concerns involve the spread of AIDS, issues of confidentiality, discrimination, and AIDS education.

TERMINOLOGY

abortion
AIDS
artificial insemination
elective sterilization
ethical dilemma
eugenic sterilization
genetic marker

institutional review board
partial birth abortion
paternalism
reasonable man standard
Roe v. Wade
stem cell research
sterilization

surrogacy
therapeutic sterilization
undue burden
Uniform Anatomical Gift Act
wrongful birth
wrongful conception
wrongful life

REVIEW QUESTIONS

1. Discuss under what circumstances ethical dilemmas arise.

2. Discuss the controversy over the Supreme Court decision in *Roe v. Wade*.

3. What ethical principles surround the abortion issue? Discuss these principles.

4. Do you agree that individual states should be able to impose reasonable restrictions or waiting periods on women seeking abortions? Who should determine what is reasonable?

5. Should a married woman be allowed to abort without her husband's consent?

6. Discuss the arguments for and against partial birth abortions.

7. Why is the medical issue of abortion an example of legislating morality?

8. What is artificial insemination? What questions should be asked when considering artificial insemination?

9. Discuss the importance of organ donations.

10. Describe the ethical considerations that should be addressed before conducting research on human subjects.

11. Why is it important that written consent be obtained from each patient who participates in a clinical trial?

12. What is sterilization, as discussed in this chapter? Do you agree that eugenic sterilization should be allowed? Explain your answer.

13. Describe the distinctions among wrongful birth, wrongful life, and wrongful conception. Discuss the moral dilemmas of these concepts.

14. Describe the controversy over surrogacy.

15. Discuss why there is controversy over genetic markers and stem cell research.

16. What is AIDS, and how is it spread?

17. Discuss the controversy that can occur when considering a patient's right to know whether a caregiver has AIDS and the caregiver's right to privacy and confidentiality.

NOTES

1. *Union Pac. Ry. Co. v. Botsford,* 141 U.S. 250, 251 (1891).
2. http://www.encyclopedia.com/doc/1G2-3406300011.html/
3. http://www.remember.org/educate/medexp.html/
4. http://www.ushmm.org/wlc/en/article.php?ModuleId=10007069.
5. http://www.wma.net/en/30publications/10policies/c8/.
6. "First Successful Kidney Transplant Performed," PBS.org, http://www.pbs.org/wgbh/aso/databank/entries/dm54ki.html.
7. http://www.ncbi.nlm.nih.gov/pmc/articles/PMC1154799/.
8. "Protection and Use of Human Subjects," Eastern Michigan University,
9. "Issues and Concepts," Ascension Health, http://www.ascensionhealth.org/ethics/public/ issues/harvard.asp.
10. https://kennedyinstitute.georgetown.edu/.
11. 464 F.2d 772 (D.C. Cir. 1972).
12. http://www.lawandbioethics.com/demo/Main/LegalResources/C5/Canterbury.htm.
13. http://caselaw.lp.findlaw.com/scripts/getcase.pl?court=us&vol=410&invol=113.
14. http://www.hhs.gov/ohrp/humansubjects/guidance/belmont.html.
15. *Id.*
16. *In re Quinlan,* 70 N.J.10, 355 A.2d 647 (N.J. 1976).
17. United States Code, Title 42—The Public Health and Welfare, Chapter 6A—Public Health Service, Subchapter XVI—President's Commission for the Study of Ethical Problems in Medicine and Biomedical and Behavior Research, Section 300v-1, http://caselaw.lp.findlaw.com/casecode/uscodes/42/chapters/6a/subchapters/xvi/sections/section_300v-1.html.
18. http://assistedsuicide.org/farewell-to-hemlock.html.
19. http://ag.ca.gov/consumers/pdf/ProbateCodeAdvancedHealthCareDirectiveForm-fillable.pdf.
20. http://www.compassionandchoices.org/who-we-are/timeline/.
21. http://www.compassionandchoices.org/who-we-are/about/.
22. 42 U.S.C. 1395cc(a)(1).
23. *Cruzan v. Director of the Mo. Dep't of Health,* 497 U.S. 261 (1990).
24. *Id.*
25. http://www.usconstitution.net/xconst_Am1.html
26. *DeGrella v. Elston,* 858 S.W.2d 698 (1993).
27. http://www.animalresearch.info/en/medical-advances/151/cloning-dolly-the-sheep/.
28. http://jama.jamanetwork.com/article.aspx?articleid=193273.
29. "Biological Sciences," Intute, http://bioresearch.ac.uk/browse/mesh/C0020125L0020125.html.
30. State of Oregon v. Ashcroft, No. 02-35587 (C.A. 9, Ore. 2004).
31. http://unesdoc.unesco.org/images/0013/001359/135928e.pdf.
32. Gonzales v. Oregon, 04-623.
33. Death with Dignity National Center, "Legal and Political Timeline in Oregon,"http://www.deathwithdignity.org/in-oregon.
34. http://donatelifecalifornia.org/livingdonationcalifornia/.

35. English Clergy, Dean of Westminster.
36. *Causeway Medical Suite v. Ieyoub,* 109 F.3d 1096 (1997).
37. 410 U.S. 113 (1973).
38. *Id.* at 164.
39. *Id.*
40. *Id.*
41. *Id.*
42. 410 U.S. 179 (1973).
43. *Id.* at 198.
44. 103 S. Ct. 2481 (1983).
45. *Planned Parenthood v. Casey,* 112 S. Ct. 2792 (1992).
46. 432 U.S. 438 (1977).
47. 432 U.S. 464 (1977).
48. 448 U.S. 297 (1980).
49. *Committee to Defend Reproductive Rights v. Myers,* 625 P.2d 779, 798 (Cal. 1981).
50. 56 P.3d 28 (Ariz. 2002).
51. 111 S. Ct. 1759 (1991).
52. Poe v. Gerstein, 517 F.2d 787 (5th Cir. 1975).
53. 405 F. Supp. 534 (M.D. Pa. 1975).
54. 486 U.S. 1308 (1988).
55. 428 U.S. 52 (1976).
56. 443 U.S. 622 (1979).
57. 533 A.2d 523 (R.I. 1987).
58. 101 S. Ct. 1164 (1981).
59. 515 So. 2d 1254 (Ala. Civ. App. 1987).
60. 107 F. Supp. 1254 (Ala. Civ. App. 1987).
61. 99 S. Ct. 675 (1979).
62. 492 U.S. 490 (1989).
63. 118 S. Ct. 1347 (1998).
64. 437 F.3d. 278 (C.A. N.Y. 2006).
65. 112 S. Ct. 2791 (1992).
66. 844 F. Supp. 1482 (D. Utah 1994).
67. 844 F. Supp. 1482 (D. Utah 1994) at 1494.
68. *American Acad. of Pediatrics v. Lungren,* 940 P.2d 797 (1997).
69. http://www.huffingtonpost.com/joseph-b-kadane/moral-persuasion-on-abortion_b_4004735.html
70. 224 U.S. 200 (1927).
71. 337 F. Supp. 671 (E.D. Ohio 1971).
72. *McKinney v. McKinney,* 805 S.W.2d 66 (Ark. 1991).
73. 165 Cal. Rptr. 477 (Cal. Ct. App. 1980).
74. *Chaffee v. Seslar,* 786 N.E.2d 705 (2003).
75. 730 A.2d 806 (N.J. 1999).
76. *Id.* at 18.
77. *Smith v. Cote,* 513 A.2d 344 (N.H. 1986).
78. *Id.* at 353.
79. 718 P.2d 635 (Kan. 1986).
80. 136 Md. App. 38 (2002).
81. *Cowe v. Forum Group, Inc.,* 575 N.E.2d 630, 631 (Ind. 1991).
82. 707 F.2d 1544 (D.C. Cir. 1983).

83. *Id.* at 1557.
84. 805 P.2d 603 (N.M. 1991).
85. *Id.* at 612.
86. 582 A.2d 1384 (Pa. Super. Ct. 1990).
87. *Id.* at 1385.
88. 11 Pa. D. & C.2d 41, 46 (Lycoming Co. Ct. Com. Pl. 1957).
89. http://www.mbc.ca.gov/About_Us/Media_Room/2011/news_releases_2011.pdf
90. Okla. Stat. Ann. 10, §§ 551–553.
91. *Id.*
92. *Id.*
93. http://www.organdonor.gov/becomingdonor/index.html?utm_source=bing&utm_medium=cpc&utm_camp.aign=2013+Sign+Up
94. U.S. Dept. of Health & Human Services, Task Force on Organ Donation and Transplantation (1986). http://www.pbs.org/wgbh/aso/databank/entries/dm54ki.html
95. 519 N.Y.S.2d 928 (N.Y. Sup. Ct. 1987).
96. http://www.fda.gov/ScienceResearch/SpecialTopics/RunningClinicalTrials/ucm155713.htm#FDARegulations.
97. Mary Ellen Stokes and Bill Stokes, "Relentless Assault on a Research Hospital," Wall Street Journal, March 15, 2004, at A17.
98. 2 C.F.R. § 488.115 (1989).
99. *Id.*
100. *Id.*
101. *Blaz v. Michael Reese Hosp. Found,* 74 F. Supp. 2d 803 (D.C. Ill. 1999).
102. http://www.cc.nih.gov/participate/patientinfo/legal/responsibilities.shtml.
103. Yuanyi S. Chun, *History of Medicine* (Wuhan, China, 1988).
104. National Human Genome Research Institute, http://www.genome.gov.
105. Cantwell, *AIDS: The Mystery and the Solution* (Los Angeles: Aries Rising Press, 1986), at 54.
106. http://www.who.int/gho/hiv/en/index.html.
107. 640 So. 2d 476 (La. App. 3d Cir. 1994).
108. http://www.usatoday.com/story/news/nation/2013/03/28/hiv-oklahoma-dentist/2028865/.
109. 592 A.2d 1251 (N.J. Super. Ct. Law Div. 1991).
110. *Id.* at 1255.
111. 592 A.2d 1251 (N.J. Super. Ct. Law Div. 1991).
112. *Id.* at 1255.
113. 734 S.W.2d 675 (Tex. Ct. App. 1987).
114. 538 N.E.2d 419 (Ohio Ct. App. 1988).
115. Application of Milton S. Hershey Med. Ctr., 639 A.2d 159, 163 (Pa. 1993).
116. 554 A.2d 954 (Pa. Super. Ct. 1989).
117. Ethics Committee of the American Academy of Dermatology, Ethics in Medical Practice, 1992, at 6.
118. *Doe v. Deer Mountain Day Camp, Inc.; Deer Mountain Basketball Academy* 682 F. Supp. 2d 324 (2010).

© makler0008/Shutterstock, Inc.

END-OF-LIFE DILEMMAS

When we finally know we are dying, and all other sentient beings are dying with us, we start to have a burning, almost heartbreaking sense of the fragility and preciousness of each moment and each being, and from this can grow a deep, clear, limitless compassion for all beings.

—SOGYAL RINPOCHE

LEARNING OBJECTIVES

Upon completion of this chapter, the reader will be able to:

- Describe the human struggle to survive.
- Discuss end-of-life issues, including:
  - Euthanasia
  - Right to self-determination
  - Defining death

- Legislative response
- Assisted suicide
- Patient Self-Determination Act of 1990
- Advance directives (e.g., living will, durable power of attorney)
- Futility of treatment
- Withholding and withdrawal of treatment

INTRODUCTION

One of the hardest lessons in life is letting go. Whether it's guilt, anger, love, loss or betrayal. Change is never easy. We fight to hold on and we fight to let go.

— SHERRY JONES

The human struggle to survive and dreams of immortality have been instrumental in pushing humankind to develop means to prevent and cure illness. Advances in medicine and related technologies that have resulted from human creativity and ingenuity have given society the power to prolong life; however, the process of dying also can be prolonged. Those victims of long-term pain and suffering, as well as patients in vegetative states and irreversible comas, are the most directly affected.

The struggle to survive and a family's inability to let go is as real today as when Methuselah, a descendant of Adam, passed away at the age of 969 (Genesis 5:27). Most likely Methuselah's family had a great deal of pain as they observed his passing. At the time of this writing, the family of 13-year-old Jahi McMath's continues their struggle to hold on, as she lapsed into a coma following a tonsillectomy and physicians determined she was brain dead.

NEWS

Brain-Dead Girl Jahi McMath Released from California Hospital

Jahi McMath is no longer inside the hospital where doctors declared her brain-dead after tonsil surgery last month.

• • •

"We're very relieved that she got safely to where she needed to be, because we were all very afraid, given the fragile condition as she wasted away at Children's, that she might not make it," attorney Chris Dolan told reporters Monday.

The move ends one chapter of a weeks-long struggle between the hospital, which sought to remove Jahi from a ventilator after doctors and a judge concluded she was brain-dead, and her relatives, who fought in court to keep her on the ventilator and contended she showed signs of life.

Ed Payne. Catherine E. Shoichet, and Jason Hanna, CNN Health, *January 7, 2014*[1]

Rather than watching hopelessly as a disease destroys a person or as a body part malfunctions, causing death to a patient, physicians now can implant artificial body organs. Exotic machines (e.g., ventilators) and antibiotics are weapons in a physician's arsenal to help extend a patient's life. Such situations have generated vigorous debate. This chapter reviews many of the issues that inevitably arise as one approaches the end of life.

End of Life or Beginning of Life?

My mother is 92 years old, and she is more active and is enjoying life more than when she was much younger. Her advanced age has actually proven to be something of an advantage, as it has given her the time and freedom to do some of the things she couldn't do while she was raising a family. It has been a joy to me, as her son, and to the rest of the family to witness her joy and vigor. Even strangers have found her stamina to be an inspiration as to the value of the end years of life. Three years ago, however, it wasn't so. Mother was critically ill, comatose on a respirator in an intensive care unit. Survival was not considered likely. I am embarrassed to say that I was making arrangements for a funeral. I am even more embarrassed because I am a physician and did not see how she could survive for long except as a vegetable. Then the unlikely occurred. She recovered! Her condition, including both physical and mental status, rapidly and surprisingly improved dramatically and she promptly resumed a life even more active than before. It would have been a tragedy to deprive her of these joyous years of her life after she worked and sacrificed so much for others most of her life. I had thought it would be an act of mercy to disconnect the respirator when her condition had looked so hopeless. I was so wrong. I learned that we must not make life and death decisions casually. Life is a beautiful mystery with many wonderful surprises if we will let them happen.

Advances in medical technology have made it possible to survive to an older age. That longer survival inevitably involves considerable cost and can therefore be a substantial financial burden to the family and the government. Is it worth it? How do we make a judgment about quality of life? What is the financial value of another day, week, or year of life? Should we assume that younger years are better than older years? Although our bodies may physically decline over time, our treasure trove of life experiences accrues over time. Our knowledge and judgment may often be better than when we were younger. Furthermore, the aged may be a source of comfort and joy to their children, grandchildren, and even great-grandchildren. As long as we are alive, we have value.

Physician

EUTHANASIA

There is nothing more sacred than life and there is nothing more natural in life to wish to cling on to it for those you love! And nothing more cruel than to play god by artificially holding onto that which god wants to bring home.

—AUTHOR UNKNOWN

When patients and their families perceive a deterioration of the quality of life with no end in sight, conflict often arises between health care professionals, who are trained to save lives, and patients and their families, who wish to hold on to their loved ones. This conflict centers on the concept of euthanasia and its place in the modern world. There seems to be an absence of controversy only when a patient who is kept alive by modern technology is still able to appreciate and maintain control over his or her life.

Any discussion of euthanasia obliges a person to confront humanity's greatest fear—death. The courts and legislatures have faced it and have made advances in setting forth some guidelines to assist decision makers in this arena; however, much more must be accomplished. Society must be protected from the risks associated with permitting the removal of life-support systems. Society cannot allow the complex issues associated with this topic to be simplified to the point where it is accepted that life can be terminated based on subjective quality-of-life considerations. The legal system must ensure that the constitutional rights of the patient are maintained, while protecting society's interests in preserving life, preventing suicide, and maintaining the integrity of the medical profession. For example, can competent adult patients who ask that no extraordinary lifesaving measures be taken recover damages for finding themselves alive after unwanted resuscitative measures? During a medical emergency, it seems unrealistic to ask a caregiver to first look in a patient's medical record for an advance directive before tending to the immediate needs of the patient. In the final analysis, the boundaries of patient rights often remain uncertain.

From its inception, euthanasia has evolved into an issue with competing legal, medical, and moral implications that continues to generate debate, confusion, and conflict. Currently, there is a strong movement advocating death with dignity, which excludes machines, monitors, and tubes.

Even the connotation of the word "euthanasia" has changed with time depending on who is attempting to define it. Euthanasia originated from the Greek word *euthanatos*, meaning "good death" or "easy death," was accepted in situations where people had what was considered to be incurable diseases. *Euthanasia* is defined broadly as "the mercy killing of the hopelessly ill, injured, or incapacitated."[2]

In the Confucian and Buddhist religions, suicide was an acceptable answer to unendurable pain and incurable disease. The Celtics went a step further, believing that those who chose to die of disease or senility, rather than committing suicide, would be condemned to Hell. Such acceptance began to change during the 1800s when Western physicians refused to lessen suffering by shortening a dying patient's life. Napoleon's physician, for example, rejected Napoleon's plea to kill plague-stricken soldiers, insisting that his obligation was to cure rather than kill people.

In the late 1870s, writings on euthanasia began to appear, mainly in England and the United States. Although such works were written, for the most part, by lay authors, the public and the medical community began to consider the issues raised by euthanasia. Then defined as "the act or practice of painlessly putting to death persons suffering from incurable conditions or diseases," it was considered to be a merciful release from incurable suffering. By the beginning of the 20th century, however, there were still no clear answers or guidelines regarding the use of euthanasia. Unlike in prior centuries when society as a whole supported or rejected euthanasia, different segments of today's society apply distinct connotations to the word, generating further confusion. Some believe euthanasia is meant to allow a painless death when one suffers from an incurable disease yet is not dying. Others, who remain in the majority, perceive euthanasia as an instrument to aid only dying people in ending their lives with as little suffering as possible.

It has been estimated that of the 2 million Americans who die each year, 80% die in hospitals or nursing homes, and 70% of those die after a decision to forgo life-sustaining treatment has been made. Although such decisions are personal in nature and based on individual moral values, they must comply with the laws applicable to the prolonging of the dying process. Courts have outlined the ways in which the government is allowed to participate in the decision-making process. Yet the misconceptions and lack of clear direction regarding the policies and procedures have resulted in wide disparity among jurisdictions, both in legislation and in judicial decisions. As a result, the American Medical Association, the American Bar Association, legislators, and judges are actively attempting to formulate and legislate clear guidelines in this sensitive, profound, and not yet fully understood area. To ensure compliance with the law while serving the needs of their patients, it is incumbent on health care providers to keep themselves informed of regulatory requirements in this ever-changing field.

ACTIVE OR PASSIVE EUTHANASIA

Active euthanasia is commonly understood to be the intentional commission of an act, such as providing a patient a lethal dose of a medication that results in death. The act, if committed by the patient, is thought of as suicide. Moreover, because in most states the patient cannot take his or her own life, any person who assists in the causing of the death could be subject to criminal sanction for aiding and abetting suicide.

Passive euthanasia occurs when lifesaving treatment (such as a respirator) is withdrawn or withheld, allowing the terminally ill patient to die a natural death. Passive euthanasia is generally accepted pursuant to legislative acts and judicial decisions. These decisions, however, generally are based on the facts of a particular case.

The distinctions are important when considering the duty and liability of a physician who must decide whether to continue or initiate treatment of a comatose or terminally ill patient. Physicians are obligated to use reasonable care to preserve health and to save lives, and, thus, unless fully protected by the law, they will be reluctant, for example, to abide by a patient's or family's wishes to terminate life-support devices.

Although there may be a duty to provide life-sustaining equipment in the immediate aftermath of cardiopulmonary arrest, there is no duty to continue its use after it has become futile and ineffective to do so in the opinion of qualified medical personnel. An example is a patient who suffered severe brain damage, placing him in a comatose and vegetative state, from which, according to tests and examinations by other specialists, he was unlikely to recover. The patient, on the written request of his family, was taken off life-support equipment. The patient's family (his wife and eight children) made the decision together after consultation with the physicians. Evidence had been presented that the patient, before his incapacitation, had expressed to his wife that he would not want to be kept alive by a machine. Decisions by family members are based on love and concern for the dignity of their loved one [*Barber v. Superior Court*, 147 Cal. App. 3d 1006 (Cal. Ct. App. 1983)].

The controversy over euthanasia is a common issue throughout the world. Belgium, for example, legalized the practice of euthanasia for adults in 2002 and is at this writing considering legalizing euthanasia for children.

Belgium Considering New Euthanasia Law for Kids

Should children have the right to ask for their own deaths?

In Belgium, where euthanasia is now legal for people over the age of 18, the government is considering extending it to children—something that no other country has done. The same bill would offer the right to die to adults with early dementia.

Advocates argue that euthanasia for children, with the consent of their parents, is necessary to give families an option in a desperately painful situation. But opponents have questioned whether children can reasonably decide to end their own lives.

Maria Cheng, News Daily, *October 31, 2013*[3]

VOLUNTARY OR INVOLUNTARY EUTHANASIA

Both active and passive euthanasia may be either voluntary or involuntary. *Voluntary euthanasia* occurs when a person suffering an incurable illness makes the decision to die. To be considered voluntary, the request or consent must be made by a legally competent adult and be based on material information concerning the possible ramifications and alternatives available.

Involuntary euthanasia, however, occurs when the decision to terminate the life of an incurable person (e.g., an incompetent or nonconsenting competent person) is made by someone other than that incurable person.

A patient's lack of consent can be due to mental impairment or a comatose state. Important value questions face courts struggling with the boundaries for making voluntary euthanasia decisions:

- Who should decide to withhold or withdraw treatment?
- On what factors should the decision be based?
- Are there viable standards to guide the courts?
- Should criminal sanctions be imposed on a person assisting in ending a life?
- When does death occur?

RIGHT TO SELF-DETERMINATION

To analyze the important questions regarding whether life-support treatment can be withheld or withdrawn from an incompetent patient, it is necessary to consider first what rights a competent patient possesses. Both statutory law and case law have presented a diversity of policies and points of view. Some courts point to common law and the early case of *Schloendorff v. Society of New York Hospital*[4] to support their belief in a patient's right to self-determination. The *Schloendorff* court stated:[5]

> Every human being of adult years has a right to determine what shall be done with his own body; and the surgeon who performs an operation without his patient's consent commits an assault for which he is liable for damages.

This right of self-determination was emphasized in *In re Storar*[6] when the court announced that every human being of adult years and sound mind has the right to determine what shall be done with his or her own body. The *Storar* case was a departure from the New Jersey Supreme Court's rationale in the case of *In re Quinlan*.[7] The *Quinlan* case was the first to address significantly the issue of whether euthanasia should be permitted when a patient is terminally ill. The *Quinlan* court, relying on *Roe v. Wade*,[8] announced that the constitutional right to privacy protects a patient's right to self-determination. The court noted that the right to privacy "is broad enough to encompass a patient's decision to decline medical treatment under certain circumstances, in much the same way as it is broad enough to encompass a woman's decision to terminate pregnancy under certain conditions."[9]

The *Quinlan* court, in reaching its decision, applied a test balancing the state's interest in preserving and maintaining the sanctity of human life against Karen Quinlan's privacy interest. It decided that, especially in light of the prognosis (physicians determined that Quinlan was in an irreversible coma), the state's interest did not justify interference with her right to refuse treatment. Thus, Karen Quinlan's father was appointed her legal guardian, and the respirator was shut off.

In the same year as the *Quinlan* decision, the case of *Superintendent of Belchertown State School v. Saikewicz*[10] was decided. There, the court, using the balancing test enunciated in *Quinlan*, approved the recommendation of a court-appointed guardian ad litem that it would be in Saikewicz's best interests to end chemotherapy treatment. Saikewicz was a mentally retarded, 67-year-old patient suffering from leukemia. The court found from the evidence that the prognosis was dim, and even though a "normal person" would probably have chosen chemotherapy, it allowed Saikewicz to die without treatment to spare him the suffering.

Although the court also followed the reasoning of the *Quinlan* opinion in giving the right to an incompetent person to refuse treatment, based on either the objective "best interests" test or the subjective "substituted judgment" test, which it favored because Saikewicz always had been incompetent, the court departed from *Quinlan* in a major way. It rejected the *Quinlan* approach of entrusting a decision concerning the continuance of artificial life support to the patient's guardian, family, attending physicians, and a hospital ethics committee. The *Saikewicz* court asserted that even though a judge might find the opinions of physicians, medical experts, or hospital ethics committees helpful in reaching a decision, there should be no requirement to seek out the advice. The court decided that questions of life and death with regard to an incompetent person should be the responsibility of the courts, which would conduct detached but passionate investigations. The court took a "dim view of any attempt to shift the ultimate decision-making responsibility away from duly established courts of proper jurisdiction to any committee, panel, or group, ad hoc or permanent."[11]

This main point of difference between the *Saikewicz* and *Quinlan* cases marked the emergence of two different policies on the incompetent person's right to refuse treatment. One line of cases has followed *Saikewicz* and supports court approval before physicians are allowed to withhold or withdraw life support. Advocates of this view argue that it makes more sense to leave the decision to an objective tribunal than to extend the right of a patient's privacy to a number of interested parties, as was done in *Quinlan*. They also attack the *Quinlan* method as being a privacy decision effectuated by popular vote.[12]

Six months after *Saikewicz*, the Massachusetts Appeals Court narrowed the need for court intervention in *In re Dinnerstein*[13] by finding that "no code" orders are valid to prevent the use of artificial resuscitative measures on incompetent terminally ill patients. The court was faced with the case of a 67-year-old woman who was suffering from Alzheimer's disease. It was determined that she was permanently comatose at the time of trial. Furthermore, the court decided that *Saikewicz*-type judicial proceedings should take place only when medical treatment could offer a reasonable expectation of effecting a permanent or temporary cure of or relief from the illness.

The Massachusetts Supreme Judicial Court attempted to clarify its *Saikewicz* opinion with regard to court orders in *In re Spring*.[14] The court here held that different factors such as the patient's mental status and his or her medical prognosis with or without treatment must be considered before judicial approval is necessary to withdraw or withhold treatment from an incompetent patient. The problem in all three cases is that there is still no clear guidance as to exactly when the court's approval of the removal of life-support systems would be necessary. *Saikewicz* seemed to demand judicial approval in every case. *Spring*, however, in partially retreating from that view, stated that it did not have to articulate what combination of the factors it discussed, thus making prior court approval necessary.

The inconsistencies presented by the Massachusetts cases led courts since 1977 to follow the parameters set by *Quinlan*, requiring judicial intervention. In cases in which physicians have certified the irreversible nature of a patient's loss of consciousness, an ethics committee (actually a neurologic team) could certify the patient's hopeless neurologic condition. Then a guardian would be free to take the legal steps necessary to remove life-support systems. The main reason for the appointment of a guardian is to ensure that incompetent patients, like all other patients, maintain their right to refuse treatment. Most holdings indicate that because a patient has the constitutional right of self-determination, those acting on the patient's behalf can exercise that right when rendering their best judgment concerning how the patient would assert the right. This substituted judgment doctrine could be argued on standing grounds, whereby a second party has the right to assert the constitutional rights of another when that second party's intervention is necessary to protect the other's constitutional rights. The guardian's decision is sounder if it is based on the known desires of a patient who was competent immediately before becoming comatose.

An advance directive, such as a living will, is persuasive evidence of an incompetent person's wishes. An incompetent patient can act as a guardian and in accordance with the terms of a living will. An agent can substitute his or her judgment for that of the patient.

A court may require the attending physician to certify that a patient is in a permanent vegetative state, with no reasonable chance for recovery, before a family member or guardian can request termination of extraordinary means of medical treatment.

The decision maker would attempt to ascertain the incompetent patient's actual interests and preferences. A court can appoint a guardian if:[15]

- family members disagree as to the incompetent person's wishes.
- physicians disagree on the prognosis.
- the patient's wishes cannot be known because he or she has always been incompetent.
- evidence exists of wrongful motives or malpractice.
- no family member can serve as a guardian.

When is a patient considered to be legally dead, and what type of treatment can be withheld or withdrawn? Most cases dealing with euthanasia speak of the necessity for a physician to diagnose a patient as being either in a persistent vegetative state or terminally ill.

Traditionally, the definition of death adopted by the courts has been according to *Black's Law Dictionary*: "cessation of respiration, heartbeat, and certain indications of central nervous system activity, such as respiration and pulsation."[16] Currently, however, modern science has the capacity to sustain vegetative functions of those in irreversible comas. Machinery can sustain heartbeat and respiration even in the face of brain death. It is now generally accepted that the irreversible cessation of brain function constitutes death.

Ethicists who advocate the prohibition on taking action to shorten life agree "where death is imminent and inevitable, it is permissible to forgo treatments that would only provide a precarious and painful prolongation of life, as long as the normal care due to the sick person in similar cases is not interrupted."[17]

Relying on the 1968 Harvard Criteria set forth by the Ad Hoc Committee of the Harvard Medical School to Examine the Definition of Brain Death, the American Medical Association in 1974 accepted that death occurs when there is "irreversible cessation of all brain functions including the brain stem."[18] Most states now recognize brain death by statute or judicial decision. New York, for example, in *People v. Eulo*,[19] in rejecting the traditional cardiopulmonary definition of death, announced that the determination of brain death can be made according to acceptable medical standards. The court also repeated its holding in *In re Storar*[20] that clear and convincing evidence of a person's desire to decline extraordinary medical care may be honored and that a third person may not exercise this judgment on behalf of a person who has not expressed or cannot express the desire to decline treatment.

Some courts hold that artificial nutrition can be withheld from a patient who is unable to converse or feed ones-self. Unequivocal proof of a patient's wishes will suffice when the decision to terminate life support is at issue. Factors for determining the existence of clear and convincing evidence of a patient's intention to reject the prolongation of life by artificial means include the:

1. persistence of statements regarding an individual's beliefs.
2. desirability of the commitment to those beliefs.
3. seriousness with which such statements were made.
4. inferences that may be drawn from the surrounding circumstances.

The family of a patient who is in a persistent vegetative state cannot necessarily order physicians to remove artificial nutrition. In 1983, Nancy Cruzan sustained injuries in a car accident in which her car overturned, after which she was found face down in a ditch without respiratory or cardiac function. Although the patient was unconscious, her breathing and heartbeat were restored at the site of the accident. After examining her at the hospital, a neurosurgeon diagnosed her as having suffered cerebral contusions and anoxia. It was estimated that she had been deprived of oxygen for 12 to 14 minutes. After remaining in a coma for 3 weeks, Cruzan went into an unconscious state. At first she was able to ingest some food orally. Thereafter, surgeons implanted a gastrostomy feeding and hydration tube, with the consent of her husband, to facilitate feeding her. She did not improve, and until December 1990, she lay in a Missouri state hospital in a persistent vegetative state that was determined to be irreversible, permanent, progressive, and ongoing. She was not dead, according to the accepted definition of death in Missouri, and physicians estimated that she could live in the vegetative state for an additional 30 years. Because of the prognosis, Cruzan's parents asked the hospital staff to cease all artificial nutrition and hydration procedures. The staff refused to comply with their wishes without court approval. The state trial court granted authorization for termination, finding that Cruzan had a fundamental right—grounded in both the state and federal constitutions—to refuse or direct the withdrawal of death-prolonging procedures. Testimony at trial from a former roommate of Cruzan indicated to the court that she had stated that if she were ever sick or injured she would not want to live unless she could live halfway normally. The court interpreted that conversation, which had taken place when Cruzan was 25 years old, as meaning that she would not want to be forced to take nutrition and hydration while in a persistent vegetative state.

The case was appealed to the Missouri Supreme Court, which reversed the lower court decision. The court not only doubted that the doctrine of informed consent applied to the circumstances of the case, it moreover would not recognize a broad privacy right from the state constitution that would support the right of a person to refuse medical treatment in every circumstance. Because Missouri recognizes living wills, the court held that Cruzan's parents were not entitled to order the termination of her treatment because "no person can assume that choice for an incompetent person in the absence of the formalities required under Missouri's Living Will statutes or the clear and convincing, inherently reliable evidence absent here."[21] The court found that Cruzan's statements to her roommate did not rise to the level of clear and convincing evidence of her desire to end nutrition and hydration.

In June 1990, the U.S. Supreme Court after hearing oral arguments held that:[22]

1. the U.S. Constitution does not forbid Missouri from requiring that there be clear and convincing evidence of an incompetent person's wishes as to the withdrawal of life-sustaining treatment.
2. the Missouri Supreme Court did not commit constitutional error in concluding that evidence adduced at trial did not amount to clear and convincing evidence of Cruzan's desire to cease hydration and nutrition.
3. due process did not require the state to accept the substituted judgment of close family members, absent substantial proof that their views reflected those of the patient.

In delivering the opinion of the court, Justice William Rehnquist noted that although most state courts have applied the common-law right to informed consent or a combination of that right and a privacy right when allowing a right to refuse treatment, the Supreme Court analyzed the issues presented in the *Cruzan* case in terms of a Fourteenth Amendment liberty interest. They found that a competent person has a constitutionally protected right grounded in the due process clause to refuse lifesaving hydration and nutrition. Missouri provided for the incompetent patient by allowing a surrogate to act for the patient in choosing to withdraw hydration and treatment. Moreover, it put into place procedures to ensure that the surrogate's action conforms to the wishes expressed by the patient when he or she was competent. Although recognizing that Missouri had enacted a restrictive law, the Supreme Court held that right-to-die issues should be decided pursuant to state law, subject to a due process liberty interest, and in keeping with state constitutional law. After the Supreme Court rendered its decision, the Cruzans returned to Missouri probate court, where on November 14, 1990,

Judge Charles Teel authorized physicians to remove the feeding tubes from Cruzan. The judge determined that testimony presented to him early in November demonstrated clear and convincing evidence that Nancy would not have wanted to live in a persistent vegetative state. Several of her coworkers had testified that she told them before her accident that she would not want to live "like a vegetable." On December 26, 1990, 2 weeks after her feeding tubes were removed, Nancy Cruzan died.

LEGISLATIVE RESPONSE

After the Cruzan decision, states began to draft new legislation in the areas of living wills, durable powers of attorney, health care proxies, and surrogate decision making. Pennsylvania and Florida were two of the first states to react to the *Cruzan* decision. Pennsylvania law is applied to terminally ill or permanently unconscious patients. The statute, the Advance Directive for Health Care Act,[23] deals mainly with individuals who have prepared living wills. It includes in its definition of life-sustaining treatment the administration of hydration and nutrition by any means if it is stated in the individual's living will. The statute mandates that a copy of the living will must be provided to the patient's physician in order to be effective. Furthermore, the patient must be incompetent or permanently unconscious. If there is no evidence of the presence of a living will, the Pennsylvania probate codes allow an attorney-in-fact who is designated in a properly executed durable-power-of-attorney document to give permission for "medical and surgical procedures to be utilized on an incompetent patient."[24] States subsequently have been addressing the problem of surrogate decision making for those who are incompetent. Evidence of an incompetent person's wishes that had been expressed when he or she was competent is required by the courts.

Unless there is some national uniformity in the legislation, some patients and their families will shop for states that will allow them to have medical treatment terminated or withdrawn with fewer legal hassles. For example, on January 18, 1991, a Missouri probate court judge authorized a father to take his 20-year-old brain-damaged daughter, Christine Busalacchi, from the Missouri Rehabilitation Center to Minnesota for testing by a proeuthanasia physician, Dr. Ronald Cranford. Cranford, who practiced at the Hennepin County Medical Center, had been at the center of controversy in Minnesota. In January 1991, Pro Life Action Ministries demanded Cranford's resignation, claiming that he "desires to make Minnesota the killing fields for the disabled."[25] He, however, viewed himself as an advocate of patients' rights. It is clear that the main reason Busalacchi sought authorization to take his daughter to Minnesota is that he believed he would have to deal with fewer legal impediments there to allow his daughter to die.

Because of continuing litigation involving the right to die, it is clear that the public must be educated as to the importance of expressing their wishes concerning medical treatment while they are competent. Uniformity with regard to the legal instruments available for demonstrating what a patient wants should be a common goal of legislators, courts, and the medical profession. If living wills, surrogates, and durable powers of attorney were to be enacted pursuant to national rather than individual state guidelines, the process of resolving end-of-life issues might be less complicated. Some states have addressed the problem by statutorily providing for these instruments, thereby enabling individuals to have a say in the medical care they would like to receive should they become unable to speak for themselves.

Chief Justice Fred Dore of the Washington Supreme Court voiced his opinion that a legislative response to right-to-die issues could be better addressed by the legislature.

The United States Supreme Court, in *Cruzan*, questioned whether a federally protected right to forgo nutrition and hydration existed. The *Cruzan* Court confronted the same philosophical issues that we face today and wisely recognized and deferred to the Legislature's superior policy-making abilities. As was the case in *Cruzan*, our legislature is far better equipped to evaluate this complex issue and should not have its power usurped by this court.[26]

ASSISTED SUICIDE

Assisted suicide presents profound questions of ethics, religious beliefs, and public policy issues. These are precisely the kinds of issues in which public input is vital, and courts are simply not equipped to conduct the type of comprehensive review required. The legislative and executive branches of government are uniquely well equipped to pursue these issues. Courts have before them only the legal arguments and although questions of law are certainly part of the equation, the core issues presented are fundamentally grounded in questions of policy and how we view ourselves as a society. Those who must answer to the people for their policy product and not those who have no accountability to the people are best suited to answer these questions.[27]

Physician-Assisted Suicide

Physician-assisted suicide is an action in which a physician voluntarily aids a patient in bringing about his or her death. Dr. Jack Kevorkian of Michigan announced in October 1989 that he had developed a device that would end one's life quickly, painlessly, and humanely. He chose to assist a 54-year-old Alzheimer's disease patient in committing suicide on June 4, 1990. In December 1990, he was charged with first-degree murder, but the charge was later dismissed because Michigan had no law against assisted suicide. He was however ordered not to assist in a patient's suicide or to give advice about it. On February 6, 1991, he violated the court order by giving advice about the preparation of a drug to a terminally ill cancer patient.[28] Additional murder charges were lodged against Kevorkian in October 1991, when he instructed two Michigan women how to use of his "suicide machine." In dismissing the charges against him, the circuit court judge stated, "Some people with intractable pain cannot benefit from treatment." Although emphasizing that Michigan has no law against assisting suicide, the judge also expressed his belief that physician-assisted suicide remains an alternative for patients experiencing "unmanageable pain."[29]

The Michigan House on November 22, 1992 approved legislation placing a temporary ban on assisted suicide. The Senate approved the temporary ban after Kevorkian helped a sixth terminally ill patient kill herself. On December 15, 1992, Michigan Governor John Engler signed the law just hours after two more women committed suicide with Kevorkian's aid.

The new law, which became effective on April 1, 1993, made assisting suicide a felony punishable by up to 4 years in prison and a $2,000 fine. Under the new law, assisted suicide was banned for 15 months. During this time, a special commission studied assisted suicide and submitted its recommendations to the Michigan legislature for review and action. The new law apparently raised constitutional questions and was challenged by the Civil Liberties Union of Michigan because of the claim that it failed to recognize that the terminally ill have the right to end their lives painlessly and with dignity.

Kevorkian faced prosecution for murdering two people and for assisting in the suicides of three others. As a result, he appealed a Michigan Supreme Court ruling that found there is no right to assisted suicide.[30] The U.S. Supreme Court rejected his argument that assisted suicide is a constitutional right. The high court's decision allowed the State of Michigan to move forward and prosecute Kevorkian on the pending charges. At the time of the high court's ruling, Kevorkian had attended his 22nd suicide, involving a retired clergyman, less than a month after he was left facing murder charges in Michigan.[31] As of March 1998, Kevorkian had aided in or witnessed 100 suicides. Kevorkian was eventually convicted of second-degree murder for physician suicide and sentenced 10 to 25 years in prison. He was released on June 1, 2007, after serving 8 years in prison.

At the time of this writing, Oregon, Washington, and Vermont have legalized physician-assisted suicide. Vermont became the third state to legalize physician-assisted suicide, when Governor Peter Shumlin signed into law a bill allowing physicians to legally prescribe lethal doses of medication for terminally ill patients.[32]

The Montana Supreme Court ruled that state law protects physicians from prosecution for assisting terminally ill patients in committing suicide. The court, however, did not address whether assisted suicide was guaranteed under the state's constitution.[33] Montana Bill "HB 505 which would have explicitly prohibited doctor-prescribed suicide was introduced by Rep. Krayton Kerns. The bill passed in the House and was sent to the Senate, where it failed on April 15, 2013 in a 27–23 vote."[34]

In 1967, the United States Supreme Court, in two unanimous and separate decisions, ruled that state laws prohibiting assisted suicide are constitutional; nevertheless, the U.S. Supreme Court ruled that states can allow physicians to assist in the suicide of terminally ill patients.[35]

The physician-assisted suicide debate, as noted in the following news clippings, continues throughout the nation.

California Gov. Signs Assisted Suicide Information Bill into Law

California Gov. Arnold Schwarzenegger has signed into law a bill that opponents say could open the door to the eventuality of physician-assisted suicide in the nation's most populous state.

AB 2747 mandates that physicians, nurse practitioners and physician assistants provide patients diagnosed with a terminal illness—or who have been given a diagnosis of one year or less to live—with "comprehensive information and counseling regarding legal end-of-life options, as specified."

Matt Hadro, CNSNews.com, *October 3, 2008*[36]

Mass. Doctor-Assisted Suicide Measure Fails

BOSTON (AP)—A Massachusetts ballot question that would have legalized physician-assisted suicide for the terminally ill has been defeated by a narrow margin.

The measure voted on Tuesday was defeated 51 percent to 49 percent with 96 percent of precincts counted, and was the closest of the three questions on the Massachusetts ballot.

"We believe the voters came to see this as a flawed approach to end of life care, lacking in the most basic safeguards," Rosanne Bacon Meade, chairwoman of the Committee Against Assisted Suicide, said in a statement.

Associated Press, Boston.com, *November 7, 2012*[37]

ASSISTED SUICIDE VERSUS REFUSAL OR WITHDRAWAL OF TREATMENT

The Supreme Court in *Quill v. Vacco*[38] found that neither the assisted suicide ban nor the law permitting patients to refuse medical treatment treats anyone differently from anyone else or draws any distinctions between persons. There is a distinction between letting a patient die and making one die. Most legislatures have allowed the former but have prohibited the latter. The Supreme Court disagreed with the respondents' claim that the distinction is arbitrary and irrational.

In its decision, the Supreme Court determined that New York had valid reasons for distinguishing between the refusal of treatment and assisting suicide. Those reasons included prohibiting intentional killing and preserving life, preventing suicide, maintaining the physician's role as his or her patient's healer, and protecting vulnerable people from indifference, prejudice, and psychological and financial pressure to end their lives. All of those reasons, the court decided, constitute valid and important public interests fulfilling the constitutional requirement that a legislative classification bear a rational relation to a legitimate end.

In the Washington case, *Washington v. Glucksberg*,[39] the U.S. Supreme Court held that assisted suicide is not a liberty protected by the Constitution's due process clause. A majority of states now ban assisted suicide. These rulings, however, do not affect the right of patients to refuse treatment. It is clear that this emotionally charged issue is not settled. Legislative, judicial, and public debates continue to rage. Ultimately, the quality of a patient's life must be improved so that physician-assisted suicide does not become the answer for those who are suffering. Society must learn to address more effectively end-of-life issues including pain management, fear of death, self-worth, and hopelessness. Thus far, progress is slow and inadequate.

OREGON'S DEATH WITH DIGNITY ACT (1994)

On October 27, 1997, physician-assisted suicide became a legal medical option for the terminally ill residents of Oregon. The *Oregon Death with Dignity Act* allows a terminally ill

Oregon resident to obtain a lethal dose of medication from his or her physician. The act legalizes physician-assisted suicide but specifically prohibits euthanasia, where a physician or other person directly administers a medication to end another's life. The following are excerpts from the Oregon Death with Dignity Act:

Or. Rev. Stat. Sects. 127.800-.897 Section 1.01. Definitions...

(12) "Terminal disease" means an incurable and irreversible disease that has been medically confirmed and will, within reasonable medical judgment, produce death within (6) months...

Section 2.01. Who may initiate a written request for medication?

An adult who is capable, is a resident of Oregon, and has been determined by the attending physician and consulting physician to be suffering from a terminal disease, and who has voluntarily expressed his or her wish to die, may make a written request for medication for the purpose of ending his or her life in a humane and dignified manner.

Section 2.02. Form of the Written Request.

(1) A valid request for medication . . . shall be in substantially the form described in ORS 127.897, signed and dated by the patient and witnessed by at least two individuals who, in the presence of the patient, attest that to the best of their knowledge and belief the patient is capable, acting voluntarily, and is not being coerced to sign the request . . .

Section 3.01. Attending physician responsibilities. The attending physician shall: and has made the request voluntarily.

(2) Inform the patient of:

(a) His or her medical diagnosis;

(b) His or her prognosis;

(c) The potential risks associated with taking the medication to be prescribed;

(d) The probable result of taking the medication to be prescribed; and

(e) The feasible alternatives, including, but not limited to, comfort care, hospice care, and pain control.

(3) Refer the patient to a consulting physician for medical confirmation of the diagnosis, and for a determination that the patient is capable and acting voluntarily...

Section 3.06. Written and oral requests.

In order to receive a prescription for medication to end his or her life in a humane and dignified manner, a qualified patient shall have made an oral request and a written request, and reiterate the oral request to his or her attending physician no less than (15) days after making the initial oral request. At the time the qualified patient makes his or her second oral request, the attending physician shall offer the patient an opportunity to rescind the request.

Section 3.07. Right to rescind request. A patient may rescind his or her request at any time and in any manner without regard to his or her mental state. . . .

Section 3.08. Waiting periods.

No less than (15) days shall elapse between the patient's initial oral request and the writing of a prescription. . . . No less than 48 hours shall elapse between the patient's written request and the writing of a prescription. . . .

Section 6.01. Form of the request.

A request for a medication . . . shall be in substantially the following form. [**Figure 1.**]

Request for Medication to End My Life in a Humane and Dignified Manner

I, _____, am an adult of sound mind.

I am suffering from _____, which my attending physician has determined is a terminal disease and which has been medically confirmed by a consulting physician.

I have been fully informed of my diagnosis, prognosis, the nature of medication to be prescribed and potential associated risks, the expected result, and the feasible alternatives, including comfort care, hospice care, and pain control.

I request that my attending physician prescribe medication that will end my life in a humane and dignified manner.

Initial One:

_____ I have informed my family of my decision and taken their opinions into consideration.

_____ I have decided not to inform my family of my decision.

_____ I have no family to inform of my decision.

I understand that I have the right to rescind this request at any time.

I understand the full import of this request and I expect to die when I take the medication to be prescribed.

I make this request voluntarily and without reservation, and I accept full moral responsibility for my actions.
Signed: _____
Dated: _____

Declaration of Witnesses
We declare that the person signing this request:

(a) Is personally known to us or has provided proof of identity;

(b) Signed the request in our presence;

(c) Appears to be of sound mind and not under duress, fraud or undue influence;

(d) Is not a patient for whom either of us is attending physician.

FIGURE   1   Oregon Request Form to End Life

The *Patient Self-Determination Act of 1990*[40] provides that patients have a right to formulate advance directives and to make decisions regarding their health care. Self-determination includes the right to accept or refuse medical treatment. Health care providers (including hospitals, nursing homes, home health agencies, health maintenance organizations, and hospices) receiving federal funds under Medicare are required to comply with the new regulations. Providers are required to:[41]

1. Provide individuals written information concerning their rights under state law (whether statutory or recognized by courts of the state) to make decisions including the right to accept or refuse medical or surgical treatment and the right to formulate advance directives.
2. Document in the individual's medical record whether the individual has executed an advance directive.
3. Not condition the provision of care or otherwise discriminate against an individual based on whether the individual has executed an advance directive.
4. Ensure compliance with requirements of state law (whether statutory or recognized by the courts of the state) regarding advance directives. The provider must inform individuals that complaints concerning the advance directive requirements may be filed with the state survey and certification agency.
5. Provide education for staff concerning its policies and procedures on advance directives.
6. Provide for community education regarding issues concerning advance directives by defining what constitutes an advance directive, emphasizing that an advance directive is designed to enhance an incapacitated individual's control over medical treatment and describe applicable state law concerning advance directives. A provider must be able to document its community education efforts.

Providers are not entitled to reimbursement under the Medicare program if they fail to meet Patient Self-Determination Act of 1990 requirements.

ADVANCE DIRECTIVES

Patients have a right to make decisions about their health care with their physician. They may agree to a proposed treatment, choose among alternative treatments, or refuse a treatment. Patients have this right even if they become incapacitated and are unable to make decisions regarding their health care. Because of the advances in modern medical technology, everyone should give serious consideration as to their health care wishes, to decide what they would want done should they become incapacitated, to execute advance directives and make their wishes known so that family and health care providers can respect their decision.

Advance directives, in the form of a "living will" or "durable power of attorney," allow the patient to state in advance the kinds of medical care that he or she considers acceptable or not acceptable. The patient can appoint an agent, a *surrogate decision maker*, to make those decisions on his or her behalf. A patient should be asked at the time of admission if he or she has an advance directive. If a patient does not have an advance directive, the health care facility should provide the patient with information about an advance directive and the opportunity to execute a directive. A patient should clearly understand that an advance directive is a guideline for caregivers describing his or her wishes for medical care—what he or she would and would not want—in the event of incapacitation and inability to make decisions. This interaction should be documented in the patient's medical record. If the patient has an advance directive, a copy should be requested for insertion into the patient's record. If the patient does not have a copy of the advance directive with him or her, the substance thereof should be documented and flagged in the patient's medical record. Documentation should include the location of the advance directive, the name and telephone number of the designated health care agent, and any information that might be helpful in the immediate care situation (e.g., patient's desire for food and hydration). The purpose of such documentation should not be considered to be a need to recreate a new directive, but should be considered a desire to adhere to a patient's wishes in the event some untoward event occurs while waiting for a copy of the directive.

The patient can execute a new directive at any time if desired. Patient and family education should be provided regarding the existence of the directive and its contents. The patient should be periodically queried about whether he or she wishes to make any changes with regard to an advance directive.

Living Will

A *living will* is the instrument or legal document that describes those treatments an individual wishes or does not wish to receive should he or she become incapacitated and unable to communicate treatment decisions. Typically, a living will allows a person, when competent, to inform caregivers in writing of his or her wishes with regard to withholding and withdrawing life-supporting treatment, including nutrition and hydration. The living will is helpful to health care professionals because it provides guidance about a patient's wishes for treatment, provides legally valid instructions about treatment, and protects the patient's rights and the provider who honors them.

The Supreme Court of Kentucky's Living Will Directive Act was determined to be constitutional in *T. Bruce Simpson, Jr., v. Commonwealth of Kentucky and Cabinet for Human Resources*, 142 S.W.3d 24 (Ky. 2004). The act allows a judicially appointed guardian or other designated surrogate to remove a ward's life support. After suffering cardiac arrest, it was agreed that the patient, Woods, would never regain consciousness. After a recommendation of the hospital's ethics committee, Wood's guardian asked for the removal of Woods's life support. If there was no legal guardian but the physicians, family, and ethics committee all agree with the surrogate's decision—in this case, the state's—there is no need for judicial approval. The Supreme Court did determine that when there is disagreement in a particular case, withdrawal of life support would be prohibited absent clear and convincing evidence that the patient is permanently unconscious or in a persistent vegetative state and that withdrawal of life support was in the patient's best interest. In support of its holding, the Supreme Court cited the ethical standards of the National Center for State Courts, the Council on Ethical and Judicial Affairs of the American Medical Association, an Address to an International Congress of Anesthesiologists by Pope Pius XII, and the Declaration on Euthanasia by Pope John Paul II:[42]

In determining the patient's best interests, courts may consider, but are not limited to considering: (1) the patient's present level of physical, sensory, emotional, and cognitive functioning and possibility of improvement thereof; (2) any relevant statements or expressions made by the patient, when competent, as to his or her own wishes with a rebuttable presumption attaching to a valid living will or a designation of a health care surrogate; (3) to the extent known, the *patient's own philosophical, religious, and moral views, life goals, values about the purpose of life and the way it should be lived, and attitudes toward sickness, medical procedures, suffering, and death;* (4) the degree of physical pain caused by the patient's condition, treatment, and termination of treatment; (5) the degree of humiliation, dependence, and loss of dignity probably resulting from the condition or treatment; (6) the life expectancy and prognosis for recovery with and without the treatment; (7) the various treatment options and their risks, benefits, and side effects; (8) whether any particular treatment would be proportionate or disproportionate in terms of the benefits gained; and (9) the impact on the patient's family (the assumption being that the patient would be concerned about the well-being and happiness of his or her own family members).

The living will should be signed and dated by two witnesses who are not blood relatives or beneficiaries of property. A living will should be discussed with the patient's physician, and a signed copy should be placed in the patient's medical record. A copy also should be given to the individual designated to make decisions in the event the patient is unable to do so. A person who executes a living will when healthy and mentally competent cannot predict how he or she will feel at the time of a terminal illness; therefore, it should be updated regularly so that it accurately reflects a patient's wishes. The written instructions become effective when a patient is either in a terminal condition, permanently unconscious, or suffering irreversible brain damage. An example of a living will is illustrated in **Figure   2**.

Right to Die Without a Living Will

In *San Juan-Torregosa v. Garcia*,[43] the evidence at trial established that Garcia suffered a cardiac arrest. Although she was later resuscitated, she suffered oxygen deprivation to her brain for more than 10 minutes and was in a chronic vegetative state. Medical opinion established that she was breathing reflexively, but there was no evidence that she would be able to recover "cortical functions." Garcia also had metastatic breast cancer. Her treating physician, Dr. Parrish, testified at trial that within a reasonable degree of medical certainty Garcia would not recover and that he had never seen anyone in her condition recover. He stated that Garcia was functioning on a low brain level, whereby the brainstem kept her blood circulating, maintained blood pressure, and maintained respiration, and that she was in a persistent vegetative state with zero chance of recovering any cortex activity. Parrish further stated that he discussed the discontinuation of artificial nutrition and hydration with the family and that they had ultimately decided to continue the fluids but stop the nutrition, which he felt was reasonable.

When asked why Garcia had been given life support in the first place, Parrish explained that although Garcia's injury initially seemed very severe, he could not say from the beginning whether she would recover and wanted to give her every chance to improve if she could.

The trial court ruled that because Garcia, who was in a chronic vegetative state, had not executed a living will, the court had no authority to authorize discontinuance of artificial

My Living Will

To my Family, Doctors, and All Those Concerned with My Care:

I, _____, being of sound mind, make this statement as a directive to be followed if for any reason I become incapacitated and unable to participate in decisions regarding my medical care.

If I should be in an incurable or irreversible mental or physical condition with no reasonable expectation of recovery, I direct my attending physician to withhold or withdraw treatment that merely prolongs my dying. I direct that my treatment in this instance be limited to comfort care and the control of and relief from pain.

Care I Want:

_____

_____

_____

_____

_____

To live as long as possible regardless of the quality of life that I may experience:

- I direct that all appropriate medical/surgical measures be provided to sustain my life regardless of my mental or physical condition.

- Upon my death, I want to donate any parts of my body that may be of benefit to others.

Care I Do Not Want:

_____

_____

_____

_____

_____

- I am permanently unconscious with and permanently connected to a ventilator.

- I am permanently unconscious with a feeding tube and/or intravenous hydration.

- I am on a ventilator when there is little or no chance of recovery.

- I am conscious but unable to communicate, being fed with a feeding tube and/or hydrated.

- I am in the end stage of a fatal irreversible mental or physical illness, disease, or condition.

- I do not want: _____ Mechanical ventilation _____ CPR _____ Dialysis _____ Feeding tubes

- Other exceptions and/or comments:

_____

_____

_____

FIGURE 2   Living Will

Additional Comments or Exceptions:

This living will describes my express wishes and legal right to accept or refuse treatment. As I am of sound mind, I expect my family, physician/s, and all those concerned with my care to regard themselves as legally and morally bound to act in accord with my wishes.

Signed _____

Date _____

Witness (Cannot be designated healthcare agent). I declare that the person who signed the document or asked another to sign this document on his/her behalf did so in my presence and that he/she appears to be of sound mind and free of duress or undue influence.

Signed _____

Date _____

Signed _____

Date _____

Note: A copy of the executed living will should be provided to the patient's physician and healthcare agent.

FIGURE   2   Living Will (*Continued*)

nutrition. On appeal, the appellants asserted that the trial court erred in refusing to allow Garcia's family to terminate the artificial nutrition and hydration that was keeping her body alive, thereby failing to honor her wishes and denying her constitutional right to bodily integrity.

The United States Supreme Court, in *Cruzan v. Director, Missouri Dept. of Health*, 497 U.S. 261, 110 S. Ct. 2841 (1990), recognized that a competent person had a constitutionally protected liberty interest in refusing unwanted medical treatment. The court stopped short of finding that an incompetent person would have the same right; however, the court said: "An incompetent person is not able to make an informed and voluntary choice to exercise a hypothetical right to refuse treatment, or any other right. Such a 'right' must be exercised for her, if at all, by some sort of surrogate."

Tennessee's public policy on this issue is set forth in the "Legislative intent" section of the Tennessee Right to Natural Death Act, codified at Tenn. Code Ann. §32-11-102. This statute reads:

> The general assembly declares it to be the law of the state of Tennessee that every person has the fundamental and inherent right to die naturally with as much dignity as circumstances permit and to accept, refuse, withdraw from, or otherwise control decisions relating to the rendering of the person's own medical care, specifically including palliative care and the use of extraordinary procedures and treatment.

This policy applies to every person and does not distinguish between those who are competent and those who are not. An individual has a right to refuse treatment so long as that individual is competent. When an individual is incompetent to make such a decision, the state has a duty to become involved by trying to determine what the desires of the patient would have been had he been conscious and competent. The initial assumption would be that the patient desired lifesaving treatment unless that assumption was contradicted by previous statements made when the patient was competent. It is clear from state court decisions that artificial nutrition and hydration are to be included in the realm of medical treatment that a patient has a right to refuse.

The appeals court concurred with the trial court's fact-finding that evidence is clear and convincing that Garcia would not want to be kept alive by artificial means and that her wishes, expressed while she was competent, would be to have these services discontinued. Courts have the duty to protect constitutional rights and when necessary enable individuals to exercise them. The appeals court ordered that a conservator be appointed to carry out Garcia's wishes, including the refusal of medical care.

DURABLE POWER OF ATTORNEY

A *durable power of attorney* is a legal device that permits one individual, known as the "principal," to give to another person, called the "attorney-in-fact," the authority to act on his or her behalf. The attorney-in-fact is authorized to handle banking and real estate affairs, incur expenses, pay bills, and handle a wide variety of legal affairs for a specified period of time. The power of attorney may continue indefinitely during the lifetime of the principal so long as that person is competent and capable of granting power of attorney. If the principal becomes comatose or mentally incompetent, the power of attorney automatically expires, just as it would if the principal dies.

Because a power of attorney is limited by the competency of the principal, some states have authorized a special legal device for the principal to express intent concerning the durability of the power of attorney, to allow it to survive disability or incompetency. The durable power of attorney is more general in scope and applies to a wider range of situations than those involving a patient in imminent danger of death, as is necessary for a living will to apply. Although it need not delineate desired medical treatment specifically, it must indicate the identity of the principal's attorney-in-fact and that the principal has communicated his or her health care wishes to the attorney-in-fact. Although the laws vary from state to state, all 50 states and the District of Columbia have durable power of attorney statutes. This legal device is an important alternative to guardianship, conservatorship, or trusteeship. Because a durable power of attorney places a considerable amount of power in the hands of the attorney-in-fact, an attorney in the state where the client resides should draw up the power of attorney. In the health care setting, a *durable power of attorney for health care* (e.g., **Figure 3**) is a legal instrument that designates and grants authority to an agent to, for example, make health care decisions for another.

SURROGATE DECISION MAKING

A surrogate decision maker is an agent who acts on behalf of a patient who lacks the capacity to participate in a particular decision. A health care agent's rights are no greater than those of a competent patient; however, the agent's rights are limited to any specific instructions included in the proxy document. An agent's decisions take priority over those of any

Durable Power of Attorney for Health Care

I, _____ , appoint:

1. Name _____   Phone _____
   Address _____

as my attorney-in-fact or agent to make my health and personal care decisions for me if I become unable to make my own decisions.

If the person I have named above is unable to act as my agent, I hereby designate the following person to serve as my agent:

2. Name _____   Phone _____
   Address _____

This *durable power of attorney* shall become effective upon my incapacity to make health or personal care decisions. (Please initial the statement/s below that best expresses your wishes.)

_____ I authorize my admission to or discharge from any medical, nursing, residential, or similar facility and to enter into agreements for my care.

_____ I authorize my agent to refuse or withdraw consent to any and all types of treatment, including, but not limited to, nutrition and hydration administered by artificial or invasive means.

I have discussed with my agent my wishes for health care. If my agent is not able to determine what I would want, I trust my agent to make his/her decision based on what he/she believes would be my wishes. This durable power of attorney is meant to replace all others.

Signed _____ Date _____

Witness (Cannot be the principal's designated healthcare agent). I declare that the person who signed this document or asked another to sign this document on his/her behalf did so in my presence and that he/she appears to be of sound mind and free of duress or undue influence.

Signed _____ Date _____

Signed _____ Date _____

Primary Agent

I, _____, have read the above durable power of attorney and am the person identified as the agent for _____. My signature below indicates that I acknowledge and accept responsibility to act as the agent and will exercise the powers herein granted in the best interest of the principal.

Signed _____ Date _____

FIGURE 3 Durable Power of Attorney for Health Care

FIGURE 3 Durable Power of Attorney for Health Care (*Continued*)

other person except the patient. The agent has the right to consent or refuse to consent to any service or treatment, routine or otherwise, to refuse life-sustaining treatment, and to access all of the patient's medical information to make informed decisions. The agent must make decisions based on the patient's moral and religious beliefs. If a patient's wishes are not known, decisions must be based on a good-faith judgment of what the patient would have wanted.

Substituted Judgment

Substituted judgment is a form of surrogate decision making where the surrogate attempts to establish what decision the patient would have made if that patient were competent to do so. This conclusion can be based on the patient's preference expressed in previous statements or the surrogate's knowledge of the patient's beliefs (e.g., religious) and values.[44]

CASE: SPOUSAL RIGHTS IN DECISION MAKING

Mr. Martin sustained debilitating injuries as the result of an automobile accident. He suffered severe subcortical brain damage, significantly impairing his physical and cognitive functioning.[45] His injuries left him totally paralyzed on the left side. He could not speak or eat and had no bladder or bowel control. Martin remained conscious and had some awareness of his surroundings. He could communicate to a very minimal degree through head nods.

The trial court determined that Martin did not have nor would he ever have the ability to have the requisite capacity to make decisions regarding the withdrawal of life-support equipment. The evidence demonstrated that Martin's preference would have been to decline life-support equipment given his medical condition and prognosis. The trial court's decision was based on the following *four-part test* for determining whether a person has the requisite capacity to make a decision: Does the person have sufficient mind to reasonably understand the condition? Is the person capable of understanding the nature and effect of the treatment choices? Is the person aware of the consequences associated with those choices? Is the person able to make an informed choice that is voluntary and not coerced?

The trial court also determined that Mrs. Martin, the patient's spouse, was a suitable guardian for him. She petitioned to withdraw her husband's life support. Martin's mother and sister counter petitioned to have Mrs. Martin removed as the patient's guardian. The Michigan Court of Appeals held that the evidence was sufficient to support a finding that the patient lacked capacity to make decisions regarding the withholding or withdrawal of life-sustaining treatment. As to the patient's desire not to be placed on life-support equipment, there was sufficient evidence to show that the patient had a medical preference to decline treatment under circumstances such as those that occurred. There was also sufficient evidence to show that the patient's spouse was a suitable guardian.

The test for determining whether Martin had the requisite capacity to make a decision regarding the withholding or withdrawal of life-supporting medical treatment was clear and convincing—he did not have sufficient decision-making capacity. The evidence was just as clear that he never would regain sufficient decision-making capacity that would enable him to make such a decision. It was the general consensus of all of the experts that Martin's condition and cognitive level of functioning would not improve in the future.

Testimony from two of Martin's friends described statements made by him that he would never want to be maintained in a coma or in a vegetative state. In addition, Mrs. Martin described numerous statements made to her by Martin prior to the accident that he would not want to be maintained alive, given the circumstances described previously here. The trial court found that Mrs. Martin was credible. The court of appeals found no reason to dispute the trial court's finding as to Mrs. Martin's credibility.

In contrast to allegations made by the patient's mother and sister, the evidence was clear that Mrs. Martin's testimony was credible. There was no evidence that Mrs. Martin had anything but her husband's best interest at heart. There were allegations, but no evidence, that financial considerations or pressure from another individual influenced Mrs. Martin's testimony.

Ethical and Legal Issues

1. Knowing that the patient had some ability to interact with his environment, discuss the four-part test for determining the patient's ability to make a decision.
2. Do you agree with the court's decision? Explain.
3. Should the concern of the mother and sister have carried more weight in removing custody from Mrs. Martin?
4. What influence do you believe the mother and sister might have had on Mrs. Martin?

Guardianship

Guardianship is a legal mechanism by which the court declares a person incompetent and appoints a guardian. The court transfers the responsibility for managing financial affairs, living arrangements, and medical care decisions to the guardian. The right to refuse medical treatment on behalf of an incompetent person is not limited to legally appointed guardians but may be exercised by health care proxies or surrogates, such as close family members or friends. When a patient has not expressed instructions concerning his or her future health care in the event of later incapacity but has merely delegated full responsibility to a proxy, designation of a proxy must have been made in writing.

Health Care Proxy

A *health care proxy* allows a person to appoint a health care agent to make treatment decisions in the event he or she becomes incompetent and is unable to make decisions for him- or herself. The agent must be made aware of the patient's wishes regarding nutrition and hydration in order to be allowed to make a decision concerning withholding or withdrawing them. In contrast to a living will, a health care proxy does not require a person to know about and consider in advance all situations and decisions that could arise. Rather, the appointed agent would know about and interpret the expressed wishes of the patient and then make decisions about the medical care and treatment to be administered or refused. The *Cruzan* decision indicates that the Supreme Court views advance directives as clear and convincing evidence of a patient's wishes regarding life-sustaining treatment.

Although most statutes fail to cover incompetence, cases such as *Quinlan* and *Saikewicz* created a constitutionally protected obligation to terminate the incurable incompetent patient's life when guardians use the doctrine of substituted judgment. Furthermore, some states provide for proxy consent in the form of durable power of attorney statutes. Generally, these involve designation of a proxy to speak on the incurable incompetent person's behalf. They represent a combination of the intimate wishes of the patient and the medical recommendations of the physicians.

Oral declarations are accepted only after the patient has been declared terminally ill. Moreover, the declarant bears the responsibility of informing the physician to ensure that the document becomes a part of the medical record. The California statute provides that the document be reexecuted after 5 years. Other statutes differ in the length of time of effectiveness. Most states allow the document to be effective until revoked by the individual. To revoke, the patient must sign and date a new writing, destroy the first document himself or herself, direct another to destroy the first document in his or her presence, or orally state to the physician an intent to revoke. The effect of the directive varies among jurisdictions; however, there is unanimity in the promulgation of regulations that specifically authorize health care personnel to honor the directives without fear of incurring liability. The highest court of New York in *In re Eichner*[46] complied with the request of a guardian to withdraw life-support systems from an 83-year-old brain-damaged priest. The court reached its result by finding the patient's previously expressed wishes to be determinative.

Before exercising an incompetent patient's right to forgo medical treatment, the surrogate decision maker must satisfy the following conditions:

- The surrogate must be satisfied that the patient executed a document (e.g., Durable Power of Attorney for Health Care and Health Care Proxy) knowingly, willingly, and without undue influence and that the evidence of the patient's oral declaration is reliable.

- The patient must not have reasonable probability of recovering competency so that the patient could exercise the right.
- The surrogate must take care to ensure that any limitations or conditions expressed either orally or in written declarations have been considered carefully and satisfied.

FUTILITY OF TREATMENT

Futility of treatment, as it relates to medical care, occurs when the physician recognizes that the effect of treatment will be of no benefit to the patient. Morally, the physician has a duty to inform the patient when there is little likelihood of success. The determination as to futility of medical care is a scientific decision.

After a diagnosis has been made that a person is terminally ill with no hope of recovery and is in a chronic vegetative state with no possibility of attaining cognitive function, a state generally has no compelling interest in maintaining life. The decision to forgo or terminate life-support measures is, at this point, simply a decision that the dying process will not be artificially extended. Although the state has an interest in the prolongation of life, it has no interest in the prolongation of dying, and although there is a moral and ethical decision to be made to end the process, that decision can be made only by the surrogate. The decision whether to end the dying process is a personal decision for family members or those who bear a legal responsibility for the patient.

A determination as to the futility of medical care is a decision that must be made by a physician. Even if death is not imminent but a patient's coma is irreversible beyond doubt and there are adequate safeguards to confirm the accuracy of the diagnosis with the concurrence of those responsible for the patient's care, it is not unethical to discontinue all means of life-prolonging medical treatment.

WITHHOLDING AND WITHDRAWAL OF TREATMENT

Withholding of treatment is a decision not to initiate treatment or medical intervention for the patient. This is a decision often made when death is imminent and no hope of recovery. *Withdrawal of treatment* is a decision to discontinue treatment or medical interventions for the patient. When death is imminent and cannot be prevented by available treatment. Withholding or withdrawing treatment should be considered when:

- the patient is in a terminal condition and there is a reasonable expectation of imminent death of the patient;
- the patient is in a noncognitive state with no reasonable possibility of regaining cognitive function; and/or
- restoration of cardiac function will last for a brief period.

Theologians and ethicists have long recognized a distinction between ordinary and extraordinary medical care. The theological distinction is based on the belief that life is a gift from God that should not be destroyed deliberately by humans. Therefore, extraordinary therapies that extend life by imposing grave burdens on the patient and family are not required.

Although the courts have accepted decisions to withhold or withdraw extraordinary care, especially the respirator, from those who are comatose or in a persistent vegetative state with no possibility of emerging, they have been unwilling until recent years to discontinue feeding, which they have considered to be ordinary care. For example, the Illinois Supreme Court, in *In re Estate of Longeway*,[47] found that the authorized guardian of a terminally ill patient in an irreversible coma or persistent vegetative state has a common-law right to refuse artificial nutrition and hydration. The court found that there must be clear and convincing evidence that the refusal is consistent with the patient's interest. The court also required the concurrence of the patient's attending physician and two other physicians. Court intervention is also necessary to guard against the possibility that greed may taint the judgment of the surrogate decision maker. Although there may be a duty to provide life-sustaining equipment in the immediate aftermath of cardiopulmonary arrest, there is no duty to continue its use when it has become futile and ineffective to do so in the opinion of qualified medical personnel.

The Texas Natural Death Act provided immunity to caregivers in the following case for what the plaintiffs claimed was a failure of caregivers to withdraw lifesaving treatment.

CASE: FAILURE TO *WITHDRAW* LIFE SAVING TREAMENT

In this medical malpractice suit, the Stolles (appellants) sought damages from physicians and hospitals (appellees) for disregard of their instructions not to use "heroic efforts" or artificial means to prolong the life of their child, Mariel, who was born with brain damage. The Stolles argued that such negligence resulted in further brain damage to Mariel, prolonged her life, and caused them extraordinary costs that will continue as long as the child lives.

The Stolles had executed a written "Directive to Physicians" on behalf of Mariel in which they made known their desire that Mariel's life not be artificially prolonged under the circumstances provided in that directive.

Mariel suffered a medical episode after regurgitating her food. An unnamed, unidentified nurse–clinician administered chest compressions for 30 to 60 seconds, and Mariel survived.

The Stolles sued, alleging the following, among other things: Appropriate medical entries were not made in the medical record to reflect the Stolles' wishes that caregivers refrain from "heroic" life-sustaining measures. Lifesaving measures were initiated in violation of the physician's orders. The hospital did not follow the physician's orders, which were in Mariel's medical chart, when chest compressions and mechanically administered breathing to artificially prolong Mariel's life were applied, and a bioethics committee meeting was not convened to consider the Stolles' wishes and the necessity of a do-not-resuscitate (DNR) order.

The central issue in this case is whether appellees are immune from liability under the Texas Natural Death Act. Section 672.016(b) of the Texas Natural Death Act provides the following: "A physician, or a health professional acting under the direction of a physician, is not civilly or criminally liable for failing to effectuate a qualified patient's directive" [Tex. Health & Safety Code Ann. A4 672.016(b) (Vernon 1992)]. A "qualified patient" is a "patient with a terminal condition that has been diagnosed and certified in writing by the attending physician and one other physician who have personally examined the patient." A "terminal condition" is an "incurable condition caused by injury, disease, or illness that would produce death regardless of the application of life-sustaining procedures, according to reasonable medical judgment, and in which the application of life-sustaining procedures serves only to postpone the moment of the patient's death."

Mariel was not in a terminal condition, as appellees alleged. The Stolles failed to cite any authority that would have allowed the withdrawal of life sustaining procedures in a lawful manner. The Texas Natural Death Act, therefore, provided immunity to the caregivers for their actions in the treatment and care of Mariel.[48]

Ethical and Legal Issues

1. Describe the ethical principles in conflict in this case.
2. Do you agree with the court's decision? Explain your answer.

PATIENT NOT IN A PERSISTENT VEGETATIVE STATE

A guardian may direct the withdrawal of life-sustaining medical treatment, including nutrition and hydration, *only* if the incompetent ward is in a persistent vegetative state and the decision to withdraw is in the best interests of the ward.

In *Spahn v. Eisenberg,* Edna's sister and court-appointed guardian, Spahn, sought permission to direct the withholding of Edna's nutrition, claiming that her sister would not want to live in this condition; however, the only testimony presented at trial regarding Edna's views on the use of life-sustaining medical treatment involved a statement made 30 years earlier. At that time, Spahn and Edna were having a conversation about their mother, who was recovering from depression, and Spahn's mother-in-law, who was dying of cancer. Spahn testified that during this conversation, Edna said to her that she would rather die of cancer than lose her mind. Spahn further testified that this was the only time that she and Edna discussed the subject and that Edna never said anything specifically about withholding or withdrawing life-sustaining medical treatment.

The ethics committee at the nursing facility where Edna lived met to discuss the issue of withholding artificial nutrition from Edna. The committee approved withholding nutrition if no family member objected; however, one of Edna's nieces refused to sign a statement approving the withdrawal of nutrition.

The record spoke very little to what Edna's desires would be, and there was no clear statement of what her desires would be today under the current conditions. Her friends and family never had any conversations or discussions with her regarding her feelings or opinions about withdrawing nutrition or hydration, and she did not execute any advance directives expressing her wishes while she was competent.

Consequently, the court held that a guardian could only direct the withdrawal of life-sustaining medical treatment, including nutrition and hydration, if the incompetent ward is in a persistent vegetative state and the decision to withdraw is in the best interests of the ward. In this case, where the only indication of Edna's desires was made at least 30 years earlier and under different circumstances, there was not a clear statement of intent such that Edna's guardian might authorize the withholding of her nutrition.

The circuit judge concluded his own questioning of one member of the ethics committee, "The way I understand it, what you really have is a liability problem, and that's why you want everybody to consent, is that correct?" Dr. Erickson answered, "That is correct."[49]

Although there may be a duty to provide life-sustaining equipment in the immediate aftermath of cardiopulmonary arrest, there is no duty to continue its use after it has become futile and ineffective to do so in the opinion of qualified medical personnel. Two physicians in *Barber v. Superior Court*[50] were charged with the crimes of murder and conspiracy to commit murder. The charges were based on their acceding to requests of the patient's family to discontinue life-support equipment and intravenous tubes. The patient had suffered a cardiopulmonary arrest in the recovery room after surgery. A team of physicians and nurses revived the patient and placed him on life-support equipment. The patient had suffered severe brain damage, placing him in a comatose and vegetative state from which, according to tests and examinations by other specialists, he was unlikely to recover. On the written request of the family, the patient was taken off life-support equipment. The family, his wife and eight children, made the decision together after consultation with the physicians. Evidence had been presented that the patient, before his incapacitation, had expressed to his wife that he would not want to be kept alive by a machine. There was no evidence indicating that the family was motivated in their decision by anything other than love and concern for the dignity of their loved one. The patient continued to breathe on his own. Because the patient showed no signs of improvement, the physicians again discussed the patient's poor prognosis with the family. The intravenous lines were removed, and the patient died sometime thereafter.

A complaint then was filed against the two physicians. The magistrate who heard the evidence determined that the physicians did not kill the deceased because their conduct was not the proximate cause of the patient's death. On motion of the prosecution, the superior court determined as a matter of law that the evidence required the magistrate to hold the physicians to answer and ordered the complaint reinstated. The physicians then filed a writ of prohibition with the court of appeals. The court of appeals held that the physicians' omission to continue treatment, although intentional and with knowledge that the patient would die, was not an unlawful failure to perform a legal duty. The evidence amply supported the magistrate's decision. The superior court erred in determining that, as a matter of law, the evidence required the magistrate to hold the physicians to answer. The preemptory writ of prohibition to restrain the Superior Court of Los Angeles from taking any further action in this matter—other than to vacate its order reinstating the complaint and to enter a new and different order denying the People's motion—was granted.

FEEDING TUBES

The New Jersey Supreme Court in 1985 heard the case of *In re Claire C. Conroy*.[51] The case involved an 84-year-old nursing home patient whose nephew petitioned the court for authority to remove the nasogastric tube that was feeding her. The court overturned the appellate division decision and held that life-sustaining treatment, including nasogastric feeding, could be withheld or withdrawn from incompetent nursing home patients who will, according to physicians, die within 1 year, in three specific circumstances. These are as follows:[52]

1. When it is clear that the particular patient would have refused the treatment under the circumstances involved (the subjective test)

2. When there is some indication of the patient's wishes (but he or she has not "unequiv-ocally expressed" his or her desires before becoming incompetent) and the treatment "would only prolong suffering" (the limited objective test)
3. When there is no evidence at all of the patient's wishes, but the treatment "clearly and markedly outweighs the benefits the patient derives from life" (the pure objective test, based on pain)

A procedure involving notification of the state Office of the Ombudsman is required before withdrawing or withholding treatment under any of the three tests. The ombudsman must make a separate recommendation.

The court also found tubal feeding to be a medical treatment, and as such, as intrusive as other life-sustaining measures. The court in its analysis emphasized duty, rather than cau-sation, with the result that medical personnel acting in good faith will be protected from liability. If physicians follow the *Quinlan/Conroy* standards and decide to end medical treat-ment of a patient, the duty to continue treatment ceases. Thus, the termination of treatment becomes a lawful act.

Although *Conroy* presents case-specific guidelines, there is concern that the opinion will have far-reaching repercussions. There is fear that decisions to discontinue treatment will not be based on the "balancing of interests" test, but rather that a "quality-of-life" test will be used to end the lives of severely senile, old, and economic burdensome people.

Those quality-of-life judgments would be most dangerous for nursing home patients whose age would be a factor in the decision-making process. "Advocates of 'the right to life' fear that the 'right to die' for the elderly and handicapped will become a 'duty to die.'"[53] In both the *Saikewicz* and *Spring* cases, age was a determining factor weighing against life-sustaining treatment. Furthermore, in *In re Hier,*[54] the court found that Mrs. Hier's age of 92 years made the "proposed gastrostomy substantially more onerous or bur-densome . . . than it would be for a younger, healthier person." Moreover, a New York Superior Court held that the burdens of an emergency amputation for an elderly patient outweighed the benefit of continued life.[55] Finding that prolonging her life would be cruel, the court stated that life had no meaning for her. Although some courts have recognized the difference, other courts must still address the difference between *Quinlan*-type patients and older, confined, and conscious patients who can interact but whose mental or physical functioning is impaired.

In a New Jersey case, however, the ombudsman denied a request to remove feeding tubes from a comatose nursing home patient.[56] In applying the *Conroy* tests, the ombudsman decided that Hilda Peterson might live more than 1 year, the period that *Conroy* used as a criterion for determining whether life support can be removed.

To complicate this issue further, on March 17, 1986, the American Medical Association (AMA) changed its code of ethics on comas. Now physicians may ethically withhold food, water, and medical treatment from patients in irreversible comas or persistent vegetative states with no hope of recovery— even if death is not imminent.[57] Although physicians can consider the wishes of the patient and family or the legal representatives, they cannot cause death intentionally. The wording is permissive, and, thus, those physicians who feel uncom-fortable withdrawing food and water may refrain from doing so. The AMA's decision does not comfort those who fear abuse or mistake in euthanasia decisions, nor does it have any legal value as such. There are physicians, nurses, and families who have their own, and not the patient's, interests in mind. Even with the *Conroy* decision and the AMA's code of ethics change, the feeding tube issue is not settled.

On April 23, 1986, the New Jersey Superior Court ruled that the husband of severely brain-damaged Nancy Jobes could order the removal of her life-sustaining feeding tube, which would ultimately cause the 31-year-old comatose patient, who had been in a vegetative state in a hospice for the past 6 years, to starve to death.[58] Dr. Fred Plum created and defined the term "persistent vegetative state" as one in which:[59]

> The body functions entirely in terms of its internal controls. It maintains temperature. It maintains digestive activity. It maintains heart beat and pulmonary ventilation. It maintains reflex activity of muscles and nerves for low-level conditioned responses. But there is no behavioral evidence of either self-awareness or awareness of the surroundings in a learned manner.

Medical experts testified that the patient could, under optimal conditions, live another 30 years. Relieving the nursing home officials from performing the act on one of its residents, the court ruled that the patient may be taken home to die (with the removal to be supervised by a physician and medical care to be provided to the patient at home).

The nursing home had petitioned the court for the appointment of a "life advocate" to fight for continuation of medical treatment for Jobes, which, it argued, would save her life. The court disallowed the appointment of a life advocate, holding that case law does not support requiring the continuation of life-support systems in all circumstances. Such a requirement, according to the court, would contradict the patient's right of privacy.

The court's decision applied "the principles enunciated in *Quinlan* and . . . *Conroy*" and the "ruling by the AMA's Council on Judicial Affairs that the provision of food and water is, under certain circumstances, a medical treatment like any other and may be discontinued when the physician and family of the patient feel it is no longer benefiting the patient."[60]

An Illinois court found that the authorized guardian of a terminally ill patient in an irreversible coma or persistent vegetative state has a common law right to refuse artificial nutrition and hydration. The court found that there must be clear and convincing evidence that the refusal is consistent with the patient's interest. The court also required the concurrence of the patient's attending physician and two other physicians. "Court intervention is also necessary to guard against the remote, yet real possibility that greed may taint the judgment of the surrogate decision maker."[61] Dissenting, Judge Ward said, "The right to refuse treatment is rooted in and dependent on the patient's capacity for informed decision, which an incompetent patient lacks."[62]

Also, Elizabeth Bouvia, a mentally competent cerebral palsy victim, won her struggle to have feeding tubes removed even though she was not terminally ill.[63] The California Court of Appeals announced on April 16, 1986, that she could go home to die. The court found that Bouvia's decision to "let nature take its course" did not amount to a choice to commit suicide with people aiding and abetting it. The court stated that it is not "illegal or immoral to prefer a natural, albeit sooner, death than a drugged life attached to a mechanical device."[64] The court's finding that it was a moral and philosophical question, not a legal or medical one, leaves one wondering whether the courts are opening the door to permitting "legal starvation" to be used by those who are not terminally ill but who do wish to commit suicide.

DO-NOT-RESUSCITATE ORDERS

Do-not-resuscitate orders (DNR) are physician orders not to resuscitate a patient in the event of cardiac or respiratory arrest. Determination as to futility of medical care is a medical decision based on scientific evidence that further treatment is futile and one's quality of life has been so diminished that "heroic" rescue methods are no longer in the patient's best interests. DNR orders must be written, signed, and dated by the physician. Appropriate consents must be obtained either from the patient or his or her health care agent. Many states have acknowledged the validity of DNR orders in cases involving terminally ill patients in which the patients' families make no objections to such orders. Such orders are generally written as the result of a patient wishes as a result of an advance directive (e.g., living will). If a patient lacks the ability to make a decision regarding a DNR order, the patient's legally *appointed decision maker* can make such decisions provided it can be demonstrated that the decision maker is following the patient's wishes. Advance directives, such as living wills, are helpful in determining a patient's wishes. DNR orders can also be made at the family's request.

DNR orders must comply with statutory requirements, be of short duration, and be reviewed periodically to determine whether the patient's condition or other circumstances (e.g., change of mind by the patient or family) surrounding the "no code" orders have changed. Currently, it is generally accepted that if a patient is competent, the DNR order is considered to be the same as other medical decisions in which a patient may choose to reject life-sustaining treatment. In the case of an incompetent patient, absent any advance written directives, the best interests of the patient would be considered.

Competent Patients Make Their Own Decisions

Should relatives of a patient agree to a no code order when the patient is competent to make his or her own decision?

In *Payne v. Marion General Hospital*,[65] the Indiana Court of Appeals overturned a lower court decision in favor of the physician. The physician had issued a no code status on Payne despite evidence given by a nurse that up to a few minutes before his death Payne could communicate. The physician had determined that Payne was incompetent, thereby rendering him unable to give informed consent to treatment. Because Payne left no written directives, the physician relied on one of Payne's relatives, who asked for the DNR order. The court found that there was evidence that Payne was not incompetent and should have been consulted before a DNR order was given.

Furthermore, the court reviewed testimony that 1 year earlier Payne had suffered and recovered from the same type of symptoms, leading to the conclusion that there was a possibility that he could have survived if resuscitation had continued. There was no DNR policy in place at the hospital to assist the physician in making his decision. To avoid this type of problem, health care providers should adopt an appropriate process with respect to issuing no code orders.

Help Me Bear the Pain

Some say, "Men don't cry." Not true! You may find yourself crying alone someday. But for now, you have to be strong for Sunshine. Sunshine was her name, as given to her by her grandmother. For purposes of this case, she remains Sunshine. Not Miss or Ms. or Mrs., for Sunshine is her name. If you were to ask Sunshine what she thought about her life, this is what she would tell you.

As a hard-charging former district attorney, Sunshine knows what it's like to be under the constant threat of death. In the notorious 1990 "Angel Gabriel" case, a key witness to a cult leader's rape spree was murdered. As a result, the district attorney ordered that a panic alarm be placed in Sunshine's home.

Still, one enemy has done more damage than all of her former enemies combined. Sunshine has been battling systemic sclerosis for more than 6 years and has beaten the long-shot odds for survival.

Early on, she lost 20 pounds in 3 weeks. One by one, from her esophagus to her bottom, her internal organs came under painful attack. Her skin hardened in patches. Her fingers became discolored and swollen. Fingernails fell off. Calcification set in, and she nearly lost several digits. At the moment, she has a mysterious edema throughout her body.

Maintaining a full-time work schedule, she bounced from physician to physician for 3 years, seeking to find a reason for the sudden illness. The clues were finally put together, and her illness was diagnosed as systemic sclerosis—a degenerative connective tissue disease.

Most people don't know she has an illness. She's always in good spirits. She hides it well. Sunshine admits to putting a mask on in the morning. "When I cannot hide the pain, I disappear—go away or go home. I don't want to be defined by my illness. You go through mourning and anger. You feel tethered by the disease. It's a sadness you have to cope with."

With her mask firmly in place, a smiling Sunshine says she is not bitter. "I had a great life. I had fun. If it ended, I had fun."

Sunshine's Prayer: Strength to Cope

O God, you know my feelings. You know that I want to feel better. I want to be better. I want to have my health restored. But the hours of testing, the days of diagnosis, and the question marks concerning my future seem nearly more than I can bear! Grant me, O God, the strength to face each hour of this and every day. In fact, when it seems that I cannot face even this hour, fill me with strength to face the next five minutes. Amen.

Wherever Sunshine goes, the sun always shines, for she, as always, recognizes the beauty of each day.

–Anonymous

1. Euthanasia
   - *Mercy killing* of the hopelessly ill, injured, or incapacitated.
   - Debate over euthanasia is complex.
     - Legal system must maintain a balance between ensuring the patient's constitutional rights are protected and protecting society's interests in preserving life, preventing suicide, and maintaining the integrity of the medical profession.
   - When there is uncertainty regarding a patient's wishes in an emergency
     - The situation should be resolved in a way that favors the preservation of life.
     - Protect the patient's right to freedom of religion and self-determination.
   - *Active euthanasia* is the intentional commission of an act that will result in death.
   - *Passive euthanasia* is when a potentially lifesaving treatment is withdrawn or withheld.
   - *Voluntary euthanasia*
     - When a competent adult patient with an incurable condition who has been informed of the possible ramifications and alternatives available gives consent.
   - *Involuntary euthanasia*
     - When the decision to terminate the life of an incurable person is made by someone other than the incurable person.
   - Supreme Court ruled there is no constitutional right to assisted suicide.
     - Decision allowed the state of Michigan to prosecute Dr. Jack Kevorkian for assisting patients in committing suicide.
2. Right to self-determination
3. Assisted suicide
   - Oregon legislates physician-assisted suicide.
4. Patient Self-Determination Act of 1990
   - Health care organizations have a responsibility to explain to patients, staff, and families that patients have legal rights to direct their medical and nursing care as it corresponds to existing state law.
5. *Advance directives*, in the form of a "living will" or "durable power of attorney," allow the patient to make end-of-life choices.
   - *Living will* is the instrument or legal document that describes those treatments an individual wishes or does not wish to receive should he or she become incapacitated and unable to communicate treatment decisions.
   - *Durable power of attorney* is a legal device that permits one individual, known as the "principal," to give to another person, called the "attorney-in-fact," the authority to act on his or her behalf.
   - *Guardianship* is a legal mechanism by which the court declares a person incompetent and appoints a guardian. The court transfers the responsibility for managing financial affairs, living arrangements, and medical care decisions to the guardian.
   - *Health care proxy* allows a person to appoint a health care agent to make treatment decisions in the event that he or she becomes incompetent and is unable to make decisions for him- or herself.

- *Surrogate decision maker* is an agent who acts on behalf of a patient who lacks the capacity to participate in a particular decision.
- *Substituted judgment* is a form of surrogate decision making where the surrogate attempts to establish what decision the patient would have made if that patient were competent to do so.

6. Futility of treatment
   - When the physician recognizes further treatment will be of no benefit to the patient.
   - Morally, the physician has a duty to inform the patient when there is little likelihood of success of further treatment.
   - Determination as to futility of medical care is a medical decision based on scientific evidence.

7. Withholding or withdrawal of treatment
   - *Withholding of treatment* is a decision not to initiate treatment or medical intervention for the patient.
   - *Withdrawal of treatment* is a decision to discontinue treatment or medical interventions for the patient.
   - *Do-not-resuscitate orders* are physician orders not to resuscitate a patient in the event of a cardiac or respiratory arrest.
     - Generally written as the result of a patient wishes or at the family's request
     - Orders must be in written form, signed and dated by the physician.

TEST YOUR UNDERSTANDING

TERMINOLOGY

active euthanasia	futility of treatment	Patient Self-Determination Act
advance directives	guardianship	
appointed decision makers	health care proxy	physician-assisted suicide
do-not-resuscitate (DNR) order	involuntary euthanasia	substituted judgment
durable power of attorney	living will	surrogate decision maker
durable power of attorney for health care	Oregon Death with Dignity Act	voluntary euthanasia
euthanasia	passive euthanasia	withdrawal of treatment
		withholding of treatment

REVIEW QUESTIONS

1. Describe why there is such a struggle when addressing end-of-life issues.

2. Describe the difference between active and passive euthanasia.

3. Describe the difference between voluntary and involuntary euthanasia.

4. What are the differences between allowing a patient to die and physician-assisted suicide?

5. Constitutionally, what gives patients the right to self-determination?

6. Describe Oregon's Death with Dignity Act.

7. What was the purpose of the Patient Self-Determination Act of 1990?

8. What are advance directives?

9. Describe how a living will differs from a durable power of attorney for health care.

NOTES

1. http://www.cnn.com/2014/01/06/health/jahi-mcmath-girl-brain-dead/index.html.
2. J. Podgers, *Matters of Life and Death*, A.B.A.J. May 1992, at 60.
3. http://www.newsdaily.com/article/b177a24caf91af300f25679219db15c1/belgium-considering-new-euthanasia-law-for-kids.
4. 105 N.E. 92 (N.Y. 1914).
5. *Id.* at 93.
6. 438 N.Y.S.2d 266, 272 (N.Y. 1981).
7. *In re Quinlan*, 355 A.2d 647 (N.J. 1976).
8. 410 U.S. 113 (1973).
9. *Quinlan*, 355 A.2d at 663.
10. 370 N.E.2d 417 (Mass. 1977).
11. *Id.* at 434.
12. Gelford, *Euthanasia and the Terminally Ill Patient*, 63 Neb. L. Rev. 741, 747 (1984).
13. 380 N.E.2d 134 (Mass. 1978).
14. 405 N.E.2d 115 (Mass. 1980).
15. *John F. Kennedy Mem'l Hosp. v. Bludworth*, 452 So. 2d 921, 925 (Fla. 1984) (citing *In re Welfare of Colyer*, 660 P.2d 738 (Wash. 1983), in which the court found prior court approval to be "unresponsive and cumbersome").
16. *Schmitt v. Pierce*, 344 S.W.2d 120 (Mo. 1961).
17. Connery, *Prolonging Life: The Duty and Its Limits, Moral Responsibility in Prolonging Life's Decisions*, in To Treat or Not To Treat, 25 (1984).
18. Statement of Medical Opinion Re: "Brain Death," A.M.A. House of Delegates Res. (June 1974).
19. 482 N.Y.S.2d 436 (1984).
20. 438 N.Y.S.2d 266 (1981).
21. *Id.* at 425.
22. *Cruzan v. Director of the Mo. Dep't of Health*, 497 U.S. 261 (1990).
23. Pa. S.646, Amendment A3506, Printer's No. 689, Oct. 1, 1990.
24. 20 Pa. Cons. Stat. Ann. § 5602(a)(9) (1988).
25. "Hospital wants to let wife die," *Newsday*, Jan. 11, 1991, at 13.
26. *Farnam v. Crista Ministries*, 807 P.2d 830, 849 (Wash. 1991).
27. *Kevorkian v. Thompson*, 947 F. Supp. 1152 (1997).
28. "Dr. Death at work," *Newsday*, February 7, 1991, at 12.
29. "Kevorkian charges dropped," *Newsday*, July 22, 1992, at 4.
30. *Hobbins v. Attorney Gen. of Mich.*, No. 94–1473 (Mich. 1994); *Kevorkian v. Michigan*, No. 94–1490 (Mich. 1994).
31. "22nd Death for 'Dr. Death,'" *USA Today*, May 9, 1995, at 2A.

32. http://townhall.com/tipsheet/danieldoherty/2013/05/21/sigh-vermont-legalizes-physicianassisted-suicide-n1602510.

33. *Baxter v. State*, 354 Mont. 234, 224 P.3d 1211 (2009)

34. http://www.patientsrightscouncil.org/site/montana/.

35. http://righttodie.uslegal.com/physician-assisted-suicide/supreme-court-rulings/.

36. http://cnsnews.com/news/article/california-gov-signs-assisted-suicide-information-bill-law.

37. http://www.myfoxboston.com/story/20027701/2012/11/07/backers-of-mass-doctor-assisted-suicide-concede>

38. 117 S. Ct. 2293 (1997).

39. *Washington v. Glucksberg*, 117 S.Ct. 2258 (1997).

40. 42 U.S.C. 1395cc(a)(1).

41. http://www.wsha.org/EOL-FedState.cfm

42. http://www.euthanasia.com/vatican.html.

43. No. E2001-02906-COA-R3-CV (2002).

44. Ascension Health, "Issues and Concepts," http://www.ascensionhealth.org/ethics/public/issues/substituted.asp.

45. *In re Martin*, 517 N.W.2d 749 (Mich. Ct. App. 1994).

46. 420 N.E.2d 64 (N.Y. 1981).

47. 549 N.E.2d 292 (Ill. 1989).

48. *Stolle v. Baylor College of Medicine*, 981 S.W.2d 709 (1998).

49. *Spahn v. Eisenberg*, 563 N.W.2d 485 (1997).

50. 195 Cal. Rptr. 484 (Cal. Ct. App. 1983).

51. 486 A.2d 1209 (N.J. Sup. Ct. 1985).

52. *Id.*

53. U.S. Congress, Off. of Technology Assessment, Pub. No. OTA-BA-306, Life-Sustaining Technologies and the Elderly 48 (1987).

54. 464 N.E.2d 959 (Mass. 1984).

55. *In re Beth Israel Med.* Ctr., 519 N.Y.S.2d 511, 517 (N.Y. Sup. Ct. 1987).

56. Ronald Sullivan, "Ombudsman bars food tube removal," *New York Times*, March 7, 1986, at 82.

57. "AMA changes code of ethics on comas," *Newsday*, March 17, 1986, at 2.

58. *In re Jobes*, 529 A.2d 434 (N.J. 1987).

59. *Id.* at 438.

60. "Man wins right to let wife die," *Newsday*, Apr. 24, 1986, at 3.

61. *Id.* at 790.

62. *Id.* at 793.

63. *Bouvia v. Superior Court (Glenchur)*, 225 Cal. Rptr. 297 (Cal. Ct. App. 1986).

64. *Id.* at 306.

65. 549 N.E.2d 1043 (Ind. Ct. App. 1990).

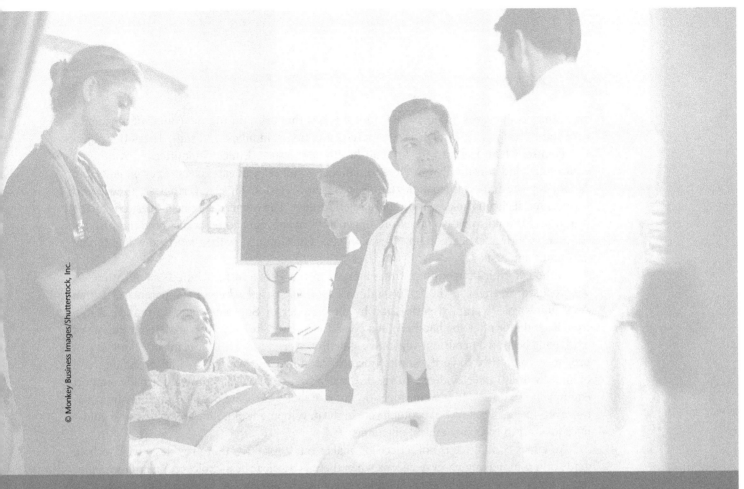

© Monkey Business Images/Shutterstock, Inc.

HEALTH CARE ETHICS COMMITTEE

LEARNING OBJECTIVES

Upon completion of this chapter, the reader will be able to:

- Describe the function and purpose of ethics committees.
- Describe the structure and goals of ethics committees.
- Explain the consultation process of ethics committees.
- Describe the expanding role of ethics committees.
- Discuss why the resolution of ethical dilemmas is no easy task.

INTRODUCTION

A *health care ethics committee* is an advisory body whose purpose is to facilitate discussion and consultation on ethical issues arising in the patient care setting. The goal of the ethics committee is to improve patient care and outcomes through recognition of the needs, interests, and rights of each patient and participants in the delivery of each patient's care. Health care ethics committees address legal–ethical issues that arise during the course of a patient's care and treatment. They serve as a resource for patients, families, and staff. They offer objective counsel when dealing with difficult health care issues. Ethics committees provide both educational and consultative services to patients, families, and caregivers. They enhance but do not replace important patient/family–physician relationships; nevertheless, they afford support for decisions made within those relationships. The numerous ethical questions facing health professionals involve the entire life span from the right to be born to the right to die. Ethics committees concern themselves with issues of morality, patient autonomy, legislation, and states' interests.

Although ethics committees first emerged in the 1960s in the United States, attention was focused on them in the 1976 landmark *Quinlan* case,[1] wherein the parents of Karen Ann Quinlan were granted permission by the New Jersey Supreme Court to remove Karen from a ventilator after she had been in a coma for a year. She died 10 years later at the age of 31, having been in a persistent vegetative state the entire time. The Quinlan court looked to a prognosis committee to verify Karen's medical condition. It then factored in the committee's opinion with all other evidence to reach the decision to allow withdrawing her life-support equipment. To date, ethics committees do not have sole surrogate decision-making authority; however, they play an ever-expanding role in the development of policy and procedural guidelines to assist in resolving ethical dilemmas.

An ethics committee is not a decision maker but a resource that provides advice to help guide others in making wiser decisions when there is no clear best choice. A unanimous opinion is not always possible when an ethics committee convenes to consider the issues of an ethical dilemma; however, consultative advice as to a course of action to follow in resolving the dilemma is a major the role of the ethics committee. Any recommendations for issue resolution reached by the ethics committee need to be communicated to those most closely involved with the patient's care. Being sensitive to each family member's values and assisting them in coping with whatever consensus decision is reached are crucial to the success of the committee. Unresolved issues often need to be addressed and a course of action followed. Each new consultation presents new opportunities for learning and teaching others how to cope with similar issues. Guidelines for resolving ethical issues will always be in a state of flux. Each new case presents new challenges and learning opportunities.

Making a decision, suggesting a course of action, recommending a path to follow, and making a choice require accepting the fact that there will be elements of right and wrong in the final decision. The idea is to cause the least pain and provide the greatest benefit.

COMMITTEE STRUCTURE

A hospital-based ethics committee should be composed of a multidisciplinary group of individuals whose membership includes representatives from the hospital (e.g., administrator, chaplain, nurse, physician, patient advocate) and community (e.g., clergy, legal counsel, ethicist). Members may also include those in positions of corporate and political stature, respect, and diversity. Appointment and rotation of new members to the ethics committee should be staggered in order to maintain continuity and stability.

Ethics committee members should be carefully vetted as to their skills in *conflict resolution*. Members of the ethics committee should complete a mandatory orientation that includes training and coaching. They should participate in continuing education programs. Committee members are expected to be active participants in committee activities. Self-study interest in the law and ethics should prove helpful. Those members of the committee who participate in consultative services involving patient care dilemmas should have appropriate medical, legal, and ethics training.

COMMITTEE GOALS

The goals of ethics committees often include the following:

- Provide a forum for review and discussion of ethical and moral issues relative to patient care.
- Provide information to patients as to the functioning of the ethics committee and how to access the committee at the time of admission. This information is generally provided in patient handbooks and/or informational brochures. The electronic media through patient room TVs is also helpful in educating patients as to their rights and responsibilities including the process for requesting a consultation.
- Serve as support and resource for hospital staff, families, and patients.
- Provide consultation, as requested, when there are conflicts in care options.
- Provide assistance in clarifying situations that are ethical, legal, or religious in nature that extend beyond the scope of daily practice.
- Clarify issues and discuss alternatives to ethical dilemmas.
- Promote patient rights.
- Assist the patient and family in coming to consensus with the options that best meet the patient's care needs.
- Review cases for educational purposes.
- Enhance the ethical tenor of both the hospital and health care professionals.

COMMITTEE FUNCTIONS

The functions of ethics committees are multifaceted and include development of policy and procedure guidelines to assist in resolving ethical dilemmas; staff and community education; conflict resolution; case reviews, support, and consultation; and political advocacy. The degree to which an ethics committee serves each of these functions varies in different health care organizations.

POLICY AND PROCEDURE DEVELOPMENT

The ethics committee is a valuable resource for assisting in the development of hospital policies and procedures pertinent to addressing ethical dilemmas (e.g., consultation procedures, confidentiality of information, staff and community education, annual review of the committee's activities and effectiveness). The following policies are a sampling of those often recommended by ethics committees.

Policy: Staff and Community Education

The director of education collaborates with hospital staff college faculty, when available, and ethicists to teach and train caregivers to resolve ethical issues that occur in the work environment. Programs are also arranged for community members interested in such topics as understanding and executing advance directives. To learn more about the community-sponsored ethics education programs, community members are encouraged to contact the hospital's department of education at xxx-xxx-xxxx.

Policy: Requests for Consultations

Ethics consultations are available to caregivers, patients, or family members who request an ethics consult. Ethics consultations are available 24 hours a day 365 days a year by calling the ethics hotline xxx-xxx-xxxx. Consultations shall be requested on a form prepared by the ethics committee and reviewed and approved by the hospital's administration, legal counsel, and board of directors.

Policy: Confidentiality of Information

Ethics committee information shall be considered confidential and shall not be used in any way except as provided herein or as required by law. Any information or case study developed for use by the committee shall not be required to become part of a patient's medical record. Committee members shall not make entries in a patient's medical record unless required by law and/or hospital policy.

Policy: Annual Review

An overall review of the ethics committee's activities will be conducted on an annual basis to determine the effectiveness of the committee and if it is accomplishing its stated goals. This review may take the form of a self-study or external review, preferably by a qualified ethicist.

EDUCATION

The ethics committee typically provides education on current ethical concepts and issues to committee members, staff, and the community at large. Some community hospitals provide ethics education to the staff at ambulatory care facilities, home health agencies, long-term care facilities, and physicians' offices. Such education helps reduce the need for emergent end-of-life consultations in acute-care settings.

The ethics committee provides resources for educational purposes to support staff in the development of the appropriate competencies for addressing ethical, legal, and spiritual issues, for example, those common to end-of-life issues (e.g., surrogate decision-making, the patient's refusal to accept recommended medical treatment, family conflict). Educational programs on ethical issues are developed for ethics committee members and staff on such topics as moral theories and principals, as well common ethical dilemmas that occur as they relate to such services common to emergency departments and critical care units. Community education often includes such topics as how to prepare and execute an advance directive.

Ethics consultations are helpful in resolving uncertainty and disagreements over health care dilemmas. Ethics committees often provide consultation services for patients, families, and caregivers struggling with difficult treatment decisions and end-of-life dilemmas. Always mindful of its basic orientation toward the patient's best interests, the committee provides options and suggestions for resolution of conflict in actual cases. Consultation with an ethics committee is not mandatory but is conducted at the request of a physician, patient, family member, or other caregiver.

The ethics committee strives to provide viable alternatives that will lead to the optimal resolution of dilemmas confronting the continuing care of the patient. It is important to remember that an ethics committee functions in an advisory capacity and should not be considered a substitute proxy for the patient.

A representative of the ethics committee is often able to intervene, when requested, in resolving ethical dilemmas. On occasion it may be necessary to request the assistance of one or more additional members of the ethics committee. An on-call roster is generally helpful when a consultation is necessary during evening, night, and weekend hours. Ethics committee members of the hospital staff generally provide on-call services.

Requests for Committee Consultations

Requests for ethics consultations often involve clarification of issues regarding decision-making capacity, informed consent, advance directives, and withdrawal of treatment. Consultations should be conducted in a timely manner considering the following information:

- Who requested the consultation?
- What are the issues?
- Is there is a problem that needs referral to another service?
- What specifically is being requested of the ethics committee (e.g., clarification of the problem or mediation)?

When conducting a consultation, all patient records must be reviewed and discussed with the attending physician, family members, and other caregivers involved in the patient's treatment. If an issue can be resolved easily, a designated member of the ethics committee should be able to consult on the case without the need for a full committee meeting. If the problem is unusual, problematic, or delicate, or has important legal ramifications, a full committee meeting may be necessary. Others who can be invited to an ethics committee case review, as appropriate, include the patient, if competent; relatives; agent or surrogate decision maker; and caregivers. Evaluation of a case consultation should take the following into consideration:

- Patient's current medical and mental status, diagnosis, and prognosis
- Patient's mental status and ability to make decisions, understand the information that is necessary to make a decision, and clearly understand the consequences of his or her choice
- Benefits and burdens of recommended treatment, or alternative treatments
- Life expectancy, treated and untreated

- Views of caregivers and consultants
- Pain and suffering
- Quality-of-life issues
- Financial burden on family (e.g., if the patient is in a comatose state with no hope of recovery, should the spouse deplete his or her finances to maintain the spouse on a respirator?)

Decisions concerning patient care must take into consideration the patient's:

- Personal assessment of the quality of life
- Current expressed choices
- Advance directives
- Competency to make decisions
- Ability to process information rationally to compare risks, benefits, and alternatives to treatment
- Ability to articulate major factors in decisions and reasons for them and ability to communicate

The patient must have all the information necessary to allow a reasonable person to make a prudent decision on his or her own behalf. The patient's choice must be voluntary and free from coercion by family, physicians, or others.

Family members must be identified and the following questions considered when making decisions:

- Do family members understand the patient's wishes?
- Is the family in agreement with the patient's wishes?
- Does the patient have an advance directive?
- Has the patient appointed an agent?
- Are there any religious proscriptions?
- Are there any financial concerns?
- Are there any legal concerns that need to be addressed (applicable state statutes and case law)?

When an ethics committee is engaged in the consulting process, its recommendations should be offered as suggestions, imposing no obligation for acceptance on the part of the patient, family, surrogate decision maker, organization, its governing body, medical staff, attending physicians, or other persons. **Figure 1** presents an ethics consultation form for documenting an ethics committee consultation.

When conducting a formal consultation, ethics committees should:

1. Identify the ethical dilemma (e.g., reasons why the consult was requested).
2. Be sure that the appropriate "Consultation Request" form has been completed.
3. Identify relevant facts.
   a. Diagnosis and prognosis.
   b. Patient goals and wishes.
   c. Regulatory and legal issues.

Ethics Consultation

Date: _____ Time: _____ Caller: _____

Reason for call _____

Action taken: _____

Patient: _____ Age: _____

Record #: _____ Consultation requested by: _____

Relationship (e.g., caregiver, spouse) _____

Attending physician: _____

Other physicians: _____

Will the patient participate in the consultation? ❑ Yes ❑ No

Does the patient have decision-making capacity? ❑ Yes ❑ No Explain _____

Surrogate decision maker? ❑ Yes ❑ No If yes, name: _____

Phone #: _____ Advance directives (e.g., living will)? _____

Availability of advance directive _____

Consultation participants:

❑ Family/relationship_____

❑ Physicians _____

❑ Nurses _____

❑ Ethics committee members (e.g., Chaplain, social worker, community representative) _____
_____
_____
_____

Medical Treatment/Care Information

Diagnoses _____ Prognosis _____

Course of illness _____

Treatment options appropriate _____

Treatment options medically beneficial: _____

Treatment options available: _____

Would the patient have wanted the treatment? _____

Ethical issues: _____

Legal issues: _____

Other persons to contact for input, if any. _____

Consultative guidance: _____

Guidance communicated? ❑ Yes ❑ No If yes, to whom? _____

Consultation noted on the medical record ❑ Yes ❑ No

Disposition: _____
_____

Form completed by: _____ Date/Time: _____

FIGURE 1 Hospital Consultation Request Form

d. Professional standards and codes of ethics.
e. Institutional policies and values.
4. Identify stakeholders.
5. Identify moral issues.
   a. Human dignity.
   b. Common good.
   c. Justice.
   d. Beneficence.
   e. Respect for autonomy.
   f. Informed consent.
   g. Medical futility and so on.
6. Identify legal issues.
7. Consider alternative options.
8. Conduct consultation.
9. Review, discuss, and provide reasoning for recommendations made.
10. Review and follow up.
11. Committee discussion includes family members.
12. Family members are queried as to their hopes and expectations.
13. Consultations are documented.

CASE: ETHICS COMMITTEE SERVES AS GUARDIAN

The Kentucky Supreme Court ruled in *Woods v. Commonwealth*, 1999-SSC0773 (August 24, 2004) that Kentucky's Living Will Directive, allowing a court-appointed guardian or other designated surrogate to remove a patient's life support systems, is constitutional. The patient in this case, Woods, had been placed on a ventilator after having a heart attack. It was generally agreed that he would never regain consciousness and would die in 2 to 10 years. After a recommendation of the hospital ethics committee, Woods's guardian at the time asked for approval to remove Woods's life support. The Kentucky Supreme Court affirmed an appeals court decision, holding that: (1) "If there is no guardian," but the family, physicians, and ethics committee all agree with the surrogate, there is no need to appoint a guardian; (2) "If there is a guardian" and all parties agree, there is no need for judicial approval; (3) "If there is disagreement," the parties may petition the courts.

Withdrawal of life support from a patient is prohibited absent clear and convincing evidence that the patient is permanently unconscious or in a persistent vegetative state and that withdrawing life support is in the patient's best interest.

Ethical and Legal Issues

1. Discuss the ethical issues of this case.
2. Discuss under what circumstances an ethics committee should serve as a legal guardian.
3. Discuss the pros and cons of an ethics committee serving as a patient's guardian.

Typically, hospital ethics committees concern themselves with biomedical issues as they relate to end-of-life issues; unfortunately, they often fail to address external decisions that affect internal operations. The role of an organization's ethics committee is evolving into more than a group of individuals who periodically gather together to meet a regulatory requirement and address advance directives and end-of-life issues. The organizational ethics committee has an ever-expanding role. This expanded role involves addressing external issues that affect internal operations (e.g., managed care, malpractice insurance, and complicated Health Insurance Portability and Accountability Act regulations that often increase legal and other financial costs). Ethics committees need to review their functions periodically and redefine themselves.

The ethics committee is health care's sleeping giant. Because of its potential to bring about change, its mission must not be limited to end-of-life issues. Its vision must not be restricted to issues internal to the organization but must include external matters that affect internal operations.

Failure to increase the good of others when one is knowingly in a position to do so is morally wrong. Preventative medicine and active public health interventions exemplify this conviction. After methods of treating yellow fever and smallpox were discovered, for example, it was universally agreed that positive steps ought to be taken to establish programs to protect public health.

The wide variety of ethical issues that an ethics committee can be involved in is somewhat formidable. Although an ethics committee cannot address every issue that one could conceivably imagine, the ethics committee should periodically reevaluate its scope of activities and effectiveness in addressing ethical issues. Some of the internal and external issues facing an organization's ethics committee are listed here.

INTERNAL ETHICAL ISSUES

1. Dilemma of blind trials: Who gets the placebo when the investigational drug looks very promising?
2. Informed consent: Are patients adequately informed as to risks, benefits, and alternative procedures that may be equally effective, knowing that one procedure may be more risky or damaging than another (e.g., lumpectomy versus a radical mastectomy)?
3. What is the physician's responsibility for informing the patient of his or her education, training, qualifications, and skill in treating a medical condition or performing an invasive procedure?
4. What is the role of the ethics committee when the medical staff is reluctant or fails to take timely action, knowing that one of its members practices questionable medicine?
5. Should a hospital's medical staff practice evidence-based medicine or follow its own best judgment?
6. To what extent should the organization participate in and/or support genetic research?
7. How should the ethics committee address confidentiality issues?
8. To what extent should medical information be shared with the patient's family?

9. To what extent should the organization's leadership control the scope of issues that the ethics committee addresses?
10. What are the demarcation lines as to what information should or should not be provided to the patient when mistakes are made relative to his or her care?

EXTERNAL ETHICAL ISSUES

1. Does the ethics committee have a role in addressing questionable reimbursement schemes?
2. Should an ethics committee have its own letterhead? What value would this serve?
3. What role, if any, should an ethics committee play in the following scenario?

CASE: CHOOSING THE RIGHT HOSPITAL

Emergency services ambulance personnel regularly transport suspected stroke patients to Hospital A. This hospital has no neurologists or neurosurgeons on its medical staff but does provide coffee and donuts to transport personnel. Ambulance personnel have an option to take the suspected stroke victim to Hospital B, which is within five blocks of Hospital A. Hospital B has a well-trained stroke team with staff neurologists and neurosurgeons readily available.

Ethical and Legal Issues

1. Describe the ethical issues in this case.
2. Describe the organizational politics that might come into play.
3. Discuss how organizational politics may prevent an ethics committee from becoming involved in many of the issues just described.

Although an ethics committee's serves in an advisory capacity, its value to an organization has yet to be fully realized.

RESOLUTION OF ETHICAL DILEMMAS

The difference between moral dilemmas and ethical ones, philosophers say, is that in moral issues the choice is between right and wrong. In ethics, the choice is between two rights.
—PAMELA WARRICK

The resolution of ethical dilemmas is a perplexing task at best, especially when two opposite answers both have elements of right and wrong—good and bad, regardless of the ultimate decision made. Finding compromise is no easy task when ethical principles, values, and morals are in conflict and vary from individual to individual. This is no easy task for members of an ethics committee, especially when the mix of opinions of caregivers, family members, and the health care entity's mission of healing collide. Although decision-making can be much easier when the patient has executed end-of-life directives, ethics committees often do not have this luxury, thus creating a need for ethics committees to help guide others in making difficult care decisions. With outcomes that often result in the decision-maker reflecting back and doubting his or her own decisions, it is important that each committee member reflect on the following thoughts prior to participating in an ethics consultation:

- I will accept the patient's wishes, if known.
- I will accept the dialogue of committee members with varying beliefs, expectations, and values, knowing some will undoubtedly challenge my own sense of right and wrong.
- I will help the ethics committee seek a morally acceptable resolution to an ethical dilemma.
- I will not be too fearful to seek clarification of issues and ask questions.
- I will contribute to making consultations meaningful and not argumentative.
- My compassion will outweigh my need to be right.
- The ultimate decision is not mine to make.
- I will provide guidance, consultation, and education.

An ethical dilemma can arise when, for example, the principles of autonomy and beneficence conflict with one another. The following cases illustrate how one's right to make his or her decisions can conflict with the principle of doing good and not harm.

CASE: PATIENT REFUSES BLOOD

Mrs. Jones has gangrene of her left leg. Her hemoglobin slipped to 6.4. She has a major infection and is diabetic. There is no spouse and no living will. The patient has decided that she does not want to be resuscitated if she should go into cardiopulmonary arrest. She may need surgery. She has agreed to surgery but refuses a blood transfusion, even though she is not a Jehovah's Witness. The surgeon will not perform the surgery, which is urgent, without Jones agreeing to a blood transfusion, if it becomes necessary. The attending physician questions the patient's capacity to make decisions. Her children have donated blood. She says she is not afraid to die.

Ethical and Legal Issues

1. Should the physician refuse to treat this patient? Explain your answer.
2. Should the family have a right to override the patient's decision to refuse blood? Explain your answer.

CASE: A SON'S GUILT, A FATHER'S WISHES

Following a massive stroke, Mr. Smith was transported from the Rope nursing facility to a local hospital by ambulance on July 4, 2004. Smith, 94 years of age, had been a resident at the Rope nursing facility for the past 12 years. Before being placed in Rope, Smith had been living with Mr. Curry, a close friend, for the previous 8 years. He had an advance directive indicating that he would never want to be placed on a respirator.

Smith's son and only child, Barry, who now lives in Los Angeles and had been estranged from his dad for more than 20 years, was notified by Curry that his dad had been admitted to the hospital in a terminal condition. Smith had mistakenly been placed on a respirator by hospital staff contrary to the directions in his advance directive, which had been placed on the front cover of Smith's medical chart. Curry, who was legally appointed by Smith to act as his health care surrogate decision maker, called Barry and explained that, according to his dad's wishes and advance directives, he was planning to ask hospital staff to have the respirator removed. Barry asked Curry to wait until he flew in from California to see his dad. Curry agreed to wait for Barry's arrival the following day, July 5. After arriving at the hospital, Barry told Curry that he would take responsibility for his dad's care and that Curry's services would no longer be needed. Barry told hospital staff that he objected to the hospital's plan to remove his father from the respirator. He said that he needed time to say goodbye to his dad, which he did by whispering his sorrows in his dad's ears. Smith, however, did not respond. Barry demanded that the hospital do everything that it could to save his dad's life, saying, "I don't know if Dad heard me. We have to wait until he wakes up so that I can tell him how sorry I am for not having stayed in touch with him over the years." Smith's physicians explained to Barry that there was no chance Smith would ever awaken out of his coma. Barry threatened legal action if the hospital did not do everything it could to keep his dad alive. Smith's physician again spoke to Barry about the futility of maintaining his dad on a respirator. Barry remained uncooperative. The hospital chaplain was called to speak to Barry, but had little success. Finally, hospital staff requested an ethics consult.

Ethical and Legal Issues

1. Discuss the ethical dilemmas in this case.
2. Discuss the issues and the role of the ethics committee in this case.

HELPFUL HINTS

The reason for studying ethical and legal issues is to understand and help guide others through the decision-making process as it relates to ethical dilemmas. The following are some helpful guidelines when faced with ethical dilemmas:

- Be aware of how everyday life is full of ethical decisions and that numerous ethical issues can arise when caring for patients.
- Help guide others to make choices.
- Ask your patient how you might help him or her.

- Be aware of why you think the way you do. Do not impose your beliefs on others.
- Ask yourself whether you agree with the things you do. If the answer is no, ask yourself how you should change.
- When you are not sure what to do, the wise thing to do is to talk it over with another person, someone whose opinion you trust.
- Do not sacrifice happiness for devotion to others.
- Do not lie to avoid hurting someone's feelings.

CHAPTER REVIEW

1. Ethics committee serves as a resource for patients, families, and staff, offering an objective counsel when dealing with difficult health care dilemmas.
2. Ethics committee should be structured to include a wide range of community leaders in positions of political stature, respect, and diversity.
3. The goals of the ethics committee are to:
    - Promote the rights of patients.
    - Promote shared decision making between patients and clinicians.
    - Assist the patient and family in coming to consensus when faced with ethical dilemmas.
4. The functions of ethics committees are multifaceted and include:
    - Policy and procedure development.
    - Staff and community education.
    - Consultation and conflict resolution.
        ○ A resource tool in resolving ethical dilemmas.
        ○ Patients and family should be encouraged to participate in addressing ethical dilemmas.
5. Decision making is difficult when there are:
    - A variety of value beliefs held by patients, family members, and caregivers.
    - Alternative choices that offer both good and bad outcomes.
    - Limited resources.
6. The resolution of ethical dilemmas is a perplexing task. Ethics committee member must be prepared to understand the challenge by actively participating in the decision-making process without bias.

TEST YOUR UNDERSTANDING

TERMINOLOGY

circular reasoning
conflict resolution
ethical decision making

health care ethics committee
ethics consultation
partial reasoning

reasoning and decision making

REVIEW QUESTIONS

1. What is the purpose of an ethics committee?

2. Discuss the functions of an ethics committee.

3. Explain the consultative role of the ethics committee.

4. Discuss the educational role of the ethics committee.

5. Discuss the ever-expanding role of ethics committees, including internal operational issues and external influences that affect internal operations.

6. Discuss what ethics members should take into consideration when addressing ethical dilemmas.

NOTES

1. *In re Quinlan*, 355 A.2d 647 (N.J. 1976).

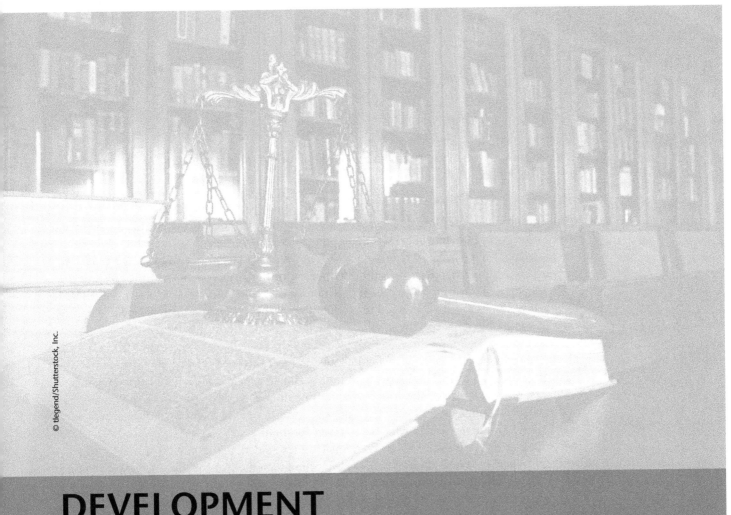

© tiegend/Shutterstock, Inc.

DEVELOPMENT OF LAW

Laws are the very bulwarks of liberty; they define every man's rights, and defend the individual liberties of all men.

–J. G. HOLLAND (1819–1881)

LEARNING OBJECTIVES

Upon completion of this chapter, the reader will be able to:

- Understand the development and sources of law.
- Describe how the government is organized through the three branches of government.
- Explain the principle *separation of powers*.
- Describe what is meant by *conflict of laws*.
- Describe the functions of the Department of Health and Human Resources and its various operating divisions.

In law a man is guilty when he violates the rights of others. In ethics he is guilty if he only thinks of doing so.

—IMMANUEL KANT

It is appropriate here to provide the reader with a background of the law, as it is the law that enables society to uphold what is right and punish those who transgress its intent—to protect the moral fiber upon which this nation was founded. This chapter introduces the reader to the development of American law, the functioning of the legal system, and the roles of the three branches of government in creating, administering, and enforcing the law in the United States. It is important to understand the foundation of the legal system before one can appreciate or comprehend the specific laws and principles relating to health care.

The law is rooted in tradition, culture, customs, and beliefs (e.g., religious influence—the Mosaic law). Laws constantly grow and change to meet the needs of the American culture, a mixture of many cultures. Familiarity with the vocabulary enables one to understand the ideas, concepts, and structure of the law. Laws continually evolve because of the ever-changing political, social, religious, and personal values of society, which is composed of many cultures that become more intertwined with each new generation.

Supreme Court Justice Oliver Wendell Holmes said that the law "is a magic mirror, wherein we see reflected not only our own lives but also the lives of those who went before us."[1] "The government of the United States has been emphatically termed a government of laws, and not of men. It will certainly cease to deserve this high appellation, if the laws furnish no remedy for the violation of a vested right."[2]

Most definitions of *law* define it as a system of principles and processes by which people in a society deal with their disputes and problems, seeking to solve or settle them without resorting to force. Laws are general rules of conduct that are enforced by government, which imposes penalties when prescribed laws are violated.

Laws govern the relationships between private individuals and organizations and between both of these parties and government. *Public law* deals with the relationships between individuals and government; *private law* deals with relationships among individuals. Laws regulate the activities and behaviors of individuals in international, federal, state, local, and municipal settings.

One important segment of public law is criminal law, which prohibits conduct deemed injurious to public order and provides for punishment of those proven to have engaged in such conduct. Public law also consists of countless regulations designed to advance societal objectives by requiring private individuals and organizations to adopt a specified courses of action in their activities and undertakings. The thrust of most public law is to attain what society deems to be valid public goals.

Private law is concerned with the recognition and enforcement of the rights and duties of private individuals and organizations. Tort and contract actions are two basic types of private law. In a tort action, one party asserts that the wrongful conduct of another has caused harm, and the injured party seeks compensation for the harm suffered. Generally, a contract action involves a claim by one party that another party has breached an agreement by failing to fulfill an obligation. Either remuneration or specific performance of the obligation may be sought as a remedy. It is clear that without an organized, clear system of laws that regulate society, anarchy would be the result.

The goal of this chapter is to help caregivers better understand the law and how it affects the difficulties they face while trying to do the right thing by making health care decisions that are both morally and legally acceptable.

SOURCES OF LAW

The basic sources of law are common law, which is derived from judicial decisions; statutory law, which emanates from the federal and state legislatures; and administrative law, prescribed by administrative agencies. In those instances in which written laws are either silent, vague, or contradictory to other laws, the judicial system often is called on to resolve those disputes until such time as appropriate legislative action can be taken to clear up a particular legal issue. In the following sections, the sources of law that formed the foundation of our legal system are discussed.

COMMON LAW

The term *common law* refers to the body of principles that have evolved and expanded from judicial decisions. Many of the legal principles and rules applied today by courts in the United States have their origins in English common law. Common law has its roots in "reason and justice" for all.

The judicial system is necessary because it is impossible to have a law that covers every potential human conflict that might occur in society. It not only serves as a mechanism for reviewing legal disputes that arise in the written law, but it also serves as an effective review mechanism for those issues on which the written law is silent or, in instances of a mixture of issues, involving both written law and common-law decisions.

During the colonial period, English common law began to be applied in the colonies. According to John Dickinson in his *Letters from a Farmer in Pennsylvania* in 1768:[3]

> The common law of England is generally received . . . but our courts *exercise a sovereign authority,* in determining what parts of the common and statute law ought to be extended: For it must be admitted, that the difference of circumstances necessarily requires us, in some cases to *reject* the determination of both. . . . Some of the English rules are adopted, others rejected.

Joseph Story, in an 1829 U.S. Supreme Court decision, wrote, "The common law of England is not to be taken in all respects to be that of America. Our ancestors brought with them its general principles, and claimed it as their birthright. But they brought with them, and adopted only that portion which was applicable to their situation."[4]

> The size of the country and the abundance of its natural resources made impossible the importation of the common law exactly as it had been developed in England. Measured by English standards, America had superabundant land, timber, and mineral wealth. American law had to serve the primary need of the new society to master the vast land areas of the American continent. The decisive facts upon which the law had to be based were the seemingly limitless expanses of land and the wealth and variety of natural resources.[5]

After the Revolution, each state, with the exception of Louisiana, adopted all or part of the existing English common law. Laws were added as needed. Louisiana civil law is based to a great extent on the French and Spanish laws and especially on the Napoleonic Code. As a result, there is no national system of common law in the United States, and common law on specific subjects may differ from state to state.

> Case law court decisions did not easily pass from colony to colony. There were no printed reports to make transfer easy, though in the 18th century some manuscript materials did circulate among lawyers. These could hardly have been very influential. No doubt custom and case law slowly seeped from colony to colony. Travelers and word of mouth spread knowledge of living law. It is hard to say how much; thus it is hard to tell to what degree there was a common legal structure.[6]
>
> Judicial review started to become part of the living law during the decade before the adoption of the federal Constitution. During that time American courts first began to assert the power to rule on the constitutionality of legislative acts and to hold unconstitutional statutes void.[7]

Cases are tried applying common-law principles unless a statute governs. Even though statutory law has affirmed many of the legal rules and principles initially established by the courts, new issues continue to arise, especially in private-law disputes that require decision making according to common-law principles. Common-law actions are initiated mainly to recover money damages and/or possession of real or personal property.

When a higher state court has enunciated a common-law principle, the lower courts within the state where the decision was rendered must follow that principle. A decision in a case that sets forth a new legal principle establishes a precedent. Trial courts or those on equal footing are not bound by the decisions of other trial courts. Also, a principle established in one state does not set precedent for another state. Rather, the rulings in one jurisdiction may be used by the courts of other jurisdictions as guides to the legal analysis of a particular legal problem. Decisions found to be reasonable will be followed.

The position of a court or agency, relative to other courts and agencies, determines the place assigned to its decision in the hierarchy of decisional law. The decisions of the Supreme Court of the United States are highest in the hierarchy of decisional law with respect to federal legal questions. Because of the parties or the legal question involved, most legal controversies do not fall within the scope of the Supreme Court's decision-making responsibilities. On questions of purely state concern—such as the interpretation of a state statute that raises no issues under the U.S. Constitution or federal law—the highest court in the state has the final word on proper interpretation. The following are explanations of some of the more important common-law principles:

- *Precedent*: A precedent is a judicial decision that can be used as a standard in subsequent similar cases. A precedent is set when a court decision is rendered that serves as a rule for future guidance when deciding similar cases.
- *Res judicata*: In common law, the term res judicata—which means "the thing is decided"— refers to that which has been previously acted on or decided by the courts. According to *Black's Law Dictionary*, it is a rule where "a final judgment rendered by a court of competent jurisdiction on the merits is conclusive as to the rights of the parties and their privies,

and, as to them, constitutes an absolute bar to subsequent action involving the same claim, demand, or cause of action."[8]

- *Stare decisis*: The common-law principle of stare decisis ("let the decision stand") provides that when a decision is rendered in a lawsuit involving a particular set of facts, another lawsuit involving an identical or substantially similar situation is to be resolved in the same manner as the first lawsuit. The resolution of future lawsuits is arrived at by applying the rules and principles of preceding cases. In this manner, courts arrive at comparable rulings. Sometimes, slight factual differences may provide a basis for recognizing distinctions between the precedent and the current case. In some cases, even when such differences are absent, a court may conclude that a particular common-law rule is no longer in accord with the needs of society and may depart from precedent. It should be understood that principles of law are subject to change, whether they originate in statutory or in common law. Common-law principles may be modified, overturned, abrogated, or created by new court decisions in a continuing process of growth and development to reflect changes in social attitudes, public needs, judicial prejudices, or contemporary political thinking.

STATUTORY LAW

Statutory law is written law emanating from federal and state legislative bodies. Although a statute can abolish any rule of common law, it can do so only by stating it in express words. States and local jurisdictions can enact and enforce only laws that do not conflict with federal law. Statutory laws may be declared void by a court; for example, a statute may be found unconstitutional because it does not comply with a state or federal constitution, because it is vague or ambiguous, or in the case of a state law, because it is in conflict with a federal law.

In many cases involving statutory law, the court is called on to interpret how a statute applies to a given set of facts. For example, a statute may state merely that no person may discriminate against another person because of race, creed, color, or gender. A court may then be called on to decide whether certain actions by a person are discriminatory and therefore violate the law.

Constitution of the United States

In civilized life, law floats on a sea of ethics.

—EARL WARREN

The principles and rules of statutory law are set in hierarchical order. The *Constitution of the United States* adopted at the Constitutional Convention in Philadelphia in 1787 is highest in the hierarchy of enacted law. Article VI of the Constitution declares:

This Constitution, and the Laws of the United States which shall be made in Pursuance thereof; and all Treaties made, or which shall be made, under the Authority of the United States, shall be the supreme Law of the Land; and the Judges in every State shall be bound thereby, any Thing in the Constitution or Laws of any State to the Contrary notwithstanding.[9]

The clear import of these words is that the U.S. Constitution, federal law, and federal treaties take precedence over the constitutions and laws of specific states and local jurisdictions. Statutory law may be amended, repealed, or expanded by action of the legislature.

Bill of Rights

The conventions of a number of the states, at the time of adopting the U.S. Constitution, expressed a desire to prevent the abuse of its powers. As a result of this concern, Congress ratified amendments to the Constitution of the United States. The *Bill of Rights,* the first 10 amendments to the constitution, was added to protect the rights of citizens. The amendments included the rights to privacy, equal protection, and freedom of speech and religion.

ADMINISTRATIVE LAW

Administrative law is the extensive body of public law issued by administrative agencies to direct the enacted laws of the federal and state governments. It is the branch of law that controls the administrative operations of government. Congress and state legislative bodies realistically cannot oversee their many laws; therefore, they delegate implementation and administration of the law to an appropriate administrative agency. Health care organizations in particular are inundated with a proliferation of administrative rules and regulations affecting every aspect of their operations.

The Administrative Procedures Act[10] describes the different procedures under which federal administrative agencies must operate.[11] The act prescribes the procedural responsibilities and authority of administrative agencies and provides for legal remedies for those wronged by agency actions. The regulatory power exercised by administrative agencies includes power to license, power of rate setting (e.g., Centers for Medicare and Medicaid Services), and power over business practices (e.g., National Labor Relations Board).

The rules and regulations established by an agency must be administered within the scope of the authority delegated to the agency by Congress. Agency regulations and decisions can be subject to judicial review.

U.S. GOVERNMENT ORGANIZATION

The government of the United States is a national constitutional republic covering 50 states, the nation's capital and its territories (e.g., Puerto Rico, Guam). The federal government is organized into three branches. The legislative, executive, and judicial branches of government are illustrated in **Figure** 1. The powers and duties of the three branches of government are described in the U.S. Constitution.

SEPARATION OF POWERS

A vital concept in the constitutional framework of government on both federal and state levels is the *separation of powers*. Essentially, this principle provides that no one branch of government is clearly dominant over the other two; however, in the exercise of its functions, each may affect and limit the activities, functions, and powers of the others. The concept of *separation of powers*—in effect, a system of checks and balances—is illustrated in the relationships

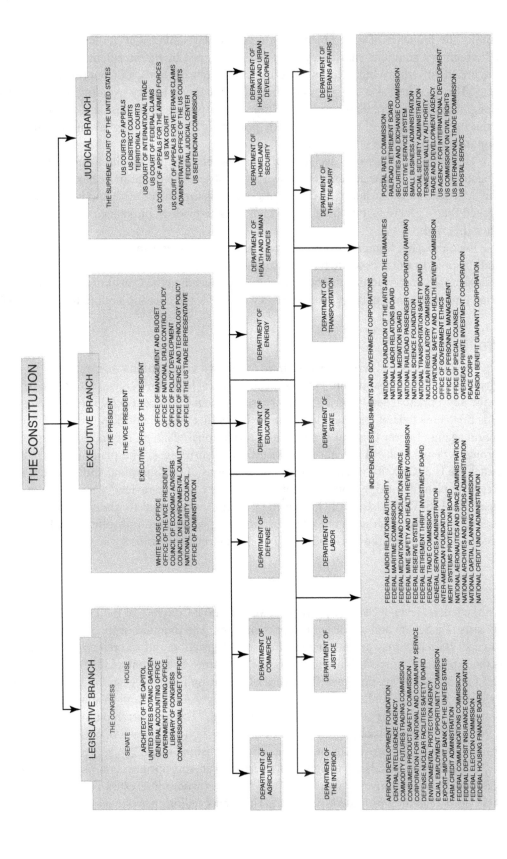

FIGURE 1 U.S. Government Organization.

among the branches of government with regard to legislation. On the federal level, when a bill creating a statute is enacted by Congress and signed by the president, it becomes law. If the president vetoes a bill, it takes a two-thirds vote of each house of Congress to override the veto. The president also can prevent a bill from becoming law by avoiding any action while Congress is in session. This procedure, known as a pocket veto, can temporarily stop a bill from becoming law and may permanently prevent it from becoming law if later sessions of Congress do not act on it favorably.

The Supreme Court may declare a bill that has become law invalid if the law violates the Constitution. "It is also not entirely unworthy of observation, that in declaring what shall be the Supreme law of the land, the Constitution itself is first mentioned; and not the laws of the United States generally, but those only which shall be made in pursuance of the Constitution, have that rank."[12]

Even though a Supreme Court decision is final regarding a specific controversy, Congress and the president may generate new, constitutionally sound legislation to replace a law that has been declared unconstitutional. The procedures for amending the Constitution are complex and often time consuming, but they can serve as a way to offset or override a Supreme Court decision.

CONFLICT OF LAWS

The various states and territories also have there own constitutions that must not be in conflict with the U.S. Constitution. When state and federal laws conflict, resolution can be sought in the appropriate federal court. The legal case, *Dorsten v. Lapeer County General Hospital*,[13] illustrates how federal and state laws can be in conflict. The plaintiff in this case brought an action against Lapeer General Hospital and certain physicians on the medical board alleging wrongful denial of her application for medical staff privileges. The plaintiff asserted claims under the U.S. Code for sex discrimination, violations of the Sherman Antitrust Act, and the like. The plaintiff filed a motion to compel discovery of peer-review reports to support her case. The U.S. District Court held that the plaintiff was entitled to discovery of peer-review reports despite a Michigan state law purporting to establish an absolute privilege barring access to peer-review reports conducted by hospital review boards.

LEGISLATIVE BRANCH

On the federal level, legislative powers are vested in the Congress of the United States, which consists of a Senate and a House of Representatives. The function of the legislative branch is to enact laws that may amend or repeal existing legislation and to create new legislation. It is the legislature's responsibility to determine the nature and extent of the need for new laws and for changes in existing laws. The work of preparing federal legislation is the responsibility of the various committees of both houses of Congress. There are 16 standing committees in the Senate and 19 in the House of Representatives. "The membership of the standing committees of each house is chosen by a vote of the entire body; members of other committees are appointed under the provisions of the measure establishing them."[14]

Legislative proposals are assigned or referred to an appropriate committee for study. The committees conduct investigations and hold hearings where interested persons may present their views regarding proposed legislation. These proceedings provide additional information to assist committee members in their consideration of proposed bills. A bill may be reported out of a committee in its original form or it may be reported out with recommended amendments, or the bill might be allowed to lie in the committee without action. Some bills eventually reach the full legislative body, where, after consideration and debate, they may be approved or rejected.

The U.S. Congress and all state legislatures are bicameral (consisting of two houses), except for the Nebraska legislature, which is unicameral. Both houses in a bicameral legislature must pass identical versions of a legislative proposal before the legislation can be brought to the chief executive.

JUDICIAL BRANCH

As I have said in the past, when government bureaus and agencies go awry, which are adjuncts of the legislative or executive branches, the people flee to the third branch, their courts, for solace and justice.

—JUSTICE J. HENDERSON, SUPREME COURT OF SOUTH DAKOTA[15]

The function of the judicial branch of government is adjudication— resolving disputes in accordance with law. As a practical matter, most disputes or controversies that are covered by legal principles or rules are resolved without resort to the courts.

Alexis de Tocqueville, a foreign observer commenting on the primordial place of the law and the legal profession, stated, "Scarcely any political question arises in the United States that is not resolved, sooner or later, into a judicial question."[16]

> It is emphatically the province and duty of the judicial branch to say what the law is. Those who apply the rule to particular cases must of necessity expound and interpret that rule. If two laws conflict with each other, the courts must decide on the operation of each.
>
> So if a law be in opposition to the constitution; if both the law and the constitution apply to a particular case, so that the court must either decide that case conformably to the law, disregarding the constitution; or conformably to the constitution, disregarding the law; the court must determine which of these conflicting rules govern the case. This is the very essence of judicial duty.
>
> . . . [I]t is apparent, that the framers of the constitution contemplated that instrument, as a rule for the government of courts, as well as of the legislature. Why otherwise does it direct the judges to take such an oath to support it?[17]

State Court System

Each state in the United States provides its own court system, which is created by the state's constitution and/or statutes. The oldest court in the United States, established in 1692, is the Supreme Judicial Court of Massachusetts.[18] Most of the nation's judicial business is reviewed and acted on in state courts. Each state maintains a level of trial courts that have original jurisdiction. This jurisdiction may exclude cases involving claims with damages less than a specified minimum, probate matters (e.g., wills and estates), and workers' compensation.

Different states have designated different names for trial courts (e.g., superior, district, circuit, or supreme courts). Also on the trial court level are minor courts such as city, small claims, and justice of the peace courts. States such as Massachusetts have consolidated their minor courts into a statewide court system.

There is at least one appellate court in each state. Many states have an intermediate appellate court between the trial courts and the court of last resort. Where this intermediate court is present, there is a provision for appeal to it, with further review in all but select cases. Because of this format, the highest appellate tribunal is seen as the final arbiter in cases that are important in themselves or for the particular state's system of jurisprudence.

Federal Court System

The trial court of the federal system is the U.S. District Court. There are 89 district courts in the 50 states (the larger states having more than one district court) and one in the District of Columbia. The Commonwealth of Puerto Rico also has a district court with jurisdiction corresponding to that of district courts in the different states. Generally, only one judge is required to sit and decide a case, although certain cases require up to three judges. The federal district courts hear civil, criminal, admiralty, and bankruptcy cases. The Bankruptcy Amendments and Federal Judgeship Act of 1984[19] provided that the bankruptcy judges for each judicial district shall constitute a unit of the district court to be known as the bankruptcy court.

The U.S. Courts of Appeals (formerly called Circuit Courts of Appeals) are appellate courts for the 11 judicial circuits. Their main purpose is to review cases tried in federal district courts within their respective circuits, but they also possess jurisdiction to review orders of designated administrative agencies and to issue original writs in appropriate cases. These intermediate appellate courts were created to relieve the U.S. Supreme Court of deciding all cases appealed from the federal trial courts.

The Supreme Court is the nation's highest court. It is the only federal court created directly by the Constitution.

> The judicial Power of the United States, shall be vested in one Supreme Court, and in such inferior Courts as the Congress may from time to time ordain and establish. The Judges, both of the supreme and inferior Courts, shall hold their Offices during good Behaviour, and shall, at stated Times, receive for their Services a Compensation, which shall not be diminished during their Continuance in Office.[20]

Eight associate justices and one chief justice sit on the Supreme Court. The court has limited original jurisdiction over the lower federal courts and the highest state courts. In a few situations, an appeal will go directly from a federal or state court to the Supreme Court, but in most cases today, review must be sought through the discretionary writ of certiorari, an appeal petition. In addition to the aforementioned courts, special federal courts have jurisdiction over particular subject matters. The U.S. Court of Claims has jurisdiction over certain claims against the government. The U.S. Court of Appeals for the Federal Circuit has appellate jurisdiction over certain customs and patent matters. The U.S. Customs Court reviews certain administrative decisions by customs officials. Also, there is a U.S. Tax Court and a U.S. Court of Military Appeals.

The primary function of the executive branch of government on the federal and state level is to administer and enforce the law. The chief executive, either the President of the United States or the governor of a state, also has a role in the creation of law through the power to approve or veto legislative proposals.

The U.S. Constitution provides that "the executive Power shall be vested in a President of the United States of America. He shall hold his Office during the Term of four Years . . . together with the Vice President, chosen for the same Term."[21] The president serves as the administrative head of the executive branch of the federal government, which includes 15 executive departments, as well as a variety of agencies, both temporary and permanent.

The Cabinet, a creation of custom and tradition dating back to George Washington's administration, functions at the pleasure of the president. Its purpose is to advise the president on any subject on which he requests information (pursuant to Article II, section 2, of the Constitution).

The Cabinet is composed of the 15 executive departments.[22] Each department is responsible for a different area of public affairs, and each enforces the law within its area of responsibility. For example, the Department of Health and Human Services (DHHS) administers much of the federal health law enacted by Congress. Most state executive branches also are organized on a departmental basis. These departments administer and enforce state law concerning public affairs.

On a state level, the governor serves as the chief executive officer. The responsibilities of a state governor are provided for in the state's constitution. The Massachusetts State Constitution, for example, describes the responsibilities of the governor as follows:[23]

- To present an annual budget to the state legislature
- To recommend new legislation
- To veto legislation
- To appoint and remove department heads
- To appoint judicial officers
- To act as commander-in-chief of the state's military forces (the Massachusetts National Guard)

DEPARTMENT OF HEALTH AND HUMAN SERVICES

The Department of Health and Human Services (DHHS), a cabinet-level department of the executive branch of the federal government (**Figure 2**) responsible for developing and implementing appropriate administrative regulations for carrying out national health and human services policy objectives. It is also the main source of regulations affecting the health care industry. The secretary of the DHHS, serving as the department's administrative head, advises the president with regard to health, welfare, and income security plans, policies, and programs. The DHHS also is responsible for many health programs designed through its operating divisions and agencies to meet the health needs of the people.[24]

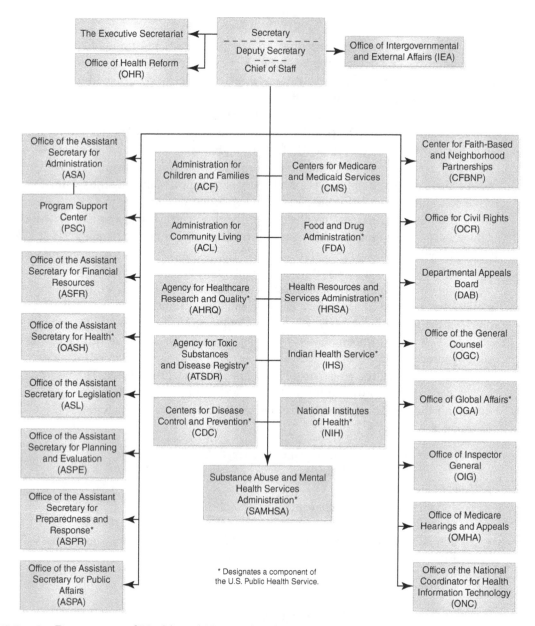

FIGURE 2 Department of Health and Human Services

CENTERS FOR MEDICARE AND MEDICAID SERVICES

The Centers for Medicare and Medicaid Services (CMS), formerly the Health Care Financing Administration, was created to combine under one administration the oversight of the Medicare program, the federal portion of the Medicaid program, the State Children's Health Insurance Program, and related quality-assurance activities.

Medicare is a federally sponsored health insurance program for persons older than 65 and certain disabled persons. It has two complementary parts: Medicare Part A helps cover the costs of inpatient hospital care and, with qualifying preadmission criteria, skilled nursing facility care, home health care, and hospice care. Medicare Part B helps pay for physicians' services and outpatient hospital services. It is funded through Social Security contributions (Federal Insurance Contributions Act payroll taxes), premiums, and general revenue. The program is administered through private contractors, referred to as intermediaries, under Part A and carriers under Part B. The financing of the Medicare program has received much attention by Congress because of its rapidly rising costs.

Medicaid, Title XIX of the Social Security Act Amendments of 1965, is a government program administered by the states that provides medical services (both institutional and outpatient) to the medically needy. Federal grants, in the form of matching funds, are issued to those states with qualifying Medicaid programs. In other words, Medicaid is jointly sponsored and financed by the federal government and several states. Medical care for needy persons of all ages is provided under the definition of need established by each state. Each state has set its own criteria for determining eligibility for services under its Medicaid program.

PUBLIC HEALTH SERVICE

The Public Health Service (PHS) is responsible for the protection of the nation's physical and mental health. The PHS accomplishes its mission by coordinating with the states in setting and implementing national health policy and pursuing effective intergovernmental relations; generating and upholding cooperative international health-related agreements, policies, and programs; conducting medical and biomedical research; sponsoring and administering programs for the development of health resources, the prevention and control of diseases, and alcohol and drug abuse; providing resources and expertise to the states and other public and private institutions in the planning, direction, and delivery of physical and mental health care services; and enforcing laws to ensure drug safety and protection from impure and unsafe foods, cosmetics, medical devices, and radiation-producing objects. Within the PHS are smaller agencies that are responsible for carrying out the purpose of the division and DHHS. The PHS is composed of the offices and agencies described next.

National Institutes of Health

The National Institutes of Health (NIH) is the principal federal biomedical research agency. It is responsible for conducting, supporting, and promoting biomedical research.

Centers for Disease Control and Prevention

The Centers for Disease Control and Prevention (CDC) is recognized as the lead federal agency for protecting the health and safety of people at home and abroad, providing credible information to enhance health decisions, and promoting health. The CDC serves as the national focus for developing and applying disease prevention and control, environmental health, and health promotion and education activities.

Food and Drug Administration

The Food and Drug Administration (FDA) supervises and controls the introduction of drugs, foods, cosmetics, and medical devices into the marketplace and protects society from impure and hazardous items. Although the intention of the FDA is to do good, as noted in the following news clipping, ethical conflicts can arise and be detrimental to the good intent of the agency.

Long Waits for Generics

Brand-name drug makers already pay hefty user fees to help speed their applications through the FDA. That money is expected to provide about a third of the agency's budget this year.

In general, we oppose user fees that allow a regulated industry to fund the regulators. A government agency can become dependent on the companies it's supposed to objectively regulate, which can influence decisions. In a 2006 survey . . . many FDA employees said they felt pressured to hastily and perhaps improperly approve user-fee drugs. And at least one felt the agency viewed industry, not the American public, as its client.

Jim Guest, Consumer Reports, *November 2010*

Discussion

1. Identify and describe the ethical issues of the FDA's funding practice.
2. Do you see any conflict in allowing private for-profit and not-for-profit hospital accreditation programs accredit hospitals on behalf of Medicare, noting that the hospitals pay the accrediting organization to conduct such surveys? Discuss your answer.

Substance Abuse and Mental Health Services Administration

The agency's mission is to reduce the impact of substance abuse and mental illness on America's communities.

Health Resources and Services Administration (HRSA)

The primary federal agency for improving access to health care services for people who are uninsured, isolated, or medically vulnerable. Its mission is to improve health and achieve health equity through access to quality services, a skilled health workforce, and innovative programs. HRSA takes a comprehensive approach to addressing HIV/AIDS with activities taking place across multiple bureaus and offices designed to deliver care to people living with HIV or AIDS, expand and strengthen the HIV care workforce, and improve access to and the quality of HIV care and treatment.

Agency for Healthcare Research and Quality

The Agency for Healthcare Research and Quality (AHRQ) provides evidence-based information on health care outcomes, quality, cost, use, and access. Information from AHRQ's research helps people make more informed decisions and improve the quality of health care services.

Agency for Toxic Substances and Disease Registry

The mission of the Agency for Toxic Substances and Disease Registry (ATSDR) is to prevent or mitigate harmful exposures and related disease by applying science, taking responsive action, and providing trustworthy health information.

Indian Health Service

Indian Health Service provides a comprehensive health service delivery system for approximately 2 million American Indians and Alaska Natives (AI/AN) who belong to 566 federally recognized tribes in 35 states.

CHAPTER REVIEW

1. A law is a general rule of conduct that is enforced by the government. When a law is violated, the government imposes a penalty.
   - *Public law* deals with the relationships between individuals and the government. Criminal law is a segment of public law.
   - *Private law* deals with relationships among individuals. Two types of private laws are tort and contract actions.
2. *Common law*
   - U.S. common law has as its roots in the English common-law system.
     - The first English royal court was established in the year 1178. There were few written laws at the time, and a collection of principles evolved from the decisions of the court. These principles, known as *common law*, were used to decide subsequent cases.
   - During the colonial period, the United States based its law on English common law, but states had the authority to modify their legal systems.
   - Lower courts must follow common-law principles established in a higher state court.
   - Trial courts or those otherwise on equal footing are not bound by the decisions of other trial courts.
   - A principle of law set in one state does not set precedent for another state.
   - Common-law principles can be modified, overturned, abrogated, or created by new court decisions.
3. *Statutory law* is written law that emanates from legislative bodies.
   - The Constitution is the highest level of enacted law.
   - Statutory law can be amended, repealed, or expanded by the legislature.
4. *Administrative law*
   - Public law issued by administrative agencies to administer the enacted laws of the federal and state governments.
   - Administrative agencies implement and administer the administrative law.
   - Rules and regulations established by an agency must be administered within the scope of the authority delegated by Congress.

5. Government organization
   - Three branches of government
     - *Legislative branch*, composed of the House of Representatives and the Senate, both enacts laws that can amend or repeal existing legislation and creates new legislation.
     - *Judicial branch* resolves disputes in accordance with the law.
     - Executive branch administers and enforces the law.
     - *Separation of powers* provides that no one branch of the government will be dominant over the other two.
     - States and local jurisdictions can enact and enforce only those laws that do not *conflict* with federal laws.
     - When state and federal laws conflict, resolution can be sought in an appropriate federal court.
6. The DHHS develops and implements administrative regulations for carrying out national health and human services policy objectives.
   - DHSS is the main source of regulations that affect the health care industry. Operating divisions of DHHS include the:
     - Centers for Medicare and Medicaid Services
     - Public Health Service
     - National Institutes of Health
     - Centers for Disease Control and Prevention
     - Food and Drug Administration
     - Substance Abuse and Mental Health Services Administration
     - Health Resources and Services Administration
     - Agency for Healthcare Research and Quality
     - Agency for Toxic Substances and Disease Registry
     - Indian Health Service

TEST YOUR UNDERSTANDING

TERMINOLOGY

administrative law
Bill of Rights
common law
Constitution of the United
   States

law
Medicare
precedent
private law
public law

res judicata
separation of powers
stare decisis
statutory law

REVIEW QUESTIONS

1. Define the term *law* and describe the sources from which law is derived.

2. Describe and contrast the legal terms *res judicata* and *stare decisis*.

3. Describe the function of each branch of government.

4. What is the meaning of separation of powers?

5. What is the function of an administrative agency?

6. Describe the various operating divisions and agencies within the DHHS.

NOTES

1. B. Schwartz, *The Law in America* 1 (1974).
2. *Marbury v. Madison,* 5 U.S. (Cranch) 137, 163 (1803).
3. Schwartz, supra note 1, at 29.
4. *Id.*
5. *Id.* at 30–31.
6. L. Friedman, *A History of American Law* 92 (1985).
7. Schwartz, supra note 1, at 51.
8. *Black's Law Dictionary* 1305 (6th. ed. 1990).
9. U.S. Const. art. VI, A4 1, cl. 2.
10. 5 U.S.C.S. A4A4 500–576 (Law. Co-op. 1989).
11. An "agency means each authority of the Government of the United States . . . but does not include (A) the Congress; the Courts of the United States . . ." 5 U.S.C.S. A4 551(1) (Law. Co-op. 1989).
12. *Marbury v. Madison,* 5 U.S. (Cranch) 137, 180 (1803).
13. 88 F.R.D. 583 (E.D. Mich. 1980).
14. Office of the Federal Register, National Archives and Records Administration, The United States Government Manual 2000/2001 29 (2000) [hereinafter Manual].
15. *Heritage of Yankton, Inc. v. South Dakota Dep't of Health*, 432 N.W.2d 68, 77 (S.D. 1988).
16. Schwartz, supra note 1, at 15.
17. *Marbury v. Madison,* 5 U.S. (Cranch) 137, 177–180 (1803).
18. Levitan, supra note 46, at 32.
19. 28 U.S.C. A4 151.
20. U.S. Const. art. III, A4 1.
21. U.S. Const. art. II, A41, cl. 1.
22. http://dir.yahoo.com/Government/U_S__Government/Executive_Branch/Departments_and_Agencies/.
23. D. Levitan, Your Massachusetts Government 14 (10th ed. 1984).
24. http://www.hhs.gov/about/foa/opdivs/.

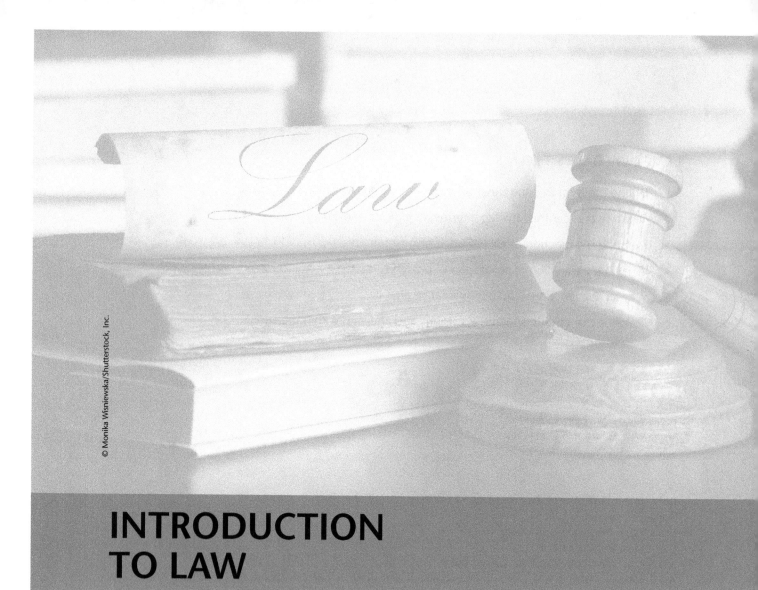

INTRODUCTION TO LAW

Every instance of a man's suffering the penalty of the law, is an instance of the failure of that penalty in effecting its purpose, which is to deter from transgression.

—WHATELY

LEARNING OBJECTIVES

Upon completion of this chapter, the reader will be able to:

- Understand the meaning and objectives of tort law.
- Define negligence and understand the distinction and similarity between negligence and malpractice.
- Explain how the commission and omission of an act differ.
- Explain the elements necessary to prove a negligence case.
- Describe the importance of foreseeability in a negligence case.

- Describe what an intentional tort is and discuss several examples of intentional torts and how they might apply in various health care settings.
- Explain what a crime is and how various crimes are not so uncommon in the health care setting.
- Explain the various elements of a contract.
- Describe the pretrial procedures and the process of a trial.

INTRODUCTION

Laws are enacted to regulate human behavior for the benefit of society. They are designed to prevent harm to others while protecting the rights of individuals. In the law we are taught that we have a duty to care and that if we breach that duty and someone is injured as a result of that breach, there will be a penalty to pay, which could be financial loss, loss of license, and/or jail time to be served. This chapter introduces the reader to tort law, criminal law, contract law, and trial procedures. These are the areas of law that most often affect providers and patients.

TORT LAW

A *tort* is a civil wrong, other than a breach of contract, committed against a person or property (real or personal) for which a court provides a remedy in the form of an action for damages. Tort actions touch an individual on both a personal and a professional level, which is why those involved in the health care field should be armed with the knowledge necessary for them to be aware of their rights and responsibilities.

The objectives of tort law are as follows: preservation of peace (between individuals by providing a substitute for retaliation); culpability (to find fault for wrongdoing); deterrence (to discourage the wrongdoer [tort-feasor] from committing future torts); and compensation (to indemnify the injured person[s] of wrongdoing).

NEGLIGENCE

Negligence is a tort, a civil or personal wrong. It is the unintentional commission or omission of an act that a reasonably prudent person would or would not perform under given circumstances. Negligence is a form of conduct caused by heedlessness or carelessness that constitutes a departure from the standard of care generally imposed on reasonable members of society. It can occur where a person has considered the consequences of an act and has exercised his or her best possible judgment, fails to guard against a risk that should be appreciated, and engages in certain behavior expected to involve unreasonable danger to others.

Commission of an act includes, for example, the following acts:

- administering the wrong medication
- administering the wrong dosage of a medication
- administering a medication to the wrong patient
- performing a surgical procedure without patient consent

- performing a surgical procedure on the wrong patient
- surgically removing the wrong body part
- failing to assess and reassess a patient's nutritional needs

Omission of an act includes the following:

- failure to administer medication[s]
- failure to order required diagnostic tests per established hospital protocol for head trauma (e.g., CT scan)
- failure to follow up on abnormal test results
- failure to perform a "time-out" to ensure the correct surgical procedure is being conducted on the correct patient at the correct site

Malpractice is the negligence or carelessness of a professional person (e.g., a nurse, pharmacist, physician, or accountant). Criminal negligence is the reckless disregard for the safety of another (e.g., willful indifference to an injury that could follow an act).

Negligence generally involves one of the following acts:

- *malfeasance* (execution of an unlawful or improper act [e.g., performing an abortion in the third trimester when such is prohibited by state law]);
- *misfeasance* (improper performance of an act, resulting in injury to another [e.g., wrong site surgery]), and
- *nonfeasance* (failure to act, when there is a duty to act as a reasonably prudent person would in similar circumstances [e.g., failing to order diagnostic tests or prescribe medications that should have been ordered or prescribed under the circumstances]).

ELEMENTS OF NEGLIGENCE

The four elements that must be present for a plaintiff to recover damages caused by negligence are (1) duty to care, (2) breach of duty, (3) injury, and (4) causation. All four elements must be present in order for a plaintiff to recover for damages suffered as a result of a negligent act.

Duty to Care

The first requirement in establishing negligence is that the plaintiff must prove the existence of a legal relationship between himself or herself and the defendant. *Duty* is defined as a legal obligation of care, performance, or observance imposed on one to safeguard the rights of others. This duty may arise from a special relationship such as that between a physician and a patient. The existence of this relationship implies that a physician–patient relationship was in effect at the time an alleged injury occurred. The duty to care can arise from a simple telephone conversation or out of a physician's voluntary act of assuming the care of a patient. Duty also can be established by statute or contract between the plaintiff and the defendant.

Duty to care is depicted in **Figure 1**, for example, where the pharmacy manager of General Hospital's pharmacy, prior to leaving work for the day, assigns responsibility to a recently hired pharmacist behind the counter, telling her, "You're in charge of the pharmacy, which includes the IV admixture room. Your duties and responsibilities are those as described in

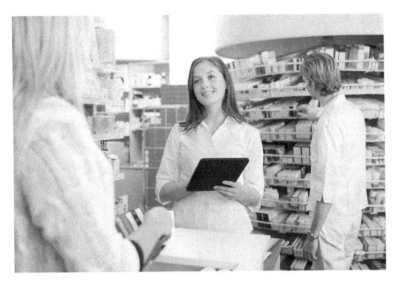

FIGURE 1 Duty to Care (© Tyler Olsen/Shutterstock, Inc.)

the pharmacy department policy and procedure manual. I will be leaving in an hour, so you should review them before I leave. If you have any questions after I leave, you can reach me on my cell phone."

This assignment established a duty on the part of the pharmacist to adhere to the policies and procedures in the department manual.

Standard of Care Expected

A duty of care carries with it a corresponding responsibility not only to provide care but also to provide it in an acceptable manner. Because of this obligation to conform to a recognized *standard of care*, the plaintiff must show that the defendant failed to meet the required standard of care. Just because an injury is suffered is not sufficient for imposing liability without proof that the defendant deviated from the practice of competent members of his or her profession.

The standard of care describes what conduct is expected of an individual in a given situation. The standard of care that must be exercised is that which a reasonably prudent person would adhere to when acting under the same or similar circumstances. A nurse, for example, who assumes the care of a patient has the duty to exercise that degree of skill, care, and knowledge ordinarily possessed and exercised by other nurses. If a patient's injury is the result of a negligent act of a physician, the standard of care required would be that degree of skill, care, and knowledge ordinarily possessed and exercised by other physicians. For an injury involving a specific specialty, the treating physician nurse, pharmacist, etc., would be expected to treat the patient in that same manner as the specialist in the field in which the caregiver is practicing.

The *reasonably prudent person* concept describes a nonexistent, hypothetical person who is put forward as the community ideal of what would be considered reasonable behavior. It is a measuring stick representing the conduct of the average person in the community under the circumstances facing the defendant at the time of the alleged negligence. The reasonableness of conduct is judged in light of the circumstances apparent at the time of injury and by reference to different characteristics of the actor (e.g., age, gender, physical condition, education, knowledge, training, and mental capacity).

The actual performance of an individual in a given situation will be measured against what a reasonably prudent person would or would not have done. Deviation from the standard of care will constitute negligence if there are resulting damages.

Ethicists and the Standard of Care

The standard of care required by a caregiver can in part be influenced by the principles of ethics that apply to the caregiver's profession. For example, a decision concerning termination of resuscitation efforts is an area in which the standard of care includes an ethical component. Under these circumstances, it occasionally may be appropriate for a medical expert to testify about the ethical aspects underlying the professional standard of care. In *Neade v. Portes,* 710 N.E.2d 418 (Ill. App. Ct. 1999), a physician expert was allowed to base an opinion on the breach of the standard of care based on violation of an ethical standard established by the American Medical Association.

Some duties are created by statute, which occurs when a statute specifies a particular standard that must be met. Many such standards are created by administrative agencies under the provisions of a statute. For liability to be established, based on a defendant's failure to follow the standard of care outlined by statute, the following elements must be present:

1. the defendant must have been within the specified class of persons outlined in the statute;
2. the plaintiff must have been injured in a way that the statute was designed to prevent; and
3. the plaintiff must show that the injury would not have occurred if the statute had not been violated.

Duty to Provide Timely Care

The surviving parents in *Hastings v. Baton Rouge Hospital*[1] brought a medical malpractice action for the wrongful death of their 19-year-old son. The action was brought against the hospital; the emergency department physician, Dr. Gerdes; and the thoracic surgeon on call, Dr. McCool. The patient had been brought to the emergency department at 11:56 p.m. because of two stab wounds and weak vital signs. Gerdes decided that a thoracotomy had to be performed. He was not qualified to perform the surgery and called McCool, who was on call that evening for thoracic surgery. Gerdes described the patient's condition, indicating that he had been stabbed in a major blood vessel. At trial, McCool claimed that he did not recall Gerdes saying that a major blood vessel could be involved. McCool asked Gerdes to transfer the patient to the Earl K. Long Hospital. Gerdes said, "I can't transfer this patient." McCool replied, "No. Transfer him." Kelly, an emergency department nurse on duty, was not comfortable with the decision to transfer the patient and offered to accompany him in the ambulance. Gerdes reexamined the patient, who exhibited marginal vital signs, was restless, and was draining blood from his chest.

The ambulance service was called at 1:03 a.m., and by 1:30 a.m. the patient had been placed in the ambulance for transfer. The patient began to fight wildly. The chest tube came out, and the bleeding increased. An attempt to revive him from a cardiac arrest was futile, and the patient died after having been moved back to the emergency department. The patient virtually bled to death.

The duty to care in this case cannot be reasonably disputed. Louisiana, by statute, imposes a duty on hospitals licensed in Louisiana to make emergency services available to all persons residing in the state regardless of insurance coverage or economic status. The hospital's own bylaws provided that no patient should be transferred without due consideration for his or her condition. Hospitals are required to stabilize the patient prior to transfer. In this case, there was a surgeon who was available to treat this patient. McCool decided to practice telephone medicine and made the unfortunate decision to transfer the patient, which resulted in risking the life of an unstable patient, resulting in his death.

Duty to Hire Competent Staff

Texas courts recognize that an employer has a duty to hire competent employees, especially if they are engaged in an occupation that could be hazardous to life and limb and requires skilled or experienced persons. For example, the appellant in *Deerings West Nursing Center v. Scott*[2] was found to have negligently hired an incompetent employee who it knew or should have known was incompetent, thereby causing unreasonable risk of harm to others.

Hopper testified that he was hired sight unseen over the telephone by the Deerings director of nursing. Even though the following day he went to the nursing facility to complete an application, he still maintained that he was hired over the phone. In his application, he falsely stated that he was a Texas-licensed vocational nurse (LVN). Additionally, he claimed that he had never been convicted of a crime. In reality, he had been previously employed by a bar, was not an LVN, had committed more than 56 criminal offenses of theft, and was on probation at the time of his testimony.

The duty of care in this case is clear. The appellant violated the very purpose of Texas licensing statutes by failing to validate whether or not Hopper had a current LVN license. The appellant then placed him in a position of authority and not only allowed him to dispense drugs but also made him a shift supervisor. This negligence eventually resulted in an inexcusable assault on an older woman.

Breach of Duty

After a duty to care has been established, the plaintiff must demonstrate that the defendant breached that duty by failing to comply with the accepted standard of care required. *Breach of duty*, the second element that must be present for a plaintiff to establish negligence, is the failure to conform to or the departure from a required obligation owed to a person. The obligation to perform according to a standard of care may encompass either performing or refraining from performing a particular act.

The court in *Hastings v. Baton Rouge Hospital*,[3] discussed earlier, found a severe breach of duty. Hospital regulations provide that when a physician cannot be reached or refuses a call, the chief of service is to be notified so that another physician can be obtained. This was not done. It is not necessary to prove that a patient would have survived if proper treatment

FIGURE   2   Breach of Duty (© Minerva Studio/Shutterstock, Inc.)

had been administered, only that the patient would have had a chance of survival. As a result of Dr. Gerdes' failure to make arrangements for another physician and Dr. McCool's failure to perform the necessary surgery, the patient had no chance of survival. The duty to provide for appropriate care under the circumstances was breached.

Breach of duty is illustrated in **Figure   2**, where the intravenous (IV) admixture room pharmacist checking the work of a pharmacy technician, fails to follow-up on his concern as to whether or not the medication in the IV bag had been diluted in the correct dosage. Failure to follow-up established a breach of duty.

Injury/Actual Damages

A defendant may be negligent and not incur liability if there is no injury or actual damages suffered by the plaintiff, the third element necessary to establish negligence. *Injury* includes more than physical harm. Without harm or injury, there is no liability. Injury is not limited to physical harm but includes loss of income or reputation and compensation for pain and suffering. The mere occurrence of an injury does not necessarily establish negligence for which the law imposes liability because the injury might be the result of an unavoidable accident or act of God, such as a lighting strike that is the direct cause of an injury.

The third element of negligence—injury—is portrayed in **Figure   3** where the death of an infant in General Hospital's nursery occurred 3 hours following administration of an improper dose of an IV medication.

In *Hastings*, the patient's death was a direct result of the breach of duty.

Causation/Proximate Cause

Causation, the fourth element necessary to establish negligence, requires that there be a reasonable, close, and causal connection between the defendant's negligent conduct and the resulting damages suffered by the plaintiff. In other words, the defendant's negligence must

FIGURE   3   Injury Established (© Paul Hakimata Photography/Shutterstock, Inc.)

be a substantial factor causing the injury. *Proximate cause* is a term referring to the relationship between a breached duty and the injury. The breach of duty must be the proximate cause of the resulting injury.

Figure   4 portrays a defense attorney successfully arguing that the cause of death of an infant in General Hospital's nursery was due to the failure of the pharmacist to properly verify that the IV medication had been properly diluted and labeled by the pharmacy technician in the hospital's pharmacy. The IV solution, containing the medication, was delivered to the nursery, where the nurse checked the label, unaware that the medication left the pharmacy mislabeled and improperly diluted, administered it to the infant who subsequently died. Thus establishing the proximate cause of the injury, the fourth element of negligence—causation.

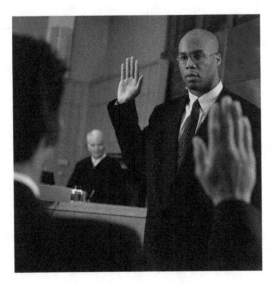

FIGURE   4   Causation Determined (© Corbis/age fotostock)

Causation in the *Hastings*[4] case was well established. In the ordinary course of events, a person does not bleed to death in a hospital emergency department over a 2-hour period without some surgical intervention to save the patient's life.

Foreseeability and Anticipation of Harm

Foreseeability is the reasonable anticipation that harm or injury is likely to result from an act or an omission of an act. As an aspect of causation in a negligence case, the test for foreseeability is whether a person of ordinary prudence and intelligence should have anticipated the danger to others caused by his or her negligent act. "The test is not what the wrongdoer believed would occur; it is whether he or she ought reasonably to have foreseen that the event in question, or some similar event, would occur."[5]

There is no expectation that a person can guard against events that cannot reasonably be foreseen. Foreseeability involves guarding against that which is probable and likely to happen, not against that which is only remotely and slightly possible. In *Hastings*, it was highly probable that the patient would die if the bleeding was not stopped. "The broad test of negligence is what a reasonably prudent person would foresee and would do in the light of this foresight under the circumstances."[6]

SUMMARY CASE

CASE: CURSORY EXAMS ARE RISKY

All of the elements necessary to establish negligence were well established in *Niles v. City of San Rafael*.[7] On June 26, 1973, at approximately 3:30 p.m., Kelly Niles, a young boy, got into an argument with another boy on the ball field. He was hit on the right side of his head. Kelly rode home on his bicycle and waited for his father, who was to pick him up for the weekend. At approximately 5:00 p.m., Kelly's father arrived. By the time they arrived in San Francisco, Kelly appeared to be in a great deal of pain. His father then decided to take him to Mount Zion Hospital, which was a short distance away. He arrived at the hospital emergency department at approximately 5:45 p.m.. On admission to the emergency department, Kelly was taken to a treatment room by a registered nurse. The nurse obtained a history of the injury and took Kelly's pulse and blood pressure. During his stay in the emergency department, he was irritable, vomited several times, and complained that his head hurt. An intern who had seen Kelly wrote "pale, diaphoretic, and groggy" on Kelly's chart. Skull X-rays were ordered and found to be negative except for soft tissue swelling that was not noted until later. The intern then decided to admit Kelly. A second-year resident was called, and he agreed with the intern's decision. An admitting clerk called the intern and indicated that Kelly had to be admitted by an attending physician. The resident went as far as to write "admit" on the chart and later crossed it out. A pediatrician who was in the emergency department at the time was asked to look at Kelly. The pediatrician was also the paid director of the Mount Zion Pediatric Out-Patient Clinic. The pediatrician asked Kelly a few questions and then decided to send him home. The physician could not recall what instructions he gave Kelly's father, but he did give the father his business card.

The pediatrician could not recall giving the father a copy of the emergency department's *Head Injury Instructions*, an information sheet that had been prepared for distribution to patients with head injuries. The sheet explained that patients should return to the emergency department should any of the following signs appear: a large, soft lump on the head, unusual drowsiness (cannot be awakened), forceful or repeated vomiting, a fit or convulsion (jerking or spells), clumsy walking, bad headache, and/or one pupil larger than the other.

Kelly was taken back to his father's apartment at about 7:00 p.m.. A psychiatrist friend stopped by and examined Kelly. He noted that one pupil was larger than the other. Kelly was taken back to the emergency department. A physician on duty noted an epidural hematoma during his examination and ordered that a neurosurgeon be called.

Today, Kelly can move only his eyes and neck. A lawsuit was brought against the hospital and pediatrician for $5 million. The city of San Rafael and public school district were included in the lawsuit as defendants. Expert testimony by two neurosurgeons during the trial indicated that Kelly's chances of recovery would have been very good if he had been admitted promptly. This testimony placed the proximate cause of the injury with the hospital. The final judgment was $4 million against the medical defendants, $2.5 million for compensatory damages, and another $1.5 million for pain and suffering.

Ethical and Legal Issues

The many lessons for discussion in *Niles v. City of San Rafael* include the following:

1. An organization can improve the quality of patient care rendered in the facility by establishing and adhering to policies, procedures, and protocols that facilitate the delivery of high-quality care across all disciplines.
2. The provision of high-quality health care requires collaboration across disciplines.
3. A physician must conduct a thorough and responsible examination and order the appropriate tests for each patient, evaluating the results of those tests before discharging the patient.
4. A patient's vital signs must be monitored closely and documented in the medical record. Corrective measures must be taken when a patient's medical condition signals a medical problem.
5. A complete review of a patient's medical record must be accomplished before discharging a patient.
6. Review of the record must include review of test results, nurses' notes, residents' and interns' notes, and the notes of any other physician or consultant who may have attended the patient.
7. Failure to fully review a patient's record can lead to an erroneous diagnosis, and the premature dismissal of a case can result in liability for both the organization and physician.

Duty to care involves a responsibility to do the "right thing." The right thing is based on an acceptable standard of care. If breaching the standard causes harm to the patient, not only is there a legal issue, there are ethical principles that have been violated. Nonmaleficence, for example, requires caregivers to avoid causing harm to patients.

INTENTIONAL TORTS

An *intentional tort* is one that is committed deliberately. Proof of intent is based on the premise that the defendant intended the harmful consequences of his or her behavior. An individual's reason to cause harm is irrelevant and does not protect him or her from responsibility for the damages suffered as the result of an intentional act.

Assault and Battery

It has long been recognized by law that a person possesses a right to be free from aggression and the threat of actual aggression against one's person. The right to expect others to respect the integrity of one's body has roots in both common and statutory law. The distinguishing feature between assault and battery is that *assault* effectuates an infringement on the mental security or tranquility of another, whereas *battery* constitutes a violation of another's physical integrity.

An assault is defined as the deliberate threat, coupled with the apparent present ability to do physical harm to another. No actual contact or damages are necessary. It is the deliberate threat or attempt to injure another or the attempt by one to make bodily contact with another without his or her consent. To commit the tort of assault, the following two conditions must be proven:

1. The person attempting to touch another unlawfully must possess the apparent present ability to commit the battery.
2. The person threatened must be aware of or have actual knowledge of an immediate threat of a battery and must fear it.

A *battery* is the intentional touching of another's person, in a socially impermissible manner, without that person's consent. It is intentional conduct that violates the physical security of another. The receiver of the battery does not have to be aware that a battery has been committed (e.g., a patient who is unconscious and has surgery performed on him or her without consent, either expressed or implied, is the object of a battery). The unwanted touching may give rise to a cause of action for any injuries brought about by the touching. No actual damages need be shown to impose liability.

False Imprisonment

False imprisonment is the unlawful restraint of an individual's personal liberty or the unlawful restraining or confining of an individual. The personal right to move freely and without hindrance is basic to our legal system. Any intentional infringement on this right may constitute false imprisonment. Actual physical force is not necessary to constitute false imprisonment. All that is necessary is that an individual who is physically confined to a given area experience a reasonable fear that force, which may be implied by words, threats, or gestures, will be used to detain the individual or to intimidate him or her without legal justification. Excessive force used to restrain a patient may produce liability for both false imprisonment and battery.

Defamation of Character

Defamation of character involves communications to someone other than the person defamed that tends to hold that person's reputation up to scorn and ridicule.

Slander is the oral form of defamation. For example, in *Eli v. Griggs County Hospital & Nursing Home*,[8] a nurse's aide was terminated as the result of an incident in the hospital dining room in which the aide, in the presence of patients and visitors, cursed at her supervisor and complained that personnel were working short staffed. Given the nature of her employment, such behavior justified her termination on a charge of reported breach of patient- and facility-specific information. No defamation resulted from the entry of such charges in the aide's personnel file because the record established that the charges were true.

Libel is the written form of defamation. Libel can be expressed in the form of signs, photographs, letters, cartoons, and various other forms of written communication. To be an actionable wrong, defamation must be communicated to a third person. Defamatory statements communicated only to the injured party are not grounds for an action. Truth of a statement is a complete defense.

Defamation on its face is actionable without proof of special damages. In certain cases, a court will presume that the words caused injury to the person's reputation. There are four generally recognized exceptions whereby no proof of actual harm to reputation is required to recover damages:

1. accusing someone of a crime
2. accusing someone of having a loathsome disease
3. using words that affect a person's profession or business
4. accusing someone of sexual misconduct

Invasion of Privacy

Invasion of privacy is a wrong that invades the right of a person to personal privacy. Absolute privacy has to be tempered with reality in the care of any patient, and the courts recognize this fact. Disregard for a patient's right to privacy is legally actionable, particularly when patients are unable to protect themselves adequately because of unconsciousness or immobility.

The *right to privacy* is implied in the Constitution. It is recognized as a right to be left alone—the right to be free from unwarranted publicity and exposure to public view, as well as the right to live one's life without having one's name, picture, or private affairs made public against one's will. Health care organizations and professionals may become liable for invasion of privacy if, for example, they divulge information from a patient's medical record to improper sources or if they commit unwarranted intrusions into a patient's personal affairs.

Patients have a right to personal privacy and a right to the confidentiality of their personal and clinical records. The information in a patient's medical record is confidential and should not be disclosed without the patient's permission. Those who come into possession of the most intimate personal information about patients have both a legal and an ethical duty not to reveal confidential communications. The legal duty arises because the law recognizes a right to privacy. An ethical duty is broader because it applies at all times. There are, however, occasions when there is a legal obligation or duty to disclose information. The law requires, for example, the reporting of communicable diseases, gunshot wounds, and the reasonable suspicion of patient abuse.

The intentional or reckless *infliction of mental distress* is characterized by conduct that is so outrageous that it goes beyond the bounds tolerated by a decent society. It is a civil wrong for which a tort-feasor can be held liable for damages. Mental distress includes mental suffering resulting from painful emotions such as grief, public humiliation, despair, shame, and wounded pride. Liability for the wrongful infliction of mental distress may be based on either intentional or negligent misconduct. A plaintiff may recover damages if he or she can show that the defendant intended to inflict mental distress and knew or should have known that his or her actions would give rise to it. Recovery generally is permitted even in the absence of physical harm.

CASE: THE COURT WAS APPALLED

In *Tomcik v. Ohio Dep't of Rehabilitation & Correction*,[9] the plaintiff, Tomcik, was in the custody of the defendant, a penal institution. Pursuant to the defendant's policy of medically evaluating all new inmates, on May 26, 1989, Dr. Evans gave Tomcik a medical examination. He testified that his physical evaluation included an examination of Tomcik's breasts; however, he stated that his examination was very cursory.

The day after her examination, Tomcik examined her own breasts. At that time, she discovered a lump in her right breast, which she characterized as being about the size of a pea. She then sought an additional medical evaluation at the defendant's medical clinic. Testimony indicated that fewer than half of the inmates who sign the clinic list are actually seen by medical personnel the next day. Also, inmates who are not examined on the day for which the list is signed are given no preference in being examined on the following day. In fact, their names are simply deleted from the daily list, and their only recourse is to continually sign the list until they are examined.

The evidence indicated that from May 27 on, Tomcik constantly signed the clinic list and provided the reason she was requesting medical care.

A nurse finally examined Tomcik on June 21. The nurse wrote in her nursing notes that Tomcik had a "moderate large mass in right breast." The nurse recognized that the proper procedure was to measure such a mass, but she testified that this was impossible because no measuring device was available. The missing "measuring device" to which she alluded was a simple ruler. The nurse concluded that Evans, the original doctor who had examined Tomcik, should examine her again.

On June 28, Evans examined Tomcik again. He recorded in the progress notes that she had "a mass on her right wrist. Will send her to hospital and give her Benadryl for allergy she has."[10] Evans meant to write "breast," not "wrist." He again failed to measure the size of the mass on Tomcik's breast.

Tomcik was transferred to the Franklin County Prerelease Center on September 28. On September 30, a nurse there examined Tomcik; the nurse recorded that she had a "golf ball–sized" lump in her right breast. Tomcik was transported to the hospital on October 27, where Dr. Walker treated her. A mammogram indicated that Tomcik's tumor was probably malignant. This diagnosis was confirmed by a biopsy performed on November 9. Tomcik was released from confinement on November 13.

On November 16, Dr. Lidsky, a surgeon employed outside of the penal institution, examined Tomcik. Lidsky noted the existence of the lump in her breast and determined that the size of the mass was approximately 4 to 5 centimeters and somewhat fixed. He performed a modified radical mastectomy on the plaintiff's right breast, removing nearly the entire breast.

Tomcik alleged that it was the delay in her examination that ultimately led to the removal of her right breast; had she been seen in a more timely manner, much of the breast could have been spared. The defendant, the corrections department, contended that even if its employees were negligent, Tomcik's cancer was so advanced when discovered that it would nevertheless have required removal of her breast.[11]

The Ohio Court of Appeals held that the delay in providing treatment to Tomcik fell below the medically acceptable standard of care. The court was *appalled* that the physician had characterized his evaluation as a medical examination and that what he described as a *cursory breast examination* should be considered medically sufficient. It seemed incredible to the court that a physician would deliberately choose not to take the additional few minutes or seconds to palpate thoroughly the sides of the breasts, which is a standard minimally intrusive cancer detection technique.

Ethical and Legal Issues

1. Do you agree with the court's decision? Discuss your answer.
2. Discuss why the court was appalled.
3. What ethical values were lacking by the caregivers?

CRIMINAL LAW

Laws were made to restrain and punish the wicked; the wise and good do not need them as a guide, but only as a shield against rapine and oppression; they can live civilly and orderly, though there were no law in the world.

—Owen Feltham (1602–1668)

What Went Wrong?

The son of a prominent Boston doctor . . . was on his way to becoming a leading surgeon in his own right when a bizarre blunder interrupted his climb: he left his patient on the operating table so he could cash his paycheck. A series of arrests followed, exposing a life of arrogance, betrayal, and wasted promise . . .

Reproduce from Neil Swidey, "What Went Wrong?" The Boston Globe, March 21, 2004.

Criminal law is society's expression of the limits of acceptable human behavior. A crime is any social harm defined and made punishable by law. The objectives of criminal law are to:

- maintain public order and safety
- protect the individual
- use punishment as a deterrent to crime
- rehabilitate the criminal for return to society

Crimes are generally classified as misdemeanors or felonies. The difference between a misdemeanor and a felony revolves around the severity of the crime committed and the punishment imposed. A *misdemeanor* is an offense punishable by less than 1 year in jail and/or a fine (e.g., petty larceny). A *felony* is a much more serious crime (e.g., rape, murder) and is generally punishable by imprisonment in a state or federal penitentiary for more than 1 year.

Peculiar to health care organizations is the fact that patients are often helpless and at the mercy of others. Health care facilities are far too often places where the morally weak and mentally deficient prey on the physically and sometimes mentally helpless. The very institutions designed to make the public well and feel safe can sometimes provide the setting for criminal conduct.

The topics in this section run counter to the ethics theory of *nonmaleficence*–to do no harm, as well as to the codes of professional ethics. For example, as noted in the grand jury indictment **Figure 5**, Dr. Gosnell snipped the spinal cords of infants delivered alive during abortion procedures. Crimes like his and others against society are not only legal wrongs, they are also ethically wrong.

The U.S. Department of Justice and state and local prosecutors are vigorously pursuing and prosecuting health care organizations and individuals for criminal conduct. Health care fraud, patient abuse, and other such crimes have caused law enforcement agencies to establish a zero-tolerance policy for such acts. This reality requires health care professionals to be observant in their environments and to report suspicious conduct, as appropriate.

CRIMINAL PROCEDURE

Criminal procedure deals with the set of rules governing the series of proceedings through which the government enforces criminal law as provided by municipalities, states, and the federal government, each of which have their own criminal codes that address and define conduct that constitute crimes. The following sections provide an overview of criminal procedure and the process for the prosecution of misdemeanors and felonies.

Arrest

Prosecutions for crimes generally begin with the arrest of a defendant by a police officer or with the filing of a formal action in a court of law and the issuance of an arrest warrant or summons. On arrest, the defendant is taken to the appropriate law enforcement agency for processing, which includes paperwork and fingerprinting. The police also prepare accusatory statements, such as misdemeanor information and felony complaints. Detectives are assigned to cases when necessary to gather evidence, interview persons suspected of committing a crime and witnesses to a crime, and assist in preparing a case for possible trial. After processing has been completed, a person is either detained or released on bond.

IN THE COURT OF COMMON PLEAS

FIRST JUDICIAL DISTRICT OF PENNSYLVANIA

CRIMINAL TRIAL DIVISION

IN RE: MISC. NO. 0009901-2008

COUNTY INVESTIGATING:

GRAND JURY XXIII: C-17

_____

REPORT OF THE GRAND JURY

_____

R. SETH WILLIAMS

District Attorney

This case is about a doctor who killed babies and endangered women. What we mean is that he regularly and illegally delivered live, viable, babies in the third trimester of pregnancy – and then murdered these newborns by severing their spinal cords with scissors. The medical practice by which he carried out this business was a filthy fraud in which he overdosed his patients with dangerous drugs, spread venereal disease among them with infected instruments, perforated their wombs and bowels – and, on at least two occasions, caused their deaths. Over the years, many people came to know that something was going on here. But no one put a stop to it.

There remained, however, a final difficulty. When you perform late-term "abortions" by inducing labor, you get babies. Live, breathing, squirming babies. By 24 weeks, most babies born prematurely will survive if they receive appropriate medical care. But that was not what the Women's Medical Society was about. Gosnell had a simple solution for the unwanted babies he delivered: he killed them. He didn't call it that. He called it "ensuring fetal demise." The way he ensured fetal demise was by sticking scissors into the back of the baby's neck and cutting the spinal cord. He called that "snipping."

❏ ❏ ❏

Gosnell's students parroted his grisly techniques. Massof himself admitted to us that, of the many spinal cords he cut, there were about 100 instances where he did so after seeing a breath or some sign of life. The shocking regularity of killing babies who were born alive, who moved and breathed, as testified to by Gosnell's employees, demonstrates that these murders were intentional and collaborative. In addition to the specific murder charges identified above, **we recommend that Kermit Gosnell, Lynda Williams, Sherry West, Adrienne Moton, and Steven Massof be charged with conspiracy to commit murder.**

❏ ❏ ❏

Section VII: Criminal Charges

Gosnell and his staff showed consistent disregard not only for the health and safety of their patients, but also for the laws of Pennsylvania. After reviewing extensive and compelling evidence of criminal wrongdoing at

FIGURE   5   Report of the Grand Jury

the clinic, the Grand Jury has issued a presentment recommending the prosecution of Gosnell and members of his staff for criminal offenses including:

- Murder of Karnamaya Mongar
- Murders of babies born alive
- Infanticide
- Violations of the Controlled Substances Act
- Hindering, Obstruction, and Tampering
- Perjury
- Illegal late-term abortions
- Violations of the Abortion Control Act
- Violations of the Controlled Substances Act
- Abuse of Corpse
- Theft by Deception
- Conspiracy
- Corrupt Organization
- Corruption of Minors

❑ ❑ ❑

15. The authorities responsible for overseeing, monitoring, or licensing Gosnell or his operation should conduct serious self-assessments to determine why their departments failed to protect the women and babies whose lives were imperiled at Gosnell's clinic. Employees who failed to perform their jobs of protecting the public should be held accountable.

The employees of the state and local health departments and the prosecutors for the Board of Medicine are charged with protecting the public health. Very few that we ran across in this investigation came even close to fulfilling that duty. These people seemed oblivious to the connection between their dereliction and the deaths and injuries that Gosnell inflicted under their watch.[i]

i http://www.phila.gov/districtattorney/pdfs/grandjurywomensmedical.pdf.

FIGURE   5   Report of the Grand Jury (*Continued*)

Arraignment

The arraignment is a formal reading of the accusatory instrument and includes the setting of bail. The accused should appear with counsel or have counsel appointed by the court if he or she cannot afford his or her own. After the charges are read, the defendant pleads guilty or not guilty. A not guilty plea is normally offered on a felony. On a plea of not guilty, the defense attorney and prosecutor make arguments regarding bail. After arraignment of the defendant, the judge sets a date for the defendant to return to court. Between the time of arraignment and the next court date, the defense attorney and the prosecutor confer about the charges and the evidence in the possession of the prosecutor. At that time, the defense will offer any mitigating circumstances that it believes will convince the prosecutor to lessen or drop the charges.

Indictment

A felony complaint or an indictment commences a criminal proceeding. An individual may be tried for a felony after indictment by a grand jury unless the defendant waives presentment to the grand jury and pleads guilty by way of a superior court. Felony cases are presented to a grand jury by a district attorney or an assistant district attorney. The grand jury is presented with the prosecution's evidence, after which the grand jury may indict the target if they find reasonable cause to believe from the evidence presented all the elements of a particular crime are present. The grand jury may request that witnesses be subpoenaed to testify. A defendant may choose to testify and offer information if he or she wishes. Actions of a grand jury are handed up to a judge, after which the defendant is notified to appear to be arraigned for the crimes charged in the indictment.

Conference

If the defendant does not plead guilty, both felony and misdemeanor cases are taken to conference, and plea-bargaining commences with the goal of an agreed-on disposition. If no disposition can be reached, the case is adjourned, motions are made, and further plea-bargaining ensues. Generally after several adjournments, a case is assigned to a trial court.

Prosecution

The role of the prosecutor in the criminal justice system is well defined in *Berger v. United States*:[12]

> The United States Attorney is the representative not of an ordinary party to a controversy, but of a sovereignty whose obligation to govern impartially is as compelling as its obligation to govern at all; and whose interest, therefore, in a criminal prosecution is not that it shall win a case, but that justice will be done. As such, he is in a peculiar and very definite sense the servant of the law, the twofold aim of which is that guilt shall not escape or innocence suffer.

The potential of the prosecutor's office is not always fully realized in many jurisdictions. In many cities, the combination of the prosecutor's staggering caseload and small staff of assistants prevents sufficient attention being given to each case.[13]

Defense

The defense attorney generally sits in the proverbial hot seat, being perceived as the bad guy. Although everyone seems to understand the attorney's function in protecting the rights of those represented, the defense attorney often is not very popular.

> There is a substantial difference in the problem of representing the "run-of-the-mill" criminal defendant and one whose alleged crimes have aroused great public outcry. The difficulties in providing representation for the ordinary criminal defendant are simple compared with the difficulties of obtaining counsel for one who is charged with a crime which by its nature or circumstances incites strong public condemnation.[14]

Trial

Most of the processes of a criminal trial are similar to those of a civil trial. They include jury selection, opening statements, presentation of witnesses and other evidence, summations, instructions to the jury by the judge, jury deliberations, verdict, and opportunity for appeal to a higher court. In a criminal trial, the jury verdict must be unanimous, and the standard of proof is that guilt must be determined beyond a reasonable doubt whereas in a civil trial the plaintiff need only prove a claim by a preponderance of the evidence.

HEALTH CARE FRAUD

Executive's Medicare Scheme Had Lobbying Effort to Support It
He Franchised Fraud With Advocacy Group

Miami health-care executive Larry Duran orchestrated one of the largest Medicare frauds in U.S. history, submitting more than $205 million in phony claims and landing a record-breaking 50-year prison sentence for his crimes.

• • •

Patients often suffered from Alzheimer's disease, dementia or other conditions unsuited for therapy and were frequently left to urinate or defecate on themselves as they waited for treatment that never came, testimony showed.

"The people that were there were just kept there and run through like cattle," the judge in the case said.

Dan Eggen, The Washington Post, *October 5, 2011*

Health care fraud involves an unlawful act, generally deception for financial gain. It "encompasses an array of irregularities and illegal acts characterized by intentional deception."[15] The Federal Bureau of Investigation (FBI) reports that:

Health care fraud costs the country an estimated $80 billion a year. And it's a rising threat, with national health care spending topping $2.7 trillion and expenses continuing to outpace inflation. *Recent cases also show that medical professionals are more willing to risk patient harm in their schemes.*[16]

The victims of health care frauds often include those who are physically and neurologically challenged. Senior citizens at the time in their life that they are most vulnerable are often the targets of perpetrators of fraud.

Investigation and Prosecution of Fraud

The primary agency for exposing and investigating health care fraud is the FBI. with jurisdiction over both federal and private insurance programs.[17] The Department of Justice-Health and Human Services Medicare Fraud Strike Force is a multiagency team of federal, state, and local investigators that is designed to combat Medicare fraud. Medicare fraud is estimated to cost the nation $80 billion dollars annually.[18] The success of cooperation of agencies on the federal and state levels was evident when the Medicare Fraud Strike Force charged 111 defendants in nine cities, including doctors, nurses, health care company owners and executives, and others, for their alleged participation in Medicare fraud schemes involving more than $225 million in false billing.[19]

> [T]he Department of Justice (DOJ) and HHS announced the expansion of Medicare Fraud Strike Force operations to two additional cities—Dallas and Chicago. Today's operation is the largest-ever federal health care fraud takedown. More than 700 law enforcement agents from the FBI, HHS-Office of Inspector General (HHS-OIG), multiple Medicaid Fraud Control Units, and other state and local law enforcement agencies participated in the operation. In addition to making arrests, agents also executed 16 search warrants across the country in connection with ongoing strike force investigations.[20]

The message is clear that those involved in health care fraud are being vigorously pursued. The federal government's initiative to investigate and prosecute health care organizations for criminal wrongdoing has resulted in the establishment of corporate compliance programs for preventing, detecting, and reporting criminal conduct. An effective corporate compliance program should include:

1. Developing appropriate policies and procedures
2. Appointing a compliance officer to oversee the compliance program
3. Communicating the organization's compliance program to employees
4. Providing for monitoring and auditing systems that are designed to detect criminal conduct by employees and other agents
5. Publicizing a reporting system whereby employees and other agents can report criminal conduct by others within the organization without fear of retribution
6. Taking appropriate steps to respond to criminal conduct and to prevent similar offenses
7. Periodically reviewing and updating the organization's corporate compliance program
8. Working with state and federal law enforcement and regulatory agencies and insurance companies to detect, prevent, and prosecute health care fraud
9. Developing appropriate policies and procedures
10. Appointing a compliance officer to oversee the compliance program
11. Communicating the organization's compliance program to employees
12. Providing for monitoring and auditing systems that are designed to detect criminal conduct by employees and other agents
13. Publicizing a reporting system whereby employees and other agents can report criminal conduct by others within the organization without fear of retribution
14. Taking appropriate steps to respond to criminal conduct and to prevent similar offenses
15. Periodically reviewing and updating the organization's corporate compliance program
16. Working with state and federal law enforcement and regulatory agencies and insurance companies to detect, prevent, and prosecute health care fraud

As noted in the following remarks by Attorney General Eric Holder, health care fraud continues to present significant risks to patient health and is a financial drain on the health care system leading to higher costs for legitimate care.

We are here to announce that Johnson & Johnson and three of its subsidiaries have agreed to pay more than $2.2 billion to resolve criminal and civil claims that they marketed prescription drugs for uses that were never approved as safe and effective—and that they paid kickbacks to both physicians and pharmacies for prescribing and promoting these drugs.

• • •

Put simply, this alleged conduct is shameful and it is unacceptable. It displayed a reckless indifference to the safety of the American people. And it constituted a clear abuse of the public trust, showing a blatant disregard for systems and laws designed to protect public health.

As our filings make clear, these are not victimless crimes. Americans trust that the medications prescribed for their parents and grandparents, for their children, and for themselves are selected because they are in the patient's best interest. Laws enacted by Congress—and the enforcement efforts of the Food and Drug Administration—provide important safeguards to ensure that drugs are approved for uses that have been demonstrated as safe and effective. Efforts by drug companies to introduce their drugs into interstate commerce for unapproved uses subvert those laws. Likewise, the payment of kickbacks undermines the independent medical judgment of health care providers. It creates financial incentives to increase the use of certain drugs, potentially putting the health of some patients at risk. Every time pharmaceutical companies engage in this type of conduct, they corrupt medical decisions by health care providers, jeopardize the public health, and take money out of taxpayers' pockets.

This settlement demonstrates that the Departments of Justice and Health and Human Services—working alongside a variety of federal, state, and local partners—will not tolerate such activities. No company is above the law. And my colleagues and I are determined to keep moving forward—guided by the facts and the law, and using every tool, resource, and authority at our disposal—to hold these corporations accountable, to safeguard the American people, and to prevent this conduct from happening in the future.[21]

Schemes to Defraud

A defendant is guilty of a scheme to defraud when he or she engages in an arrangement establishing a systematic ongoing course of conduct with intent to defraud more than one person or to obtain property from more than one person by false or fraudulent pretenses, representations, or promises, and so obtains property from one or more of such persons. To show intent in a scheme to defraud, one needs to establish the following elements:

- That on or about (date), in the county of (county), the defendant (defendant's name), engaged in a scheme constituting a systematic ongoing course of conduct;
- That the defendant did so with intent to defraud more than one person or to obtain property from more than one person by false or fraudulent pretenses, representations, or promises; and

- That the defendant so obtained property from one or more of such persons, at least one of whom has been identified.[22]

Health care fraud is committed when a dishonest provider or consumer intentionally submits or causes someone else to submit false or misleading information for use in determining the amount of health care benefits payable. Some examples of provider health care fraud include the following:

- *Billing for services not rendered*
- *Falsifying a patient's diagnosis* to justify tests, surgeries, or other procedures that are not medically necessary
- *Misrepresenting procedures performed* to obtain payment for noncovered services, such as cosmetic surgery
- *Upcoding services* (billing for a more costly service than the one actually performed)
- *Upcoding medical supplies and equipment* (billing for more expensive equipment than what was delivered to the patient)
- *Unbundling* (billing each stage of a procedure as if it were a separate procedure)
- *Billing for unnecessary* services (services that are not medically indicated)
- *Accepting kickbacks* for patient referrals
- *Waiving patient copays or deductibles*
- *Overbilling* the insurance carrier or benefit plan

Schemes to defraud are rampant on the Internet. Internet pharmacy is a risky business as noted in the next news clipping.

$12 Million in Medicaid Funds Went to Deceased in Illinois

The Illinois Medicaid program paid an estimated 12 million for medical services for people listed as the deceased in other state records, according to the internal state government memo.

• • •

Auditors identified overpayments for services to roughly 2,900 people after the date of their deaths.

Carla K. Johnson and Sara Burnett, The Washington Post, *April 20, 2014*

Renewed Criticism for Google Over Drug Sites

Several state attorneys general are pressing Google to make it harder for its users to find counterfeit prescription medicine and illegal drugs online, marking the second time in the past three years that the firm has drawn government scrutiny for its policies on rogue Internet pharmacies.

• • •

Google, which failed to persuade a California judge to dismiss the suits, entered settlement talks last month after attorneys for the shareholders obtained e-mails showing that top executives warned then-chief executive Eric Schmidt and co-founder Larry Page more than a decade ago about the risks of accepting such ads.

Matea Gold and Tom Hamburger, The Washington Post, *April 16, 2014*

Although Google reached a settlement to pay $500 million to avoid prosecution for aiding illegal online pharmaceutical ads, some state prosecutors want to see more from Google in preventing ads from unlicensed pharmacies. "Google acknowledged in the settlement that it had improperly and knowingly assisted online pharmacy advertisers allegedly based in Canada to run advertisements for illicit pharmacy sales targeting U.S. customers."[23]

A variety of schemes to defraud are noted in the following news clippings.

Medicare Fraud Crackdown Nabs 91 in 8 Cities Across U.S.

Among those charged in the coordinated series of arrests was a doctor in Detroit who allegedly billed Medicare for services provided to dead people and claimed that he performed psychotherapy treatments more than 24 hours a day. Other doctors, nurses and health-care company owners were charged in various schemes to get paid for services that were medically unnecessary or never provided, officials said.

"From Brooklyn to Miami to Los Angeles, the defendants allegedly treated the Medicare program like a personal piggy bank," Lanny A. Breuer, assistant attorney general for the Justice Department's criminal division, said at a news conference in Washington.

Jerry Markon, The Washington Post, *September 8, 2011*

Medicare Bilked of $77M "Like an ATM"

Over 7 years, the federal program for the elderly and disabled paid at least about $77 million—and possibly as much as $92 million—to purported medical equipment suppliers who used Medicare ID numbers of deceased physicians, says a report out today by congressional investigators. . . .

Despite learning of the problem in 2001, the government failed to fix it, the report says. Investigators reviewing billing data submitted by equipment suppliers from 2000 to 2007 using the ID numbers of 1,500 deceased doctors.

Julie Appleby, USA Today, *July 9, 2008*

Woman Guilty of Health Care Fraud

A Severna Park woman pleaded guilty yesterday to health care fraud, admitting she billed the government and insurance companies for more than $200,000 in services she never rendered. . . . A state-licensed clinical specialist in child and adolescent psychiatric and mental health, [she] now faces the possibility of 10 years in prison and $250,000 in fines.

To conceal the fraud, she used false information on medical forms and patient logs.

Scott Daugherty, The Capital, *July 3, 2008*

Healthy Dose of Fraud

In one example of fraud, patients were allegedly brought to California, where they were paid to undergo surgeries that they did not need. In the scam, agents say, recruiters bring "patients from across the nation to surgery centers in California where they give phony or exaggerated symptoms and doctors perform unnecessary operations on them. Then the surgery centers send inflated claims for the unnecessary procedures to the patients' insurance companies. When the insurers pay up, federal authorities say, the recruiters, the surgery centers and the patients split the proceeds."[24] Corporate fraud has become so rampant that the level of trust in and reputation of organizational leadership has reached an all-time low.

Home Care Fraud

Today, more Americans are living longer than ever before. As medicine has advanced, the average life expectancy has increased by 50%. An increasing number of older persons receive in-home care, dependent on family and health care providers to attend to their physical, financial, emotional, and health care needs. Medicare home health benefits allow individuals with restricted mobility to remain home, outside an institutional setting, by providing home care benefits. Home care services and supplies are generally provided by nurses, home nursing aides, speech therapists, and physical therapists under a physician-certified plan of care.

Home care is rapidly being recognized as a breeding ground for abuse. The numerous scams in home care fraud are caused by the difficulty in supervising services provided in the home, Medicare's failure to monitor the number of visits per patient, beneficiaries paying no copayments except for medical equipment, and the lack of accountability to the patient by failing to explain services provided.

Home care fraud is generally not easy to detect. It involves charging insurers for more services than patients received, billing for more hours of care than were provided, falsifying records, and charging higher nurses' rates for care given by aides. The trend toward shorter hospital stays has created a multibillion-dollar market in home care services. This new market brings many opportunities for fraud.

Manslaughter

Manslaughter is the commission of an unintentional act that results in the death of another person. It can be either voluntary or involuntary. Voluntary manslaughter is the intentional killing of another person in what is commonly referred to as the "heat of passion," which is caused by the provocation of the victim (e.g., found having an affair with the defendant's spouse). Involuntary manslaughter is the result of a negligent act (e.g., reckless driving).

MURDER

Murder is the unlawful killing of a person. It is a homicide, and it involves malice aforethought and the premeditated intent to kill another human being. First-degree murder involves the deliberate and premeditated killing of another with malice aforethought. Second-degree murder is not deliberate, nor is it premeditated; however, it is the killing of another with malice aforethought. The tragedy of murder in health care settings that are dedicated to the healing of the sick has all too frequently occurred, as noted in the following examples.

- In a highly publicized case, Dr. Kermit Gosnell was convicted of murdering newborn babies by snipping their spinal cords shortly after delivery. Following a 2-month trial and 10 days of deliberation the jury convicted Gosnell of murder. Although it was expected that prosecutors would seek the death penalty, Gosnell made a deal with prosecutors promising not to appeal the jury's decision in exchange for life in prison without parole.
- Cullen, a former nurse, pleaded guilty to 13 murders and attempting to kill two others in New Jersey and Pennsylvania.[25] Cullen had refused to cooperate with prosecutors unless they promised not to seek the death penalty. Cullen claimed responsibility for the deaths of 30 to 40 patients over a 16-year nursing career. "The case raises concerns about hospital oversight of medical errors, narcotics security, and background checks on prospective employees. Cullen was fired from five hospitals and resigned from two amid questions about his job performance."[26] Cullen had been found violating nursing standards from the beginning of his career. He had problems in every one of the 10 institutions that he worked for in New Jersey and Pennsylvania. Apparently not one of the institutions in which Cullen worked gave him a bad reference. "It amounted to a policy of 'see no evil, speak no evil'— one that gave Cullen, in effect, a license to kill."[27]
- Richard Angelo, an Eagle Scout and voluntary fireman, gained national attention as the "angel of death." He was a registered nurse on the cardiac/ intensive care unit at a Long Island hospital, where he murdered patients by injecting them with the drug Pavulon. Angelo was ultimately convicted of two counts of depraved indifference murder (second-degree murder), one count of second-degree manslaughter, one count of criminally negligent homicide, and six counts of assault with respect to five of the patients and was sentenced to 61 years to life.[28] Angelo had committed the murders in a bizarre scheme to revive the patients and be thought of as a hero. The attorney for the estate of one of the alleged victims had filed a wrongful death suit against Angelo and the hospital a day before the verdict was rendered by the jury.[29]

THEFT

Theft is the illegal taking of another person or organization's property. Health care organizations must be alert to the potential ongoing threat of theft by unscrupulous employees, physicians, patients, visitors, and trespassers. The theft of patient or resident valuables, supplies, drugs, and medical equipment is substantial and costs health care organizations millions of dollars each year.

Drug Theft by Employee

One day in October, the night shift charge nurse began to reconcile the narcotics inventory on the patient care unit with the evening charge nurse. All appeared to be okay and the reconciliation sheet was signed off by both charge nurses. An evening shift staff nurse walked over to the two charge nurses and reported suspicious activity as to the usage of Demerol and Percocet during the day shift. She reported that one of the day shift nurses had been signing out two narcotic medications for a 3-day postoperative C-section patient. The patient's medication record showed that the patient was administered Demerol at 8:30 a.m., 10:30 a.m., and 1:00 p.m.. The nurse also had written that Percocet and Tylenol 3 had been administered every 2 hours. The charge nurses recognized that it would be unusual for a patient to be administered both an injection and oral narcotic at the same time and unlikely every 2 hours. When three other evening shift nurses were queried about the suspicion of medication theft, they responded:

Nurse 1: "This has been going on for a long time."
Nurse 2: "I am not getting involved."
Nurse 3: "Do you think we should report this?"

The two charge nurses spoke to the hospital's night supervising nurse who reported the possibility of medication theft to the VP of nursing. The nurse in question had been suspected of medication theft in the past, but no one ever established sufficient evidence to confront her. The VP for nursing questioned the suspected RN the following day when she arrived for work. She denied involvement in the theft of drugs. The nurse was asked to undergo a drug test, which she refused. She was then suspended for a week. When she returned, she was not permitted to carry the narcotics lock keys for a week. Later, after she regained access to narcotic drugs, she was observed giving a patient two Motrin when Percocet had been prescribed. Although an incident report had been filed against her, she continued to work into January. As other nurses eventually became concerned that they might be implicated in drug theft, they went to the VP of nursing and reported their observations. Finally, the suspected nurse was terminated. Eventually she was listed in the state professional newsletter as having a suspended license.

Sadly, this young nurse (39 years of age) was in a vehicle accident 6 months later with two other passengers. They were speeding 75 mph around a 35-mph curve without seat belts. They hit the embankment and were thrown from the car. The nurse and one passenger died instantly. The nurse had drugs in her possession, and an autopsy confirmed the presence of alcohol and drugs in all three passengers.

If action had been taken sooner, this tragedy may never have occurred. Management had the opportunity to explain the responsibility of nurses to report suspicious activity but failed to do so.

This same scenario was reported to have occurred in another state when an LPN was caught stealing medications. Within 24 hours of being caught, she had a choice of admitting to the theft and her chemical dependency or walking out of the hospital in handcuffs with the police.

Distraught Nurse (edited)

The evidence presented in *People v. Lancaster*[30] was found to have provided a probable cause foundation for information charging felony theft of nursing home residents' money by the office manager. Evidence showed that on repeated occasions the residents' income checks were cashed or cash was otherwise received on behalf of residents; that the defendant, by virtue of her office, had sole responsibility for maintaining the residents' ledger accounts; and that cash receipts frequently were never posted to the residents' accounts.

In another case, *Miller v. Dunn*,[31] there was sufficient evidence to hold that a nurse assistant had misappropriated $15,000 from an 83-year-old nursing home resident. The record indicated that the funds were taken during those times when the resident made visits to the hospital for respiratory problems. The patient had been diagnosed with dementia, and the resident's confusion was increasing. The nursing assistant actively procured the check in question, filling in the date, amount, and her name as payee. As a result, the nursing assistant was placed on the Employee Disqualification List for misappropriating funds.

The following news clippings illustrate how rampant theft is in the health care industry.

Virginia Court Rules Identity Theft Victim to Get $532,000 from . . .

Sloane delivered her second child . . . unaware that her last name would prove too big a temptation for an employee of the hospital's accounting department, Shovana Sloan.

Sloan, who was hired for the department even though she was a felon, appropriated Sloane's identification and went on a $35,000 spending spree.

Alan Cooper, Daily Record and the Kansas City Daily News-Press, *September 23, 2006*[32]

Medical Theft Trend Sweeps Pennsylvania

A slew of hospital thefts nationwide—including close to $75,000 of equipment from Mount Nittany Medical Center in 2005—has opened investigators' eyes to a black market specializing in the swap of used medical instruments.

Krystle Kopacz, The Daily Collegian Online, *January 13, 2006*[33]

NHS Hospital Thefts Cost Millions

National Health Service (NHS) hospital wards in the UK are being targeted by thieves who steal tens of millions of pounds worth of medical equipment every year.

Hospital Healthcare.com, *June 26, 2008*[34]

Millions of Patient Billing Records Stolen from UT Hospital

Billing records for about 2.2 million patients and guarantors were stolen last week from the University of Utah Hospitals & Clinics, just one more in what appears to be a rapidly growing flood of identity theft incidents.

Anne Zieger, Fierce HealthIT, *June 14, 2008*[35]

Grady Hospital Battles Patient Thefts

"It's got to be clearly 180 degrees from what we expect in an institution of care and shelter," said Atlanta attorney Mark Spix, who says he represented a man whose wife lost an engagement ring after being flown to Grady in October 2004 with fatal injuries. "I just think that is unacceptable."

There were 260 thefts involving patients, employees and visitors in 2007, compared with 262 in 2006 and 279 in 2005, Grady spokeswoman Denise Simpson said.

Tim Eberly, The Atlanta Journal-Constitution, *July 24, 2008*[36]

CONTRACTS

A *contract* is a special kind of agreement, either written **(Figure 6)**, or oral, that involves legally binding obligations between two or more parties. A contract can also be implied such as when one or more persons provide emergency care and treatment to a comatose patient injured during an automobile accident. The major purpose of a contract is to specify, limit, and define the agreements that are legally enforceable.

ELEMENTS OF A CONTRACT

Whether contracts are executed in writing or agreed to orally, they must contain the following elements to be enforceable: (1) offer/communication, (2) consideration, and (3) acceptance.

Offer/Communication

An offer must be communicated to the other party so that it can be accepted or rejected. Unless the offeror specifically requires that the acceptance be received before a contract is formed, communication of the acceptance to the offeror is not necessary.

Consideration

An offer is a promise by one party to do (or not to do) something if the other party agrees to do (or not do) something. Not all statements or promises are offers. Generally, advertisements

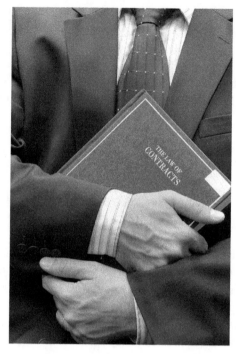

FIGURE 6   The Law of Contracts (© corgarashu/Shutterstock, Inc.)

of goods for sale are not offers but are invitations to the public to come to the place of business, view the merchandise, and be made an offer. An opinion is not an offer. Preliminary negotiations are not offers.

Acceptance

On proper acceptance of an offer, a contract is formed. It involves:

- *Meeting of the minds:* Acceptance requires a "meeting of the minds" (mutual assent). The parties must understand and then agree on the terms of the contract.
- *Definite and complete:* Acceptance requires mutual assent to be found between the parties. The terms must be so complete that both parties understand and agree to what has been proposed.
- *Duration:* Generally, the other party may revoke an offer at any time prior to a valid acceptance. When the offeror does revoke the proposal, the revocation is not effective until the offeree (the person to whom the offer is made) receives it. After the offeree has accepted the offer, any attempt to revoke the agreement is too late and is invalid.
- *Complete and conforming:* The traditional rule is that the acceptance must be the mirror image of the offer. In other words, the acceptance must comply with all the terms of the offer.

EMPLOYMENT CONTRACTS

An employer's right to terminate an employee can be limited by express agreement with the employee or through a collective bargaining agreement to which the employee is a beneficiary.

No such agreement was found to exist in *O'Connor v. Eastman Kodak Co.,*[37] in which the court held that an employer had a right to terminate an employee at will at any time, and for any reason or no reason. The plaintiff did not rely on any specific representation made to him during the course of his employment interviews, nor did he rely on any documentation in the employee handbook, which would have limited the defendant's common-law right to discharge at will. The employee had relied on a popular perception of Kodak as a "womb-to-tomb" employer.

EXCLUSIVE CONTRACTS

An *exclusive contract*, in the context of a hospital, is an agreement between two or more entities to deal only with each other regarding a specific area of business (e.g., hospital[s] and radiology physician[s] group). The essential feature of an exclusivity contract is the covenant not to engage in a particular business activity with other parties for a specified period of time.

An organization often enters into an exclusive contract with physicians and/or medical groups for the purpose of providing a specific service to the organization. Exclusive contracts generally occur within the organization's ancillary service departments (e.g., radiology, anesthesiology, and pathology). Physicians who seek to practice at organizations in these ancillary areas but who are not part of the exclusive group have attempted to invoke the federal antitrust laws to challenge these exclusive contracts. These challenges generally have been unsuccessful.

Exclusive Contract with Radiology Group

Tennessee code permitted the hospital authority to enter into an exclusive contract with a radiology group. The governing body's decision to close the staff of the imaging department did not violate medical staff bylaws, and the defendant radiologists were not legally or constitutionally entitled to a hearing if their privileges were terminated on entry of the hospital authority into an exclusive provider contract.[38]

Commercial Ethics and Noncompetition Agreements

The purpose in allowing noncompetition agreements is to foster "commercial ethics" and to protect the employer's legitimate interests by preventing unfair competition, not ordinary competition.

The respondent hospital in *Washington County Memorial Hospital v. Sidebottom*[39] employed the appellant/nurse practitioner from October 1993 through April 1998. Before beginning her employment, the nurse entered into an employment agreement with the hospital. The agreement included a noncompetition clause providing in part that the nurse "during the term of [the] Agreement and for a period of one (1) year after the termination of her employment . . . will not, anywhere within a fifty (50) mile radius . . . directly or indirectly engage in the practice of nursing . . . without the express direction or consent" of the hospital. In February 1994, the nurse requested the hospital's permission to work for the Washington County Health Department doing prenatal nursing care. Because the hospital was not then doing prenatal care, the hospital gave her permission to accept that employment but reserved the ability to withdraw the permission if the services the nurse was providing later came to be provided by the hospital. In January 1996, the nurse and the hospital entered into a second employment agreement that continued the parties' employment relationship through January

9, 1998. This agreement included a noncompetition clause identical to the 1993 employment agreement. It also provided for automatic renewal for an additional 2 years unless either party gave written termination notice no less than 90 days prior to the expiration of the agreement.

The hospital's interest lies in protecting its patient base as a primary source of revenue. The specific enforcement of the nurse's noncompetition clause is reasonably necessary to protect the hospital's interest. Actual damage need not be proven to enforce a covenant not to compete. Rather, the employee's opportunity to influence customers justifies enforcement of the covenant. Thus, the quality, frequency, and duration of an employee's exposure to an employer's customers are crucial in determining the covenant's reasonableness. The nurse had opportunity to influence the hospital's patients. Before her employment with the hospital, the nurse had never worked in Washington County, nor did she have a patient base there. The nurse helped to establish two rural health care clinics for the hospital, one of which she managed during her first year of employment. During almost 5 years of employment with the hospital, the nurse saw more than 3,000 patients. Pursuant to a collaborative practice agreement with a physician, the nurse treated patients, diagnosed illnesses and injuries, prescribed and dispensed medications, and ordered and interpreted laboratory tests. The nurse got to know the patients and families to whom she provided these services. At the clinic, she had her own telephone number, receptionist, appointment book, medical assistant, patient charts, laboratory, and examination rooms. Her offices were physically separated from those of the other medical practitioner at the clinic. Furthermore, during her employment, the hospital promoted the nurse as a nurse practitioner in the community by paying for advertisements with her picture and telephone number in the newspaper. In general, the nurse had a good rapport with her patients, and she had patients who requested her for medical services.

TRIAL PROCEDURE AND THE COURTROOM

This next section presents a brief review of the law as applied in the courtroom **(Figure 7)**. Although many of the procedures leading up to and followed during a trial are discussed in

FIGURE 7 The Courtroom (© Everett Collection/Shutterstock, Inc.)

this chapter, civil procedure and trial practice are governed by each state's statutory requirements. Federal statutes govern cases on the federal level.

PLEADINGS

The pleadings of a case (e.g., summons and complaint), which include all the allegations of each party to a lawsuit, are filed with a court. The pleadings may raise questions of both law and fact. If only questions of law are at issue, the judge will decide the case based on the pleadings alone. If questions of fact are involved, the purpose of a trial is to determine those facts.

Summons and Complaint

The parties to a controversy are the plaintiff and the defendant. The plaintiff is the person who initiates an action by filing a complaint; the defendant is the person against whom a suit is brought. Many cases have multiple plaintiffs and defendants. Filing an order with a court clerk to issue a writ or summons commences an action.

Although the procedures for beginning an action vary according to jurisdiction, there are procedural common denominators. All jurisdictions require service of process on the defendant (usually through a summons) and a return to the court of that process by the person who served it. When a summons is not required to be issued directly by a court, an attorney, as an officer of the court, may prepare and cause a summons to be served without direct notice to or approval of a court. Notice to a court occurs when an attorney files a summons and complaint in a court, thereby indicating to the court that an action has been commenced.

The first pleading filed with the court in a negligence action is the complaint. The complaint identifies the parties to a suit, states a cause of action, and includes a demand for damages. It is filed by the plaintiff and is the first statement of a case by the plaintiff against the defendant. In some jurisdictions, a complaint must accompany a summons (an announcement to the defendant that a case has been commenced).

Answer

After service of a complaint, a response is required from the defendant in a document called the answer. In the answer, the defendant responds to each of the allegations contained in the complaint by stating his or her defense and by admitting to or denying each of the plaintiff's allegations. If the defendant fails to answer the complaint within the prescribed time, the plaintiff can seek judgment by default against the defendant.

Bill of Particulars

A bill of particulars in a civil case is a written demand for more detailed information concerning the alleged claim/s by the defendant/s. A bill of particulars is requested when there is generally insufficient information provided in the complaint to file an answer. If a counterclaim is filed, the plaintiff's attorney may request a bill of particulars from the defense attorney. In a criminal case the defendant/s attorney may request a bill of particulars in order to prepare their case.

Discovery is the process of investigating the facts of a case before trial. The objectives of discovery are to:

- obtain evidence that might not be obtainable at the time of trial
- isolate and narrow the issues for trial
- gather knowledge of the existence of additional evidence that may be admissible at trial
- obtain leads to enable the discovering party to gather further evidence

The parties to a lawsuit have the right to discovery and to examine witnesses before trial. Examination before trial (EBT) is one of several discovery techniques used to enable the parties of a lawsuit to learn more regarding the nature and substance of each other's case. An EBT consists of oral testimony under oath and includes cross-examination. A deposition, taken at an EBT, is the testimony of a witness that has been recorded in a written format. Testimony given at a deposition becomes part of the permanent record of the case. Each question and answer is transcribed by a court stenographer and may be used at the subsequent trial. Truthfulness and consistency are important because answers that differ from those given at trial will be used to attack the credibility of the witness.

PREPARATION OF WITNESSES

The manner in which a witness handles questioning at a deposition or trial is often as important as the facts of the case. Each witness should be well prepared before testifying. Preparation should include a review of all pertinent records. Helpful guidelines for witnesses undergoing examination in a trial or a court hearing include the following:

- Review the records (e.g., medical records and other business records) on which you might be questioned.
- Do not be antagonistic when answering the questions. The jury may already be somewhat sympathetic toward a particular party to the lawsuit; antagonism may serve only to reinforce such an impression.
- Be organized in your thinking and recollection of the facts regarding the incident.
- Answer only the questions asked.
- Explain your testimony in simple, succinct terminology.
- Do not overdramatize the facts you are relating.
- Do not allow yourself to become overpowered by the cross-examiner.
- Be polite, sincere, and courteous at all times.
- Dress appropriately and be neatly groomed.
- Pay close attention to any objections your attorney may have as to the line of questioning being conducted by the opposing counsel.
- Be sure to have reviewed any oral deposition in which you may have participated.
- Be straightforward with the examiner. Any answers designed to cover up or cloud an issue or fact will, if discovered, serve only to discredit any previous testimony that you may have given. Do not show any visible signs of displeasure regarding any testimony with which you are in disagreement.

- Be sure to have questions that you did not hear repeated and questions that you did not understand rephrased.
- If you are not sure of an answer, indicate that you are not sure or that you just do not know the answer.
- Remember that lawyers often get the answers they want by how they frame the questions they ask.

THE COURT

A case is heard in the court that has jurisdiction over the subject of controversy. The judge decides questions of law and is responsible for ensuring that a trial is conducted properly in an impartial atmosphere and that it is fair to both parties of a lawsuit. He or she determines what constitutes the general standard of conduct required for the exercise of due care. The judge informs the jury of what the defendant's conduct should have been, thereby making a determination of the existence of a legal duty.

The judge decides whether evidence is admissible, charges the jury (defines the jurors' responsibility in relation to existing law), and may take a case away from the jury (by directed verdict or judgment notwithstanding the verdict) if he or she believes that there are no issues for the jury to consider or that the jury has erred in its decision. This right on the part of the judge with respect to the role of the jury narrows the jury's responsibility with regard to the facts of the case. The judge maintains order throughout the suit, determines issues of procedure, and is generally responsible for the conduct of the trial.

Mother Loses Custody of Her Children—Because She Has Breast Cancer

A woman with terminal breast cancer says she has lost custody of her children because doctors do not know how long she will live.

A judge ruled that 37-year-old Alaina Giordano, from Durham, North Carolina, must give up both her children to her estranged husband after she was diagnosed with stage four breast cancer.

Durham County Family Court judge Nancy Gordon ruled that Mr. Snyder should get the children after a psychiatrist recommended that they should live with him because of the "deteriorating condition of the mother's health."

John Stevens, Daily Mail, *May 10, 2011*

A Facebook account was set up for Alaina, and within several weeks, 18,743 people linked to her page. The following is a sampling of the numerous posts on her Facebook page:

D.D. MAY GOD HAVE MERCY ON YOU AND I WILL PRAY FOR YOU AND YOUR CHILDREN. NO ONE HAS THE RIGHT TO TAKE WHAT GOD HAS GIVEN YOU . . . "YOUR CHILDREN"

M.A.B. she should not lose her family because she feel ill. Falling ill is not a lifestyle choice she made—it is a circumstance she is forced to endure she should not endure it without her children. mothers in prison may have their children with them for God's sake.

S.X. Came home to NC after a business trip to see this report. SHAMEFUL that a court and an "expert witness" could have so little compassion and rule like this. I'm shocked. I know the family. These kids belong with Mom!

"We have learned that the North Carolina Supreme Court has denied my motion for a stay—this means that now, my children will be moving to Chicago to start the school year with their father.

As I write today, I deal with the difficult recognition that my children will have to live 800 miles away from me, until my appeal can be heard. In the wake of this legal decision, my children and I now must grieve the pending loss of each other."

http://www.facebook.com/friendsofalaina

Comments by Danny

Alaina, I have been a hospital administrator and later inspected more that 500 hospitals and 100 ambulatory sites from Alaska to Puerto Rico. I have never experienced such a travesty by a Judge who apparently has little knowledge of the law or an understanding of the horrors you have been put through. Judges of this sort need some major training in ethics. I quote Earl Warren, Chief Justice of the United States (1891-1974), "In civilized life, law floats on a sea of ethics." The Judge in your case failed to understand and practice the teachings of this most Honorable judge—Earl Warren. I wish you love and happiness always . . . and know that you are loved.

Danny

Mother With Terminal Cancer Can Retain Child Custody, Judge Holds

In a case of first impression, a New Jersey judge has refused to strip a divorced mother of primary custody of her children even though she has terminal and inoperable breast cancer.

Ocean County Superior Court Judge Lawrence Jones said granting the father's motion for an emergency change in the children's primary residential status could cause them emotional harm.

"It would be fundamentally inequitable and inappropriate for this court to conclude that a person's illness, disability, or condition, even a condition as serious as Stage IV cancer, automatically renders a person unfit per se to continue serving as a custodial parent . . . ."

Michael Booth, New Jersey Law Journal, *November 22, 2013*[40]

Discussion

1. Make an argument supporting the judge's decision and one that opposes her decision.
2. Discuss both the moral and legal issues (e.g., the best interests of the child) you believe the judge may have failed to consider in this case.

The Jury

The right to a trial by jury is a constitutional right in certain cases. Not all cases entitle the parties to a jury trial as a matter of right. For example, in many jurisdictions, a case in equity (a case seeking a specific course of conduct rather than monetary damages) may not entitle the parties to a trial by a jury. An example of an equity case is one that seeks a declaration as to the title to real property. Members of a jury are selected from a jury list. They are summoned to court by a paper known as the jury process. Impartiality is a prerequisite of all jurors. The number of jurors who sit at trial is 12 in common law. If there are fewer than 12, the number must be established by statute.

An individual may waive the right to a jury trial. If this right is waived, the judge acts as judge and jury, becomes the trier of facts, and decides issues of law.

Counsel for both parties of a lawsuit may question each prospective jury member for impartiality, bias, and prejudicial thinking. This process is referred to as the *voir dire*, the examination of jurors. After members of the jury are selected, they are sworn in to try the case.

The jury makes a determination of the facts that have occurred, evaluating whether the plaintiff's damages were caused by the defendant's negligence and whether the defendant exercised due care. The jury makes a determination of the particular standard of conduct required in all cases in which the judgment of reasonable people might differ. The jury must pay close attention to the evidence presented by both sides of a suit in order to render a fair and impartial verdict.

The jury also determines the extent of damages, if any, and the degree to which the plaintiff's conduct may have contributed to any injuries suffered.

Subpoenas

A *subpoena* is a legal order requiring the appearance of a person and/or the presentation of documents to a court or administrative body. Attorneys, judges, and certain law enforcement and administrative officials, depending on the jurisdiction, may issue subpoenas.

- A *subpoena ad testificandum* orders the appearance of a person at a trial or other investigative proceeding to give testimony. Witnesses have a duty to appear and may suffer a penalty for contempt of court should they fail to appear.
- A *subpoena duces tecum* is a written command to bring records, documents, or other evidence described in the subpoena to a trial or other investigative proceeding. The subpoena is served on a person able to produce such records.

Opening Statements

During the opening statement, the plaintiff's attorney outlines what he or she intends to prove. The opening statement by the plaintiff's attorney provides in capsule form the facts of the case, what he or she intends to prove by means of a summary of the evidence to be presented, and a description of the damages to his or her client.

The defense attorney makes his or her opening statement indicating the position of the defendant and the points of the plaintiff's case he or she intends to refute. The defense attorney summarizes the facts as they apply to the case for the defendant.

BURDEN OF PROOF

The *burden of proof* requires that the plaintiff's attorney show that the defendant violated a legal duty by not following an acceptable standard of care and that the plaintiff suffered injury because of the defendant's breach. If the evidence presented does not support the allegations made, the case is dismissed.

EVIDENCE

Evidence consists of the facts proved or disproved during a lawsuit. The law of evidence is a body of rules under which facts are proved. To be admitted at trial, evidence must be competent, relevant, and material.

Direct Evidence

Direct evidence is proof offered through direct testimony. It is the jury's function to receive testimony presented by witnesses and to draw conclusions in the determination of facts.

Demonstrative Evidence

Demonstrative (real) evidence is evidence furnished by things themselves. It is considered the most trustworthy and preferred type of evidence. It consists of tangible objects to which testimony refers (e.g., medical instruments and broken infusion needles) that can be requested by a jury. Demonstrative evidence is admissible in court if it is relevant, has probative value, and serves the interest of justice. It is not admissible if it will prejudice, mislead, confuse, offend, inflame, or arouse the sympathy or passion of the jury. Other forms of demonstrative evidence include photographs, motion pictures, computer generated information, drawings, human bodies as exhibits, pathology slides, fetal monitoring strips, safety committee minutes, infection committee reports, medical staff bylaws, rules and regulations, nursing policy and procedure manuals, census data, and staffing patterns.

A plaintiff's injuries are admissible as an exhibit if the physical condition of the body is material to the complaint. The human body is considered the best evidence as to the nature and extent of the alleged injury/injuries. If there is no controversy about either the nature or the extent of an injury, presenting such evidence could be considered prejudicial and an objection can be made as to its presentation to a jury.

Documentary Evidence

Documentary evidence is written evidence capable of making a truthful statement (e.g., drug manufacturer inserts, autopsy reports, birth certificates, and medical records). Documentary evidence must satisfy the jury as to authenticity. Proof of authenticity is not necessary if the opposing party accepts its genuineness. In some instances, concerning wills, for example, witnesses are necessary. In the case of documentation, the original of a document must be produced unless it can be demonstrated that the original has been lost or destroyed, in which case a properly authenticated copy may be substituted.

After conclusion of the opening statements, the judge calls for the plaintiff's witnesses. An officer of the court administers an oath to each witness, and direct examination begins. On cross-examination by the defense, an attempt is made to challenge or discredit the plaintiff's witness. The plaintiff's attorney may ask the same witness more questions in an effort to overcome the effect of the cross-examination. Re-cross-examination may also take place if necessary for the defense of the defendant.

Expert Witness

Laypersons are quite able to render opinions about a great variety of general subjects, but for technical questions, the opinion of an expert is necessary. At the time of testifying, each expert's training, experience, and special qualifications are explained to the jury. The experts are asked to give an opinion concerning hypothetical questions based on the facts of the case. Should the testimony of two experts conflict, the jury will determine which expert opinion to accept. Expert witnesses may be used to assist a plaintiff in proving the wrongful act of a defendant or to assist a defendant in refuting such evidence. In addition, expert testimony may be used to show the extent of the plaintiff's damages or to show the lack of such damages.

DEFENSE OF ONE'S ACTIONS

The defendant's case is presented to discredit the plaintiff's cause of action and prevent recovery of damages. Principles of law that may relieve a defendant from liability include assumption of a risk, comparative negligence, contributory negligence, Good Samaritan laws, ignorance of fact, unintentional wrongs, the statute of limitations, and sovereign immunity.

Assumption of a Risk

Assumption of a risk is knowing that a danger exists and voluntarily accepting the risk by exposing oneself to it, knowing that harm might occur. Assumption of a risk may be implicitly assumed, as in alcohol consumption, or expressly assumed, as in relation to warnings found on cigarette packaging.

This defense provides that the plaintiff expressly has given consent in advance, relieving the defendant of an obligation of conduct toward the plaintiff and taking the chances of injury from a known risk arising from the defendant's conduct. For example, one who agrees to care for a patient with a communicable disease and then contracts the disease would not be entitled to recover from the patient for damages suffered. In taking the job, the individual agreed to assume the risk of infection, thereby releasing the patient from all legal obligations.

The following two requirements must be established in order for a defendant to be successful in an assumption of risk defense:

1. the plaintiff must know and understand the risk that is being incurred; and,
2. the choice to incur the risk must be free and voluntary.

Comparative Negligence

A defense of *comparative negligence* provides that the degree of negligence or carelessness of each party to a lawsuit must be established by the finder of fact and that each party then is responsible for his or her proportional share of any damages awarded. For example, if a plaintiff suffers injuries of $10,000 from an accident and is found to be 20% negligent and the defendant is found to be 80% negligent, the defendant would be required to pay $8,000 to the plaintiff. Thus, with comparative negligence, the plaintiff can collect for 80% of the injuries, whereas an application of contributory negligence would deprive the plaintiff of any monetary judgment. This doctrine relieves the plaintiff from the hardship of losing an entire claim when a defendant has been successful in establishing that the plaintiff has contributed to his or her own injuries.

Contributory Negligence

Contributory negligence can be defined as any lack of ordinary care on the part of the person injured that, combined with the negligent act of another, caused the injury. A person is contributorily negligent when that person does not exercise reasonable care for his or her own safety. As a general proposition, if a person has knowledge of a dangerous situation and disregards the danger, then that person is contributorily negligent.

Good Samaritan Laws

The various states have enacted *Good Samaritan laws* that relieve health care professionals, and in some instances laypersons, from liability in certain emergency situations. Good Samaritan legislation encourages health care professionals to render assistance at the scene of emergencies. Good Samaritan statutes provide a standard of care that delineates the scope of immunity for those persons eligible under the law.

Ignorance of the Law and Unintentional Wrongs

 Ignorance of the law excuses no man; not that all men know the law, but because 'tis an excuse every man will plead, and no man can tell how to confute him.

—John Selden (1584–1654)

The defendant cannot use ignorance of the law to excuse his or her negligent actions; otherwise, pleading ignorance would reward an individual. Arguing that a negligent act is unintentional is no defense. If such a defense were acceptable, all defendants would use it.

Because a defense of ignorance or "I didn't know what I was doing" is not an acceptable answer in a courtroom, you need to learn and understand the potential consequences of your actions in the health care setting. This text lays the foundation for understanding your legal and ethical rights and responsibilities.

Statute of Limitations

The *statute of limitations* refers to legislatively imposed time constraints that restrict the period of time after an injury occurs during which a legal action must be commenced. Should a cause of action be initiated later than the period of time prescribed, the case cannot proceed. The statutory period begins when an injury occurs, although in some cases (usually involving foreign objects left in the body during surgery) the statutory period commences when the injured person discovers or should have discovered the injury.

Many technical rules are associated with statutes of limitations. Computation of the period when the statute begins to run in a particular state may be based on any of the following factors:

- The date that the physician terminated treatment
- The time of the wrongful act
- The time when the patient should have reasonably discovered the injury
- The date that the injury is discovered
- The date when the contract between the patient and the physician ended

Sovereign Immunity

Sovereign immunity refers to the common-law doctrine by which federal and state governments historically have been immune from liability for harm suffered from the tortious conduct of employees. For the most part, both federal and state governments have abolished sovereign immunity.

CLOSING STATEMENTS

Closing statements give attorneys an opportunity to summarize for the jury and the court what they have proven. They may point out faults in their opponent's case and emphasize points they want the jury to remember.

JUDGE'S CHARGE TO THE JURY

After the attorneys' summations, the court charges the jury before the jurors recess to deliberate. Because the jury determines issues of fact, it is necessary for the court to instruct the jury with regard to applicable law. This is done by means of a charge. The charge defines the responsibility of the jury, describes the applicable law, and advises the jury of the alternatives available to it.

JURY DELIBERATION

After the judge's charge, the jury retires to the jury room and deliberates as to whether or not the defendant is liable. The jury returns to the courtroom upon reaching a verdict, and its determinations are presented to the court.

If a verdict is against the weight of the evidence, a judge may dismiss the case, order a new trial, or set his or her own verdict. At the time judgment is rendered, the losing party has an opportunity to motion for a new trial. If a new trial is granted, the entire process is repeated; if not, the judgment becomes final, subject to review of the trial record by an appellate court.

DAMAGES

Damages suffered by plaintiffs can be awarded as compensation for loss or injury as a result of the negligence of the defendants.. Damages can be sought for emotional distress, physical pain and suffering, and economic loss. *Punitive damages* are sometimes awarded over and above that which is intended to compensate the plaintiff for economic losses resulting from the injury. Punitive damages cover such items as physical disability, mental anguish, loss of a spouse's services, physical suffering, injury to one's reputation, and loss of companionship. Punitive damages are referred to as "that mighty engine of deterrence" in *Johnson v. Terry*.[41] In *Estes Health Care Centers v. Bonnerman,* it was found that:[42]

> While human life is incapable of translation into a compensatory measurement, the amount of an award of punitive damages may be measured by the gravity of the wrong done, the punishment called for by the act of the wrongdoer, and the need to discourage similar wrongs.

APPEALS

An appellate court reviews a case on the basis of the trial record as well as written briefs and, if requested, concise oral arguments by the attorneys. A brief summarizes the facts of a case, testimony of the witnesses, laws affecting the case, and arguments of counsel. The party making the appeal is the appellant. The party answering the appeal is the appellee. After hearing the oral arguments, the court takes the case under advisement until such time as the judges consider it and agree on a decision. An opinion is then prepared, explaining the reasons for a decision. The appellate court may modify, affirm, or reverse the judgment or may order a new trial on appeal.

CHAPTER REVIEW

1. *Tort* is a civil wrong committed against a person or property for which a court provides a correction in the form of an action for damages.
   - Objectives of tort law
     - Preservation of peace (between individuals by providing a substitute for retaliation)
     - Culpability—find fault for wrongdoing.
     - Deterrence—to discourage the wrongdoer (tort-feasor) from committing future torts.
     - Compensation—to indemnify the injured person[s] of wrongdoing.
2. *Negligence* is the unintentional *commission* or *omission* of an act that a reasonably prudent person would *or would not perform under given circumstances.*
   - *Malpractice*
     - Negligence or carelessness of a professional person
   - Forms of negligence
     - *Malfeasance,* execution of an unlawful or improper act
     - *Misfeasance,* improper performance of an act that results in injury to another
     - *Nonfeasance,* failure to act when there is a duty to do so

- Elements of negligence
  - *Duty to care*—obligation to conform to a recognized standard of care
  - *Breach of duty*—failure to meet a prevailing standard of care
  - *Injury*—actual damages must be established
  - *Causation*—defendant's departure from the standard of care must be the cause of the plaintiff's injury.
    - *Foreseeability*—reasonable anticipation that harm or injury will result from an act or a failure to act.
    - The test for foreseeability is whether or not one should have reasonably anticipated that the event in question or a similar event would occur.
3. *Intentional tort* is a wrong involves an act that violates another person's interests.
   - Assault and battery
     - *Assault* is the infringement on the mental security or tranquility of another person.
     - *Battery* is the violation of another person's physical integrity.
   - False imprisonment
     - The unlawful restraint of an individual's personal liberty or the unlawful restraint or confinement of an individual
   - Defamation of character
     - A false oral or written communication to someone other than the individual defamed, subjecting that individual's reputation to scorn and ridicule
       - *Libel*—written defamation
       - *Slander*—spoken defamation
   - Invasion of privacy
   - Infliction of mental distress
     - Characterized by conduct that is so outrageous that it goes beyond the bounds tolerated by a decent society
4. *Criminal law* is society's expression of the limits of acceptable human behavior.
   - *Crime*, a social harm defined and made punishable by law
     - *Misdemeanor* is an offense punishable by less than 1 year in jail and/or a fine.
     - *Felony* is generally punishable by imprisonment in a state or federal prison for a period of more than 1 year.
     - *Criminal negligence*, the reckless disregard for the safety of others and willful indifference to an injury that could result from an act. It differs from tort liability in that it provides for a more specific lack of care commonly characterized as "gross negligence" and "recklessness."
   - Objectives of criminal law
     - Maintain public order and safety
     - Protect individuals and society from harm
     - Provide punishment as a deterrent to crime
     - Rehabilitate criminals for return to society
   - Criminal procedure
     - Arrest
     - Arraignment
     - Indictment
     - Conference

- Prosecution
- Defense
- Trial
- Health care fraud
- Manslaughter
- Murder
- Theft
5. *Contract*, a written or oral agreement that involves legally binding obligations between two or more parties.
   - Elements of a contract
     - Offer/communication
     - Consideration
     - Acceptance
   - *Exclusive contracts* allow organizations to contract with physicians and/or medical groups to provide specific services to the organization.
     - Employment contracts
     - Exclusive contracts
     - Commercial ethics and noncompetitive agreements
6. Trial procedures
   - Pleadings
     - *Summons and complaint*
     - *Answer*
     - *Bill of particulars*
     - Discovery
       - Investigation of facts.
       - Examination Before Trial (EBT).
     - Process that allows for witnesses to be examined prior to trial
   - Preparation of witnesses
   - Court
   - Jury
     - Determines the facts in a case.
     - Makes a determination of the particular standards of conduct required in which the judgment of reasonable people might differ.
   - Subpoenas
   - Opening statements
   - Burden of proof
   - Evidence
     - *Direct evidence*, proof offered via direct testimony
     - *Demonstrative evidence*, proof offered by objects themselves
     - *Documentary evidence*, written evidence capable of making a truthful statement
   - Examination of witnesses
     - *Expert witness* used to resolve issues in a case outside the understanding or experience of the average juror
   - Defending one's actions in a negligence case
     - *Assumption of a risk*

- ○ *Comparative negligence*
- ○ *Contributory negligence*
- ○ *Good Samaritan laws*
- ○ *Ignorance of the law and unintentional wrongs*
- ○ *Statute of limitations*
- ○ *Sovereign Immunity*
- Closing statements
- Judge's charge to the jury
- Jury deliberation
- Damages
  - ○ Nominal damages,
  - ○ Compensatory damages,
  - ○ Punitive damages.
- Appeals process

TEST YOUR UNDERSTANDING

TERMINOLOGY

assault	evidence	murder
assumption of a risk	exclusive contract	negligence
battery	false imprisonment	nonfeasance
breach of duty	felony	nonmaleficence
burden of proof	foreseeability	omission
causation	Good Samaritan laws	proximate cause
commission	infliction of mental distress	punitive damages
comparative negligence	injury	reasonably prudent person
contract	intentional tort	right to privacy
contributory negligence	invasion of privacy	slander
damages	libel	sovereign immunity
defamation of character	malfeasance	standard of care
demonstrative evidence	malpractice	statute of limitations
direct evidence	manslaughter	subpoena
documentary evidence	misdemeanor	theft
duty to care	misfeasance	tort

REVIEW QUESTIONS

1. Describe the objectives of tort law.

2. Discuss the distinctions among negligent torts, intentional torts, and strict liability.

3. Explain the difference between a *commission* and *omission* of a negligent act.

4. Explain the difference between negligence and malpractice.

5. What are the elements that must be proven in order to be successful in a negligence suit? Illustrate your answer with a case. (The facts of the case can be hypothetical.)

6. Describe the categories of intentional torts.

7. How does slander differ from libel? Give an example of each.

8. Describe the objectives of criminal law.

9. Describe the difference between a misdemeanor and a felony. Give an example of each.

10. Discuss why physicians have been so reluctant to remove a patient's life-support systems.

11. Describe a scheme to defraud.

12. Explain the elements of a contract.

13. Describe why exclusive contracts are so controversial.

14. Describe the trial process, including pretrial motions and the functions of the judge, jury, and attorneys.

15. Describe the kinds of evidence that a plaintiff can present in order to establish a negligent act.

16. What defenses can a defendant present in order to refute a plaintiff's evidence?

17. Describe how statutes of limitations favor defendants in a lawsuit.

18. Describe the various types of damages that can be awarded a plaintiff.

19. Explain why either the plaintiff or defendant may wish to appeal a jury's verdict.

NOTES

1. 498 So. 2d 713 (La. Ct. App. 1986).
2. 787 S.W.2d 494 (Tex. Ct. App. 1990).
3. 498 So. 2d 713 (La. Ct. App. 1986).
4. 498 So. 2d 713 (La. Ct. App. 1986).
5. *Clark v. Wagoner,* 452 S.W.2d 437, 440 (Tex. 1970).
6. 57A Am. Jur.2d Torts § 134 (1989).
7. 116 Cal. Rptr. 733 (Cal. Ct. App. 1974).
8. 385 N.W.2d 99 (N.D. 1986).
9. *Tomcik v. Ohio Dep't of Rehabilitation & Correction,* 598 N.E.2d 900 (Ohio Ct. App. 1991).
10. *Id.* at 904.
11. *Id.*

12. 295 U.S. 78, 88 (1935).

13. J. Kaplan, *Criminal Justice Introductory Cases and Materials* 228 (1973).

14. *Id.* at 259.

15. http://www.osc.state.ny.us/localgov/pubs/red_flags_fraud.pdf.

16. http://www.fbi.gov/about-us/investigate/white_collar/health-care-fraud/.

17. *Id.*

18. *Id.*

19. *U.S. Department of Health and Human Services*, News Release, *February 17, 2011.*

20. *Id.*

21. *Attorney General Eric Holder*, Attorney General Eric Holder Delivers Remarks at the Johnson and Johnson Press Conference, The United States Department of Justice, *November 4, 2013.* http://www.justice.gov/iso/opa/ag/speeches/2013/ag-speech-131104.html.

22. New York State Unified Court System, "Scheme to Defraud in the Second Degree," http:// www.nycourts.gov/cji/2-PenalLaw/190/190.60.pdf.

23. Thomas Catan, *Con Artist Starred in Sting That Cost Google Millions, The Wall Street Journal*, January 25, 2012. http://online.wsj.com/news/articles/SB10001424052970204624204577176964003660658.

24. Huge Medical Insurance Scam Alleged, ABC News, *March 18*; http://abcnews.go.com/Primetime/story?id=131894&page=1#.TswWoWB-Tbp.

25. *USA Today*, November 30, 2004, at 3A.

26. *USA Today*, November 29, 2004, at 3A.

27. http://www.cbsnews.com/stories/2004/08/13/60minutes/main635860.shtml.

28. Charles Montaldo, "Profile of serial killer Richard Angelo," About.com; http://crime.about.com/od/serial/a/richardangelo.htm.

29. Collwell, *The Verdict of Angelo*, 50(103) *Newsday* 1989, at 3.

30. 683 P.2d 1202 (Colo. 1984).

31. 184 S.W.3d 122 (Mo. App. 2006).

32. Alan Cooper, "Virginia court rules identity theft victim to get $532,000 from credit agency," CBS Interactive Business Network Resource Library.

33. http://www.collegian.psu.edu/archives/article_a90522a0-e00a-57bc-9c67-2eb64b1018ba.html.

34. HospitalHealthcare.com, "NHS hospital theft costs millions," June 6, 2008; http:// www.hospitalhealthcare.com/default.asp?page=article.display&title=NHShospital theftscostmillions&article.id=11504.

35. Anne Zieger, "Millions of patient billing records stolen from UT hospital," FierceHealthIT, June 14, 2008; http://www.fiercehealthit.com/story/millions-patient-billing-records-stolen-uthospital/2008-06-14-0.

36. Tim Eberly, "Grady Hospital battles patient thefts," *Atlanta Journal-Constitution,* July 24, 2008.

37. 492 N.Y.S.2d 9 (N.Y. 1985).

38. *City of Cookeville*, No. M2001-00695-SC-R11-CV (Tenn. 2004).

39. 7 S.W.3d 542 (Mo. App. 1999).

40. http://www.njlawjournal.com/id=1202629427960&Mother_With_Terminal_Cancer_Can_Retain_Child_Custody_Judge_Holds.

41. No. 537-907 (Wis. Cir. Ct. Mar. 18, 1983).

42. 411 So. 2d 109, 113 (Ala. 1982).

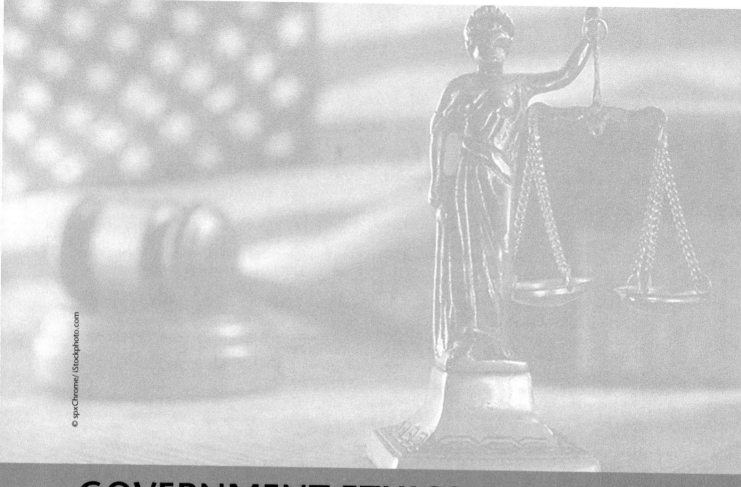

GOVERNMENT ETHICS AND THE LAW

Nothing is politically right which is morally wrong.

–Daniel O'Connell (1775–1847)[1]

LEARNING OBJECTIVES

Upon completion of this chapter, the reader will be able to:

- Describe some of the reasons why there has been a loss of trust in government.
- Explain the purpose of various government committees on ethics.
- Discuss how public policy protects the rights of citizens.
- Describe federal laws designed to protect each individual's rights.
- Explain the concept of political malpractice.
- Understand the importance of ethics in public service.

Let every American, every lover of liberty, every well wisher to his posterity, swear by the blood of the Revolution, never to violate in the least particular, the laws of the country; and never to tolerate their violation by others. As the patriots of seventy-six did to the support of the Declaration of Independence, so to the support of the Constitution and Laws, let every American pledge his life, his property, and his sacred honor—let every man remember that to violate the law, is to trample on the blood of his father, and to tear the character of his own, and his children's liberty. Let reverence for the laws, be breathed by every American mother, to the lisping babe, that prattles on her lap—let it be taught in schools, in seminaries, and in colleges; let it be written in Primers, spelling books, and in Almanacs—let it be preached from the pulpit, proclaimed in legislative halls, and enforced in courts of justice. And, in short, let it become the political religion of the nation; and let the old and the young, the rich and the poor, the grave and the gay, of all sexes and tongues, and colors and conditions, sacrifice unceasingly upon its altars.[2]

—ABRAHAM LINCOLN

The words of Abraham Lincoln, so passionately spoken, resonate true today. Political corruption, antisocial behavior, declining civility, Veterans Administration hospitals misrepresenting wait times for veterans to get doctors' appointments, and rampant unethical conduct have heightened discussions over the nation's moral decline and decaying value systems. The numerous instances of questionable political decisions, executives with shocking salaries, dishonesty at work and school, sexually explicit websites, and the entertainment media have contributed to this decline. Legislators, investigators, prosecutors, and the courts have been quick to speak moral truths but continue to be slow in action. Can this boat be turned around, or are we just plugging the holes with new laws and creating more leaks in a misguided sinking ship?

The question remains: Can the decline in ethical behavior be reversed as citizens struggle with a broken legal system inundated with new laws? The answer is more likely to be a return to practicing the virtues and values upon which this nation was founded. Ethics and the law are not mutually exclusive—they are intertwined throughout the text, providing an overview of government agencies designed to protect each individual's rights (e.g., the right to privacy and self-determination).

U.S. OFFICE OF GOVERNMENT ETHICS

The *Office of Government Ethics* (OGE) is an agency within the executive branch of government whose mission and goals is to foster high ethical standards for employees in the executive branch of government. Common ethical issues that come under the committee's purview include gifts from outside sources, gifts between employees, conflicting financial interests, remedies for financial conflicts of interest, impartiality in performing official duties, seeking other employment, misuse of position, outside activities, postemployment, representation to government agencies and courts, supplementation of salary, financial disclosure, informal advisory letters and memoranda and formal opinions, DAEOgrams (memoranda to Designated Agency Ethics Officials providing guidance on how to interpret and comply with modifications or new issuances of ethics laws, policies, and procedures; copies of the memoranda released since 1992 are available in the DAEOgrams section of the OGE website), and contractors in the workplace.[3]

HOUSE OF REPRESENTATIVES COMMITTEE ON ETHICS

I weep for the liberty of my country when I see at this early day of its successful experiment that corruption has been imputed to many members of the House of Representatives, and the rights of the people have been bartered for promises of office.

—Andrew Jackson

The Committee on Ethics is designated the "supervising ethics office" for the House of Representatives. The jurisdiction of the Committee on Ethics is derived from authority granted under House Rules and federal statutes.

> The Committee on Ethics is unique in the House of Representatives. Consistent with the duty to carry out its advisory and enforcement responsibilities in an impartial manner, the Committee is the only standing committee of the House of Representatives with its membership divided evenly by party. These rules are intended to provide a fair procedural framework for the conduct of the Committee's activities and to help ensure that the Committee serves the people of the United States, the House of Representatives, and the Members, officers, and employees of the House of Representatives.[4]

The scope of the committee's jurisdiction under the various authorizing rules and statutes involves duties and responsibilities related to:

- Jurisdiction over all bills, resolutions, and other matters relating to the Code of Official Conduct.
- Recommendations of administrative actions to establish or enforce standards of official conduct.
- Investigation of alleged violations of the Code of Official Conduct or of any applicable rules, laws, or regulations governing the performance of official duties or the discharge of official responsibilities.
- Reports to appropriate federal or state authorities substantial evidence of a violation of any law applicable to the performance of official duties that may have been disclosed in a committee investigation.
- Consideration of requests for written waivers of the gift rule.
- Oversight over foreign gifts and gifts to superiors and other federal employees.
- Prohibition of members, officers, and employees of the House of Representatives from soliciting or receiving gifts.[5]

(a) The ideal concept of public office, expressed by the words, "a public office is a public trust," signifies that the officer has been entrusted with public power by the people; that the officer holds this power in trust to be used only for their benefit and never for the benefit of himself or of a few; and that the officer must never conduct his own affairs so as to infringe on the public interest. All official conduct of Members of the Senate should be guided by this paramount concept of public office.[6]

The U.S. Senate Select Committee on Ethics consists of six members of the Senate, of whom three shall be selected from members of the majority party and three shall be selected from members of the minority party.[7] The committee is responsible for investigating complaints involving a violation of the Franking statute, Financial Disclosure Statements and for Outside Employment with respect to members, officers, and employees of the Senate, foreign gifts and decorations, gifts to an official superior or receiving gifts from employees with a lower salary level, prohibitions against members, officers, and employees of the Senate soliciting or receiving gifts.[8]

The Senate Select Committee on Ethics is authorized to receive and investigate allegations of improper conduct which may reflect upon the Senate, violations of law, violations of the Senate Code of Official Conduct, and violations of rules and regulations of the Senate; recommend disciplinary action; recommend additional Senate rules or regulations to insure proper standards of conduct; and report violations of law to the proper federal and state authorities.[9]

OFFICE OF CONGRESSIONAL ETHICS

The Office of Congressional Ethics (OCE) was created in March 2008 as an independent, nonpartisan office governed by a board composed of private citizens that provides more public review and insight into the ethical conduct of members of the House of Representatives. The OCE reviews allegations of misconduct against members, officers, and staff of the House and, when appropriate, refers matters to the House Committee on Ethics. The OCE is not authorized to determine if a violation occurred nor it is it authorized to sanction members, officers, or employees of the House or to recommend sanctions. The OCE is not able to provide advice or education on the rules and standards of conduct applicable to members, officers, and employees of the House.[10] The mission of the OCE and its board is to assist the House in upholding high standards of ethical conduct for its members, officers, and staff and, in so doing, to serve the American people. The board of directors consists of eight members, which are private citizens and cannot serve as members of Congress or work for the federal government.[11] As the reader will note, there are a variety of laws and agencies that provide oversight and regulations that are designed to protect the right and safety of all citizens. Government is a reflection of the people it serves. Failure of the many to participate in the political process leads to government for the few who do.

As with other branches of government federal judges are expected to abide by a code of conduct that includes ethical principles and guidelines. "The Code of Conduct provides guidance for judges on issues of judicial integrity and independence, judicial diligence and impartiality, permissible extra-judicial activities, and the avoidance of impropriety or even its appearance."[12]

PUBLIC POLICY

Public policy is the principle of law that holds that no one can lawfully do that which tends to be injurious to the public or against the public good. The sources of public policy "include legislation; administrative rules, regulations, or decisions; and judicial decisions. In certain instances, a professional code of ethics may contain an expression of public policy."[13]

Ethics and the law are not mutually exclusive—they are intertwined. Without the two, we would become a lawless land. The following pages present an overview of laws, influenced by ethical principles, designed to protect each individual's rights (e.g., the right to privacy and self-determination).

VETERANS ADMINISTRATION

The House Committee on Veterans' Affairs reviews veteran programs, examines current laws, and reports bills and amendments to strengthen existing laws concerning veterans and the Department of Veterans Affairs (VA), such as health care and disability compensation. Jeff Miller (R-FL) chairs the committee.[14] The news clippings below describe a variety of concerns with care veterans are receiving in Veterans Hospitals. Although there is undoubtedly excellent care in the VA system, there is a need to improve the care for every veteran, as noted by committee chairman Jeff Miller:

A pattern of heartbreaking veteran deaths, suicides and a host of other patient safety issues have cast a dark shadow over VA medical centers around the country. For months we have tried in vain to compel VA leaders to take meaningful steps to prevent future adverse incidents by holding accountable VA employees and managers responsible for letting patients fall through the cracks. Unfortunately, department officials seem more intent on issuing bureaucratic slaps on the wrist than the sort of serious punishments required to send a message that substandard care for veterans will not be tolerated. What's more, patient deaths apparently aren't even enough to prevent failing VA executives from receiving huge performance bonuses and glowing performance reviews. Because these issues are long-standing, systemic, and evidently immune to the current structure of accountability within VA, I believe President Obama's direct involvement and leadership is required to help us end the culture of complacency that is engulfing the Veterans Health Administration and compromising patient safety." [15]

With growing concerns that certain VA hospitals have been misrepresenting wait times for veterans to schedule medical appointments, Veterans Affairs Secretary Eric Shinseki, under increasing pressure by Congress, resigned his position. President Obama nominated Robert A. McDonald for the position, which was confirmed by Congress on July 29, 2014.[16]

VA, Heal Thyself, Agency is Told at Hearing Filled with Pained Testimony

The House Committee on Veteran's Affairs met in Pittsburgh on Monday to hear testimony about problems with health care at agency facilities in that city and others.

• • •

Miller said the "the vast majority of the departments more than 300,000 employees are dedicated and hard-working, and many veterans are satisfied with the medical care they received from the VA."

But he and others sharply doubted the ability of the department's leadership to avoid "heartbreaking situations" like those reported to the committee.

"By now," he said, "It's abundantly clear to most people that a culture change at VA is in order."

Joe Davidson, The Washington Post, *September 13, 2013*

Atlanta VA Exec Scored Bonuses While Audits Found Lapses

The former top administrator at the Atlanta VA Medical Center received $65,000 in performance bonuses over a four-year span as internal audits revealed lengthy wait times for mental health care and mismanagement that led to three deaths.

Daniel Malloy, The Atlanta Journal – Constitution, *April 26, 2013*

"Too trapped in a war to be at peace"

Shortly before his death on June 10, Army veteran Daniel Somers wrote a note for his family, asking his wife, Angel, to share it as she saw fit.

"I am left with basically nothing," he typed on his laptop at their Phoenix townhouse. "Too trapped in a war to be at peace, too damaged to be at war."

His service in Iraq, including multiple combat missions as a turret gunner, left him with severe post–traumatic stress disorder and traumatic brain injury. But the government, he wrote, had "turned around and abandoned me."

Steve Vogel, The Washington Post, *August 24, 2013*

Daniel Somers eventually saw a caregiver. Unfortunately for Daniel, the caregiver retired. He attempted to make a new appointment. That is when he ran into the all too common roadblock, being told that there was a shortage of caregivers and that he would be notified when he could be scheduled for his next appointment.

The following *reality check* is believed by some to be an all too common experience by inspectors of not only VA hospitals but many hospitals across the country.

VA Hospital

And so there we were in a VA hospital, sent to survey the quality of patient care services provided to veterans. During the survey, there seemed to be a lack of interest in constructive suggestions as to how the hospital could improve services. Survey team members who wrote negative findings had been watched closely as though they were the ones being surveyed throughout the process. The real concern of management seemed to be more how the surveyors would score the hospital's delivery of care to veterans, then how they could improve services. They seemed pleasant when things were going well, argumentative when they were not. The surveyors were between a rock and a hard place. Not only do the surveyors score the hospital, the hospital scores the surveyors as required by the surveyors' employer. Down score the hospital and the inspectors could often expect to be down scored. The problem comes down to the integrity of the surveyor and the hospital. If a hospital views a survey as an opportunity to learn and improve patient care services, it is likely that it can be a win-win situation for both the surveyors and the hospital, ultimately benefiting the patient.

Anonymous

The next *reality check* illustrates how the majority of veterans standing outside a major VA hospital waiting for the clinics to open viewed their care. As I approached them and inquired about their care, it was reassuring that these veterans were extremely positive as to the care they were receiving.

Veterans Lack Insurance Benefits

Marc had a chat with some veterans about their health care benefits. Most seemed satisfied. Joe, one of the veterans, opening his mouth wide to show me, said, "Look at my teeth. [He had but a few teeth in his mouth.] They won't fix them because they are not considered a war-related injury." He turned his head sideways, and Marc noticed that an ear was missing. Joe continued, "Now this ear is gone. I lost it during the Viet Nam war. I was, however, able to get a prosthesis. It needs some work, so I didn't wear it. I guess they will provide me with a new one. I am able to get care for it because it is a war-related injury, but I really could use some teeth."

Marc queried the hospital about Joe's teeth. They said that because of policy and the fact that Joe's teeth were not related to a war injury, there was nothing that they could do for him. They did however suggest Joe could go to the University Hospital and get a set of false teeth that should be relatively inexpensive. Marc asked to see the hospital's dental area. Following a tour of the dental suite, Marc commented, "This is the most modern dental facility I have ever seen." The staff was happy that Marc was pleased with the facility. After observing ample staff, workspace, modern equipment, top of the line dental chairs, and unoccupied rooms, he asked, "Are you open? Where are the patients?" The staff in unison responded, "Oh yes, we are open but we don't have any patients at the moment. We should have a few later." The staff proceeded to discuss with enthusiasm the wide variety of dental procedures they could provide, including complicated extractions, implants, preparation of dentures, and so on.

Discussion

1. Would you consider this to be a form of political malpractice? Discuss your answer.
2. Because hospital staff was able to make suggestions to a veteran for care outside the Veterans Administration health care system, how would you respond if you were the veteran?

FOURTEENTH AMENDMENT TO THE CONSTITUTION

According to the Fourteenth Amendment to the Constitution, a state cannot act to deny any person equal protection of the laws. If a state or a political subdivision of a state, whether through its executive, judicial, or legislative branch, acts in such a way as to deny unfairly to any person the rights accorded to another, the amendment has been violated.

Section 1. All persons born or naturalized in the United States, and subject to the jurisdiction thereof, are citizens of the United States and of the state wherein they reside. No State shall make or enforce any law, which shall abridge the privileges or immunities of citizens of the United States; nor shall any State deprive any person of life, liberty, or property, without due process of law; nor deny to any person within its jurisdiction the equal protection of the laws

Section 5. The Congress shall have power to enforce, by appropriate legislation, the provisions of this article.

TITLE VI: CIVIL RIGHTS ACT

Civil rights are those rights ensured by the U.S. Constitution and by the acts of Congress and the state legislatures. Generally, the term includes all the rights of each individual in a free society.

Congress and the federal courts have dealt with discriminatory practices in health care organizations. Discrimination in the admission of patients and segregation of patients on racial grounds are prohibited in any organization receiving federal financial assistance. Pursuant to Title VI of the *Civil Rights Act* of 1964, the guidelines of the Department of Health and

Human Services (HHS) prohibit the practice of racial discrimination by any organization or agency receiving money under any program supported by HHS. This includes all "providers of service" receiving federal funds under Medicare legislation.

SHERMAN ANTITRUST ACT

The *Sherman Antitrust Act*, named for its author, Senator John Sherman of Ohio, prescribes that every contract, combination in the form of trust or otherwise, or conspiracy in restraint of trade or commerce among the several states is declared to be illegal. Those who attempt to monopolize, combine, or conspire with any other person or persons to monopolize any part of the trade or commerce can be deemed guilty of a felony.[17] Areas of concern for health care organizations include reduced market competition, price fixing, actions that bar or limit new entrants to the field, preferred provider arrangements, and exclusive contracts.

A health care organization must be cognizant of the potential problems that may exist when limiting the number of physicians that it will admit to its medical staff. Because closed staff determinations can effectively limit competition from other physicians, the governing body must ensure that the decision-making process in granting privileges is based on legislative, objective criteria and is not dominated by those who have the most to gain competitively by denying privileges. Physicians have attempted to use state and federal antitrust laws to challenge determinations denying or limiting medical staff privileges. Generally, these actions claim that the organization conspired with its medical staff to ensure that the complaining physician would not obtain privileges in order to reduce competition.

PRIVACY ACT

The *Privacy Act of 1974*, Title 5 United States Code (U.S.C.) 552, was enacted to safeguard individual privacy from the misuse of federal records, to give individuals access to records concerning themselves that are maintained by federal agencies, and to establish a Privacy Protection Safety Commission. Section 2 of the Privacy Act reads as follows:

[a] The Congress finds that (1) the privacy of an individual is directly affected by the collection, maintenance, use, and dissemination of personal information by Federal agencies; (2) the increasing use of computers and sophisticated information technology, while essential to the efficient operations of the Government, has greatly magnified the harm to individual privacy that can occur from any collection, maintenance, use, or dissemination of personal information; (3) the opportunities for an individual to secure employment, insurance, and credit, and his right to due process, and other legal protections are endangered by the misuse of certain information systems; (4) the right to privacy is a personal and fundamental right protected by the Constitution of the United States; and (5) in order to protect the privacy of individuals identified in information systems maintained by Federal agencies, it is necessary and proper for the Congress to regulate the collection, maintenance, use, and dissemination of information by such agencies. [b] The purpose of this Act is to provide certain safeguards for an individual against an invasion of personal privacy by requiring Federal agencies, except as otherwise provided by law, to (1) permit an individual to determine what records pertaining to him are collected, maintained, used, or disseminated by such agencies; (2) permit an individual to prevent records pertaining to him

obtained by such agencies for a particular purpose from being used or made available for another purpose without his consent; (3) permit an individual to gain access to information pertaining to him in Federal agency records, to have a copy made of all or any portion thereof, and to correct or amend such records; (4) collect, maintain, use, or disseminate any record of identifiable personal information in a manner that assures that such action is for a necessary and lawful purpose, that the information is current and accurate for its intended use, and that adequate safeguards are provided to prevent misuse of such information . . .

HEALTH INSURANCE PORTABILITY AND ACCOUNTABILITY ACT (HIPAA)

The *Health Insurance Portability and Accountability Act* (HIPAA) of 1996 (Public Law 104–191) was designed to protect the privacy, confidentiality, and security of patient information. HIPAA standards are applicable to all health information in all of its formats (e.g., electronic, paper, verbal). It applies to both electronically maintained and transmitted information. HIPAA privacy standards include restrictions on access to individually identifiable health information and the use and disclosure of that information, as well as requirements for administrative activities such as training, compliance, and enforcement of HIPAA mandates.

EMERGENCY MEDICAL TREATMENT AND ACTIVE LABOR ACT (EMTALA)

In 1986, Congress passed the *Emergency Medical Treatment and Active Labor Act* (EMTALA), which forbids Medicare-participating hospitals from "dumping" patients out of emergency departments. The act provides that:

> In the case of a hospital that has a hospital emergency department, if any individual (whether or not eligible for benefits under this subchapter) comes to the emergency department and a request is made on the individual's behalf for examination or treatment for a medical condition, the hospital must provide for an appropriate medical screening examination within the capability of the hospital emergency department, including ancillary services routinely available to the emergency department, to determine whether or not an emergency medical condition . . . exists.[18]

EMTALA was clearly violated in the *Burditt* case reviewed next.

CASE: EMTALA VIOLATED

In *Burditt v. U.S. Department of Health and Human Services*,[19] EMTALA was violated by a physician when he ordered a woman with dangerously high blood pressure (210/130) and in active labor with ruptured membranes transferred from the emergency department of one hospital to another hospital 170 miles away. The physician was assessed a penalty of $20,000. Dr. Louis Sullivan, secretary of HHS at that time, issued a statement: "This decision sends a message to physicians everywhere that they need to provide quality care to everyone in need of emergency treatment who comes to a hospital. This is a significant opinion and we are pleased with the result."[20] The American Public Health Association, in filing an amicus curiae brief, advised the appeals court that "if Burditt wants to ensure that he will never be asked to treat a patient not of his choosing, then he ought to vote with his feet by affiliating only with hospitals that do not accept Medicare funds or do not have an emergency department."[21]

Ethical and Legal Issues

1. What are the main issues in this case?
2. What ethical theories, principles, and values are of concern? Describe them.
3. What action can be taken to prevent similar occurrences in the future?
4. What could have been done to prevent the ethical and legal issues from occurring in the first place?
5. If you were the judge in this case, what would you do in light of the American Public Health Association's comments?
6. Describe both the hospital and physician's ethical and legal responsibilities.

HEALTH CARE QUALITY IMPROVEMENT ACT

The *Health Care Quality Improvement Act* of 1986 (HCQIA) was enacted in part to provide those persons giving information to professional review bodies and those assisting in review activities limited immunity from damages that may arise as a result of adverse decisions that affect a physician's medical staff privileges. Before enacting the HCQIA, Congress found that "[t]he increasing occurrence of medical malpractice and the need to improve the quality of medical care . . . [had] become nationwide problems," especially in light of "the ability of incompetent physicians to move from State to State without disclosure or discovery of the physician's previous damaging or incompetent performance" (42 U.S.C. § 11101). The problem, however, could be remedied through effective professional peer review combined with a national reporting system that made information about adverse professional actions against physicians more widely available. HCQIA was enacted by Congress to "facilitate the frank exchange of information among professionals conducting peer review inquiries without the fear of reprisals in civil lawsuits. The statute attempts to balance the chilling effect of litigation on peer review with concerns for protecting physicians improperly subjected to disciplinary action."

CASE: FAILURE TO MEET ETHICAL STANDARDS

Meyers applied for medical staff privileges at a hospital. Shortly thereafter, the Credentials Committee and the Medical Executive Committee (MEC) and the board of the hospital approved Meyers for appointment to the medical staff. All initial appointments to the medical staff were provisional for 1 year. At the end of that year, the physician was required to be reevaluated for advancement from associate to active staff.

The Credentials Committee began to evaluate Meyers for advancement to active staff privileges. The committee was concerned about Meyers's history: moving from hospital to hospital after disputes with hospital staff, his failure to disclose timely and fully disciplinary and corrective action taken against him in another state, and the quality of his patient care. The MEC voted to accept a Credentials Committee recommendation to revoke Meyers's staff privileges. The MEC was to consider the recommendation from the Credentials Committee and make a recommendation to the board, which had the ultimate authority to grant or deny advancement, or terminate Meyers's privileges.

The board informed Meyers that it was assuming responsibility for determining his reappointment and advancement to active staff because of concerns with the manner in which the peer review process was being handled. Three members of the board, acting as a Credentials Committee, conducted an independent review. This committee discussed concerns about Meyers's behavior and his inability to get along with others, in addition to questions about his surgical technique. The committee questioned Meyers about several incident reports concerning disruptive behavior, his history of problems at other hospitals, his failure to complete medical records timely, his hostility toward the operation room staff, reports of breaking the sterile field, and his failure to provide appropriate coverage for patients while he was away. Meyers acknowledged that he had a personality problem.

The three-member committee of the board voted to deny Meyers's appointment to active staff. The reasons cited for the committee's decision were Meyers's failure to satisfy requirements that he "abide by the ethics of the profession," work cooperatively with others, timely complete medical records, and abide by hospital standards. The committee outlined Meyers's pattern of rude, abusive, and disruptive behavior that included, but was not limited to, temper tantrums, attempted interference with the right of an attending physician to refer a patient to the surgeon of his choice or to transfer the patient, condescending remarks toward women, refusal to speak to a member of his surgical team during surgical procedures, and several instances of throwing a scalpel during surgery. The committee informed Meyers that this behavior could have an adverse effect on the quality of patient care. As for his failure to complete medical records timely, the committee stated "delinquent medical records can put patients at risk by being inaccurate or incomplete if needed to assist in later diagnosis and treatment of a patient."

A Fair Hearing Committee issued its recommendation that Meyers not be reappointed to the hospital's staff because of his failure to meet "ethical standards" and his inability to work cooperatively with others. In May, the board adopted and affirmed the Fair Hearing Committee's recommendation. Ultimately, after further appeals the board revoked Meyers's privileges.

Meyers brought suit in seeking a permanent injunction to require the hospital to reinstate him to staff. The court denied the motion for an injunction that would require the hospital to reinstate Meyers's privileges.

The court agreed with hospital defendants that the behavior of Meyers had the potential of affecting the health and welfare of patients, despite the fact that no patients were actually injured. High-quality patient care demands that doctors possess at least a reasonable ability to work with others. Clearly, the hospital defendants were acting with a reasonable belief that the professional review action was in the furtherance of quality health care. They were concerned that Meyers's behavior would continue until a patient was injured as a result of his actions.[22]

Ethical and Legal Issues

1. Describe the ethical theories, principles, and values of concern in this case.
2. Describe what steps the organization could take to prevent similar occurrences in the future.

Agency for Healthcare Research and Quality

The *Agency for Healthcare Research and Quality* (AHRQ), established in 1989, is charged with researching ways to improve the quality of health care, reduce its costs, and broaden access to essential services. The AHRQ was created as a result of the mistakes that have occurred and continue to occur in the delivery of care. The pain, misery, and financial drain on the injured, their families, and society have taken its toll. The numerous ethical and legal issues that have evolved spawned the need for the AHRQ.

Ethics in Patient Referral Act

In 1989, the *Ethics in Patient Referral Act* was enacted, prohibiting physicians who have ownership interest or compensation arrangements with a clinical laboratory from referring Medicare patients to that laboratory. The law also requires all Medicare providers to report the names and provider numbers of all physicians or their immediate relatives with ownership interests in the provider entity prior to October 1, 1991.

Patient Self-Determination Act

The *Patient Self-Determination Act* of 1990 (PSDA)[23] was enacted to ensure that patients are informed of their rights to execute advance directives and accept or refuse medical care. On December 1, 1991, the PSDA[24] took effect in hospitals, skilled nursing facilities, home health agencies, hospice organizations, and health maintenance organizations serving Medicare and Medicaid patients. As a result of implementation of the PSDA,[25] health care organizations participating in the Medicare and Medicaid reimbursement programs must address patient rights regarding life-sustaining decisions and other advance directives. Health care organizations have a responsibility to explain to patients, staff, and families that patients have a legal right to direct their own medical and nursing care as it corresponds to existing state law, including right-to-die directives. A person's right to refuse medical treatment is not lost when his or her mental or physical status changes. When a person is no longer competent to exercise his or her right of self-determination, the right still exists, but the decision must be delegated to a surrogate decision maker. Those organizations that do not comply with a patient's medical directives or those of a legally authorized decision maker are exposing themselves to the risk of a lawsuit.

Each state is required under the PSDA to provide a description of the law in the state regarding advance directives to providers, whether such directives are based on state statutes or judicial decisions. Providers must ensure that written policies and procedures with respect to all adult individuals regarding advance directives are established as follows:[26]

(A) to provide written information to each such individual concerning

(i) an individual's rights under State law (whether statutory or as recognized by the courts of the State) to make decisions concerning such medical care, including the right to accept or refuse medical or surgical treatment and the right to formulate advance directives . . . and

(ii) written policies of the provider organization respecting the implementation of such rights;

(B) to document in the individual's medical record whether or not the individual has executed an advance directive;

(C) not to condition the provision of care or otherwise discriminate against an individual based on whether or not the individual has executed an advance directive;

(D) to ensure compliance with requirements of State law (whether statutory or recognized by the courts of the State) respecting advance directives at the facilities of the provider or organization; and

(E) to provide (individually or with others) for education for staff and the community on issues concerning advance directives.

Although the PSDA is being cheered as a major advancement in clarifying and nationally regulating this often obscure area of law and medicine, there are continuing problems and new issues that must be addressed.

SARBANES-OXLEY ACT

The sense of somehow me beating up on Wall Street, I think most folks on Main Street feel like they got beat up on. . . . There's a big chunk of the country that thinks that I have been too soft on Wall Street. That's probably the majority, not the minority.

If you're making a billion dollars a year after a very bad financial crisis where eight million people lost their jobs and small businesses can't get loans, then I think that you shouldn't be feeling put upon.

The notion that somehow me saying maybe you should be taxed more like your secretary when you're pulling home a billion dollars or a hundred million dollars a year, I don't think is me being extremist or being anti-business.

—PRESIDENT BARACK OBAMA

The *Sarbanes-Oxley Act* was signed by President George W. Bush on July 30, 2002, in response to the Enron debacle and high-profile cases of corporate financial mismanagement. The act requires top executives of public corporations to vouch for the financial reports of their companies. The act encourages self regulation and the need to promote due diligence, select a leader with morals and core values, examine incentives, constantly monitor the organization's culture, build a strong, knowledgeable governing body, be on the alert for conflicts of interest, focus attention on the right things, and have the courage to speak out.

PATIENT PROTECTION AND AFFORDABLE CARE ACT (2010)

The *Patient Protection and Affordable Care Act* (PPACA) is a federal statute that contains a set of health care reforms passed by Congress and signed into law by President Barack Obama on March 23, 2010. After several challenges as to the constitutionally of the PPACA, the United States Supreme Court determined in 2012 that the PPACA was constitutional.

The PPACA was designed to expand medical insurance coverage to Americans that did not already have it by offering affordable and competitive rates through a newly created Health Insurance Marketplace, providing subsidies to individuals based on ability to pay.

The law was set to bring insurance coverage to over 30 million Americans who never had coverage. The PPACA includes provisions for reform of the private health insurance market, providing better coverage for people with preexisting conditions, improving prescription drug coverage in Medicare, and extending the life of the Medicare trust fund by at least 12 years.

The website www.healthcare.gov has been set up to assist those who wish to purchase health insurance. The website has been fraught with problems in connecting and signing up for insurance. Glitches in the system should come as no surprise with such a far-reaching program considering a population of over 317 million. As with a wedding of 300 people, there are glitches and often times a lot of angry people who were invited to the church but not the reception, food was cold, the wedding was on an island in the South Pacific, you preferred to sit at a different table then the one you were assigned, you were placed to far away from the bride and groom's table, you were forgotten when the family picture was taken, and yet you were the grandparents, etc. In the end there is a happily married couple. The plan for the PPACA is to provide a more affordable and accessible health care system. Unfortunately, the political battles over the PPACA continue to disrupt the democratic process.

Congress continues to make decisions on a bipartisan basis, often, seemingly, without regard to the needs of the people. There are those who consider health care a right and others who consider it a privilege. Many believe, for Congress, it seems, health care is a right, as noted by their superior health insurance plans at reduced costs due to lucrative subsidized health insurance premiums paid by the people. The costs associated with PPACA are without question fraught with numerous ethical dilemmas. Responsibility for reducing the costs associated with PPACA lies in part with each individual and their chosen style of life, which includes the abuse of addictive substances.

POLITICAL MALPRACTICE

I hate all the bungling as I do sin, but particularly bungling in politics, which leads to the misery and ruin of many thousands and millions of people.

–Johann Wolfgang von Goethe

Political malpractice is negligent conduct by an elected or appointed political official. Ronald Brownstein wrote in a news column in the *St. Petersburg Times*, "Practical steps are possible to help millions of low income families live healthier lives and receive more effective care when they need it. Ignoring that opportunity, while waiting for consensus on coverage, would be a form of political malpractice."[27]

The likelihood of a successful negligence case against a member of Congress is doubtful. If such a case ever got through a courtroom door the following four elements of negligence would have to be proven:

1. The first element necessary to prove political malpractice requires that the plaintiff/s be able to establish there is *a duty to care*. Establishing this first element of negligence for a senator, for example, would be a difficult hurdle to jump. The oath of office for a senator is so amorphous that it would be difficult to establish a duty to care, as illustrated in the following quotes.

Oath of Office

I do solemnly swear (or affirm) that I will support and defend the Constitution of the United States against all enemies, foreign and domestic; that I will bear true faith and allegiance to the same; that I take this obligation freely, without any mental reservation or purpose of evasion; and that I will well and faithfully discharge the duties of the office on which I am about to enter: So help me God.[28]

Looking beyond the oath of office:

For nearly three-quarters of a century, that oath served nicely, although to the modern ear it sounds woefully incomplete. Missing are the soaring references to bearing "true faith and allegiance"; to taking "this obligation freely, without any mental reservation or purpose of evasion"; and to "well and faithfully" discharging the duties of the office.[29]

> Should a plaintiff be able to overcome this first element of negligence, thus proving a duty to care, the remaining elements could be just as difficult to establish.

2. The second element of political malpractice requires the plaintiff to prove that the *duty to care was breached*. Arguably, politicians, for example, who agree to veto any program the President supports while he is in office is contrary to the spirit of the law. The dilemma here requires the plaintiff/s to prove what specific duty to care was breached.

3. The third element of political malpractice requires proof of harm.

4. The fourth element requires proof of a *causal connection* between the politician's breach of duty and harm suffered. In other words, the plaintiff/s must prove that the breach of duty was the proximate cause of the plaintiff's injury.

Like medical malpractice, political malpractice involves a failure to offer professional services to help prevent the travesties that take place daily, as illustrated by the following anonymous true story.

The Coal Miner

Jimmy was a coal miner who had black lung disease. I had introduced myself to him as the administrator. Jimmy introduced himself to me and then turned to a man who was on the opposite side of his bed and said, "This is my brother Bill." I asked, as he turned looking back at me, "Are we taking good care of you?" He said, "Yes." Bill, looking at me, choked up and asked, "Can you help my brother? He has given up the will to live. Please help my brother want to live." I looked at Jimmy lying there in his bed, fragile and struggling to breathe between each word, as he said, "I can no longer carry on this way. I am ready to move on. I'm a tired old man. I have fought so long. I've needed benefits for so many years for my family and myself. No one was able to help me. You see, I have black lung disease. I can barely breathe." He then turned, looking over to Bill, and said, "My brother also has black lung disease. We worked together in the coalmines for many years. This is our reward." I looked at Jimmy and slowly back to Bill and said, "I will help you." As we said our goodbyes, I thought to myself, as I left the room, this man has fought so long. He has asked for so little, a man forgotten by a cruel system of corrupt government and greedy corporations. I remember this day all too well. It brings tears to my eyes as I recall the sadness of that day.

Administrator

Discussion

1. Explain what action you would take to help Jimmy.
2. Describe the ethical principles that apply to this case.

CHAPTER REVIEW

1. Government Ethics Committees
   - U.S. Office of Government Ethics
     - Agency within the executive branch of government.
   - House of Representatives Committee on Ethics
   - Senate Select Committee on Ethics
   - Office of Congressional Ethics
   - U.S. Judicial Code of Conduct
2. Public Policy Protecting the Rights of Citizens—Principle of law that holds that no one can lawfully do that which tends to be injurious to the public or against the public good.
   - Veterans Administration
   - Fourteenth Amendment to the Constitution
     - A state cannot act to deny any person equal protection of the laws.
   - Title VI of the Civil Rights Act of 1964
     - HHS prohibits the practice of racial discrimination by any organization or agency receiving money under any program supported by HHS.
   - Sherman Antitrust Act
   - The Privacy Act of 1974, Title 5 United States Code (U.S.C.) 552
     - Enacted to safeguard individual privacy from the misuse of federal records.
     - Provide individuals access to records concerning themselves that are maintained by federal agencies.
     - Establish a Privacy Protection Safety Commission.
   - HIPAA (Public Law 104-191)
     - Designed to protect the privacy, confidentiality, and security of patient information.
     - HIPAA standards are applicable to all health information in all of its formats (e.g., electronic, paper, verbal). It applies to both electronically maintained and transmitted information.
   - EMTALA
     - Forbids Medicare-participating hospitals from "dumping" patients out of emergency departments.

- HCQIA
  - Enacted in part to provide those persons giving information to professional review bodies and those assisting in review activities limited immunity from damages that may arise as a result of adverse decisions that affect a physician's medical staff privileges.
- AHRQ
  - Charged with researching ways to improve the quality of health care, reduce its costs, and broaden access to essential services.
- Ethics in Patient Referral Act of 1989
  - Prohibits physicians who have ownership interest or compensation arrangements with a clinical laboratory from referring Medicare patients to that laboratory.
- PSDA
  - Enacted to ensure that patients are informed of their rights to execute advance directives and accept or refuse medical care. Each state is required under the PSDA to provide a description of the law in the state regarding advance directives to providers, whether such directives are based on state statutes or judicial decisions.
- Sarbanes-Oxley Act
  - Executives of public corporations to vouch for the financial reports and encourages self-regulation.
3. Political malpractice
  - Negligent or unethical conduct on the part of an elected official.

TEST YOUR UNDERSTANDING

TERMINOLOGY

Agency for Healthcare Research and Quality
Civil Rights Act
Emergency Medical Treatment and Active Labor Act
Ethics in Patient Referral Act
Health Care Quality Improvement Act

Health Insurance Portability and Accountability Act
Office of Government Ethics
Patient Protection and Affordable Care Act
Patient Self-Determination Act
political malpractice
Privacy Act of 1974

public policy
Sarbanes-Oxley Act
Sherman Antitrust Act

REVIEW QUESTIONS

1. Discuss how the various branches of government address ethical issues.

2. Discuss how public policy protects individual rights (e.g., privacy and self-determination).

3. Discuss the legal and ethical implications of the public policy acts presented here.

4. Describe how the concept of "political malpractice" is similar to "medical malpractice" as discussed in this chapter.

NOTES

1. Irish politician.
2. http://www.abrahamlincolnonline.org/lincoln/speeches/lyceum.htm.
3. http://oge.gov/About/Mission-and-Responsibilities/Mission—Responsibilities/.
4. Committee on Ethics, Committee Rules, http://ethics. house.gov/about/committee-rules.
5. Committee on Ethics, Jurisdiction, http://ethics.house.gov/jurisdiction.
6. U.S. Senate Select Committee on Ethics, Jurisdiction, http://www.ethics.senate.gov/public/index.cfm/jurisdiction.
7. U.S. Senate Select Committee on Ethics, Rules of Procedure, http://www.ethics.senate.gov/public/index.cfm/files/serve?File_id=551b39fc-30ed-4b14-b0d3-1706608a6fcb.
8. U.S. Senate Select Committee on Ethics, Jurisdiction, http://www.ethics.senate.gov/public/index.cfm/jurisdiction.
9. *Id.*
10. Office of Congressional Ethics, Frequently Asked Questions, http://oce.house.gov/faq.html.
11. *Id.*
12. http://www.uscourts.gov/RulesAndPolicies/CodesOfConduct.aspx.
13. *Pierce v. Ortho Pharmaceutical Corp.*, 417 A.2d 505, 512 (N.J. 1980).
14. http://veterans.house.gov/about.
15. Rep. Jeff Miller, Chairman, House Committee on Veterans Affairs, *July 11, 2013* http://veterans.house.gov/press-release/miller-president-obama-must-help-stop-patient-deaths-bring-accountability-to-va.
16. http://www.va.gov/opa/bios/secretary.asp.
17. 15 U.S.C. § 1 (1982).
18. 42 U.S.C.A. § 1395dd(a) (1992).
19. 934 F.2d 1362 (5th Cir. Tex. 1991).
20. Courts Uphold Law, *Regulations against Patient Dumping,* Nation's Health, August 1991, at 1.
21. *Id.* at 17.
22. *Meyers v. Logan Mem. Hosp.*, 82 F. Supp. 2d 707 (2000).
23. 42 U.S.C. 1395cc(a)(1).
24. Public Law 101–508, November 5, 1990, sections 4206 and 4751 of the Omnibus Budget Reconciliation Act.
25. 42 U.S.C. § 1395 (1992).
26. 42 U.S.C. § 1395cc (1992).
27. *Health Care Safety Net Stretched Thin*, Ronald Brownstein, *St. Petersburg Times*, June 4, 2004, Section A, at 13a.
28. http://www.senate.gov/artandhistory/history/common/briefing/Oath_Office.htm.
29. *Id.*

ORGANIZATIONAL ETHICS AND THE LAW

It is of utmost importance that each organization recognizes that its success lies with its ability to assure the staff, community and patients that it holds itself accountable to ensuring the highest standards of quality professional care and the well-being of all that enter its hallowed halls.

—Gᴘ

LEARNING OBJECTIVES

Upon completion of this chapter, the reader will be able to:

- Describe corporate structure.
- Describe a code of ethics for organizations.
- Discuss organizational misconduct.
- Explain *respondeat superior* and *corporate negligence*.
- Describe corporate duties and responsibilities.
- Describe strategies to restore organizational trust.

INTRODUCTION

Legal and ethical issues in the health care setting are being carefully scrutinized across the nation by state and federal regulatory agencies. Organizations, like individuals, must comply with rules of law and ethical conduct. This chapter introduces the reader to corporate authority, contents for codes of ethics for organizations, and the ethical and legal risks to which health care organizations and their governing bodies can be exposed. There is an overview of corporate negligence, respondeat superior, and independent contractor. The emphasis of this chapter is on the duties and responsibilities of health care organizations.

CORPORATE AUTHORITY

The typical health care organization is incorporated under state law as a freestanding for-profit or not-for-profit corporation. The corporation has a governing body that has ultimate responsibility for the decisions made in the organization. The existence of this authority creates certain duties and liabilities. The governing body, having ultimate responsibility for the operation and management of the organization, generally delegates responsibility for the day-to-day operations of the organization to the organization's chief executive officer.

Although health care organizations may operate as sole proprietorships or partnerships, most function as corporations. Thus, an important source of law applicable to governing boards and to the duties and responsibilities of their members is state corporation laws. An incorporated health care organization is a legal person with recognized rights, duties, powers, and responsibilities. Because the legal "person" is in reality a "fictitious person," there is a requirement that certain people are designated to exercise the corporate powers and that they are held accountable for corporate decision making.

Health care corporations—governmental, charitable, or proprietary— have certain powers expressly or implicitly granted to them by state statutes. Generally, the authority of a corporation is expressed in the law under which the corporation is chartered and in the corporation's articles of incorporation. The existence of this authority creates certain duties and liabilities for governing bodies and their individual members. Members of the governing body have both express and implied *corporate authority*.

EXPRESS CORPORATE AUTHORITY

Express corporate authority is authority specifically delegated by statute. Health care corporations derive authority to act from the laws of the state in which they are incorporated. The articles of incorporation set forth the purposes of each corporation's existence and the powers that the corporation is authorized to exercise to carry out its purposes.

IMPLIED CORPORATE AUTHORITY

Implied corporate authority is the authority to perform any and all acts necessary to exercise a corporation's expressly conferred authority and to accomplish the purposes for which it was created. Generally, implied corporate authority arises where there is a need for corporate powers not specifically granted in the articles of incorporation. A governing body, at its own discretion, may enact new bylaws, rules, and regulations; purchase or mortgage property; borrow money; purchase equipment; select personnel; adopt corporate resolutions that delineate decision-making responsibilities; and so forth. These powers can be enumerated in the articles of incorporation and, in such cases, would be categorized as express rather than implied corporate authority.

ULTRA VIRES ACTS

Ultra vires is a Latin term meaning "beyond the powers." *Ultra vires acts* are those acts conducted by a corporation that lies beyond its scope of authority to perform. A governing body can be held liable for acting beyond its scope of authority, which is either expressed (e.g., in its articles of incorporation) or implied in law. The governing body acts on behalf of the corporation. If any action is in violation of a statute or regulation, it is illegal. An example of an illegal act would be the "known" employment of an unlicensed person in a position that by law requires a license. The state, through its attorney general, has the power to prevent the performance of an *ultra vires act* by means of an injunction.

CODE OF ETHICS FOR ORGANIZATIONS

Codes of ethics for organizations provide guidelines for behavior that help carry out an organization's mission, vision, and values. Organizational codes of ethics build trust, increase awareness of ethical issues, guide decision-making, and encourage staff to seek advice and report misconduct when appropriate. The following list provides some value statements that should be considered when preparing an organization's code of ethics.

1. Employees and staff members will comply with the organization's code of ethics, which includes compassionate care; an understanding and acceptance of the organization's mission, vision, and values; and adherence to one's professional code of conduct.
2. Ethics training will be provided as required training for all employees.
3. Ethics competencies will be reviewed at the time of each employee's initial ethics training and scheduled evaluation.
4. The organization will be honest and fair in dealings with employees.
5. The organization will develop and maintain an environment that fosters the highest ethical and legal standards.
6. Corporate officers, managers, and employees will be impartial when personal interests conflict with those of the organization and fellow employees.
7. Employees will be free to speak up without fear of retribution or retaliation.
8. A compliance officer will be available to protect employees who wish to speak-up as to unprofessional practices he or she observes in the organization. The compliance officer will be held accountable for maintaining the confidentiality of the employee's identity. Failure to do so will result in the immediate termination of the compliance officer.

9. The pitfalls of groupthink will not be acceptable conduct in the organization. The preservation of harmony will not become more important than the critical evaluation of ideas by *all* employees.

10. Employees and patients will be provided with a safe environment (e.g., freedom from sexual harassment) within which to work.

11. The drive to increase revenues will not be tied to unethical activities, such as work-force cutbacks as a means to discharge employees when they are encouraged to speak up and then blacklisted because of their honesty.

12. Employees will avoid conflict-of-interest situations by not favoring one's own interests over those of others, including the organization.

13. Patients will be provided with care that is of the highest quality regardless of the setting.

14. All patients will be treated with honesty, dignity, respect, and courtesy.

15. Patients will be informed as to the risks, benefits, and alternatives to care.

16. Patients will be treated in a manner that preserves their rights, dignity, autonomy, self-esteem, privacy, and involvement in their care.

17. Each patient's culture, religion, and heritage will be respected and addressed as appropriate.

18. The organization will provide for a patient advocacy program.

19. The organization will provide appropriate support services for those with physical disabilities (e.g., those with language barriers and those who are hearing- or seeing-impaired).

20. Patients will be provided with a "Patient's Bill of Rights and Responsibilities" on admission to the hospital.

21. Each patient's right to execute advance directives will be honored.

UNPROFESSIONAL CONDUCT

Unprofessional conduct continues to plague the health care system. Complex health care fraud schemes, for example, resulting in losses of billions of dollars annually impede advances in medicine and deny high-quality health care to the people. Enforcing and bringing to justice the number of individuals and organizations who defraud the government simply add to the losses. This section introduces the reader to a variety of ethical and legal risks associated with such conduct. Unprincipled behavior and conduct includes: lack of trust and integrity; false advertising; failure to disclose financial incentives, and concealing mistakes.

TRUST AND INTEGRITY

Trust and integrity cannot always be presumed. Organizations must encourage patients to ask questions and seek second opinions both for peace of mind and to aid in determining the best course of treatment. As noted in the next news clipping, some health care providers consider their financial interests more important then the welfare of their patients.

Settlement Reached in St. Joe's Medical Malpractice Case

A federal investigation and hospital review that began in 2010 found hundreds of cases between 2007 and 2009 in which Midei allegedly profited by placing stents in patients' arteries that weren't medically necessary.

• • •

During opening statements in the case, lawyers for the plaintiffs said the coronary unit at St. Joe's was completely out of control and that patients were given stents they did not need. They said Midei and the hospital consciously decided to break the rules and look the other way, profiting from an abnormally high number of procedures.

WBAL TV 11, *May 3, 2013*[1]

FALSE ADVERTISING

False or misleading advertising by health care entities continues to confuse and mislead the public in the search for high-quality care. Hospitals, for example, at a time when the Joint Commission provided hospitals with numerical scores advertised their perfect or nearly perfect accreditation scores. Scores as high as 100 were often posted on billboards and/or in local newspapers. The intent of such advertisements was to associate high scores with a higher quality of care then hospitals receiving lower scores. Following numerous complaints by health care organizations and surveyors, numerical scoring was discontinued, arguably due in part to the misuse of scores for advertising purposes. Some hospitals seemed to be more concerned with scores than complying with the standards required for accreditation purposes. From both an ethical and legal point of view, health care organizations should not advertise misleading information to encourage public confidence in the quality of care provided by the organization over that of another.

Advertising Unintentionally Misleading

Imagine you are an off-duty EMT on vacation driving down a four-lane highway and suddenly you observe a car swerving off the road and flipping onto its side. You stop and see a young man lying on the grass and a young lady hysterical and afraid. Her friend appears to have hit his head on the windshield. There are no streetlights or cell phone connections, and there are no car lights in the distance. Not knowing the extent of the injuries, you gently place the victims in the car and start driving to the nearest exit. You observe a sign advertising "Anytown Hospital—Accreditation Survey Score 100, Exit 11-A" and another billboard advertising "General Medical Center—Accreditation Survey Score 89, Exit 11-B." You just passed exit 10. Luck was on your side. Knowing that a score of 100 sounded better than a score of 88, you decided to take Exit 11-A. You followed the emergency sign.

You stopped the car in front of the emergency department entrance, jumped out and ran to the door. There was a sign that said ring bell if you need help. You quickly learned that you just arrived at a behavioral health hospital. General Medical Center Exit-B turned out to be a major teaching hospital. Anytown Hospital's advertisement was not intended to mislead the public but to advertise how well they did during their survey. After all, the community was well aware of the services each hospital offered.

Discussion

1. Discuss what action the hospitals should take to prevent confusion in advertising.
2. Describe a principle of ethics that has been violated if no action is taken to prevent similar incidents.

CASE: BAIT AND SWITCH ADVERTISING

An action was filed against the defendant, Managed Care, alleging claims of false advertising in connection with Managed Care's sale, marketing, and rendering of medical services. The plaintiff alleged that he was an enrollee in Managed Care's health plan. He also alleged that through misleading and deceptive material representations and omissions, Managed Care had employed a fraudulent, unfair scheme to induce people to enroll in its plan by misrepresenting that its primary commitment was to maintain and improve the quality of health care. The plaintiff alleged that Managed Care had been aggressively engaged in implementing undisclosed systemic internal policies that were designed to discourage its primary care physicians from delivering medical services and to interfere with the medical judgment of its health care providers. The result of these policies, he alleged, was a reduction in the quality of health care that is directly contrary to Managed Care's representations.

The plaintiff claimed that Managed Care's false advertising reduced the quality of medical services available to the enrollees and decreased the monetary value of their health coverage. The plaintiff requested restitution, refund, or reimbursement of monies paid by or on behalf of enrollees that resulted from excessive and ill-gotten monies obtained by Managed Care as a result of its unlawful, fraudulent, and unfair business practices and misleading advertisements.

Ethical and Legal Issues

1. Describe the ethical issues in this case.
2. Describe the value of a corporate compliance program and how it could help prevent false advertising.

CONCEALING MISTAKES

Mistakes in medicine are common occurrences that often result in extended hospital stays, higher costs, injury, disability, or death. The Joint Commission in its accreditation process requires that patients be informed when a mistake has been made.

22. The licensed independent practitioner responsible for managing the patient's care, treatment, and services, or his or her designee, informs the patient about unanticipated outcomes of care, treatment, and services related to sentinel events when the patient is not already aware of the occurrence or when further discussion is needed. [2014] Hospital Accreditation Standards, Standard RI.01.02.01.]

Unfortunately for patients, organizations sometimes cover up their mistakes as noted in the following case.

CASE: WRONG SURGICAL PROCEDURE COVER-UP

The physician–petitioner in *In re Muncan*[2] did not review either the patient's CT or MRI images prior to surgery. In addition, he did not have the images with him in the operating room on the day of surgery. Had he done so, he would have discovered that the CT scan report erroneously stated there was a mass in the patient's left kidney when in fact the mass was located in the patient's right kidney. During surgery, the physician did not observe any gross abnormalities or deformities in the left kidney and was unable to palpate any masses. Nonetheless, he removed the left kidney.

The Supreme Court of New York, Appellate Division, Third Department held that the evidence was sufficient to support an inference of fraud. The physician knew he removed the wrong kidney and instead of taking steps to rectify the situation, intentionally concealed his mistake.

Statistical reports can knowingly be inaccurate and give patients a false sense of comfort when selecting a hospital for care, as noted in the following *reality check*.

Appearance May Not Be Reality

General Hospital's staff aggregated its infection rate data for comparison purposes with four other hospitals in the community. The staff members were aware that the data were flawed. They presented a false perception that General Hospital's postoperative infection rates were lower than those of peer hospitals. The comparison data were published in the local newspaper.

The Jones family, believing the data to be correct and concerned about the number of deaths related to hospital-acquired infections, relied on the data in selecting General Hospital as their preferred hospital.

Anonymous

Ethical and Legal Issues

1. Describe how organizational and professional codes of ethics were violated in this case.
2. Describe what role an organization's ethics committee could play in addressing this or similar issues.

Corporate negligence occurs when a corporation fails to perform those duties it owes directly to a patient or to anyone else to whom a duty may extend. If such a duty is breached and a patient is injured as a result of that breach, the organization can be held culpable under the theory of corporate negligence.

> Corporate negligence is a doctrine under which the hospital is liable if it fails to uphold the proper standard of care owed the patient, which is to ensure the patient's safety and well-being while at the hospital. This theory of liability creates a nondelegable duty which the hospital owes directly to a patient. Therefore, an injured party does not have to rely on and establish the negligence of a third party.[3]

Liability extends to nonemployees who act as a hospital's ostensible agents. For example, in *Thompson v. Nason Hospital,*[4] a Pennsylvania court recognized that hospitals are more than mere conduits through which health care professionals are brought into contact with patients. Hospitals owe some nondelegable duties directly to their patients independent of the negligence of their employees, such as duties to use reasonable care in the maintenance of safe and adequate facilities and equipment; select and retain only competent physicians; oversee all persons who practice medicine within their walls as to patient care; and formulate, adopt, and enforce adequate rules and policies to ensure the best quality care for their patients. *Darling v. Charleston Community Memorial Hospital*, discussed next, has had a major impact on the liability of health care organizations for patient injuries suffered within their walls. The immunity status of nonprofit hospitals was no longer an acceptable defense against a plaintiff's negligence claims.

CASE: DARLING—HEALTH CARE'S BENCHMARK CASE

In 1965, the landmark case *Darling v. Charleston Community Memorial Hospital*[5] had a major impact on the liability of health care organizations. The court enunciated a "corporate negligence doctrine" under which hospitals have a duty to provide adequately trained medical and nursing staff. A hospital is responsible, in conjunction with its medical staff, for establishing policies and procedures for monitoring the quality of medicine practiced within the hospital.

Darling involved an 18-year-old college football player who was preparing for a career as a teacher and coach. The patient, a defensive halfback for his college football team, was injured during a play. He was rushed to the emergency department of a small, accredited community hospital where the only physician on emergency duty that day was Dr. Alexander, a general practitioner. Alexander had not treated a major leg fracture for 3 years.

The physician examined the patient and ordered an X-ray that revealed that the tibia and the fibula of the right leg had been fractured. The physician reduced the fracture and applied a plaster cast from a point 3 or 4 inches below the groin to the toes. Shortly after the cast had been applied, the patient began to complain continually of pain. The physician split the cast and continued to visit the patient frequently while the patient remained in the hospital. Not thinking that it was necessary, the emergency department physician did not call in a specialist for consultation.

After 2 weeks, the student was transferred to a larger hospital and placed under the care of an orthopedic surgeon. The specialist found a considerable amount of dead tissue in the fractured leg. During the next 2 months, the specialist removed increasing amounts of tissue in a futile attempt to save the leg until it became necessary to amputate the leg 8 inches below the knee. The student's father did not agree to a settlement and filed suit against the emergency department physician and the hospital. Although the physician later settled out of court for $40,000, the case continued against the hospital.

The documentary evidence relied on to establish the standard of care included the rules and regulations of the Illinois Department of Public Health under the Hospital Licensing Act; the standards for hospital accreditation, today known as the Joint Commission; and the bylaws, rules, and regulations of Charleston Hospital. These documents were admitted into evidence without objection. No specific evidence was offered that the hospital had failed to conform to the usual and customary practices of hospitals in the community.

The trial court instructed the jury to consider those documents, along with all other evidence, in determining the hospital's liability. Under the circumstances in which the case reached the Illinois Supreme Court, it was held that the verdict against the hospital should be sustained if the evidence supported the verdict on any one or more of the 20 allegations of negligence. Allegations asserted that the hospital was negligent in its failure to (1) provide a sufficient number of trained nurses for bedside care of all patients at all times, in this case, nurses who were capable of recognizing the progressive gangrenous condition of the plaintiff's right leg, and (2) failure of its nurses to bring the patient's condition to the attention of the hospital administration and staff so that adequate consultation could be secured and the condition rectified.

Although these generalities provided the jury with no practical guidance for determining what constitutes reasonable care, they were considered relevant to helping the jury decide what was feasible and what the hospital knew or should have known concerning hospital responsibilities for the proper care of a patient. There was no expert testimony characterizing when the professional care rendered by the attending physician should have been reviewed, who should have reviewed it, or whether the case required consultation.

Evidence relating to the hospital's failure to review Alexander's work, to require consultation or examination by specialists, and to require proper nursing care was found to be sufficient to support a verdict for the patient. Judgment was eventually returned against the hospital in the amount of $100,000.

The Illinois Supreme Court held that the hospital could not limit its liability as a charitable corporation to the amount of its liability insurance.

[T]he doctrine of charitable immunity can no longer stand . . . a doctrine which limits the liability of charitable corporations to the amount of liability insurance that they see fit to carry permits them to determine whether or not they will be liable for their torts and the amount of that liability, if any.[6]

In effect, the hospital was liable as a corporate entity for the negligent acts of its employees and physicians. Among other things, the Darling case indicates the importance of instituting effective credentialing and continuing medical evaluation and review programs for all members of a professional staff.

Ethical and Legal Issues

1. Describe the legal issues in this case.
2. Describe how the hospital failed in its ethical duty to the patient.

Respondeat superior (let the master respond) is a legal doctrine holding employers liable, in certain cases, for the wrongful acts of their agents (employees). This doctrine has also been referred to as vicarious liability, whereby an employer is answerable for the torts committed by employees. In the health care setting, an organization, for example, is liable for the negligent acts of its employees, even though there has been no wrongful conduct on the part of the organization. For liability to be imputed to the employer:

1. A master–servant relationship must exist between the employer and the employee; and
2. The wrongful act of the employee must have occurred within the scope of his or her employment.

The question of liability frequently rests on whether persons treating a patient are independent agents (responsible for their own acts) or employees of the organization. The answer to this depends on whether the organization can exercise control over the particular act that was the proximate cause of the injury. The basic rationale for imposing liability on an employer developed because of the employer's right to control the physical acts of its employees. It is not necessary that the employer actually exercise control, only that it possesses the right, power, and authority to do so.

When filing a lawsuit, the plaintiff's attorney generally names both the employer and employee. This occurs because the employer is generally in a better financial condition to cover the judgment. The employer is not without remedy if liability has been imposed against the organization due to an employee's negligent act. The employer can seek indemnification from the employee. Although it would be highly unlikely for a hospital to seek recovery from an employee, the ever-increasing number of employed physicians could give rise to a hospital to seek indemnification from a physician who is the cause of a negligent injury and carries his own malpractice insurance policy.

INDEPENDENT CONTRACTOR

Independent contractors are responsible for their own negligent acts. The independent contractor relationship is established when the principal has no right of control over the manner in which the agent's work is to be performed. However, some cases indicate that an organization can be held liable for an independent contractor's negligence. For example, in *Mehlman v. Powell,*[7] the court held that a hospital could be found vicariously liable for the negligence of an emergency department physician who was not a hospital employee but who worked in the emergency department in the capacity of an independent contractor. The court reasoned that the hospital maintained control over billing procedures, maintained an emergency department, and represented to the patient that the members of the emergency department staff were its employees, which might have caused the patient to rely on the skill and competence of the staff.

CORPORATE DUTIES AND RESPONSIBILITIES

Along with the corporate authority that is granted to the governing body, duties are attached to its individual members. These responsibilities are considered duties because they are imposed by law and can be enforced in legal proceedings. Governing body members are considered by law to have the highest measure of accountability. They have a fiduciary duty that requires acting primarily for the benefit of the corporation. The general duties of a governing body are both implied and express. Failure of a governing body to perform its duties may constitute mismanagement to such a degree that the appointment of a receiver to manage the affairs of the corporation could be warranted.

The duty to supervise and manage is applicable to the trustees as it is to the managers of any other business corporation. In both instances, there is a duty to act as a reasonably prudent person would act under similar circumstances. The governing body must act prudently in administering the affairs of the organization and exercise its powers in good faith. Various duties and responsibilities of hospital organizations are reviewed here.

APPOINTMENT OF A CEO

The governing body is responsible for appointing a chief executive officer (CEO) to act as its agent in the management of the organization. The CEO is responsible for the day-to-day operations. The individual selected as CEO must possess the competence and the character necessary to maintain satisfactory standards of patient care.

The responsibilities and authority of the CEO should be expressed in an appropriate job description, as well as in any formal agreement or contract that the organization has with the CEO. Some state health codes describe the responsibilities of administrators in broad terms. They generally provide that the CEO/administrator shall be responsible for the overall management of the organization.

The general duty of a governing body is to exercise due care and diligence in supervising and managing the organization. This duty does not cease with the selection of a CEO. A governing body can be liable if the level of patient care becomes inadequate because of the governing body's failure to supervise properly the management of the organization. CEOs, like board members, can be personally liable for their own acts of negligence that injure others.

CEO CHALLENGES AND RESPONSIBILITIES

Among the many responsibilities that apply to CEOs are the following:

- Uphold the organization's and one's professional code of ethics.
- Show support and respect to all physicians and staff, knowing that as a team they are the ones who provide bedside care.
- Make daily rounds in the organization. Fix the things they can and find a way to fix the things they think they cannot.
- Develop friendships and supporters who can help the organization to meet those extraordinary goals.
- Implement community outreach programs. Reach out, teach, and educate members of the community on preventative care.
- Not be influenced by power brokers simply because of their position. CEOs and managers must do the right thing, all the time—not in a vacuum, but as a team.
- Show respect to all persons. Treat consultants, accreditation representatives, and inspectors on all levels (e.g., federal, state, local, and private) with respect, knowing that they are all there to help the organization become better in its delivery of patient care.

The following is the preamble to the Code of Ethics of the American College of Healthcare Executives (ACHE):[8]

> The purpose of the Code of Ethics of the American College of Healthcare Executives is to serve as a standard of conduct for members. It contains standards of ethical behavior for health care executives in their professional relationships. These relationships include colleagues, patients, or others served; members of the health care executive's organization and other organizations, the community, and society as a whole.
>
> The Code of Ethics also incorporates standards of ethical behavior governing individual behavior, particularly when that conduct directly relates to the role and identity of the health care executive.
>
> The fundamental objectives of the health care management profession are to maintain or enhance the overall quality of life, dignity, and well-being of every individual needing health care service and to create a more equitable, accessible, effective, and efficient health care system.
>
> Health care executives have an obligation to act in ways that will merit the trust, confidence, and respect of health care professionals and the general public. Therefore, health care executives should lead lives that embody an exemplary system of values and ethics.

Maintain Moral Integrity

The CEO must reflect moral integrity in fulfilling the duties and responsibilities of his or her position. There will often be decisions that may be costly to one's career path, as noted in the following *reality checks*.

Ensuring Integrity

Jim, the administrator of General Hospital, was reviewing his mail and reports placed in his inbox by Carol, his secretary. He noticed a copy of correspondence that had been forwarded to him from the corporate office. The letter, describing a donation that had been made, read:

Dear John,

The care received at your East campus was outstanding. As a result, I am forwarding to your offices a check in the amount of $500,000.

Sincerely,

After reading his morning mail and reports, Jim placed the letter in his outbox for filing. Carol later picked up Jim's mail and other reports from his outbox. Later that afternoon, Carol walked back into Jim's office and inquired, "Did you read this letter forwarded to you from the corporate office?" Handing it to Jim, he replied, "Yes, I read it." Carol then asked, "Do you see anything that piqued your curiosity in this letter?" Jim replied that he had not. Carol, pointing at a strip of whiteout tape, urged Jim to look more closely. She then asked Jim to turn the letter over and read the words the tape was covering. He turned the letter over, noting what the letter had said. It appeared that only a copy had been meant for Jim, not the original correspondence. With the missing words inserted, the correspondence read:

Dear John,

The care received at your East campus was outstanding. As a result, I am forwarding to your offices a check in the amount of $500,000, earmarked for capital projects at your
East campus.

Sincerely,

Anonymous

Discussion

1. Discuss why the whiteout tape might have been placed over the words, "earmarked for capital projects at your East campus." Take into account the comma placed prior to the word "earmarked."
2. What action should Jim take? Remember that Jim could not absolutely determine who placed the whiteout tape on the correspondence, the letter's author or some other unknown person.
3. Assuming Jim sent a memo to the corporate chief financial officer (CFO) to inquire what happened to the donated funds, should the CFO respond to Jim? In what way?
4. Assuming that the CFO failed to respond to Jim, should Jim take any further action, and, if so, what action should he consider?

Discrimination: Behind Closed Doors

It was a Monday morning. Jack remembers it well. As an administrator of a hospital in a multihospital system, Jack was settling into his office when his secretary put through a call from Gerard, the system CEO who was in the corporate office. Gerald asked Jack about interviews of candidates for the emergency department director. Jack replied that the emergency department director search committee has three interviews scheduled for that afternoon. Gerard replied, "The director has to be Christian." Jack interrupted saying, "Are you serious?" Gerard responded, "This is what the board wants. There are too many Jewish medical directors." Jack replied, "This is what the board wants?" Gerard, again quickly interrupting, "Well no, it's what I want." Jack, not believing that Gerard made this decision on his own, replied, "First of all, the selection of director is being conducted by a search committee that includes myself and the other medical directors as well as representatives from the general medical staff. The final decision is the consensus of that committee." Gerard replied, "You are the administrator, and you can pick who you want." Jack responded, "Who I want is the most qualified person for the position." Gerard replied, "You got my message," and abruptly hung up the phone.

That afternoon after interviewing the final candidates, the entire search committee unanimously agreed to select the physician they considered most qualified, a person who happened to be Jewish.

Later that week, Jack decided to take a vacation day to celebrate the Feast of San Gennaro in New York City. He received a call on his cell phone. Jack answered, and his secretary said, "Gerard wants to see you in his office on Monday morning." Jack said, "I can tell from your voice: it sounds ominous?" She said, "I think it is."

On Monday morning, Gerard said, "I am planning to move you to the corporate office. I need your skills here." The corporate office often was jokingly referred to as the deep dark hole. This was a place where people seemed to disappear from the face of the earth, never to be heard from again.

Jack said, "I really prefer to stay at the hospital as the administrator." Gerard replied, "That's not an option." Jack said, "Is this about the selection of the emergency department director? Because the doctor is Jewish?" Gerard said, "Now why would you think that?" Gerard, pausing for a moment, continued, "I really need your skills here." Jack replied, "Do you remember the previous administrator recorded all his telephone calls?" Gerard replied, "What are you getting at?" Jack continued, "I never disconnected the recorder. Your conversation about the selection of an emergency room director was very clear." Gerard replied angrily, "Are you threatening me." Jack said, "No, I just wanted you to understand that the recorder was never disconnected."

Anonymous

Discussion

1. Discuss what you believe are the ethical issues of this case.
2. What should Jack do, assuming he really did tape the conversation?
3. If Jack had not taped the conversation, would that change your mind as to what he should do?

Truthfulness Can Shed Light on Character

A CEO rudely left a briefing being conducted by a group of consultants. The consultants had been contracted by the governing body to review the quality of care being delivered at the hospital where he was employed. The CEO was unhappy with the report because it contained a list of things that needed to be addressed to improve the quality of patient care. As the CEO started to leave the room, he abruptly turned and said, "This is not just about the hospital! This is about my job!" His managers then rose and followed him out of the room, without looking back—no goodbyes with stone-cold faces.

Anonymous

Discussion

1. Discuss what codes of ethics were violated in this case.
2. Explain how you would handle this incident if you were a member of the board.

All job applicants must be closely screened prior to employment, regardless of the responsibilities for which they are seeking employment. The screening process is generally the responsibility of the human resources department and hospital managers. As noted in the news clippings that follow, failure to adequately screen applicants can lead to damaging consequences for both patients and the hospital.

Job Applicants Not Always Screened

Despite the danger of hiring an employee who might jeopardize assisted living residents, some facilities neglect background screening of new workers.

More than 1 in 10 facilities inspected by state regulators in seven states during a two-year period within 2000–2002 picked up at least one citation for neglecting background checks on prospective caregivers. . . .

Kevin McCoy, USA Today, *May 26, 2004*

Did Hospitals "See No Evil"?

When police in New Jersey arrested a male nurse named Charles Cullen last year, he made a terrible claim. He said he'd killed as many as 40 patients during the course of his nursing career.

The question remains: How could Cullen have worked at 10 different hospitals in New Jersey and Pennsylvania, over a period of 16 years—despite the fact that at seven of those hospitals, he was under investigation, fired or forced to resign?

Apparently, not one of those institutions gave Cullen a bad reference, or told other hospitals he was trouble. It amounted to a policy of "See no evil-speak no evil"—one that gave Cullen, in effect, a license to kill.

Rebecca Leung, CBSNews.com, *April 4, 2004*[9]

CREDENTIALING, APPOINTMENT, AND PRIVILEGING

The governing body is ultimately responsible for the credentialing, appointment, and privileging process of the organization's professional staff. The duty to select members of the professional staff is legally vested in the governing body charged with managing the organization. Although cognizant of the importance of professional staff membership, the governing body must meet its obligation to maintain high standards of practice and fairness. The governing board of a hospital must therefore be given great latitude in prescribing the necessary qualifications for potential applicants. Because no court should substitute its evaluation of professional competency for that of a hospital board, a court's review should be limited to ensuring that the qualifications imposed by a board are reasonably related to the operation of the hospital and fairly administered. Moreover, courts are generally reluctant to get involved with the internal affairs of a hospital or professional society unless any sanctions they impose violate public policy.

Credentialing is a process for validating the background of health care professionals and assessing their qualifications to provide health care services. The process is an objective evaluation of a professional's current licensure, training, or experience; competence; and ability to perform the services or procedures requested. Credentialing occurs during both the initial appointment and reappointment process. The *delineation of clinical privileges* is the process by which the medical staff determines precisely what procedures a physician is authorized to perform. This determination is based on the credentials necessary to competently perform the privileges requested.

The medical staff is responsible to the governing body for the quality of care rendered by members of the medical staff. The hospital's governing body has a duty to ensure that a mechanism is in place for the medical staff to evaluate, counsel, and when necessary take disciplinary action against physicians who pose an unreasonable risk of harm to patients.

Ensure Competency

Hospitals have a responsibility to take reasonable steps to ensure that physicians are qualified for the privileges granted. Failure to screen a medical staff applicant's credentials properly can lead to liability for injuries suffered by patients as a result of that omission. Hospitals must adhere to procedures established under both their own bylaws and state statutes. The measure of quality and the degree of quality control exercised in a hospital are the direct responsibilities of the medical staff. Hospital supervision of the manner of appointment of physicians to its staff is mandatory, not optional.

False Statements

In *Hoxie v. Ohio State Med. Bd.*, it was determined that a physician had made false statements concerning his criminal history when he stated in a deposition that he had never been arrested. There was sufficient evidence presented to support permanent revocation of his license to practice medicine. Certified records held by the state of California indicated that the physician had been arrested or detained by the Los Angeles Police Department multiple times in the 1970s and 1980s for possessing marijuana and PCP, for driving under the influence of alcohol and/or drugs, and for driving with a suspended license. Although the physician asserted that documentation of his criminal past had been fabricated by police and was not credible, law enforcement investigation reports are generally admissible. The physician himself added to the reliability of the records by verifying all significant identifying information contained within the documents and records.[10]

Masquerading as a Physician

An action was brought against Canton (who was masquerading as a physician, Dr. LaBella), the hospital, and others in *Insinga v. LaBella*[11] for the wrongful death of a 68-year-old woman whom Canton had admitted. The patient died while she was in the hospital. Canton was found to be a fugitive from justice in Canada, where he was under indictment for the manufacture and sale of illegal drugs. He fraudulently obtained a medical license from the state of Florida and staff privileges at the hospital by using the name of LaBella, a deceased physician. Canton was extradited to Canada without being served process. The U.S. District Court for the Southern District of Florida directed a verdict in favor of the hospital. On appeal, the Florida Supreme Court held that the corporate negligence doctrine imposes on hospitals an implied duty to patients to select competent physicians who, although they are independent practitioners, would be providing in-hospital care to their patients through staff privileges. Hospitals are in the best position to protect their patients and consequently have an independent duty to select competent independent physicians.

DISCIPLINE OF PHYSICIANS

Although the governing body has ultimate responsibility for disciplining members of the professional staff (e.g., disruptive behavior, incompetence, psychological problems, substance abuse), responsibility for disciplinary actions are generally delegated to the administrator and various department directors and managers. Depending on the seriousness of alleged misconduct, disciplinary action may require board involvement for resolution, such as those occurrences noted in the following news clipping.

The Joint Commission as far back as 2008 responded to complaints of disruptive physician behavior that can place patient care at risk and increase medical errors. The standards made it mandatory for hospitals to establish written policies designed to address behavior that is demeaning, aggressive, uncivil, or hostile in the patient care setting.[12] The American Medical Association (AMA) has defined disruptive behavior as a style of interaction with physicians, hospital personnel, patients, family members, or others that interferes with patient care.[13]

The discipline of a physician is sometimes difficult without adequate support of the medical staff, as noted in the following *reality check*.

Physicians Reluctant to Discipline Physicians

Anytown Hospital has an outstanding reputation for surgical services. The operating room supervisor and a surgical nurse told Bob Wright that Dr. Flipton, an anesthesiologist, is abusing the use of anesthesia gases in the hospital's dental suite. He was reportedly seen by operating staff administering nitrous oxide (laughing gas) by holding a mask against his face for short periods of time. This scene would be followed by a string of silly, seemingly meaningless jokes. Bob has repeatedly discussed this matter with the medical executive committee. The medical executive committee refused to take any action without definitive action by the department chair. Bob suspects that if he pursues the matter further with the governing board, he could end up without a job. The governing body is generally unable to resolve disciplinary actions against a physician without support of the medical executive committee.

Ethical and Legal Issues

1. What do you believe the ethical issues are for Bob? For Bob, doing the right thing and survival are competing concerns.
2. Which of the following would you do if you were in Bob's position, with two children in college and hefty mortgage payments?
   - Voluntarily leave my job
   - Aggressively pursue the problem
   - Secretly enlist the aid of the medical staff
   - Confront Dr. Flipton
   - Other option (explain)

A hospital and its governing body were determined to be immune from liability under the federal Health Care Quality Improvement Act of 1986 in *Taylor v. Kennestone Hosp.*,[14] for claims arising out of their decision to deny a physician's application to renew his medical staff privileges. A peer review board found that reasonable investigation had adduced evidence demonstrating that the physician had a history of sexual misconduct toward both nurses and patients. He admitted that he had sexual harassment problems, that he stopped seeing patients at the hospital, and that he sought psychiatric treatment. He admitted that he failed to comply fully with his own psychiatrist's plan of care before he resumed seeing patients in the hospital. The evidence established that the peer reviewers could reasonably believe that their actions were warranted and that those actions furthered the quality of health care.

CASE: PHYSICIAN PRIVILEGES SUSPENDED

A physician received a letter from a hospital informing him that his clinical privileges at the hospital had been summarily suspended. The medical executive committee reviewed the suspension and recommended that it be upheld. The hospital board ultimately revoked the physician's staff privileges. The physician received a hearing before a fair hearing panel, which recommended that he be reinstated. The board, however, upheld the revocation.

The physician alleged, among other things, wrongful termination and intentional infliction of emotional distress. The defendants argued that the courts do not have jurisdiction to review staffing decisions made by private, nonprofit hospitals.

The Court of Civil Appeals of Oklahoma, Division II, found that judicial tribunals are not equipped to review the action of hospital boards in selecting or refusing to appoint physicians to their medical staffs. The authorities of hospitals endeavor to serve in the best possible manner the sick and the afflicted. Not all professionals have identical ability, competence, experience, character, and standards of ethics. The mere fact that a physician is licensed to practice a profession does not justify any inference beyond the conclusion that a physician has met the minimum requirements for that purpose.

Without regard to the absence of any legal liability, the hospital in granting a physician privileges to practice in its facilities extends a moral or official approval to him in the eyes of the public. Not all professionals have personalities that enable them to work in harmony with others, and to inspire confidence in their peers and in patients. Courts should not substitute their evaluation in such matters. It is the board, not the court, that is charged with the responsibility of providing a competent staff of physicians. The board has chosen to rely on the advice of its medical staff, and the court cannot surrogate for the medical staff in executing this responsibility. Human lives are at stake, and the board must be given discretion in its selection so that it can have confidence in the competence and moral commitment of its staff.[15]

Ethical and Legal Issues

1. Do you agree with the court's decision? Explain.
2. Discuss under what circumstances you believe a court should become involved in an organization's disciplinary processes (e.g., age discrimination).

PROVIDE ADEQUATE STAFF

Staffing shortages for both hospitals and nursing homes continue to plague the health care industry. Because the quality of care provided by nursing homes is subject to substantial scrutiny, American families face difficult decisions about whether to move a loved one into such a setting.

Under federal law, nursing facilities must have sufficient nursing staff to provide nursing and related services adequate to attain and maintain the highest practicable physical, mental, and psychosocial well-being of each resident, as determined by resident assessments and individual plans of care. As nursing facilities are increasingly filled with older, disabled residents with complex care needs, the demands for highly educated and trained nursing personnel continue to grow.

PROVIDE ADEQUATE SUPPLIES AND EQUIPMENT

The governing body must ensure that there are adequate supplies and equipment on hand in each of its facilities. If the board is unable to provide the necessary supplies and equipment, it must consider finding the funds necessary to fulfill its mission or scaling back operations and, if necessary, consider other options, such as filing for bankruptcy or selling the organization's assets to a competing organization.

Hospital's Challenge to Survive

Brad was concerned with what he considered little opportunity for advancement at Blooming Hospital. He had been there for 8 years and there were two administrators in line for Woody's position as chief executive officer. As far as Brad knew, Woody had no plans to leave Blooming Hospital. He was well liked, competent, and to this day the best boss anyone could hope to have.

Because of financial needs, Brad discussed his concerns with Margaret, the chief operating officer at Hope Hospital, one of several hospitals in a multihospital system. A few months later Margaret called Brad and said, "I am leaving Hope Hospital and moving to another hospital in the system as CEO. Are you interested in applying for my job?" Brad replied that he was interested. He applied and was offered the job.

Brad found it difficult to approach Woody. As he walked towards Woody's office, he felt a veil of despair and second thoughts but knew it would be financially difficult not to accept the position at Hope Hospital. Woody had an open door policy and Brad entered his office unannounced. Woody said, "Hi Brad." Brad replied, "Hi Woody. I find it hard to tell you but I was offered a job at Hope Hospital in the number two position." Woody asked, "Are you sure this is what you want to do?" Brad replied that it was. Woody appeared disappointed as Brad left his office. Later that afternoon Woody went to Brad's office and described how the system Brad was about to enter could be problematic for him. As Woody stood in the doorway, he continued, "Hope Hospital has a reputation of being intensely political." Woody was not one to use many words but again he looked disappointed. After a few moment of silence, Woody turned and left the room. Brad could have asked for a raise but was uncomfortable to ask and felt Woody might have misgivings towards him.

Brad, after giving a months notice, had left Blooming Hospital. The CEO at Hope Hospital was a kind gentleman. He, however, resigned his position just 9 months after Brad's arrival. Brad was appointed the interim CEO as the board conducted a search for a new CEO. Brad threw his resume into the mix. Following a lengthy search and interviews, Brad was appointed CEO of Hope Hospital.

Brad was happy to be managing a profitable hospital, however he quickly faced challenges on many fronts, including a continuing battle to obtain supplies from vendors due to the transfer of funds from his hospital by corporate leadership to prop up other failing entities in the system outside the state where his hospital was located. The following timeline documents his struggle to keep the hospital afloat:

July 2010—Phone Message from the Director of Procurement
Proctor and Gamble has cut us off from all delivery of supplies. Johnson & Johnson has cut off all deliveries of supplies. Scott Labs and Anthony Medical have cut us off from all deliveries. If we don't soon get supplies, the lab will be forced to close.

August 2010—Lack of OR Sutures
Dr. Plastics entered Brad's office and said, "I can't perform surgery without the proper suture materials. I have a patient on the table and they don't have the sutures I prefer to close the surgical incision." He then turned to return to the OR, looking back and apologizing, "I know you don't control where the money goes."

Brad discussed the lack of sutures material with Marcy, the OR supervisor. Marcy, in tears, said, "Brad, supply shortages are making my job difficult enough and now the physicians are taking out their frustrations on me. Dr. Plastics, who complained to you, had other suture options, but like all surgeons, he had his own preferences, probably, I suspect, based on a salesman's pressure." Brad replied, "I can't second-guess the surgeon's selection of sutures; however, I understand your frustrations and I will continue to bring them up with the corporate CEO. I can assure you that the board members are well aware of the continuing supply shortages."

August 2010—Lack of X-ray Film
One Friday at 5:00 p.m. a radiologist went to Brad's office to report, "I know you are under a lot of pressure, but we do not have sufficient X-ray film to get through the weekend!" After Brad arranged to borrow X-ray film from a local state hospital, he called the

corporate accounts payable department to inquire about payment of the vendor—a task that was beginning to be a daily occurrence for Brad.

September 2010—Message Relayed from Administrative Secretary

"Dr. Wild stormed in. He is furious! The fetal monitor machine is out of commission. He was lied to and told it was working but it wasn't. This is a life-saving instrument and failure to have it fixed is intolerable (and a few more adjectives I couldn't get down in shorthand) and inexcusable *and a legal matter*—this is just the tip of the iceberg. If things don't start to improve he will pull his entire practice out of the hospital."

April 2011—Memo from the President of the Medical/Dental Staff

We have been reduced to using menstrual pads for abdominal dressings. On two occasions last week a major disaster was narrowly averted in the Operating Room only because of the proximity of . . . City Hospital and their willingness to supply us with emergency equipment.

March 2012—Input from Department of Supply Procurement

The director of supply procurement wrote a memo stating that the acute shortages of OR material and X-ray film were putting patients at risk at this facility. The memo recommended considering an orderly closing of the facility. Those present at a meeting to discuss the issue unanimously agreed that without immediate intervention regarding the specific needs, closing of the hospital should begin on a specified date. Ms. Nurse added that ensuring an adequate supply of sutures was critical.

June 2012—Phone Message from Dr. Orthopedics

Dr. Orthopedics called at noon today (6/12). He said about a week ago he was here at night and there were no finger splints. Dr. Orthopedics said he had to resort to the use of popsicle sticks that he obtained in the hospital coffee shop for splints.

September 2012—Memo from Dr. ER

Over the past 3 to 4 weeks the supply of orthopedic-related supplies in the emergency room has dwindled to a dangerous level. Something must be done soon.

October 2012—Letter from Dr. Peds

I was on call for the emergency room . . . on Friday, October 23, 2012. I was disappointed to note that important casting materials were not available. . . . I can repeat what others have said: if the hospital is to continue to provide high-quality care, a certain minimum level of supplies must be available.

January 2013—Memo from Dr. Orthopedics

Once again, I am forced to bring to your attention the abysmal state of affairs with reference to your credit ratings with various surgical vendors. It is a continual source of embarrassment to me to have to call in personal favors with salesmen and vendors so as to provide my patients with prostheses and equipment they need for their optimal health care.

April 2013—Board Minutes

Father Smith (board member who chaired the physicians relations committee) requested that Brad and the president of the medical staff work together in locating the areas of greatest concern with regard to supply shortages. Father Smith asked that this information be available at the next board meeting.

May 2013—Brad speaks with the Corporate CEO

Brad called the corporate office to discuss the ongoing seriousness of the supply issues. The purchase, storage, and distribution of supplies had been centralized in a corporate location off site. At the same time, Accounts Payable was also centralized and was accused of paying vendors on the basis of who screamed the loudest rather than on patient need.

June 2013—Administrator and Medical Staff President Joint Memo to the Board

We sincerely believe that as a result of the supply shortages, the negative impact on morale of patients and employees during the past 5 years is substantial. The serious nature of these concerns are noted in the following paragraphs.

Major Vendors requiring advance payment

2010	18
2011	53
2012	129
2013	350

The system CEO was distressed that Brad had provided this information to the board, complaining to him, "You're out to get me." Brad responded, "I am complying with the board's request, and it's in the board minutes. Besides, I gave you an advance copy of the memorandum."

Discussion

1. Discuss the ethical issues that this case raises.
2. Are there any circumstances in which CEOs should attempt to keep information from their boards?
3. Brad is in a multihospital system making major profits but cannot control the flow of funds out of the community hospital. The governing body is aware of the serious nature of the supply crisis. What should the board do?
4. If you were Brad or on the board, what action would you take?

ALLOCATE SCARCE RESOURCES

It is the responsibility of the governing body, and not the legal system, to provide appropriate staffing and provide adequate supplies and equipment for patients. Although the courts do not overlook the importance of maintaining adequate levels of patient care, it is not the job of the courts to referee disagreements. For example, a disagreement between the governing body and the local community as to how to allocate limited resources is not a question for the courts to settle. Questions of this sort often involve ethical principles and values. How to spend limited resources that provide good for the many is a value judgment, not a legal decision. Hospitals are in the business of serving patients with many kinds of illnesses and disabilities. Recognizing that the medical community is best equipped to conduct the balancing that medical resource allocations inevitably require, Congress has declined to give courts a mandate to arbitrate allocation disputes.[16]

The following news clippings describe how some hospitals have been negatively affected when resources are not wisely distributed.

MDs Weigh Action Over Hospital $$

A suit may be in the offing blocking the . . . [multi-system corporation] from pumping profits made by its [community hospital] into the . . . [system's] two financially-ailing sister hospitals....

"It's a matter of going to the operating room and finding that a particular piece of equipment isn't working, or finding that certain items are not up to date."

Although . . . [system] officials would not comment, sources close to the scene say the . . . [system] will maintain that it has the right to spend as it sees fit.

Vicky Penner Katz, Smithtown News, *July 24, 1980*

. . . Says Hospitals Won't Fail

The . . . [system] has been siphoning funds from the financially stable . . . hospital to make up deficits at the two other hospitals, which have a large volume of charity cases. The drain has angered . . . [community] physicians, who complain that it has caused staff and supply shortages.

Nearly 100 vendors have stopped dealing with the hospital. . . .

Neil S. Rosenfeld, Newsday, *January 22, 1981*

Multihospital System's Allocation of Scarce Resources

At a time when many hospitals were on the brink of bankruptcy and struggling to survive, Brad, the administrator of a hospital in a multihospital system had a positive bottom line in the millions. The hospital was located in an upscale, affluent community. Unfortunately, the money was siphoned off to support the operations and capital projects of other hospitals in the system. Meanwhile, Brad's hospital was suffering from lack of supplies and funds for local capital projects.

Physicians and many community members, aware of the positive bottom line, were disturbed that the hospital's funds from operations and donations were being earmarked to fund the day-to-day operations of the system's failing hospitals. In addition, at a time when these hospitals were losing money, funds from Brad's hospital were being earmarked for major building projects in these hospitals, as well as corporate office projects.

It was like trying to squeeze blood out of a stone to get people to donate to their own community hospital. The community had no trust their donations would stay in the community.

Corporate leadership was expanding its capital projects, expanding nonrevenue-producing projects, relocating corporate offices to a more expensive site, building lavish suites, adding staff with vague job descriptions that served only to burden and penalize the revenue-producing entities, and jeopardizing patient care with their pet projects by deluging hospital staff with paperwork so they could produce even more paperwork to justify their own existence. Hospital staff felt that corporate staff had become an obstacle to the provision of high-quality patient care. No relief from battlefield fatigue seemed to be on the horizon.

Brad was able to work with some local community leaders (e.g., banker, lawyer, physician, newspaper editor, real estate agent) to establish a fundraising board whose mission was to oversee the local fundraising process and ensure the proper allocation of community funds to the local hospital. Although many corporate leaders privately objected to the concept, the corporate board reluctantly recognized the community board's existence, hoping to make inroads into the pockets of the wealthy. With half-hearted support by the corporation's leadership, the death of many of the founding fathers of the community board, and the resignation of Brad, who had developed the trust and provided the leadership, the community board slowly faded out of existence under the leadership of the administrators that followed him.

Anonymous

Discussion

1. Discuss the ethical issues related to Brad's dilemma regarding cash flow to other entities in the corporation. Do you consider this an isolated incident or an all too frequent occurrence with the rise of multihospital systems? Explain your answer.
2. Discuss what steps you would take to resolve the resource allocation issues if you were in Brad's position.
3. Discuss the community's reluctance to donate to the local hospital. What would you do?

COMPLY WITH RULES AND REGULATIONS

The governing body in general and its agents are responsible for compliance with federal, state, and local rules and regulations regarding the operation of the organization. Depending on the scope of the wrong committed and the intent of the governing body, failure to comply could subject board members and/or their agents to civil liability and, in some instances, to criminal prosecution. The following *reality check* describes what can happen when an organization fails to comply with the provisions of the Family Medical Leave Act (FMLA).

Noncompliance with the FMLA

The FMLA of 1993 was enacted to grant temporary medical leave to employees up to a total of 12 workweeks of unpaid leave during any 12-month period for such things as the birth and care of an employee's child, the care of an immediate family member with a serious health condition, or inability to work because of a serious health condition. After an FMLA leave, the employee's job—or an equivalent job with equivalent pay, benefits, and other terms and conditions of employment—must be restored.

Ten CEOs and human resource directors were randomly queried to determine their compliance with the FMLA. Specifically, in 9 of the 10 organizations queried, a nurse, for example, would be returned to the same or similar position without financial penalty (e.g., prorated salary increase) after her return from family leave.

One organization chose to penalize an employee's employment status by removing the employee's part-time status for the remainder of the year in which family leave had been granted and taken. In addition, this same organization's leaders prorated the employee's salary increase. In effect, this was a penalty that would be compounded each year the employee worked in the organization.

On appeal by the employee to the United States Department of Labor, this organization was required to reimburse the employee for lost wages unlawfully withheld from the employee during the year in which family leave had been taken.

Discussion

1. Discuss what recourse the employee has when faced with discriminatory practices, both within the corporation (e.g., register a complaint with the human resources department and/or corporate compliance officer) and outside the organization (e.g., file a complaint with the Department of Labor).
2. Such activities raise both legal (e.g., interpretation of the law) and ethical issues (e.g., nonmaleficence).

COMPLY WITH ACCREDITATION STANDARDS

Accredited hospitals are responsible for compliance with their accrediting body's standards (e.g., the Joint Commission). Failure to follow safe practices identified in accreditation standards can result in patient injuries such as noted in the following news clipping where patient equipment was disconnected because alarms were annoying to staff who became desensitized to the alarms—often as a result of frequent false alarms.

"Alarm Fatigue" Poses Risk for Hospital Patients

The sheer number—several hundred alarms per patient per day—can cause alarm fatigue. Nurses and other workers, overwhelmed or desensitized by the constant barrage, sometimes respond by turning down the volume on the devices, shutting them off or simply ignoring them—actions that can have serious, potentially fatal, consequences.

Clinicians and patient-safety advocates have warned of alarm fatigue for years, but the issue is taking on greater urgency as hospitals invest in more-complex, often-noisy devices meant to save lives. Last month, the Joint Commission, which accredits hospitals, directed facilities to make alarm safety a top priority or risk losing their accreditation.

Lena H. Sun, The Washington Post, *July 8, 2013*

Noncompliance with accreditation standards can lead to an organization's loss of accreditation, which in turn would provide grounds for third-party reimbursement agencies (e.g., Medicare) to deny payment for treatment. The following case describes how a patient alarm was disabled, resulting in the death of a patient.

CASE: MONITOR ALARM DISCONNECTED

In *Odom v. State Department of Health and Hospitals*,[17] the appeals court held that the decedent's cause of death was directly related to the absence of a heart monitor. Jojo was born 12 weeks prematurely at the HPL Medical Center. Jojo remained in a premature infant's nursery and was eventually placed into two different foster homes prior to his admission to Pinecrest foster home. While Jojo was a Pinecrest resident, Mr. and Mrs. Odom adopted Jojo. He was unable to feed himself and was nourished via a gastrostomy tube. Because he suffered from obstructive apnea, he became dependent on a tracheostomy (trach) tube.

At Pinecrest, Jojo was assigned to Home 501. While making patient rounds, Ms. Means found Jojo with his trach tube out of the stoma. She called for help, and Ms. Wiley, among others, responded. Wiley immediately took the CPR efforts under her control. She noticed that Jojo was breathless and immediately reinserted the trach tube. She then noticed that Jojo was still hooked to a monitor.

No one had heard the heart monitor's alarm sound. Means asserts that the monitor was on, because she saw that the monitor's red lights were blinking, indicating the heart rate and breathing rate. She stated that she took the monitor's leads off of Jojo to put the monitor out of the way, but the alarm did not sound. CPR efforts continued while Jojo was placed on a stretcher and sent by ambulance to HPL. Jojo was pronounced dead at HPL's emergency department at 7:02 p.m.

The Odoms filed a petition against Pinecrest, alleging that Jojo's death was caused by the negligence and fault of Pinecrest, its servants, and employees. Judgment was for the plaintiffs. The trial court's reasons for judgment were enlightening because it stated that the monitor should have been on but was, however, disconnected by the staff and that this was the cause, in fact, of Jojo's injury. The appeals court found that the record supported the trial court's findings. There was overwhelming evidence upon which the trial court relied to find that the monitor was turned off, in breach of the various physicians' orders with which the nurses should have complied. The monitor was supposed to be on Jojo to warn the nurses of any respiratory distress episodes that he might experience. A forensic pathologist's report showed the cause of Jojo's death to be hypoxia, secondary to respiratory insufficiency, secondary to apnea episodes. Thus, Jojo's cause of death was directly related to the absence of a heart monitor.

The accreditation process of a health care organization is a major event in its day-to-day operations. Organizations are expected to maintain a culture that supports patient safety and an environment that fosters respect, honesty, and compassionate care. The accreditation process is one of many tools that help ensure that high-quality care is being provided. As the following *reality check* illustrates, there are times when a wake-up call is necessary to alert leadership that the provision of high-quality care is no trivial event when your goal is to heal another human being.

Accreditation is Serious Business

Three field consultants were assigned by their employer, the National Accreditation Association (NAA), to review the quality of care being delivered at Newtown Medical Center and its three outpatient centers. Newtown was larger and even more complex than the consultants had anticipated, offering multiple services. On the first day of the consulting assignment, only three of the six assigned consultants reported to the medical center for duty. Patrick, the team leader, called the corporate office to discuss the need for additional help. Mike, the manager responsible for addressing field requests, did not return Patrick's call. Despite the lack of a follow-up call from Mike, the team covered the assigned task.

On the fourth day of the 5-day survey Cheri, Newtown's survey coordinator, asked Patrick if there was anything that needed to be covered prior to the exit conference to be held the following afternoon. Patrick replied, "Yes there is. At the leadership conference this morning there was no representation from the governing body. I find it difficult to score the various aspects of leadership since no one attended the scheduled interview."Somewhat concerned about the outcome of the quality review the following day when the consultants presented their report, Cheri said, "The medical center's leadership has not taken these surveys very seriously in the past. It has been an uphill battle to get them involved. Let me see what I can do to arrange for a leadership conference in the morning. We have 36 members on our board, hopefully I can find a few to attend." The following morning Cheri approached Michael and said, "I was able to convince two board members to meet with you at 11:00 a.m."

Michael met with the two board members along with the CEO. After the meeting had ended, a board member approached Michael and said, "You sure are persistent. But I must say it was truly a worthwhile meeting."

Discussion

1. Do you agree with Michael's persistence in conducting the leadership interview? Discuss your answer.
2. Because the survey team was short three consultants, would you consider this a meaningful survey as to the quality of care being rendered at Newtown Medical Center? Discuss your answer.
3. Do you think the CEO would complain about being billed for six consultants when only three were present to conduct the survey? Discuss your answer knowing that the results of the survey were positive and that three additional consultants could have added to the number of findings resulting in a more negative report and an unhappy board.

ACCREDITATION AND CONFLICT OF INTEREST

The mission of accrediting bodies is to improve the quality of care rendered in the nation's hospitals through its survey process. Accrediting bodies depend upon the hospitals they survey to reimburse them for the costs of those surveys. This obligates the accrediting body to maintain satisfied clients, and in so doing, a *conflict of interest* arises. How credible can a survey be when the accrediting body is dependent upon satisfied customers for financial survival? Further, hospitals evaluate the performance of the surveyors. Surveyors are expected to score an organization's performance knowing that organizations often challenge a surveyor's findings, which can lead to character assassination in the worst case scenario and/or a poor performance review of the surveyor by the organization. Conflicting interests here encourage surveyors/inspectors to be cautious about what they score because of fear of retaliation by both the organizations surveyed and the accrediting body that may side with the organization. Because of the financial implications for both the accrediting body and the surveyed organization, surveys are far from effective in protecting the consumer from human errors that result in more than 100,000 deaths and injuries annually in the nation's hospitals.

The food inspection process is remarkably similar to the hospital accreditation surveys:

- Food makers often know when inspectors will audit their facilities, and they vigorously prepare for those inspections. This was also true with hospitals until the Joint Commission, for example, decided to conduct unannounced surveys. This change occurred mostly because of criticism from surveyors, the Centers for Medicare and Medicaid, the public, and some of the surveyed organizations. But the wheels of change move slowly; more than a decade passed before the Joint Commission submitted to the long overdue change.
- Most food makers score high in their inspections and still have recalls and outbreaks.
- As with hospitals, the food companies typically pay food industry inspectors, creating a conflict of interest for inspectors who might fear they will lose business if they do not hand out high ratings.

Hospital scores were eventually discontinued in the accreditation process because of criticism on numerous occasions from both its own surveyors and accredited hospitals. Because of the competition among hospitals, the surveyors were pressured to provide high scores by the organizations it surveyed. As noted in the following *reality check* patients who passed away in high-scoring hospitals were not all pleased with the scores some hospitals were receiving.

One Family's Experience

It was early winter and Mary Ann had continuous headaches for more than a year. Dr. Fastrack, her family physician, examined her and diagnosed her with migraines. Handing her a prescription for ibuprofen, Dr. Fastrack said, "Mary Ann, it is stress related. Maybe some meditation would be helpful." That following summer Mary Ann went to the Jersey shore, where she had been going on vacation for several years. While she was there she experienced excruciating headaches. She went to a local emergency room where they also diagnosed her with a severe migraine. Mary Ann returned home and was eventually examined by a neurologist who ordered a brain scan. She was diagnosed with a brain tumor in her right frontal lobe, the same area of the head she hit when she went through a car window 17 years earlier. About a year following radiation treatment she was told she was in remission. It was Christmas and she immediately called her brother who was at his in-laws, to tell him the good news. Mary Ann never saw another Christmas. Several years following her death, her daughter, my niece said, "Can you believe the hospital where my mom died had advertised in our local newspaper that it scored 100 on a hospital accreditation survey. There wasn't even a physician on duty in the emergency room. I wouldn't take my dog to that hospital. They killed my mom."

Anonymous

Clearly, the banking industry, food industry, and health care industry all share one major disturbing characteristic: there is a blatant conflict of interest between the inspecting agencies and the entities they are inspecting. As noted in the following *reality check*, someone needs to regulate the regulators.

Integrity Can Be Lost Through Greed

Forever Anonymous, Inc. (FA) employees are prohibited from consulting with accredited health care organizations during their employment with FA. In addition, employees are prohibited, for 3 years following termination, from consulting with any organizations they may have surveyed during their tenure with FA.

It is believed that not all members of FA's leadership have been following this policy after termination of their employment. Employees were questioning among themselves, does this policy apply only to rank-and-file employees, or does it include FA's leadership? Should the FA board investigate what organizations former FA leaders have been consulting with and in what capacity? Should FA's board investigate what members of leadership have consulted and/or continue to consult? And what is the propriety of such consultations?

The importance of this policy is apparent. During a survey, some hospitals through their leadership, often let it be known to the inspectors, accidentally of course, what former members of FA's leadership they have been consulting with to prepare for their survey, expecting some leniency will be shown by the surveyors during the survey process. Yes, unfortunately, there are often some members of an organization's leadership who are more concerned about the results of a survey and how it might affect their jobs than about how it affects the quality of patient care in their organization.

Anonymous

Discussion

1. Describe how the FA board could address this issue.
2. Identify the ethical issues in this *reality check*.

PROVIDE TIMELY TREATMENT

VA, Heal Thyself, Agency Is Told at Hearing Filled with Pained Testimony

VA officials in Pittsburgh knew of an outbreak of Legionnaires' disease, "but they kept it a secret for more than a year."

VA staff in Buffalo potentially exposed patients to hepatitis and HIV by reusing disposable insulin injection pens. "At least 18 veteran patients have tested positive for hepatitis so far."

VA workers, patients and family members had "a series of allegations" regarding "poor care" at the Dallas VA medical center.

Employee whistleblowers at the VA medical center in Jackson, Miss., reported "poor sterilization procedures, understaffing and misdiagnoses" to the Office of Special Counsel, an independent federal watchdog.

Joe Davidson, The Washington Post, *September 13, 2013*

Health care organizations are expected to provide timely treatment to patients. Hospitals can be liable for delays in treatment that result in injuries to their patients. For example, the patient in *Heddinger v. Ashford Memorial Community Hospital*[18] filed a malpractice action against a hospital and its insurer, alleging that a delay in treating her left hand resulted in the loss of her little finger. Medical testimony presented at trial indicated that if proper and timely treatment had been rendered, the finger would have been saved. The U.S. District Court entered judgment on a jury verdict for the plaintiff in the amount of $175,000. The hospital appealed, and the U.S. Court of Appeals held that even if the physicians who attended the patient were not employees of the hospital but were independent contractors, the risk of negligent treatment was clearly foreseeable by the hospital.

The following *reality check* describes one consultant's experience in the VA hospital system.

Veterans' Care Unconscionably Delayed

I surveyed more than 500 hospitals. At one point I asked not to be placed on Veterans hospital accreditation surveys. Not all but some of the Veterans Administration (VA) hospitals were very argumentative fearing the possibility of written citations. So much so that on a ride from one VA hospital in Pennsylvania to a Pittsburgh VA the referring VA hospital sent three staff members to chauffeur me to the Pittsburgh VA. They all argued my concerns that a veteran on a 6-month waiting list for a neurological consult was too long. They kept arguing, not discussing, that if he needed immediate attention he would have been referred to a local civilian hospital for care. I said, "In my opinion, if he needs a neurological consult, he needs it now. Not 6 months from now."

Anonymous

Discussion

1. Based on this *reality check*, what action should the VA leadership take in order to prevent such occurrences in the future?
2. Discuss how this situation might have been different if the veteran was a relative of one of the employees accompanying the surveyor in the car.

AVOID CONFLICTS OF INTEREST

Suspicious Consulting Fees

About 800,000 Americans will get a new hip or knee this year, up 63% from 491,000 in 2001. Now a U.S. Department of Justice investigation reveals that many orthopedic surgeons have been pocketing hundreds of thousands of dollars in "consulting fees" with the understanding that they would implant a particular company's device—even if it wasn't the best choice for a patient.

The country's top five medical device makers, which account for nearly 95% of the knee and hip implants on the market, have been implicated.

Catherine Guthrie, Oprah Magazine, *May 2008*

A conflict of interest involves situations where a person has the opportunity to promote self-interests that could have a detrimental effect on an organization with which he or she has a special relationship (e.g., employee, board member). The potential for conflict of interest exists for individuals at all levels within an organization. Disclosure of potential conflicts of interest should be made so that appropriate action may be taken to ensure that such conflict does not inappropriately influence important organization and health care decisions. Board members, physicians, and employees are required by most organizations to submit a form disclosing potential conflicts of interest that might negatively affect the organization's reputation or financial resources.

CASE: CORPORATE COVER-UP

The case of *Advocat, Inc. v. Sauer*[19] involved the care of Mrs. Sauer, a 93-year-old nursing facility patient. On July 19, 1998, her vital signs began to decline, and the nursing staff reported this to her treating physician, who ordered that she be taken to the emergency department at a nearby medical center. She arrived at the hospital in a semicomatose condition and died about 16 hours later.

Nursing notes indicated that Sauer had lost 15 pounds in the previous month and was in need of a feeding tube. There were signs of bedsores on her body caused by lying in urine and excrement. Sauer's estate sued for damages.

The trial began and lasted 8 days, with 28 witnesses testifying and 24 binders of exhibits. At the trial's conclusion, the jury retired to consider four counts: ordinary negligence, medical malpractice, breach of contract, and wrongful death. The jury returned a verdict for the Sauer Estate on all counts. Total damages amounted to more than $78 million. On appeal, the appellants argued that the damage awards for negligence and medical malpractice were grossly excessive.

The appellants argued that long-term care surveys conducted at the facility had been admitted into evidence over their objection. They claimed that the survey results inflamed the jury because the surveys were replete with statements that there was not enough help in the nursing home to feed, bathe, or clean residents.

They further argued that testimony submitted by witnesses that the nursing home had engaged in "false charting" to show more staff than were actually present was prejudicial, because it suggested that the appellants had staffing inadequacies that they tried to conceal from the state.

Sauer died of severe malnutrition and dehydration. There was evidence presented that she was found at times with dried feces under her fingernails from scratching herself while lying in her own excrement. At other times, staff did not get her out of her bed as they should have. Often, Sauer's food tray was found in her room, untouched, because there was no staff member at the nursing home available to feed her. She was not provided with range-of-motion assistance when the facility was short of staff.

Sauer had pressure sores on her back, lower buttock, and arms. A former staff member remembered seeing Sauer at one time with an open pressure sore the size of a softball. At times, she had no water pitcher in her room, nor did she receive a bath for a week or more because of shortage of staff. Sauer was found to suffer from poor oral hygiene, having caked food and debris in her mouth.

The appellate court found that the jury verdicts were not based on passion or prejudice. There was ample testimony and evidence to demonstrate that plaintiff's decedent suffered considerably and was not properly cared for in the nursing home, that the home was short-staffed, and that the home tried to cover this up by "false charting" and by bringing in additional employees on state inspection days. All of that served to support the estate's case that the nursing home knew it had staffing problems and committed negligence as to the decedent because it was short-staffed due to cutbacks.

The appellate court found that the circuit court abused its discretion by not granting a new trial due to excessive damages.

Ethical and Legal Issues

1. Describe the legal and ethical issues presented this case.
2. According to a federal study, nearly 90% of the nation's nursing homes are poorly staffed and find it difficult to provide basic services, such as cleaning, dressing, grooming, and feeding their residents.[20] Assuming the accuracy of this number, discuss how you would distribute limited dollars to address this issue. Consider how your decision may affect the allocation of funds to other health-related programs (e.g., immunizations, prenatal care, and preventative medicine). Assume that no new dollars can be allocated for the new health care budget year.

PROVIDE A SAFE ENVIRONMENT

Hospitals are required to provide a safe environment for patients, visitors, and staff. Safety concerns in hospitals flow from general mechanical safety to direct patient care in the operating room.

Efforts to End Surgeries on Wrong Patient or Body Part Falters

"Health care has far too little accountability for results. . . . All the pressures are on the side of production; that's how you get paid," said Hopkins's [Peter] Pronovost [safety expert and medical director of the John Hopkins Center for Innovation in Quality Patient Care], who adds that increased pressure to turn over operating rooms quickly has trumped patient safety, increasing the chance of error.

Sandra G. Boodman, Kaiser Health News, *June 20, 2011*[21]

Employers are required by law and accreditation standards to provide a safe environment for patients, visitors, and employees. Although one cannot guard against the unforeseeable, a health care organization is liable, as noted in the next case, for injuries resulting from dangers that it knowingly failed to guard against or those that it should have known about and failed to guard against. An organization has a duty to safeguard the welfare of its patients, even from harm by third persons, and that duty is measured by the ability of the patient to provide for his or her own safety.

Approximately 100 years ago, the Maryland Court of Appeals held that one who "is engaged in the undertaking of running an elevator as a means of personal transportation" is required to use the "highest degree of care and diligence practicable under the circumstances," which is the same standard that common carriers are required to meet.

On August 30, 2000, Jane Correia was a passenger in an elevator owned and operated by Johns Hopkins Health Services Company and Johns Hopkins Hospital. The elevator came to a sudden stop because of a mechanical defect. Due to injuries allegedly caused by this malfunction, Mrs. Correia and her husband sued Johns Hopkins, and others, in the Circuit Court for Baltimore City for negligence. A jury considered the matter in October 2005.

The Correias introduced evidence that showed that, in the 6 months prior to the accident, Johns Hopkins had received 32 complaints about the elevator Mrs. Correia was in when the accident occurred. The 32 complaints, if accurate, indicated that at various times prior to the accident the elevator was dropping, jumping, jerking, skipping, and sometimes trapping passengers.

At the end of a 9-day trial, the court gave the jury the following instruction:

The owner of a passenger elevator, in this case . . . Johns Hopkins is the owner of the passenger elevator, is bound to exercise to the highest degree of care and skill and diligence . . . practicable under the circumstances to guard against injury to individuals riding on those elevators. This rule of law applies to the owner of the elevator only. It does not apply to the service company [codefendant] Schindler [Elevator Company].

The jury returned a verdict in favor of Mrs. Correia in the amount of $264,500 and a separate $35,500 verdict in favor of Mr. and Mrs. Correia, jointly, for loss of consortium. Both verdicts were against Johns Hopkins; the jury found that codefendant Schindler Elevator Company was not negligent.

Johns Hopkins appealed, contending, among other things, that the trial judge committed reversible error in giving the instruction quoted previously.

On appeal, the Maryland Court of Appeals held that, from the record, it did not appear that this was a "close case" as to whether Johns Hopkins exercised the highest degree of care for Mrs. Correia's safety. There was strong evidence that it had not met its duty, especially in light of the numerous complaints about the elevator in the 6 months prior to the accident. The case, it appears, was "close" as to the issue of causation in that there was room for doubt as to whether an abrupt stop of a low-speed elevator could have caused the extensive injuries claimed.

The Court of Special Appeals of Maryland determined that the trial judge did not abuse his discretion in denying the motion for mistrial. The judgment was affirmed, with costs to be paid by Johns Hopkins Hospital and John Hopkins Health Service Company.[22]

Ethical and Legal Issues

1. Do you believe that this case should have been settled out of court? Discuss your answer.
2. Explain how would you have handled this case. Discuss your answer.

The patient in *Thomas v. Sisters of Charity of the Incarnate Word*[23] fell three stories to his death after he became locked out on the hospital roof and sat on a ledge in an apparent attempt to attract someone to get assistance. The trial court found that the fire exit configuration that allowed the patient access to the roof created an unreasonable risk of harm that was in fact the cause of his death.

There was testimony that the lack of signage violated both the Life Safety and 1988 Standard Building Codes. Standard building code required that signs direct an individual to the exit discharge or ultimate exit to the outside of the building. A lack of signage also violated hospital policy requiring that the roof should have been marked as a restricted area. The exit configuration was unsafe for either ordinary or emergency use because of the confusion encountered by an individual locked out of the building without any direction or instruction on where to go. Given the hospital's duty regarding this exit, its breach of that duty was clear. The door to the roof contained no warning that it would lock the patient out of the building if he exited. Whether the patient exited the building voluntarily or out of momentary confusion, the hospital breached its duty to warn him that he would be locked out and to direct him across the catwalk to the fire exit stairwell.

PROTECT PATIENTS AND STAFF FROM SEXUAL ASSAULT

Hospitals are expected to protect patients and staff from sexual assault. A claim that a hospital was negligent in preventing such an assault will succeed only if such an assault is foreseeable. Such was not the case in following example.

CASE: SEXUAL ASSAULT IN THE RECOVERY ROOM

The plaintiff was recovering from vaginal surgery. A surgical resident, employed by the hospital sexually assaulted her during her recovery. There is no dispute about the assault or the resident's liability. The question here is whether the hospital may be liable under a theory of vicarious liability or for negligence in its duty to protect the plaintiff.

The plaintiff, under the effects of anesthesia following surgery, was placed in a small four-bed recovery room. Nurse R, accompanied by another nurse, admitted the plaintiff to the unit and monitored her vital signs. Minutes later, the nurses turned their attention to a second patient who had been placed on an adjacent bed two feet away and were soon joined by Nurse G, their supervisor. Privacy curtains between the plaintiff and the second patient had not been drawn.

A surgical resident wearing hospital scrubs and an identification badge entered the recovery room and went to the plaintiff's bed. He was not one of the physicians listed on the plaintiff's chart, and none of the nurses knew him. According to the plaintiff, she awoke to find the resident pulling up her hospital gown and performing an "internal pelvic exam," which was contraindicated in light of the nature of the plaintiff's surgery. The plaintiff tried to sit up and cover herself with the gown and repeatedly asked him to stop. On her third plea, the physician hastily began to leave the recovery room. After the plaintiff complained to the nurses about what had taken place, the supervising nurse confronted the resident, who admitted that he had examined the plaintiff without the presence of a female witness, as required by hospital policy. The hospital terminated the resident following an investigation.

The Appellate Division Majority reasoned that a direct negligence claim must fail because the resident's misconduct was not foreseeable. The court also dismissed the vicarious liability claim against the hospital because the physician was acting outside the scope of his authority.

Two dissenting judges disagreed with the majority. They noted that the majority's holding on the direct negligence cause of action failed to consider the actual foreseeability of harm, indicated by observations the hospital staff could or should have made at the time immediately preceding the actual wrongdoing.

Nurse R had acknowledged that residents were not directly assigned to the recovery room. Her deposition testimony further indicated that she was aware of the identity of all of the plaintiff's physicians and that the resident was not one of those assigned to the plaintiff's care. In fact, all of the nurses in the recovery room were unacquainted with the resident. All of the nurses knew of the hospital's policy requiring the presence of a female staff member during a male physician's pelvic examination of a female patient.

Despite the nurses' assertions that they saw or heard nothing, an additional key question of credibility arises from the inference created by the undisputed close proximity of all of the nurses to the plaintiff's bed.

In contrast to the Appellate Division majority opinion, the dissenting judges considered that this confluence of factors provided a sufficient basis from which a jury could determine that the nurses unreasonably disregarded that which was readily there to be seen and heard, alerting them to the risk of misconduct against the plaintiff by the resident, which could have been prevented. Accordingly, the Appellate Division order was modified by remitting the case to the Supreme Court (trial court in New York) for further proceedings.[24]

Ethical and Legal Issues

1. Describe the ethical and legal issues presented in this case.
2. Describe how the physician's professional code of ethics was breached.

DECISIONS THAT COLLIDE WITH PROFESSIONAL ETHICS

Management's financial decisions can at times be on a collision course with practice and professional codes of ethics. The principles of autonomy, beneficence, and justice and the ability to practice what is right according to such principles often collide when organizations have to, for example, ration scarce resources. Such rationing may require managers to cut costs at the expense of quality.

A LIFE NEEDLESSLY SHORTENED

An action filed against a health insurance company alleged that the way the insurer handled the insured's chemotherapy needlessly shortened her life, causing her last days to be more painful than they should have been. The jury awarded the plaintiff $49 million. The punitive damages award was considered excessive under Ohio law, and the trial court's failure to find as such was so unreasonable as to constitute abuse of discretion. A $30 million award was appropriate given the profits of the corporations involved and appropriate in the scheme of past punitive damages awards in Ohio.[25]

FINANCIAL INCENTIVE SCHEMES

The managed care industry has historically failed to acknowledge the practice of denying medical claims at the expense of the patient's health, while at the same time benefiting managed care organizations. Dr. Linda Peeno, a Medical Reviewer for Humana, exposed this practice during her testimony before Congress, which stated in part:[26]

> I wish to begin by making a public confession: In the spring of 1987, as a physician, I caused the death of a man.
>
> Although this was known to many people, I have not been taken before any court of law or called to account for this in any professional or public forum. In fact, just the opposite occurred: I was "rewarded" for this. It bought me an improved reputation in my job, and contributed to my advancement afterwards. Not only did I demonstrate I could indeed do what was expected of me, I exemplified the "good" company doctor: I saved a half million dollars!
>
> Since that day, I have lived with this act, and many others, eating into my heart and soul. For me, a physician is a professional charged with the care, or healing, of his or her fellow human beings. The primary ethical norm is: do no harm. I did worse: I caused a death. Instead of using a clumsy, bloody weapon, I used the simplest, cleanest of tools: my words. The man died because I denied him a necessary operation to save his heart. I felt little pain or remorse at the time. The man's faceless distance soothed my conscience. Like a skilled soldier, I was trained for this moment. When any moral qualms arose, I was to remember: I am not denying care; I am only denying payment.

· · ·

> For me, "ethics" must be done close range. Distance blurs the complexities of human experiences. Those who argue that "the further removed, the clearer the thinking" are those who too often use "ethics" as legalism, public relations, or high-sounding rationalization. I would argue that, at least in medicine, one's ethical "authority" diminishes the further one is from the frontlines of patient experiences.[27]

Dr. Peeno came forward with her story and dedicated her career to helping others in a compassionate manner working in the field of health care ethics.

> As part of this effort, I chair a hospital ethics committee (University of Louisville Hospital), for which I do consultation, education and policy development. I am the executive director of an international academic society (International Society for the Systems Sciences), and as chair of its Medicine and Healthcare group, I work on ethical issues in international health care systems. I serve on the national board of Citizen Action, a nonpartisan consumer organization, through which I work toward equitable health reform. I am the founder of the CARE Foundation, a nonprofit group organized to promote consumer education, public accountability, and ethical responsibility in managed care. I am here to represent the largest interest group in our health care system: those affected by its design and operations, those who validate its consequences within their lives.[28]

Greg Ganske addressed the House of Representative on March 28, 2000:

Let me give my colleagues one example out of many of a health plan's definition of medically necessary services. "Medical necessity means the shortest, least expensive or least intense level of treatment, care or service rendered or supply provided as determined by us." Well, Mr. Speaker, contracts like this demonstrate that some health plans are manipulating the definition of medical necessity to deny appropriate patient care by arbitrarily linking it to saving money, not the patient's medical needs.[29]

Recently, the medical community has turned its attention to the authority of state medical boards to police improper physician expert testimony in medical malpractice actions. The discussion has been broadened to consider whether the presentation of testimony constitutes the carrying out of the practice of medicine. Depending on the state, some cases have held that the "carrying out" requirement means that the medical judgment must affect or have the possibility of affecting the patient. For example, in *Murphy v. Board of Medical Examiners*,[30] an Arizona court held that a physician performing prospective utilization review was practicing medicine because his decisions "could affect" a patient's health. Dr. Peeno was engaging in prospective utilization review; however, several federal courts have held that neither prospective nor retrospective review constituted the practice of medicine.[31] The public does, however, have the right to expect expert physicians to be accurate and truthful when giving testimony. If the profession cannot police itself, then the states will be forced to intervene in order to protect the public.

The patient in *Shea v. Esensten*[32] died after suffering a heart attack. Although the patient had recently visited his primary care physician and presented with symptoms of cardiac problems and the patient also had a family history of cardiac trouble, the physician did not refer the patient to a cardiologist. The patient's widow sued the health management organization for failing to disclose the financial incentive system it provided to its physicians to minimize referrals to specialists. The United States Court of Appeals for the Eighth Circuit agreed that knowledge of financial incentives that affect a physician's decisions to refer patients to specialists is material information requiring disclosure. The appeals court reversed a lower court's dismissal of the claim.

RESTORING TRUST

The lack of trust is slowly deteriorating the people's faith in the nation's health care system. A lack of trust in the physician, hospital, and insurer is pervasive throughout the health care system. The horror stories in newspapers, malpractice suits, and the Institute of Medicine's report on health care mistakes identify problems and provide a catalyst for encouraging lawsuits.

Organizations need to make a concerted effort to develop strategies to build and restore trust in the health care industry. The following strategies assist in building consumer trust:

* Conduct business in compliance with applicable laws, rules, and regulations.
* Adhere to ethical standards.

- Provide cost-effective care.
- Fairly and accurately represent the organization's capabilities when treating a patient's ailments.
- Maintain a uniform standard of care throughout the organization, regardless of a person's ability to pay, race, creed, color, and/or national origin.
- Consider patient values and preferences as part of recognizing the organization's legal responsibilities.
- Inform patients of their rights and responsibilities.
- Develop and recommend guidelines that assist and support patients and their families in exercising their rights.
- Describe the process to patients by which hospital staff interact and care for them.

Trust must begin within the organization between management and employees. As the following *reality check* describes, organizations can often become dysfunctional and cause employee turnover and resentment among employees.

Equal Pay for Equal Work?

The annual Health Systems Consulting conference was held at the New York City Hilton. During the closing session on Friday, the company's leadership sat onstage summarizing the week's training and conducting a question-and-answer period. Prior to the session, Frank, an administrator consultant, had asked his manager, "The grapevine is telling me that nurses have been placed at a higher pay rate than administrators. Is that true?" His manager replied, "You asked a direct question, so I will answer it, even though per company policy we don't generally share such information.

The answer is yes. It was implemented several weeks ago. The consulting process is more and more clinical and therefore nurses are getting a higher starting salary." Frank answered, "That is true, but we still all do the same work." His manager replied, "That's the way it is," and walked away.

Anonymous

Discussion

1. Because employment law requires equal pay for equal work, what ethical concerns do you see in this case?
2. If you were Frank, what action would you pursue, if any?

Questions Solicited Not Always Welcomed

When you question a company policy, even after company insistence that all questions are welcomed, there can be a price to be paid. Gerard asked anyway, "Since the health survey process is leaning more toward the clinical side of care and we are attempting to get more physician involvement in the patient care review process, why aren't physicians the team leaders? After all, they have the best clinical judgment."

The leadership were basically at a loss about what to say but in the end gave the usual response by stating they would look into it. One physician stood and said, "Nurses are better at this process than physicians." The room became silent and the physician received some glares from his colleagues. The leadership quickly moved on to the next question.

Gerard later received several conflicting comments from his colleagues in the lobby:

Nurse Consultant 1: "I knew you were an ****. Now, I know you are an ****. I will give you the dirtiest work on the survey when you are on a consulting job with me!"

Nurse 2: "You're senile!"

Nurse 3: "You had the courage to say what you think."

AF Nurse practitioner/Consultant 4: "You stood up for something you believed in. I admire you for that."

Nurse Consultant 5: "Nurses are more clinically adept than physicians."

Nurse 6: "Gerard, some of those nurses were pretty awful to you. Why don't you join us for something to eat?"

Nurse 7: "We don't agree with all you said, but we respect your opinion."

Nurse 8: "You had the courage to say what you think."

Physician Consultant 1: "You will most likely find a horse's head in your bed in the morning."

Physician Consultant 3: "Gerard, I agreed with you, but was it really worth it?"

Physician Consultant 4: "I see you're still alive."

Gerard, somewhat despondent, walked away and into the lobby gift shop. He spotted an article in the *Washington Post*.

The Role of Nurses Extends Beyond the Hospital Ward

A nurse is a doctor's best friend, according to Marvin M. Lipman, Consumers Union's chief medical adviser. This advice was given to him by a hospital ward's head nurse when he was a third-year medical student making contact with patients for the first time, along with the suggestion that he'd do well not to forget it.

Over the years, those words continued to echo in Lipman's mind. In part because hospital nurses work for the institution and many doctors work for themselves, occasional conflicts between the two are inevitable. When encountering such situations, he has generally tended to take the side of the nurses, sometimes to the chagrin of his fellow physicians. But he explains that his loyalty comes from the many times he has seen nurses go that extra step to make a patient more comfortable or more at ease.

Consumers Union of United States Inc., The Washington Post, *May 30, 2011*

Discussion

1. Gerard is a congenial, humorous, and respected person. His colleagues know that he does give his opinion if he sees a wrong that should be righted, whether it is for him or others. Should he have spoken up or remained silent? Discuss your answer.
2. Based on the *Washington Post* article, do you think Gerard might have had second thoughts about his concerns?
3. Describe the actions of Gerard's colleagues and what ethical theories might apply.

Effective Communication Builds Trust

Effective communication spawns trust and is commonly acknowledged as a deciding factor in building a harmonious organization. All the players must work together and understand the role each plays. As in an orchestra **(Figure 1)**, the instruments must work together to produce harmony. The better the musicians play, the more satisfied the audience. Even if you were able to play all the instruments in the orchestra, you can play only one at a time. During an interview with PBS Dr. William Edwards Deming, an American author, professor, and consultant, stated that in a "140 piece orchestra, everybody supports the other 139. He's not there to play a solo. He's not to play as loud as he can play to attract attention. He's there to support the other 139. The job of the conductor is to optimize their talents, their abilities."[33] And so it is with health care workers; they are there to support one another and *each caregiver trusts the other to play his or her part well.* The better the teamwork in the health care setting the better the care, which in turn breeds satisfied patients, families, and staff.

FIGURE 1   Together, the orchestra creates harmony. (© Martin Good/Shutterstock, Inc.)

1. This chapter introduces the reader to the ethical responsibilities and legal risks of health care organizations.
2. Authority of a corporation is expressed in the law under which the corporation is chartered.
    *   Governing body
        *   *Express* corporate authority
            *   *Verbal*
            *   *Written*
        *   *Implied* corporate authority
        *   *Ultra vires acts*
            *   Acts violate a corporation's scope of authority.
3. Organization code of ethics
    *   Provides guidelines for behavior that help carry out an organization's mission, vision, and values.
    *   Builds trust.
    *   Increases awareness of ethical issues.
    *   Guides decision making.
    *   Encourages staff to seek advice and report organizational misconduct.
4. Unethical organizational conduct
    *   Trust and Integrity
    *   False Advertising
    *   Concealing Mistakes
    *   Financial Incentive Schemes
5. Corporate negligence
    *   Failure to perform duties owed directly to a patient or anyone else to whom a duty may extend.
    *   *Theory of corporate negligence*—if a corporate duty is breached and a patient is injured as a result of that breach, the organization can be held liable for the injuries suffered.
6. Doctrine of *Respondeat superior*
    *   A legal doctrine holding an employer liable for the wrongful acts of its agents (employees).
    *   *Respondeat superior* has also been referred to as *vicarious liability*, whereby an employer is answerable for the torts committed by its employees.
    *   *Darling v. Charleston Community Memorial Hospital*[34] is the benchmark case, which has had a major impact on the liability of health care organizations.
    *   The court here enunciated a "corporate negligence doctrine," under which hospitals have a duty to provide adequately trained medical and nursing staff.
7. Independent contractors
    *   Responsible for their own negligent acts.
    *   Occurs when the principal has no right of control over the manner in which the agent's work is to be performed.

8. Corporate duties and responsibilities
   - Appointment of a CEO
   - Credentialing, appointments, and privileging of professional staff
   - Provide adequate staff
   - Provide adequate supplies and equipment
   - Allocation of scarce resources
   - Comply with rules and regulations
   - Comply with accreditation standards
   - Provide timely treatment
   - Avoid conflicts of interest
   - Provide a safe environment
   - Protect patients and staff from sexual assault
9. Build and restore trust through effective communications.

TEST YOUR UNDERSTANDING

TERMINOLOGY

codes of ethics for
   organizations
conflict of interest
corporate authority
corporate negligence

credentialing
Darling v. Charleston Community Memorial Hosp.
delineation of clinical
   privileges

express corporate authority
implied corporate authority
independent contractor
respondeat superior
ultra vires acts

REVIEW QUESTIONS

1. Discuss the governing body's decision-making authority.

2. Explain what an *ultra varies act* is.

3. Describe the important aspects of a code of ethics for organizations.

4. Discuss the various forms of professional misconduct discussed here.

5. Describe the relationship between *corporate negligence, respondeat superior,* and *independent contractor.*

6. Describe the duties and responsibilities of health care organizations and how the failure to adhere those duties and responsibilities can result in both legal and ethical issues.

7. Discuss how an organization's decisions can collide with professional ethics.

8. Discuss the importance of effective communications in building trust in the health care setting.

NOTES

1. http://www.wbaltv.com/news/maryland/baltimore-county/settlement-reached-in-st-joes-medical-malpractice-case/-/10136486/19985154/-/91thi9z/-/index.html
2. 745 N.Y.S.2d 304 (N.Y. App. Div. 2002).
3. *Thompson v. Nason Hosp.*, 591 A.2d 703, 707 (Pa. 1991).
4. *Id.*
5. 211 N.E.2d 253 (Ill. 1965).
6. Id. at 260.
7. 46 U.S.I.W. 2227 (Md. 1977).
8. http://www.ache.org/abt_ache/code.cfm.
9. CBSNews.com, "Did hospitals 'see no evil'?" April 4, 2004; http://www.cbsnews.com/stories/2004/04/02/60minutes/main610047.shtml
10. No. 05AP-681 (Ohio App. 2006).
11. 543 So. 2d 209 (Fla. 1989).
12. http://www.jointcommission.org/jc_physician_blog/revisiting_disruptive_and_inappropriate_behavior/.
13. http://www.ama-assn.org/ama/pub/physician-resources/medical-ethics/code-medical-ethics/opinion9045.page.
14. No. A03A2308 (Ga. App. 2004).
15. *Medcalf v. Coleman,* No. 98906 (2003).
16. *Freilich v. Upper Chesapeake Health, Inc.,* 313 F.3d 205 (2002).
17. 733 So. 2d 91 (La. App. 3 Cir. 1999).
18. 734 F.2d 81 (1st Cir. 1984).
19. 111 S.W.3d 346 (2003).
20. Christopher Newton, "90% of nursing homes providing substandard care–federal report," *Seattle Times,* February 20, 2002, at A1.
21. Sandra G. Boodman, "Effort to end surgeries on wrong patient or body part falters," June 20, 2011; http://www.kaiserhealthnews.org/Stories/2011/June/21/wrong-site-surgery-errors.aspx.
22. *The Johns Hopkins Hospital, et al. v. Jane E.S. Correia, et ux.*, 174 Md. App. 359, 921 A.2d 837 (2007).
23. No. 38,170 (La. App. 2004).
24. *N.X. v. Cabrini Med. Ctr.,* 765 N.E.2d 844 (2002).
25. 107 F.3d 625 & 8th Circuit (1997).
26. Available at http://wn.com/Linda_Peeno.
27. http://www.thenationalcoalition.org/DrPeenotestimory.html#c6.
28. http://www.thenationalcoalition.org/DrPeenotestimory.html#c6.
29. House of Representatives, "Important issue facing House-Senate Conference on Health Care Reform," March 28, 2000; http://www.fenichel.com/Ganske.shtml.
30. 949 P2d 530,535 (Ariz. Ct. App. 1997).
31. *Adnan Varol, M.D., P.C. v. Blue Cross Blue Shield of Mich.,* 708 F. Supp. 826 (E.D. Mich. 1989); *Corcoran v. United Health Care,* 956 F.2d 1321 (5th Cir. 1992).
32. http://biotech.law.lsu.edu/cases/hmo/shea_v_esensten.htm
33. http://www.getbig.com/boards/index.php?topic=179701.0.
34. *Dardinger, Exr. v. Anthem Blue Cross and Blue Shield,* 2002 Ohio 7113 (Ohio 2002).

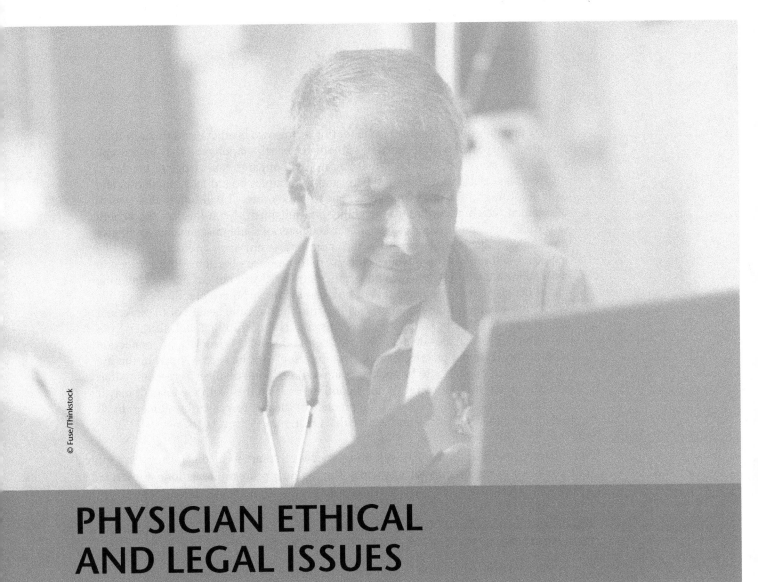

PHYSICIAN ETHICAL AND LEGAL ISSUES

LEARNING OBJECTIVES

Upon completion of this chapter, the reader will be able to:

- Apply the *Hippocratic Oath* to modern codes of medical ethics.
- Understand how the law and ethics intertwine in patient care.
- Describe common medical errors and ethical issues relative to physician practice.
- Describe important guidelines for developing positive physician–patient relations.

INTRODUCTION

The Hippocratic Oath

I SWEAR by Apollo the physician, and Aesculapius, and Health, and All-heal, and all the gods and goddesses, that, according to my ability and judgment, I will keep this Oath and this stipulation—to reckon him who taught me this Art equally dear to me as my parents, to share my substance with him, and relieve his necessities if required;

to look upon his offspring in the same footing as my own brothers, and to teach them this art, if they shall wish to learn it, without fee or stipulation; and that by precept, lecture, and every other mode of instruction, I will impart a knowledge of the Art to my own sons, and those of my teachers, and to disciples bound by a stipulation and oath according to the law of medicine, but to none others. I will follow that system of regimen which, according to my ability and judgment, I consider for the benefit of my patients, and abstain from whatever is deleterious and mischievous. I will give no deadly medicine to any one if asked, nor suggest any such counsel; and in like manner I will not give to a woman a pessary to produce abortion. With purity and with holiness I will pass my life and practice my Art. I will not cut persons laboring under the stone, but will leave this to be done by men who are practitioners of this work. Into whatever houses I enter, I will go into them for the benefit of the sick, and will abstain from every voluntary act of mischief and corruption; and, further from the seduction of females or males, of freemen and slaves. Whatever, in connection with my professional practice or not, in connection with it, I see or hear, in the life of men, which ought not to be spoken of abroad, I will not divulge, as reckoning that all such should be kept secret. While I continue to keep this Oath unviolated, may it be granted to me to enjoy life and the practice of the art, respected by all men, in all times! But should I trespass and violate this Oath, may the reverse be my lot![1]

This chapter provides the reader with an overview of common medical errors and ethical issues relative to the practice of medicine. The medical profession has long subscribed to a body of ethical principals. One of Hippocrates' gifts to medicine, among many, was the *Hippocratic Oath* for physicians, which has been modified and adopted by various medical schools such as John Baylor College of Medicine, Johns Hopkins Medical School, and Tufts University School of Medicine[2] as noted in the following extract:

I swear to fulfill, to the best of my ability and judgment, this covenant:

I will respect the hard-won scientific gains of those physicians in whose steps I walk, and gladly share such knowledge as is mine with those who are to follow.

I will apply, for the benefit of the sick, all measures which are required, avoiding those twin traps of overtreatment and therapeutic nihilism.

I will remember that there is art to medicine as well as science, and that warmth, sympathy, and understanding may outweigh the surgeon's knife or the chemist's drug.

I will not be ashamed to say "I know not," nor will I fail to call in my colleagues when the skills of another are needed for a patient's recovery.

I will respect the privacy of my patients, for their problems are not disclosed to me that the world may know. Most especially must I tread with care in matters of life and death. If it is given me to save a life, all thanks. But it may also be within my power to take a life; this awesome responsibility must be faced with great humbleness and awareness of my own frailty. Above all, I must not play at God.

I will remember that I do not treat a fever chart, a cancerous growth, but a sick human being, whose illness may affect the person's family and economic stability. My responsibility includes these related problems, if I am to care adequately for the sick.

I will prevent disease whenever I can, for prevention is preferable to cure.

I will remember that I remain a member of society, with special obligations to all my fellow human beings, those sound of mind and body as well as the infirm. If I do not violate this oath, may I enjoy life and art, respected while I live and remembered with affection thereafter. May I always act so as to preserve the finest traditions of my calling and may I long experience the joy of healing those who seek my help.

Source: *Louis Lasagna, 1964, Academic Dean of the School of Medicine at Tufts University, and used in many medical schools today.*

Although there is no direct punishment for violating the Hippocratic oath, medical malpractice suits often involve a physician's failure to adhere to the oath and/or other applicable medical codes of ethics. Malpractice suits can lead to financial awards to the injured party.

CODE OF MEDICAL ETHICS

The American Medical Association in the footsteps of Hippocrates describes the code of ethical conduct for physicians:

I. A physician shall be dedicated to providing competent medical care, with compassion and respect for human dignity and rights.

II. A physician shall uphold the standards of professionalism, be honest in all professional interactions, and strive to report physicians deficient in character or competence, or engaging in fraud or deception, to appropriate entities.

III. A physician shall respect the law and also recognize a responsibility to seek changes in those requirements that are contrary to the best interests of the patient.

IV. A physician shall respect the rights of patients, colleagues, and other health professionals, and shall safeguard patient confidences and privacy within the constraints of the law.

V. A physician shall continue to study, apply, and advance scientific knowledge; maintain a commitment to medical education; make relevant information available to patients, colleagues, and the public; obtain consultation; and use the talents of other health professionals when indicated.

VI. A physician shall, in the provision of appropriate patient care, except in emergencies, be free to choose whom to serve, with whom to associate, and the environment in which to provide medical care.

VII. A physician shall recognize a responsibility to participate in activities contributing to the improvement of the community and the betterment of public health.

VIII. A physician shall, while caring for a patient, regard responsibility to the patient as paramount.

IX. A physician shall support access to medical care for all people.

Source: Code of Medical Ethics, A9 2001, American Medical Association.[3]

This section introduces the reader to how the law and ethics intertwine in patient care. The law provides that injury to a patient due to a negligent act can result in financial penalties imposed by the courts to compensate the injured party and hopefully deter similar acts. *Non-maleficence* in medical ethics is a central guiding principle of the ethical practice of medicine; first expressed by Hippocrates, and translated into Latin as *primum non nocere*, first do no harm. It is medicine's most fundamental axiom that aptly describes where the law and ethics unite—*first do no harm*. The injury of a patient due to an avoidable negligent act often involves both principles of law and ethics.

HIPPOCRATIC OATH AND AMA CODE OF ETHICS VIOLATED

The Thompsons in *Scripps Clinic v. Superior Ct.*[4] alleged negligent treatment of Patricia Thompson's broken clavicle. A medical malpractice claim was filed against Dr. Thorne and Dr. Carpenter, both of whom were affiliated with Scripps, a group medical practice. At the time the malpractice action was filed, Patricia was no longer being treated by Thorne and Carpenter, but was being treated by other Scripps physicians: Drs. Botte and Froenke for the broken clavicle and Dr. Harkey for endometriosis.

Binford, a Scripps employee, sent a letter to the Thompsons informing them that Scripps had been notified about the legal action the Thompsons had taken against the group. Because of the legal action, the Scripps Clinic requested that Health Net immediately terminate the Thompsons with the Scripps Clinic and transfer their membership to another medical group.

When Patricia received Binford's letter, she immediately requested Health Net to reassign the couple to a new medical group. Health Net transferred the Thompsons to the San Diego Medical Group. As the result of Scripps's actions, Patricia had to cancel a follow-up visit with Dr. Harkey that had been scheduled near the end of June even though Patricia was still suffering severe pain and bleeding. Before Patricia could be referred to a new gynecologist at University of California, San Diego Medical Group, she had to schedule a visit with her new primary care physician and receive authorization. Patricia's care was also delayed until the San Diego Medical Group received her medical records from Scripps.

Scripps contends that it gave adequate notice to the Thompsons. The court disagreed. There was a 2-week hiatus between the time Scripps denied the Thompsons access to its physicians for nonemergency services and the time the Thompsons were assigned to the San Diego Medical Group.

The court rejected Scripps's contention the court should have granted summary adjudication of the negligent infliction of emotional distress and breach of fiduciary duty causes of action. The court denied the motion because the Thompsons raised a triable issue of fact as to breach, based upon the declaration of Dr. David Goldstein, the Thompsons' expert. Goldstein declared Scripps breached the standard of care and its fiduciary duty by violating the AMA Code of Medical Ethics 1.3.10 and the Hippocratic Oath, because its policy is retaliatory and "promotes the self-interest of physicians over that of patients."[5]

Physicians have both a legal and ethical obligation to attend to their patients' needs. Physicians licensed in Illinois, for example, are specifically prohibited from abandoning their patients.[6] Furthermore, the American Medical Association's Council on Ethical and Judicial

Affairs mandates that "once having undertaken a case, the physician should not neglect the patient."[7]

The relationship between a physician and a patient, once established, continues until it is ended by the mutual consent of the parties, the patient's dismissal of the physician, the physician's withdrawal from the case, or the fact that the physician's services are no longer required. A physician who decides to withdraw his or her services must provide the patient with reasonable notice so that the services of another physician can be obtained. Premature termination of treatment is often the subject of a legal action for abandonment, the unilateral termination of a physician–patient relationship by the physician without notice to the patient. The following elements must be established in order for a patient to recover damages for abandonment:

- Medical care was unreasonably discontinued.
- The discontinuance of medical care was against the patient's will. Termination of the physician–patient relationship must have been brought about by a unilateral act of the physician. There can be no issue of abandonment if the relationship is terminated by mutual consent or by dismissal of the physician by the patient.
- The physician failed to arrange for care by another physician. Refusal by a physician to enter into a physician–patient relationship by failing to respond to a call or render treatment is not considered a case of abandonment. A plaintiff will not recover for damages unless he or she can show that a physician–patient relationship had been established.
- Foresight indicated that discontinuance might result in physical harm.
- The patient as a result of the physician's abandonment suffered actual harm.

Physicians must, as provided in the Hippocratic oath and codes of ethics, make care decisions for the benefit of their patients and not for their hurt or for any wrong. Terminating a physician–patient relationship must be done within legal guidelines, otherwise the physician can be held liable for abandonment. As noted next, compassion, trust, justice, and respect for patient privacy are all ethical principles and values that are intertwined with law.

COMPASSION

Compassion is a moral value hoped for in all caregivers. Those who truly possess it will have a more rewarding career and at the end of life be able to say, "I have not only lived, but I have lived for something, it was worthwhile, I had a reason for living and a reason for leaving. I led a purpose-fulfilled life." The following news clipping succinctly illustrates how one physician's experience when faced with a dying patient can spring forth compassion and a time for reflection.

Suddenly, unexpectedly, he grabs my shirt.

"Don't let me die!" he says, spraying me with blood.
He turns with effort, his yellow eyes searing into mine.

• • •

Hours later, my pager beeps again. It's the head nurse once more, summoning me back to "pronounce him dead."

• • •

"The family is waiting to see you," she says, as if I should've known.

• • •

The woman I take to be the deceased's mother reaches into a purse on the floor and unfurls a rumpled handkerchief. She buries her face in it. *Memento mori*, the ancient Romans said. Remember that you will die. This scene will be a permanent meditation throughout the rest of my career.

Richard E. Cytowic, Washingtonian, *March 2014*

Not all physicians possess the degree of compassion noted in the news clipping. The following *reality check* describes the world of Mrs. Smith who during an interview stated that she found in over 15 years of being passed from physician to physician only 4 of 26 physicians (15.83%) that she would describe as compassionate and empathetic to her as the pain racked her body from the top of her head to the soles of her feet.

Physician Lacks Compassion

Mrs. Smith arranged for an appointment to see Dr. Mean, a rheumatologist, who was a specialist in her particular disease process, systemic scleroderma. After scheduling her appointment, Mrs. Smith was asked to have her medical records faxed to Mean's office before her scheduled appointment on March 27. Two days before her scheduled appointment with Mean, Mrs. Smith called Mean's office to confirm that her records had arrived. She was told at that time that she was on Mean's calendar for March 23, not March 27. She had missed her appointment. Mrs. Smith had waited 2 months for this date, and her illness had gotten progressively worse. Mrs. Smith, desperate for help, pleaded with the scheduler to reschedule her as soon as possible. The scheduler explained to Mrs. Smith that Mean was a busy physician and that she could not schedule a new appointment until April 27, a month later.

Discussion

1. Describe how Dr. Mean violated the professional code of ethics for a physician.
2. Discuss what role a hospital ethics committee could play in addressing Dr. Mean's insensitivity to Mrs. Smith's needs? Explain your answer.

It is not only important for the physician to show compassion, but also the office staff that works with patients from the time they walk in the office door until the time they leave, as the following *reality check* illustrates.

Staff Affects Physician Practice Image

Mark was waiting to be seen by his physician in a multispecialty physician office practice. As Mark was waiting to see his physician, he observed a woman, most likely in her late 70s, limping into the office. She had a large leg brace that ran from her thigh to the calf of her leg. She struggled to push her husband in a wheelchair into the office. She carefully parked the wheelchair and approached the check-in counter. She apologized for being late for her appointment as she was late getting out of another physician's office. The patient was told, "You are late for your appointment. The office has a 15-minute late arrival rule. You will have to reschedule your appointment." She apologized for being late but said that she did tell the office staff she would be late. She was then told, "You can wait, and I will try to squeeze you into the schedule, but I don't know how long you will have to wait." The lady said, "I don't want to bother anyone. I will reschedule my appointment." She was directed around the corner to another desk to reschedule her appointment. Mark got up out of his chair, walked over to the scheduler, and said, "I don't believe this. Her husband is sitting in a wheelchair, and she is having difficulty walking. She can have my appointment, and I can reschedule." The lady suddenly turned to Mark and gave him a big hug. The scheduler asked, "Who is your physician?" Mark told her, and she said, "I am sorry, but this lady has a different physician." The lady, now a bit teary eyed, continued to make her appointment.

Discussion

1. Describe the ethical issues involved in this observation.
2. Consider and discuss how this event could have had a more pleasant outcome.

TRUST

Patients trust their physicians to provide them the necessary medical information to assist them in making the right treatment choices. The use of risky and unproven procedures that a patient's injury can result in a lawsuit. However, a physician will not be held liable for exercising his or her judgment in applying a course of treatment supported by a reputable and respected body of medical experts even if another body of expert medical opinion would favor a different course of treatment.

Surgeons and Medical Center Breach Trust

A young woman went to a medical center for removal of a benign fibroid tumor in her uterus, an outpatient procedure. By the end of the day, she was dead.

> The surgery was performed by two doctors—one on probation—who used equipment they were neither familiar with nor authorized to use, the Health Department said. In a highly unusual violation, the agency said, a salesman from Johnson & Johnson, which made the piece of equipment used in the surgery, operated its controls while the doctors performed their procedure on the woman. And the patient was never given the chance to consent to the use of the equipment or the presence of the salesman, the agency said.[8]

The actions of the surgeons and medical center in this case clearly place the spotlight on trust and the ability of health care organizations to competently monitor their professional staff. The community of patients across the nation trust that the physicians appointed and credentialed by hospitals are closely monitored and privileged strictly according to their proven capabilities. This trust must not falter.

Failure to Read Nurses' Notes

On October 17, the medical record indicated that Todd's sternotomy wound and the mid-lower left leg incision were reddened and his temperature was 99.6 degrees F. Dr. Sauls did not commonly read the nurses' notes but instead preferred to rely on his own observations of the patient. In his October 18 notes, he indicated that there was no drainage. The nurses' notes, however, show that there was drainage at the chest tube site. In contrast to the medical records showing that Todd had a temperature of 101.2 degrees F, Dr. Sauls noted that the patient was afebrile (normal, without fever).

On October 19, Dr. Sauls noted that Todd's wounds were improving, and he did not have a fever. Nurses' notes indicated redness at the surgical wounds and a temperature of 100 degrees F. No white blood count had been ordered. Again on October 20, the nurses' notes indicated redness at the site of the wound and a temperature of 100.8 degrees F. No wound culture had yet been ordered. Dr. Kamil, one of Todd's treating physicians, noted that Todd's nutritional status needed to be seriously confronted and suggested that Dr. Sauls consider supplemental feeding. Despite this, no follow-up to his recommendation appeared and the record is void of any action by Dr. Sauls to obtain a nutritional consult.

Todd was transferred to the intensive care unit on October 21 because he was gravely ill with profoundly depressed ventricular function. The following day the nurses' notes described the chest tube site as draining foul-smelling bloody purulence. The patient's temperature was recorded to have reached 100.6 degrees F. This was the first time that Dr. Sauls had the test tube site cultured. On October 23, the culture report from the laboratory indicated a staph infection, and Todd was started on antibiotics for treatment of the infection.

On October 25, at the request of family, Todd was transferred to St. Luke's Hospital. At St. Luke's, Dr. Leatherman, an internist and invasive cardiologist, treated Todd. Dr. Zeluff, an infectious disease specialist, examined Todd's surgical wounds and prescribed antibiotic treatment. On his admission to St. Luke's, every one of Todd's surgical wounds was infected. Despite the care given at St. Luke's, Todd died on November 2, 1988. The family brought a malpractice suit against the surgeon. The District Court entered judgment on a jury verdict for the defendant, and the plaintiff appealed, claiming the surgeon breached his duty of care owed to the patient by failing to (1) aggressively treat the surgical wound infections, (2) read the nurses' observations of infections, and (3) provide adequate nourishment, allowing the patient's body weight to waste away rapidly.

Dr. Sauls committed medical malpractice when he breached the standard of care he owed to Todd. Todd was effectively ineligible for a heart transplant, which was his only chance of survival because of the infections and malnourishment caused by Dr. Sauls's negligent care. Sauls's testimony convinced the Louisiana Court of Appeals that he failed to treat the surgical wound infections aggressively, that he chose not to take advantage of the nurses' observations of infection, and that he allowed Todd's body weight to waste away, knowing that extreme vigilance was required because of Todd's already severely impaired heart.

In cases in which a patient has died, the plaintiff need not demonstrate that the patient would have survived if properly treated. Rather, he need only prove that the patient had a chance of survival and that his chance of survival was lost as a result of the defendant/physician's negligence. The defendant/physician's conduct must increase the risk of a patient's harm to the extent of being a substantial factor in causing the result, but need not be the only cause. Dr. Sauls's medical malpractice exacerbated an already critical condition and deprived Mr. Todd of a chance of survival.

Todd trusted Dr. Sauls to do the right thing. Instead he failed to follow Todd's care closely enough to identify his declining health as a result of an infection—that was clearly indicated in the nurses' notes.

Failure to Refer for Consultation

1 in 4 Cancer Cases Missed: GPs Send Away Alarming Number of Patients, Delaying Vital Treatment

Tens of thousands of patients are initially told that their symptoms are "nothing to worry about" or advised to take painkillers or antibiotics for months.

They have to make repeated trips to their doctor before being given a correct diagnosis, the report concludes. Britain has one of the lowest cancer survival rates in Europe despite billions being invested in treatment over the last decade.

Experts blame late diagnosis for the alarmingly high death rates and say many tumors are spotted only when it is too late for successful treatment.

Sophie Borland and David Wilkes, Daily Mail, *March 1, 2011*[9]

When a practitioner determines or should have determined that a patient's ailment is beyond his or her scope of knowledge, technical skill or ability, or capacity to treat with a likelihood of reasonable success, he or she is under a duty to disclose such determination to the patient. The patient should be advised of the necessity of other or different treatments.

A physician has a duty to consult and/or refer a patient whom he or she knows or should know needs referral to a physician familiar with and clinically capable of treating the patient's particular ailments. Whether the failure to refer constitutes negligence depends on whether referral is demanded by accepted standards of practice. To recover damages, the plaintiff must show that the physician deviated from the standard of care and that the failure to refer resulted in injury.

The California Court of Appeals found that expert testimony is not necessary where good medical practice would require a general physician to suggest a specialist's consultation.[10] The court ruled that because specialists were called in after the patient's condition grew worse, it is reasonable to assume that they could have been called in sooner. The jury was instructed by the court that a general practitioner has a duty to seek consultation by a specialist if a reasonably prudent general practitioner would do so under similar circumstances.

A physician is in a position of trust, and it is his or her duty to act in good faith. If a preferred treatment in a given situation is outside a physician's field of expertise, it is his or her duty to advise the patient. Failure to do so could constitute a breach of duty. Today, with the rapid methods of transportation and easy means of communication, the duty of a physician is not fulfilled merely by using the means at hand in a particular area of practice.

Falsification of Records

The intentional alteration, falsification, or destruction of medical records to avoid liability for one's medical negligence is generally sufficient to show actual malice, and punitive damages may be awarded whether or not the act of altering, falsifying, or destroying records directly causes compensable harm. The evidence in *Dimora v. Cleveland Clinic Foundation*[11] had shown that the patient had fallen and broken five or six ribs; nevertheless, on examination, the physician noted in the progress notes that the patient was smiling and laughing pleasantly, exhibiting no pain on deep palpation of the area. Other testimony indicated that she was in pain and crying. This discrepancy between the written progress notes and the testimony of the witnesses who observed the patient was sufficient to raise a question of fact as to the possible falsification of documents by the physician to minimize the nature of the incident and the injury of the patient because of the possible negligence of the hospital personnel. The testimony of the witnesses, if believed, would have been sufficient to show that the physician falsified the record or intentionally reported the incident inaccurately in order to avoid liability for the negligent care of the patient.

Tampering with records sends the wrong signal to jurors and can shatter one's credibility. Altered records can create a presumption of negligence. The court in *Matter of Jascalevich*[12] held that "a physician's duty to a patient cannot but encompass his affirmative obligation to maintain the integrity, accuracy, truth, and reliability of the patient's medical record. His obligation in this regard is no less compelling than his duties respecting diagnosis and treatment of the patient because the medical community must, of necessity be able to rely on those records in the continuing care of that patient. The rendering of good care must not be jeopardized or prejudiced by false, misleading, or inaccurate entries in the patient's medical record. A deliberate falsification by a physician of a patient's medical record in order to protect one's own personal interests at the expense of the patient's is regarded as gross malpractice endangering the health or life of his patient.[13] The physician's oath to first do no harm was violated in this case.

Post-Cath Note Written Prior to Procedure

Dr. Benjamin, a physician consultant, noted that a cardiologist had documented a postprocedure catheterization note before the procedure was completed. The physician consultant discussed with the cardiologist the inappropriate record entry and had a peer-to-peer discussion to help the surgeon understand the ramifications of his actions. The organization was most grateful for the way the physician surveyor managed the situation as it made their job much easier in addressing the issue with the surgeon, whose nonadherence to hospital and medical staff policy the organization had difficulty trying to handle over the past year. They were pleased with the process.

Discussion

1. Who should have handled the discipline issues with the physician? Explain your answer. Consider in forming your answer: The surveyor had 3 days to survey the hospital to determine its compliance with accreditation standards and now the surveyor is involved in a counseling session taking valuable time out of his duties.
2. How should the hospital have dealt with the cardiologist?

JUSTICE

Does the value of life diminish with age? Do you see me? Do you hear me? Am I less valuable because I am older? We are all created equal in God's sight. But then, when it comes to supply and demand, everything we thought we learned about ethics is put to the test. Who gets the new lung when there is a limited supply? Are there criteria for determining what the right thing to do is? If so who decided what the criteria should be? The questions as to justice and the distribution of scare resources are numerous and the answers are not easily sorted out, as noted in the following *reality check*.

Care Based on Age

I was undergoing some minor revisions to a surgical procedure that I had 5 years earlier. I distinctly remember the surgeon speaking to one of his assistants during the surgery, as he wielded a scalpel in his hand, "I definitely take more time with younger patients, especially children, than older patients." As I lie there on a small surgical table, I thought what do I say? I could've smacked him for being so rude. What an uncomfortable situation for me to be in, knowing that the surgeon had already made an incision under a local anesthetic. He spoke as though I wasn't there. I thought I better just act as though I had not heard him. Afterwards I thought that was a stupid thought. It wasn't like he was whispering. He was actually somewhat loud as though I was under a general anesthetic. If a friend told me that this happened to him, I would most likely have found it hard to believe. A surgeon should always do his best, regardless of the patient's age. But then maybe I am living in La La land.

Anonymous

Discussion

1. Discuss what, if anything, the patient should have said to the surgeon. Consider when framing your answer the patient is thinking to himself, "Unfortunately I have to come back to have the stitches taken out."
2. Describe what action you would take, if any, as a board member. Assume you had been sitting outside the treatment room and you had overheard the surgeon's remarks. Further assume you were a friend of the patient and had dropped in the surgeon's office to pick him up to take him home.

RESPECT FOR PRIVACY

Respect for the privacy of medical information is a central feature of the physician–patient relationship. Under the Hippocratic Oath and modern principles of medical ethics derived from it, physicians are ethically bound to maintain patient confidences.

The physician–patient privilege imposes on a physician an obligation to maintain the confidentiality of each patient's communications. This obligation applies to all health care professionals. An exception to the rule of confidentiality of patient communications is the implied right to make necessary information available to others involved in the patient's care. Information received by a physician in a confidential capacity relating to a patient's health should not be disclosed without the patient's consent. Disclosure may be made under compelling circumstances (e.g., suspected child abuse) to a person with a legitimate interest in the patient's health.

The Code of Medical Ethics requires that patient information remain confidential and that physicians who violate that confidentiality be reported to the appropriate regulatory body as provided for in federal and state statutes and regulations. Section 6530 (23) of the New York State Education Law, for example, defines professional misconduct as the "revealing of personally identifiable facts, data or information obtained in a professional capacity without the consent of the patient." The State of New York Department of Health has set forth a penalty of censure, reprimand, suspension of license, revocation of license, annulment of license, limitation on further license, or fine for a person found guilty of professional misconduct (Public Health Law A4 230-a), which includes revealing patient information without consent or failing to maintain accurate information. The Department of Health is responsible for maintaining the standards and ethics of the profession and for enforcing those standards. In addition, the Principles of Medical Ethics of the American Medical Association states that physicians, including physicians employed by industry, have an ethical and legal duty to protect patient confidentiality.[14]

PHYSICIAN NEGLIGENCE

This section provides an overview of common medical mistakes. The reader should keep in mind when reading this section that "ethical values and legal principles are usually closely related, but ethical obligations typically exceed legal duties . . . The fact that a physician charged with allegedly illegal conduct is acquitted or exonerated in civil or criminal proceedings does not necessarily mean that the physician acted ethically."[15]

TWO SCHOOLS OF THOUGHT

Under the *two-schools-of-thought doctrine* a physician is not be liable for medical malpractice if he or she follows a course of treatment supported by reputable, respected, and reasonable medical experts. The doctrine is applicable only in medical malpractice cases in which there is more than one method of accepted treatment for a patient's disease or injury. A physician's treatment that results in a patient's injury does not constitute negligence merely because it was unsuccessful in a particular case. A physician cannot be required to guarantee the results of treatment. The mere fact that an adverse result may occur following treatment is not in and of itself evidence of professional negligence.

Patient assessments involve the systematic collection and analysis of patient–specific data necessary to determine patient care and treatment plans. The patient's plan of care is only as good as assessments conducted by the practitioners of the various disciplines (e.g., physicians, nurses, dietitians, physical therapists).

The physician's assessment involves an evaluation of the patient's history, symptoms, and physical examination results. It must be conducted within 24 hours of a patient's admission to the hospital. The findings of the clinical examination are used to determine the patient's plan of care. The assessment is the process by which a doctor investigates the patient's state of health, looking for signs of trauma and disease. It sets the stage for accurately diagnosing the patient's medical problems. A cursory and negligent assessment can lead to a misdiagnosis of the patient's health problems and/or care needs and, consequently, to poor care.

Failure to Respond to Emergency Call

Physicians on call for a specific service in an emergency department are expected to respond to requests for emergency assistance when such is requested. Failure to respond can result in a successful lawsuit should a patient suffer injury as a result of a physician's refusal to fulfill that known duty. Such decisions are both legally and morally wrong.

Family Medical History

When reviewing a patient's family history, the physician must not be indifferent or dismissive of the patient's complaints and thoughts as to the possible cause of his or her illness. Such was the case in the following news clipping.

FIGURE   1   Family History (© Aleksandar Grozdanovski/Shutterstock, Inc.)

Bonded by Blood

A brother's history provides a clue to a woman's frightening and dangerous symptoms

Stein, who lives in Arlington, said she kept telling doctors and nurses about an odd coincidence involving her oldest brother—one she increasingly believed was relevant to her medical problems—but no one seemed to pay much attention.

"They were all sort of scratching their heads about what might be wrong, and I was getting so frustrated . . . ."

At her brother's suggestion, Stein said, she kept telling doctors about his CVID diagnosis, but no one seemed to follow up. "They'd say, 'Yeah that's interesting.'"

Sandra G. Boodman, The Washington Post, *February 25, 2014*

Patient Medical History

It is questionable in some cases as to whether a physician actually completes the process of obtaining a patient's medical history when the physician simply draws a diagonal line from the top right to the bottom left of the form and writes through the line "unremarkable" as noted in the following *reality check.*

Questionable Medical History Conducted

Smith was admitted to Community Hospital for surgery. Community Hospital medical staff bylaws require that a history and physical (H&P) exam be completed prior to patients' undergoing surgery. Smith's attending physician did not complete the H&P form. He simply drew a diagonal line from the top right to the bottom left of the H&P, indicating that the patient had no history of or current disease processes.

The patient's nurse, per hospital policy, completed a nursing assessment. The nurse documented on the patient admission assessment form that the patient had a history of transient ischemic attacks, diabetes, and hypothyroidism.

The anesthesiologist did not perform an anesthesia assessment before surgery. General anesthesia was administered without knowing the patient's previous experiences, if any, with anesthesia.

Failure of the attending physician to complete an appropriate H&P examination and the anesthesiologist's failure to perform a preanesthesia assessment placed the patient's life and health at risk. The physician did not complete the H&P. He merely went through the motions of completing a H&P examination because it was mandated that the patient have an H&P in his medical record prior to surgery.

Ethical and Legal Issues

1. Discuss the ethical issues and principles violated in this case.
2. What are the potential legal issues of concern in this case?
3. Discuss what actions the organization should consider to improve the quality of H&P documentation.

FIGURE 2 Patient Medical History (© Maksym Dykha/Shutterstock, Inc.)

Failure to obtain an adequate patient history and physical examination violates the standard of care owed to the patient. In *Foley v. Bishop Clarkson Memorial Hospital*,[16] Mr. Foley sued the hospital for the death of his wife. During her pregnancy, the patient was under the care of a private physician. She gave birth in the hospital on August 20, 1964, and died the following day. During July and August, her physician had treated her for a sore throat. Several days after her death, one of her children was treated in the hospital for a strep throat infection. There was no evidence in the hospital record that the patient had complained about a sore throat while in the hospital. The hospital rules required that an H&P had to be written promptly (within 24 hours of admission). No history had been taken, although the patient had been examined several times in regard to the progress of her labor. The trial judge directed a verdict in favor of the hospital. On appeal, the appellate court held that the case should have been submitted to the jury for determination. A jury might reasonably have inferred that if the patient's condition had been treated properly, the infection could have been combated successfully and her life saved. It also might have been reasonably inferred that if an H&P had been taken promptly when she was admitted to the hospital the throat condition would have been discovered and hospital personnel alerted to watch for possible complications of the nature that later developed. Quite possibly, this attention also would have helped in diagnosing the patient's condition, especially if it had been apparent that she had been exposed to a strep throat infection. The court held that a hospital must guard not only against known physical and mental conditions of patients, but also against conditions that reasonable care should have uncovered.

PATIENT DIAGNOSIS

Patient diagnosis refers to the process of identifying a possible disease or disease process, thus providing the physician with treatment options. Screens, assessments, reassessments, and the results of medical diagnostic testing such as electroencephalography (EEG),

FIGURE   3   Patient Diagnostic Imaging Study (© bikeriderlondon/Shutterstock, Inc.)

electrocardiography (ECG), imaging, and laboratory findings are some of the tools of medicine that assists providers (e.g., physicians, osteopaths, dentists, podiatrists, nurse practitioners, physician's assistants) in diagnosing the possible causes of a patient's symptoms and medical problems from which a treatment plan is developed. The cases presented here describe some of the lawsuits that have occurred due to misdiagnoses and failure to properly treat the patient based on the results of diagnostic testing.

As Hands-On Doctoring Fades Away, Patients Lose

"In most hospitals today, the average amount of time a busy intern spends with a patient is four minutes," said Brendan Reilly, who until recently was the executive vice chair of medicine at New York Presbyterian Hospital. No longer are tests ordered based on the results of a careful physical exam and history, Reilly said, but the "technological tests become the primary source of information on the patient. It's backwards now," and the process is driving up health-care costs posed by sometimes unnecessary, risky procedures.

Sandra G. Boodman, The Washington Post, *May 20, 2014*

Even with all the diagnostic tools available to physicians, if they order the tests and fail to review or interpret them in conjunction with a patient's physical complaints and medical history, they are of little or no value. Tests results from imaging studies and laboratory results are useless if they are merely filed away after a cursory review as to their importance in arriving at an accurate diagnosis and appropriate treatment plan.

Concern Is Growing That the Elderly Get Too Many Medical Tests

Increasingly, questions are being raised about the over testing of older patients, part of a growing skepticism about the widespread practice of routine screening for cancer and other ailments of people in their 70s, 80s, and even 90s. Critics say there is little evidence of benefit—and considerable risk—from common tests for colon, breast, and prostate cancer, particularly for those with serious problems such as heart disease or dementia that are more likely to kill them.

• • •

Telling someone that screening is no longer necessary can be dicey, as California family physician Pamela Davis discovered when she advised her robust 86-year-old mother to stop getting mammograms and routine colon tests.

Her mother was incensed.

Sandra G. Boodman, Kaiser Health News, *September 12, 2011*

Discussion

1. There are some whose age is well hidden beneath their skin. As care and treatment options become safer (e.g., robotic surgery), should age alone be the sole criterion for determining the extent of medical care one should receive?
2. Do one's rights to care and treatment diminish with age?
3. Regardless of age, who should decide whether a particular diagnostic test or treatment is warranted?

Misdiagnosis

Her Doctor Dismissed the Lump in Her Breast

Many express anger at the practice where I had my breast exams. A few people even suggested that I look into legal action.

I choose not to walk down that political path, though. Sure, sometimes I allow the thought to creep into my head. What if it had been caught earlier? Would it still be in my lymph nodes? Would my prognosis be better? As soon as they pop up, I try to kick these thoughts to the curb. I will never know the answers, and blaming someone won't change my current reality. I choose to focus my energy on a path toward healing, not fault.

Kathryn Petrides, The Washington Post, *May 14, 2014*

Misdiagnosis is the most frequently cited injury event in malpractice suits against physicians. Although diagnosis is a medical art and not an exact science, early detection can be critical to a patient's recovery. Misdiagnosis may involve the diagnosis and treatment of a disease different from that which the patient actually suffers or the diagnosis and treatment of a disease that the patient does not have. Misdiagnosis in and of itself will not necessarily impose liability on a physician, unless deviation from the accepted standard of care and injury can be established.

My Physician Would Not Listen

I was left undiagnosed for over a year and a half. I had to endure extended chemotherapy for a stage III cancer because my GP would not listen to my concerns at first and then again 1.5 years later when the cancer had spread throughout my body to my lungs causing a nasty cough. I should've taken him to the GMC [Britain's General Medical Council] at the time but was more interested in getting better first! I made a diary all about it, just google my name; it's easy to find. I'm very grateful to be alive but it has left me broke, nothing or no one can fix that.

Tim Stollery

Fractured Skull, Not Intoxication

In *Ramberg v. Morgan*,[17] a police department physician at the scene of an accident examined an unconscious man who had been struck by an automobile. The physician concluded that the patient's insensibility was a result of alcohol intoxication, not the accident, and ordered the police to remove him to jail instead of the hospital. The man, to the physician's knowledge, remained semiconscious for several days and finally was taken from the cell to the hospital at the insistence of his family. The patient subsequently died, and the autopsy revealed massive skull fractures. The court found that any physician should reasonably anticipate the presence of head injuries when a car strikes a person. Failure to refer an accident victim to another physician or a hospital was actionable neglect of the physician's duty.

Although the presence of a physician does not ensure the correctness of the diagnosis or treatment, a patient is entitled to such thorough and careful examination as his or her condition and attending circumstances permit, with such diligence and methods of diagnosis as usually are approved and practiced by medical people of ordinary or average learning, judgment, and skill in the community or similar localities.

PATIENT TREATMENT

This section focuses on negligence cases that relate to medical treatment and various legal and ethical issues that health care professionals encounter when treating patients. *Patient treatment* is the attempt to restore the patient to health following a diagnosis. It is the application of various remedies and medical techniques, including the use of medications for the purpose of treating an illness or trauma. Treatment can be *active*, directed immediately to the cure of the disease or injury; *causal*, directed against the cause of a disease; *conservative*, designed to avoid radical medical therapeutic measures or operative procedures; *expectant*, directed toward relief of untoward symptoms but leaving cure of the disease to natural forces; *palliative*, designed to relieve pain and distress with no attempt to cure; *preventive/prophylactic*,

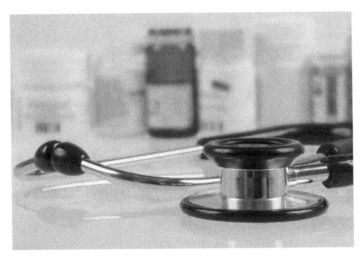

FIGURE   4   Patient Medications (© piotr_pabijan/Shutterstock, Inc.)

aimed at the prevention of disease and illness; *specific*, targeted specifically at the disease being treated; *supportive*, directed mainly to sustaining the strength of the patient; or *symptomatic*, meant to relieve symptoms without effecting a cure (i.e., intended to address the symptoms of an illness but not its underlying cause, as in scleroderma, lupus, or multiple sclerosis, for example).[18]

Medical practice guidelines are evidence-based best practices that are developed to assist physicians in the diagnosis and treatment of their patients. It should be remembered that best practices are not iron-clad rules. Skillful medical judgment demands that the physician determine how to use best practices and interpret the information.

Online Medical Treatment Advisor is a treatment program that uses medical specialists to accurately select the best and newest treatment for each patient, based on the individual patient's characteristics. Online Medical Treatment Advisor assesses each patient's symptoms with a knowledge base created by 1,500 specialist physicians. Online Medical Treatment Advisor includes treatments for 1,200 diseases.[19]

Autonomy and Informed Consent

Patients have a right to make their own treatment choices. When there are two or more medically acceptable treatment alternatives, a competent patient has the right to choose which option he or she wants after being informed of the risks, benefits, and alternatives of each option. The physician has a legal, ethical, and moral duty to respect a patient's *autonomy* and to provide only authorized medical treatment. It is inappropriate for physicians to pursue a treatment alternative other than the one to which their patient has given consent. Unless the patient consents to the physician's recommended treatment approach, the physician may not proceed with that approach even if the physician personally believes the recommended approach to be in the patient's best interests.[20]

The doctrine of *informed consent* is a theory of professional liability independent from malpractice. A physician's duty is to disclose known and existing dangers associated with a proposed course of treatment. The patient in *Leggett v. Kumar*[21] was awarded $675,000 for pain and disfigurement resulting from a mastectomy procedure. The physician in this case failed to advise the patient of treatment alternatives. He also failed to perform the surgery properly.

It is the physician's role to provide the necessary medical facts and the patient's role to make a subjective decision concerning treatment based on his or her understanding of those facts. Before subjecting a patient to a course of treatment, the physician has a duty to disclose information that will enable the patient to evaluate options and the risks attendant to a specific procedure. A failure to disclose any known and existing risks of a proposed treatment when such risks might affect a patient's decision to forgo treatment constitutes a prima facie violation of a physician's duty to disclose. If a patient can establish that a physician withheld information concerning the inherent and potential hazards of a proposed treatment, consent is abrogated. Consent for a medical procedure may be withdrawn at any time before the act consented to is accomplished.

With thousands of brand-name and generic drugs in use, it is no surprise that drug errors are one of the leading causes of patient injuries. Physicians should encourage the limited and judicious use of all medications and should document periodically the reason for their continuation. They should be alert to any contraindications and incompatibilities among prescription and over-the-counter drugs, and herbal supplements. Medication errors are often due to: administration of the wrong medication to the wrong patient; of the wrong dosage; at the wrong site; by the wrong route; or a combination of the aforementioned errors.

Medications

The Board of Regents in *Moyo v. Ambach*[22] determined that a physician had prescribed methaqualone fraudulently and with gross negligence to 20 patients. The Board of Regents found that the physician did not prescribe methaqualone in good faith or for sound medical reasons. His abuse in prescribing controlled substances constituted the fraudulent practice of medicine. Expert testimony established that it was common knowledge in the medical community that methaqualone was a widely abused and addictive drug. Methaqualone should not have been used for insomnia without first trying other means of treatment. On appeal, the court found that there was sufficient evidence to support the board's finding.

Damages were awarded in *Argus v. Scheppegrell*[23] for the wrongful death of a teenage patient with a preexisting drug addiction. It was determined that the physician had wrongfully supplied the patient with prescriptions for controlled substances in excessive amounts, with the result that the patient's preexisting drug addiction had worsened, causing her death from a drug overdose. The Louisiana Court of Appeal held that the suffering of the patient caused by drug addiction and deterioration of her mental and physical condition warranted an award of $175,000. Damages of $120,000 were to be awarded for the wrongful death claims of the parents, who not only suffered during their daughter's drug addiction caused by the physician's wrongfully supplying the prescription, but who also were forced to endure the torment of their daughter's slow death in the hospital.

Surgery

As noted in the following news clipping, surgical instruments inadvertently left in patients are reported by hospitals accredited by the Joint Commission. The various states also require the reporting of surgical errors, such as wrong patient, wrong surgery, and wrong site.

Joint Commission Alert: Preventing Retained Surgical Items

The Joint Commission today issued a Sentinel Event Alert urging hospitals and ambulatory surgery centers to take a new look at how to avoid mistakenly leaving items such as sponges, towels and instruments in a patient's body after surgery.

Known in medical terminology as the unintended retention of foreign objects (URFOs) or retained surgical items (RSIs), this is a serious patient safety issue that can cause death or harm patients physically and emotionally. The Joint Commission has received more than 770 voluntary reports of URFOs in the past seven years.

Elizabeth Eaken Zhani, The Joint Commission, *October 17, 2013*[24]

Wrong-site surgical mistakes have multiple causes, including draping the wrong surgical site, marking the wrong surgical site, and failing to mark the surgical site as required by hospital policy.

The Pain of Wrong-Site Surgery

Hospitals find it hard to protect patients from wrong-site surgery

"It's disheartening that we haven't moved the needle on this," said Peter Pronovost, a prominent safety expert and medical director of the John Hopkins Center for Innovation in Quality Patient Care. "I think we made national policy with a relatively superficial understanding of the problem." Pronovost suggests that doctors' lip service to the rules, which he calls "ritualized compliance," may be a key factor. Studies of wrong-site errors have consistently revealed a failure by physicians to participate in a timeout.

Sandra G. Boodman, Kaiser Health News, *June 20, 2011*[25]

Pregnant Woman Dies After Horrifying Medical Mixup

(Newser)—As far as medical mix-ups go, it's a horrifying one. In October 2011, a 32-year-old woman underwent an operation at Queen's Hospital outside of London; Maria De Jesus was suffering from appendicitis and needed to have her appendix removed. Instead, her right ovary was taken out, and De Jesus, who was 21 weeks pregnant with her fourth child at the time, ended up dying roughly three weeks later. The case is now in front of a medical tribunal, which is weighing the medical fates of the two doctors involved . . . .

Newser, Yahoo Shine, *April 17, 2014*[26]

Aggravation of Patient's Condition

Aggravation of a preexisting condition through negligence can result in a physician being liable for malpractice. If the original injury is aggravated by treatment or the failure to treat, liability can be imposed for injuries suffered as a result of the aggravation of the patient's condition.

Patient Infections

Physicians are increasingly at risk for lawsuits related to hospital-acquired infections (HAIs). According to the CDC over 700,000 HAIs occur each year in acute care hospital settings.[27] The serious nature of surgical site infections are all too common occurrences requiring intensive and costly care, as is illustrated in **Figure** 5. Both physicians and hospitals are at a greater risk of lawsuits when there are failures to implement and enforce recognized infection control practices, policies, and procedures.

The District Court of Appeals of Florida held in *Gill v. Hartford Accident & Indemnity Co.*[28] that the physician who performed surgery on a patient in the same room as the plaintiff should have known that the infection the patient had was highly contagious. The failure of the physician to undertake steps to prevent the spread of the infection to the plaintiff and his failure to warn the plaintiff led the court to find that hospital authorities and the plaintiff's physician caused an unreasonable increase in the risk of injury. As a result, the plaintiff suffered injuries causally related to the negligence of the defendant. The court held that the plaintiff's complaint does state a cause of action and alleges a duty and a breach of that duty.

FIGURE   5   Patient Room (© Monkey Business Images/Shutterstock, Inc.)

Pain

I have been with Angie, my wife, on many of her appointments. One such appointment I vividly remember was at the university hospital pain center, described by some as one of the top medical centers in the country. Here, after several residents poked her, they left the room. They later returned with their supervising attending physician. He stood over my Angie as she lay on the examination table. Looking down at her, he said, "We treat bone pain here." Angie replied, "You advertise yourself as a pain-management center. I don't understand." The attending physician replied, "Anything we do for you would be very risky and most likely will not work." Angie described a new implantable device being used at Duke University Medical Center. The attending responded, "We never heard of that; however, we can suggest other procedures, but they do have associated risks." The attending then proceeded to describe the procedures to Angie. Both Angie and I thought, "This is a major teaching hospital? Why won't the physicians suggest looking into Duke's procedure as to the potential risks and benefits for Angie?" The attending suggested, "Why don't you think about the procedures we have discussed. Just schedule a new appointment before you leave."

Spouse

Discussion

1. Should the physicians have conducted research to determine if the Duke device might be helpful to Angie? Explain your answer.
2. What would you do, if you were Angie?

PHYSICIAN–PATIENT RELATIONSHIP

The physician–patient relationship entails special obligations for the physician to provide care to his or her patient. The physician's primary commitment must always be the patient's welfare and best interests, whether the physician is preventing or treating illness or helping the patient to cope with illness, disability, and death. It has long been recognized that the health and welfare of the patient depends on a collaborative effort between the physician and the patient. The physician must support the dignity of all patients and respect their uniqueness. The following guidelines serve to improve physician–patient relationships and help decrease the likelihood of malpractice suits:

- *Provide personalized treatment.* A patient is more inclined to sue an impersonal physician than one with whom he or she has developed a good relationship.
- *Conduct a thorough assessment*/history and physical examination that includes a review of all body systems.

- *Do not be dismissive* as to the patient's thoughts as to the cause of his or her ailments.
- *Develop a problems list* and comprehensive treatment plan that addresses the patient's problems.
- *Provide sufficient time* and care to each patient. Take the time to explain treatment plans and follow-up care to the patient, his or her family, and other professionals who are caring for your patient.
- *Request consultations* when indicated and refer if necessary.
- *Closely monitor* the patient's progress and, as necessary, make adjustments to the treatment plan as the patient's condition warrants.
- *Maintain timely*, legible, complete, and accurate records. Do not make erasures.
- *Do not guarantee* treatment outcome.
- *Provide for cross-coverage* during days off.
- *Do not overextend* your practice.
- *Avoid prescribing* over the telephone.
- *Do not become careless* because you know the patient. Seek the advice of counsel should you suspect the possibility of a malpractice claim.

CHAPTER REVIEW

1. The medical profession has long subscribed to a body of ethical statements developed primarily for the benefit of the patient.
   - *Hippocratic Oath* dates back to 400 BC.
   - Modified version of the *Hippocratic Oath* has been used by such medical schools as Johns Hopkins, Baylor College of Medicine, Tufts University School of Medicine.
   - American Medical Association code of ethical conduct for physicians.
2. Law and ethics interweave in patient care.
   - Hippocratic Oath and AMA Code of Ethics were violated when the physicians in *Scripps Clinic v. Superior Ct.* terminated a patient's care before ensuring the patient had continuing medical care.
   - Compassion, trust, justice, and respect for patient privacy are all ethical principles and values that are intertwined with law.
3. Physician negligence often involves one or more of the following:
   - Patient assessments
   - Medical diagnosis
   - Treatment

TEST YOUR UNDERSTANDING

TERMINOLOGY

autonomy	medical treatment	patient diagnosis
Hippocratic oath	misdiagnosis	patient treatment
informed consent	nonmaleficence	two-schools-of-thought
medical diagnosis	patient assessment	doctrine

REVIEW QUESTIONS

1. Describe how the *Hippocratic Oath* and modern codes of medical ethics apply to the practice of medicine.

2. Explain how the law and ethics intertwine in patient care.

3. Describe common medical errors relative to physician practice involving assessment, diagnosis, and treatment.

4. Discuss common guidelines that would be helpful in improving the physician–patient relationships.

NOTES

1. Hippocrates, written 400 BC, Translated by Francis Adams.
2. http://guides.library.jhu.edu/content.php?pid=23699&sid=190964.
3. http://www.ama-assn.org/ama/pub/physician-resources/medical-ethics/code-medical-ethics/principles-medical-ethics.page.
4. *Scripps Clinic v. Superior Ct.,* 134 Cal. Rptr. 2d 101 (2003).
5. *Id.*
6. *Bloomington Urological Associates v. Scaglia,* 686 N.E.2d 389 (1997).
7. American Medical Association Code of Medical Ethics: Current Opinions with Annotations, 8.11 (1996).
8. Jennifer Steinhauer, "Fatal Surgery Leads to Fine for Hospital," *The New York Times,* November 6, 1998. http://www.nytimes.com/1998/11/06/nyregion/fatal-surgery-leads-to-fine-for-hospital.html.
9. Sophie Borland and David Wilkes, "1 in 4 cancer cases missed: GPs send away alarming number of patients, delaying vital treatment," *MailOnline,* March 1, 2001; http://www.dailymail.co.uk/health/article-1361269/1-4-cancer-cases-missed-GPs-delaying-vital-treatment.html.
10. *Valentine v. Kaiser Found. Hosps.,* 15 Cal. Rptr. 26 (Cal. Ct. App. 1961) (dictum).
11. 683 N.E.2d 1175 (Ohio App. 1996).
12. 442 A.2d 635 (N.J. Super. Ct. 1982).
13. *Id.* at 644–45.
14. *Horn v. New York Times,* 100 N.Y.2d 85 (2003).
15. AMA, "Opinion 1.02 - The Relation of Law and Ethics," http://www.ama-assn.org/ama/pub/physician-resources/medical-ethics/code-medical-ethics/opinion102.page?
16. 173 N.W.2d 881 (Neb. 1970).
17. 218 N.W.2d 492 (Iowa 1928).
18. http://www.medical-dictionary.thefreedictionary.com/treatment.
19. http://www.ccspublishing.com/online_medical_treatment.htm.
20. See *Bankert v. United States,* 937 F. Supp. 1169, 1173 (D. Md. 1996).
21. 570 N.E.2d 1249 (Ill. App. Ct. 1991).
22. 23 N.Y.S.2d 645 (N.Y. App. Div. 1988).
23. 489 So. 2d 392 (La. Ct. App. 1986).
24. http://www.jointcommission.org/joint_commission_alert_preventing_retained_surgical_items/
25. Sandra G. Boodman, "Effort to end surgeries on wrong patient or body part falters," Kaiser Health News, June 20, 2011; http://www.kaiserhealthnews.org/Stories/2011/June/21/wrongsite-surgery-errors.aspx
26. https://shine.yahoo.com/parenting/pregnant-woman-dies-horrifying-medical-mixup-200700512.html.
27. Magill SS et al. Multistate Point-Prevalence Survey of Health Care-Associated Infections. *N Engl J Med* 2014;370:1198–1208.
28. 337 So. 2d 420 (Fla. Dist. Ct. App. 1976).

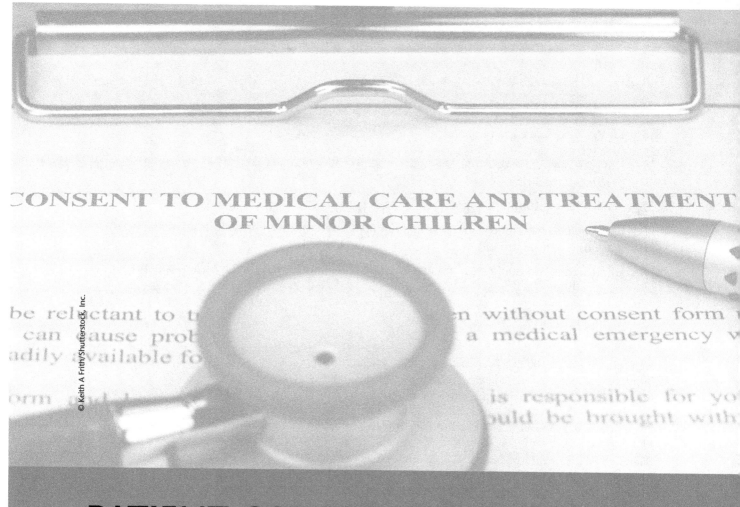

PATIENT CONSENT

LEARNING OBJECTIVES

Upon completion of this chapter, the reader will be able to:

- Discuss informed consent and how it applies the patient's right to self-determination.
- Describe how various codes of professional ethics address a patient's right to informed consent and self-determination.
- Explain and give examples of verbal, written, and implied consent.
- Describe under what circumstances statutory consent can be inferred.
- Describe how caregivers can determine a patient's capacity to consent and what action should be taken if the patient is unable to consent to recommended care choices.
- Describe what factors the courts could take into consideration when determining the adequacy of consent.
- Explain why a patient has a right to refuse treatment.
- Understand the importance of state interests when a parent refuses life saving treatment for a child.

INTRODUCTION

. . . no right is held more sacred, or is more carefully guarded, by the common law, than the right of every individual to the possession and control of his own person.

—Union Pacific Ry. Co. v. Botsford[1]

Consent is the voluntary agreement by a person who possesses sufficient mental capacity to make an intelligent choice to allow something proposed by another to be performed on himself or herself. Consent changes touching that otherwise would be nonconsensual to touching that is consensual. Consent can be either express or implied.

Express consent can take the form of either a verbal agreement or can be accomplished through the execution of a written document authorizing medical care. *Implied consent* is determined by some act of silence, which raises a presumption that consent has been authorized.

Consent must be obtained from the patient or from a person authorized to consent on the patient's behalf before any medical procedure can be performed. Every individual has a right to refuse to authorize a touching. This chapter reviews many of the issues surrounding consent in the health care setting.

INFORMED CONSENT

Informed consent is a legal concept that provides that a patient has a right to know the potential risks, benefits, and alternatives of a proposed procedure. The right to be free of unwanted medical treatment has long been recognized in this country. An "individual's right to make decisions vitally affecting his private life according to his own conscience . . . is difficult to overstate . . . because it is, without exaggeration, the very bedrock on which this country was founded."[2]

The right to control the integrity of one's own body spawned the doctrine of informed consent.[3] The United States Supreme Court has held that a competent adult patient has the right to decline any and all forms of medical intervention, including lifesaving or life-prolonging treatment.[4]

Informed consent is predicated on the duty of the physician to disclose to the patient sufficient information to enable the patient to evaluate a proposed medical or surgical procedure before submitting to it. Informed consent requires that a patient have a full understanding of that to which he or she has consented. An authorization from a patient who does not understand to what he or she is consenting is not effective consent.

Unreported Robot Surgery Injuries Open New Questions for FDA

When Sheena Wilson, 45, underwent robotic surgery for a hysterectomy in May, she didn't know the Intuitive Surgical Inc. system used by her doctor was previously tied to a variety of injuries for the same procedure.

Her rectum was badly burned in the operation, said Wilson, a mother of two from Parlin, New Jersey. Now she is on long-term disability, fearful of losing her job and facing a third corrective surgery, she said in a telephone interview.

"If I had known there were other people who had injuries, I would never have done this surgery," said Wilson, who has filed suit against Intuitive and her doctor. "Whatever they have in place is not working."

Robert Langreth, Bloomberg, *December 30, 2013*[5]

Hospitals generally do not have an independent duty to obtain informed consent or to warn patients of the risks of a procedure to be performed by a physician who is not an agent of the hospital. It is the treating physician who has the education, expertise, skill, and training necessary to treat a patient and determine what information a patient should have in order to give informed consent.

CODES OF ETHICS

The first American Medical Association Code of Medical Ethics was written in 1847. Section I of the 1998–1999 edition, titled "Fundamental Elements of the Patient–Physician Relationship," provides "the patient has the right to receive information from physicians and to discuss the benefits, risks, and costs of appropriate treatment alternatives." Because the American Medical Association is an organization composed of experts in the field of medicine, its code of ethics and the duties of physicians prescribed therein should be understood to reflect the standard of care of the profession on the issue of informed consent. Social policy does not accept the "paternalistic" view that the physician may remain silent because divulgence might prompt the patient to forgo needed therapy.

The American Dental Association Code of Ethics also reflects the standard of care for the dental profession. Part III, Section 1, of the American Dental Association Code of Ethics, titled "Principle: Patient Autonomy," provides "the dentist has a duty to respect the patient's rights to self-determination and confidentiality," and Section 1A provides that "the dentist should inform the patient of the proposed treatment, and any reasonable alternatives, in a manner that allows the patient to become involved in treatment decisions." These American Medical Association and American Dental Association ethical standards embrace the doctrine of informed consent.

The American Nurses Association code of ethics for nurses provides in part in Provision 1.4 the following as to a patient's right to self-determination:

> . . . Patients have the moral and legal right to determine what will be done with their own person; to be giving accurate, complete, and understandable information in a manner that facilitates that facilitates an informed judgment; to be assisted with weighing the benefits, burdens, and available options in their treatment, including the choice of no treatment; to accept, refuse, or terminate treatment without deceit, undue influence, duress, coercion, or penalty; and to be given necessary support throughout the decision-making and treatment process.[6]

Consent can be verbal, written, or implied. The law requires verbal or written consent for the intentional touching that involves medical or surgical procedures. Consent can also be implied in emergency situations.

Oral consent is as binding as written consent. There is no legal requirement that a patient's consent be in writing; however, oral consent is more difficult to corroborate.

Written consent provides visible proof of a patient's wishes. Because the function of a written consent form is to preserve evidence of informed consent, the nature of the treatment, the risks, benefits, and consequences involved should be incorporated into the consent form. States have taken the view that consent, to be effective, must be "informed consent." An informed consent form should include the following elements:

- The nature of the patient's illness or injury
- The name of the proposed procedure or treatment
- The purpose of the proposed treatment
- The risks and probable consequences of the proposed treatment
- The probability that the proposed treatment will be successful
- Any alternative methods of treatment along with their associated risks and benefits
- The risks and prognosis if no treatment is rendered
- An indication that the patient understands the nature of any proposed treatment, the alternatives, the risks involved, and the probable consequences of the proposed treatment
- The signatures of the patient, physician, and witnesses
- The date the consent is signed

Health care professionals have an important role in the realm of informed consent. They can be instrumental in averting major lawsuits by being observant as to a patient's doubts, changes of mind or confusion, or misunderstandings expressed by a patient regarding any proposed procedures he or she is about to undergo.

Implied consent can be assumed when immediate treatment is required to preserve the life of a patient or to prevent an impairment of the patient's health and it is impossible to obtain the consent of the patient or representative legally authorized to consent for him or her, an emergency exists, and consent is implied. This privilege to proceed in emergencies without consent is accorded to physicians because inaction at this time may cause greater injury to the patient and would be contrary to good medical practice; however, if possible, consultation should be undertaken before a procedure is commenced, and every effort must be made to document the medical need for proceeding with treatment without consent. The patient's record should clearly indicate the nature of the threat to life or health, its immediacy, and its magnitude.

Unconscious patients are presumed under law to approve treatment that appears to be necessary. It is assumed that such patients would have consented if they were conscious and competent; however, if a patient expressly refuses to consent to certain treatment, such treatment may not be instituted after the patient becomes unconscious. Similarly, conscious patients suffering from emergency conditions retain the right to refuse consent. If a procedure is necessary to protect one's life or health, every effort must be made to document the medical necessity for proceeding with medical treatment without consent. It must be shown that the emergency situation constituted an immediate threat to life or health.

In *Luka v. Lowrie,*[7] involving a 15-year-old boy whose left foot had been run over and crushed by a train, consultation by the treating physician with other physicians was an important factor in determining the outcome of the case. On the boy's arrival at the hospital, the defending physician and four house surgeons decided that it was necessary to amputate the foot. The court said that it was inconceivable that had they been present, the parents would have refused consent in the face of a determination by five physicians that amputation would save the boy's life. Thus, despite testimony at the trial that the amputation may not have been necessary, professional consultation before the operation supported the assertion that a genuine emergency existed and could have implied consent.

Consent also can be implied in nonemergency situations. For example, a patient may voluntarily submit to a procedure, implying consent, without any explicitly spoken or written expression of consent. In the Massachusetts case of *O'Brien v. Cunard Steam Ship Co.,*[8] a ship's passenger who joined a line of people receiving injections was held to have implied his consent to a vaccination. The rationale for this decision is that individuals who observe a line of people and who notice that injections are being administered to those at the head of the line should expect that if they join and remain in the line they will receive an injection. The plaintiff entered the line voluntarily. The plaintiff had opportunity to see what was taking place at the head of the line and could have exited the line but chose not to do so. The jury appropriately determined this to be consent to the injection. The *O'Brien* case contains all of the elements necessary to imply consent to a voluntary act: The procedure was a simple vaccination. The proceedings were visible at all times, and the plaintiff was free to withdraw up to the instant of the injection.

Whether a patient's consent can be implied is frequently asked when the condition of a patient requires some deviation from an agreed-on procedure. If a patient expressly prohibits a specific medical or surgical procedure, consent to the procedure cannot be implied. The same consent rule applies if a patient expressly prohibits a particular extension of a procedure even though the patient voluntarily submitted to the original procedure.

STATUTORY CONSENT

The age of consent is the minimum age at which a person is considered to be legally competent to consent to medical care. Many states have adopted legislation concerning emergency care. An emergency in most states eliminates the need for consent. When a patient is clinically unable to give consent to a lifesaving emergency treatment, the law implies consent on the presumption that a reasonable person would consent to lifesaving medical intervention; this is defined as *statutory consent*. When an emergency situation does arise, there may be little opportunity to contact the attending physician, much less a consultant. The patient's records, therefore, must be complete with respect to the description of the patient's illness and condition, the attempts made to contact the physician as well as relatives, and the emergency measures taken and procedures performed. If time does not permit a court order to be obtained, a second medical opinion, when practicable, is advisable.

Any glimmer of uncertainty as to a patient's desires in an emergency situation should be resolved "in favor of preserving life." The patient in *Matter of Hughes*[9] signed a standard blank hospital form titled "Refusal to Permit Blood Transfusion." There was no indication on the form that the consequences of her refusal had been explained to her in the context of the elective surgical procedure she was about to undergo. The form should have contained an unequivocal statement that under any and all circumstances blood is not to be used and an acknowledgment that the consequences of the refusal were fully explained. The form should fully release the physician, all medical personnel, and the hospital from liability should complications arise from the failure to administer blood, thereby resolving any doubt as to the physician's responsibility to his patient. If Hughes had refused to sign such a form, her physician could then have decided whether to continue with Hughes's treatment or to aid her in finding a physician who would carry out her wishes.

The court emphasized that this case arose in the context of elective surgery. This was not an emergency situation where the physician and patient did not have time to discuss fully the potential risks, benefits, and alternatives of the planned surgery and the conflict arising over the patient's religious beliefs. Patients have an obligation to make medical preferences known to the treating physician, including the course to follow if life-threatening complications should arise. This protects the patient's right to freedom of religion and self-determination. In addition, it is helpful to the hospital when faced with the dilemma of trying to preserve life whenever possible and honoring the patient's wishes to forgo life-sustaining treatment.

Ethical and Legal Issues

1. Describe the relevant ethical principles violated in this case.
2. Describe the relevant legal issues in this case. What actions could the parties to this lawsuit have taken beforehand to prevent this case from becoming a legal issue?

CAPACITY TO CONSENT

A patient is considered competent to make medical decisions regarding his or her care unless a court determines otherwise. Generally speaking, medical personnel make the determination of a patient's decision-making capacity. The clinical assessment of decision-making capacity should include the patient's ability to understand the risks, benefits, and alternatives of a proposed test or procedure; evaluate the information provided by the physician; express his or her treatment options/plan; and voluntarily make decisions regarding his or her treatment plan without undue influence by family, friends, or medical personnel.

If a patient is unable to make decisions by reason of age or incapacity, a patient appointed decision maker may "substitute his or her judgment" on behalf of the patient. Before declaring an individual incapacitated, the attending physician must find with a reasonable degree of medical certainty that the patient lacks capacity. A notation should be placed in the patient's medical record describing the cause, nature, extent, and probable duration of incapacity.

Before withholding or withdrawing life-sustaining treatment, a second physician must confirm the incapacity determination and make an appropriate entry on the medical record before honoring any new decisions by a health care agent.

CASE: LACK OF CONSENT AND PATIENT DEATH

Four siblings, in *Riser v. American Medical Int'l, Inc.,*[10] brought a medical malpractice action against Dr. Lang, a physician who performed a femoral arteriogram on their 69-year-old mother, who died due to the procedure.

Riser had been admitted to Hospital A experiencing impaired circulation in her lower arms and hands. She had multiple medical diagnoses, including diabetes mellitus, end-stage renal failure, and arteriosclerosis. Her physician, Dr. Sottiurai, ordered bilateral arteriograms to determine the cause of the patient's impaired circulation. Hospital A could not accommodate Sottiurai's request, and Riser was transferred to Dr. Lang, a radiologist at Hospital B. Lang performed a femoral arteriogram rather than the bilateral brachial arteriogram ordered by Sottiurai. The procedure seemed to go well, and the patient was prepared for transfer back to the hospital; however, shortly after the ambulance departed the hospital, the patient suffered a seizure in the ambulance and was returned to Hospital B. Riser's condition deteriorated, and she died 11 days later. The plaintiffs claimed in their lawsuit that Riser was a poor risk for the procedure. The district court ruled for the plaintiffs, awarding damages in the amount of $50,000 for Riser's pain and suffering and $100,000 to each of Riser's children. Lang appealed.

The Louisiana Court of Appeal held that Lang failed to obtain consent from the patient. Riser was under the impression that she was about to undergo a brachial arteriogram, not a femoral arteriogram. Two consent forms were signed; neither form authorized the performance of a femoral arteriogram. O'Neil, one of Riser's daughters, claimed that her mother said, following the arteriogram, "Why did you let them do that to me?"[11]

Ethical and Legal Issues

1. Describe how the physician violated his professional duty to the patient.
2. Should the hospital have intervened and prevented the femoral arteriogram? Explain your answer.

ADEQUACY OF CONSENT

A physician should provide as much information about treatment options as is necessary based on a patient's personal understanding of the physician's explanation of the risks of treatment and the probable consequences of the treatment. The needs of each patient can vary depending on age, maturity, and mental status.

Some courts have recognized that the condition of the patient may be taken into account to determine whether the patient has received sufficient information to give consent. The individual responsible for obtaining consent must weigh the importance of giving full disclosure to the patient against the likelihood that such disclosure will seriously and adversely affect the condition of the patient.

When questions do arise as to whether adequate consent has been given, some courts take into consideration the information that is ordinarily provided by other physicians. A physician must reveal to his or her patient information just as a skilled practitioner of good standing would provide under similar circumstances. A physician must disclose to the patient the potential of death, serious harm, and other complications associated with a proposed procedure.

Failure to Inform—Alternative Procedures

The operation you get often depends on where you live. One patient underwent a mastectomy only to learn that a less destructive alternative procedure was available in a region near her home. The procedure, a lumpectomy, has the same survival rate as a mastectomy. The patient claims that the surgeon never informed her about the alternative.

Discussion

1. Describe the ethical and legal issues involved in failing to discuss alternative treatments with a patient.
2. Should a physician describe every possible alternative treatment procedure with his or her patient? Explain your answer.

COMPETENT PATIENT

A competent adult patient's wishes concerning his or her person may not be disregarded. The court in *In re Melideo*[12] held that every human being of adult years has a right to determine what shall be done with his or her own body and cannot be subjected to medical treatment without his or her consent. When there is no compelling state interest that justifies overriding an adult patient's decision, that decision should be respected. State interests include preserving life, preventing suicide, safeguarding the integrity of the medical profession, and protecting innocent third parties.

SPOUSE

The patient in *Greynolds v. Kurman*[13] suffered a transient ischemic attack, a sudden loss of neurological function caused by vascular impairment to the brain. He was taken to an emergency department. Because of the patient's prior medical history, which included transient ischemic attacks, he was at high risk for a stroke. After receiving the results of noninvasive tests, Dr. Rafecas, a consulting physician, ordered a cerebral angiogram. Dr. Kurman performed the angiogram, and the patient suffered a stroke during the procedure that left him severely disabled.

The patient and his wife filed a medical malpractice action against Rafecas and Kurman, asserting that Rafecas had negligently recommended the procedure and that Kurman had performed the procedure without obtaining informed consent. The court of appeals held that the evidence was sufficient to support a judgment in favor of the patient and his wife.

The jury needed to determine that the risks involved in the cerebral angiogram were not disclosed, that the risks involved in the procedure materialized and caused the stroke, and that a reasonable person in the position of the patient would have decided against having the angiogram had the risks associated with the procedure been disclosed. The jury concluded that the patient did not consent to the angiogram because he "was not . . . capable of comprehending the consent form" and further noted that Kurman should have sought consent from the next of kin, specifically the spouse. Given the evidence of the patient's condition when he signed the consent forms, his past medical history, and his increased risk of suffering complications during an angiogram, the court found that evidence supported a finding of lack of informed consent.

PARENTAL CONSENT

Parents generally have the right to authorize medical care for minor children, generally under the age of 18. Consent laws for minors often vary from state to sate and should be referenced as necessary. Children who are emancipated have a right to make their own medical care decisions. Although parents may have a right to refuse medical care in certain instances, such refusal is reportable by the caregiver to the state if such refusal can result in harm to the child.

CASE: PARENTS REFUSE TREATMENT

When parents in *In re Guardianship of L.S.*[14] refused to consent to medically necessary care for their minor child based on their religious convictions, the trial court appointed the hospital as a temporary guardian to make decisions to provide medically necessary, lifesaving treatment for the child. The evidence presented to the trial court in the form of an affidavit from a hospital physician stated that the parents were refusing medically necessary blood transfusions, that the child would require blood transfusions to survive, and that the child was unable to respond to this risk. The trial court reasonably concluded from this information that the child was at risk of substantial and immediate physical harm. The trial court's decision to appoint a temporary guardian was based on the child's best interest and protected the state's interest in the welfare of children within the state.

In the midst of an emergency, the district court was confronted with the task of balancing the competing interests of the child, the parents, the hospital, and the state. Throughout the proceedings, the district court took numerous steps to protect the interests of the child and the parents, including requiring notice and a hearing within 24 hours after the original order, allowing the parents time to obtain counsel before reaching a final determination.

"Substantive due process guarantees that no person shall be deprived of life, liberty, or property for arbitrary reasons." The due process clause of the Fourteenth Amendment protects those liberty interests that are deemed fundamental and are "deeply rooted in this Nation's history and tradition." Certain family privacy rights, including the parent–child relationship, have therefore been recognized as fundamental rights. The Nevada Supreme Court adopted a "reasonableness test" to address family privacy cases involving "competing interests within the family."

Although a parent has a fundamental liberty interest in the "care, custody, and management" of his or her child, that interest is not absolute. "The state also has an interest in the welfare of children and may limit parental authority," even permanently depriving parents of their children; therefore, although the parents have a parental interest in the care of their son, both the state and L.S. have an interest in preserving the child's life. As L.S. is unable to make decisions for himself, the state's interest is heightened. The parents' liberty interest in practicing their religion must also give way to the child's welfare. Hence, the district court found that the parents' refusal to consent to treatment put L.S.'s life at substantial risk. Additionally, the state has an interest in protecting "the ethical integrity of the medical profession" and in allowing hospitals the full opportunity to care for patients under their control, especially when medical science is available to save that patient's life.

Here, the child's interest in self-preservation and the state's interests in protecting the welfare of children and the integrity of medical care outweigh the parents' interests in the care, custody, and management of their children, as well as their religious freedom. The combined weight of the interests of the child and the state are great and therefore mandate interference with parental rights.

The Supreme Court of Nevada affirmed the order of the district court appointing Valley Hospital as temporary guardian.

CONSENT BY MINORS

Parental consent is not required when a minor is married or otherwise emancipated. Most states have enacted statutes making it valid for married and emancipated minors to provide effective consent. Several courts have held the consent of a minor to be sufficient authorization for treatment in certain situations. In any specific case, a court's determination that the consent of a minor is effective and that parental consent is unnecessary will depend on such factors as the minor's age, maturity, mental status, and emancipation and the procedure involved, as well as public policy considerations.

The courts have held, as a general proposition, that the consent of a minor to medical or surgical treatment is ineffective and that the physician must secure the consent of the minor's parent or someone standing in loco parentis; otherwise, he or she will risk liability. Although parental consent should be obtained before treating a minor, treatment should not be delayed to the detriment of the child. The various states have laws allowing children to be treated without consent in order to protect the minor (e.g., provision of emergency care, protect the minor from child abuse, abortion, treat venereal diseases) and safeguard the public health of the community (e.g., communicable and venereal diseases).

INCOMPETENT PATIENTS

The attending physician, who is in the best position to determine if a patient is incompetent, should become familiar with his or her state's definition of legal incompetence. In any case in which a physician doubts a patient's capacity to consent, the consent of the legal guardian or next of kin should be obtained. If there are no relatives to consult, application should be made for a court order that would allow the procedure. It may be the duty of the court to assume responsibility of guardianship for a patient who is non compos mentis. The most frequently cited conditions indicative of incompetence are mental illness, mental retardation, senility, physical incapacity, and chronic alcohol or drug abuse.

A person who is mentally incompetent cannot legally consent to medical or surgical treatment; therefore, consent of the patient's legal guardian must be obtained. When no legal guardian is available, a court that handles such matters must be petitioned to permit treatment.

Subject to applicable statutory provisions, when a physician doubts a patient's capacity to consent, even though the patient has not been judged legally incompetent, the consent of the nearest relative should be obtained. If a patient is conscious and mentally capable of giving consent for treatment, the consent of a relative without the consent of the competent patient would not protect the physician from liability.

GUARDIAN

Consent of the patient ordinarily is required before treatment. When a patient is either physically unable or legally incompetent to consent and no emergency exists, consent must be obtained from a person who is empowered to consent on the patient's behalf. A guardian is an individual who by law is invested with the power and charged with the duty of taking care of a patient by protecting the patient's rights and managing the patient's estate. *Guardianship* is often necessary in those instances in which a patient is incapable of managing or administering his or her private affairs because of physical and/or mental disabilities or because he or she is under the age of majority.

Temporary Guardian

The courts can grant temporary guardianship if it is determined necessary for the well being of the patient.

CASE: PHYSICIAN AND ADMINISTRATOR FILE FOR TEMPORARY GUARDIANSHIP

The court in *In re Estate of Dorone* granted temporary guardianship.[15] In this case, the physician and administrator petitioned the court on two occasions for authority to administer blood. A 22-year-old male patient brought to the Hospital Center by helicopter after an automobile accident was diagnosed as suffering from an acute subdural hematoma with a brain contusion.

It was determined that the patient would die unless he underwent a cranial operation. The operation required the administration of blood, to which the parents would not consent because of their religious beliefs. After a hearing by telephone, the court of common pleas appointed the hospital's administrator as temporary guardian, authorizing him to consent to the performance of blood transfusions during emergency surgery. A more formal hearing did not take place because of the emergency situation that existed. Surgery was required a second time to remove a blood clot, and the court once again granted the administrator authority to authorize administration of blood. The superior court affirmed the orders, and the parents appealed. The Pennsylvania Supreme Court held that the judge's failure to obtain direct testimony from the patient's parents and others concerning the patient's religious beliefs were not in error when death was likely to result from withholding blood. The judge's decisions granting guardianship and the authority to consent to the administration of blood were considered absolutely necessary in the light of the facts of this case. Nothing less than a fully conscious contemporary decision by the patient himself would have been sufficient to override the evidence of medical necessity.

Ethical and Legal Issues

1. Should a hospital act to save a patient's life if he or she has not given written consent to a procedure?
2. What types of monetary awards should the court give the plaintiff, if any? Why?

RIGHT TO REFUSE TREATMENT

The individual's right to make decisions vitally affecting his private life according to his own conscience . . . is difficult to overstate . . . because it is, without exaggeration, the very bedrock on which this country was founded.

—WONS V. PUBLIC HEALTH TRUST[16]

Adult patients who are conscious and mentally competent have the right to refuse medical care to the extent permitted by law, even when the best medical opinion deems it essential to life. A patient's right to make decisions regarding his own health care is addressed in the Patient Self-Determination Act of 1990.[17] The act provides that each person has a right under state law (whether statutory or as recognized by the courts of the state) to make decisions concerning his or her medical care, including the right to accept or refuse medical or surgical treatment.

A competent patient's refusal to consent to a medical or surgical procedure must be adhered to, whether the refusal is grounded in lack of confidence in the physician, fear of the procedure, doubt as to the value of a particular procedure, or mere whim. The U.S. Supreme Court stated that the "notion of bodily integrity has been embodied in the requirement that informed consent is generally required for medical treatment" and the "logical corollary of the doctrine of informed consent is that the patient generally possesses the right not to consent, that is, to refuse treatment."[18] The common-law doctrine of informed consent is viewed as generally encompassing the right of a competent individual to refuse medical treatment.

The question of liability for performing a medical or surgical procedure without consent is separate and distinct from any question of negligence or malpractice in performing a procedure. Liability can be imposed for a nonconsensual touching of a patient, even if the procedure improved the patient's health.

The courts perform a balancing test to determine whether or not to override a competent adult's decision to refuse medical treatment. The courts balance state interests, such as preservation of life, protection of third parties, prevention of suicide, and the integrity of the medical profession, against a patient's rights of bodily integrity and religious freedom. The most frequently used state right to intervene in a patient's decision-making process is for the protection of third parties. In *In re Fetus Brown*,[19] the state of Illinois asserted that its interest in the well-being of a viable fetus outweighed the patient's right to refuse medical treatment. The state argued that a balancing test should be used to weigh state interests against patient rights. The appellate court held that it could not impose a legal obligation on a pregnant woman to consent to an invasive medical procedure for the benefit of her viable fetus.

Adult patients who are conscious and mentally competent have the right to refuse medical care to the extent permitted by law even when the best medical opinion deems it essential to life. Such a refusal must be honored whether it is grounded in religious belief or straightforward objection to the procedure. Every person has the legal right to refuse to permit a touching of his or her body. Failure to respect this right can result in a legal action for assault and battery. If a patient refuses consent, every effort should be made to explain the importance of the procedure. Coercion through threat, duress, or intimidation must be avoided.

A hospital generally has no common-law right or obligation to thrust unwanted medical care on a patient who, having been sufficiently informed of the consequences, competently and clearly declines such care. A patient's common-law right of bodily self-determination is entitled to respect and protection. Before a patient leaves a health care facility against medical advice, every attempt should be made to have a release form completed (**Figure** 1) and included in the patient's permanent record.

All reasonable steps should be taken to (1) inform the patient of the benefits and risks of treatment and (2) secure the patient's written informed consent to refuse examination and treatment. If the patient refuses to sign the "refusal to consent form," documentation of a patient's refusal of care should be placed in the patient's medical record.

REFUSAL OF CARE BASED ON RELIGIOUS BELIEFS

As part of their religious beliefs, Jehovah's Witnesses generally have refused the administration of blood, even in emergency situations. Case law over the past several decades has developed to a point where any person, regardless of religious beliefs, has the right to refuse medical treatment.

CASE: A MOTHER'S RIGHT, A CHILD'S DEATH

Harrell, a Jehovah's Witness, was 6 months pregnant when physicians discovered a life-threatening blood condition that could rapidly deteriorate, placing both her life and the life of the fetus in jeopardy. Because of her religious beliefs, Harrell objected to a blood transfusion. After an emergency hearing during which the Harrells could not summon an attorney, the court ruled that a blood transfusion could be given to Harrell if it was necessary to save the life of the fetus and that after the child was born a blood transfusion could be given to the child if necessary to save the child's life. The Harrells appealed. The child was delivered by Caesarean section and died 2 days later. No blood transfusion was given to Harrell or to the child. As a result, the hospital and the state claimed that the *appeal* of the trial court's order was moot. Because of the hospital's serious misunderstanding about its standing to bring

Hospital _____

Address _____

Phone _____

Refusal of Care and Treatment

(Leave Against Medical Advice)

The patient meets all of the following criteria:

1. The patient is over the age of 18 years of age.

2. The patient exhibits no evidence of:

_____ Altered level of consciousness

_____ Alcohol or drug ingestion that would impair judgment

3. The patient understands the nature of his or her medical condition, including the risks, benefits, and of alternative treatments, as well as, the consequences of refusing care treatment alternatives.

Acknowledgement of Information (initial each of the following lines)

_____ I have been advised that medical care on my behalf is necessary, and that refusal of care and assistance could be hazardous to my health, and under certain circumstances, including disability or death.

_____ I acknowledge that I may have a medical problem which may require additional medical attention, and that NDSP or an ambulance is available to transport me to the hospital. Instead, I elect to seek alternative medical care and/or refuse further evaluation, treatment and/or transport.

Release of Liability (initial on line)

_____ By signing this form, I am releasing _____ (name of hospital or healthcare facility) of any liability or medical claims resulting from my decision to refuse care against medical advice.

_____ I have read and understand the Acknowledgement ofInformation and Release of Liability.

_____ If I change my mind, or my condition changes, I will call 911 in an emergency and request that I be taken to the _____ Hospital emergency room or call my private doctor, for follow-up care as appropriate.

Signature _____   Date _____

Witness Information

Signature: _____   Name Printed: _____   Date: _____

Signature: _____   Name Printed: _____   Date: _____

FIGURE   1   Refusal of Care and Treatment

such proceedings, the Florida District Court of Appeal addressed the issue as capable of repetition yet evading review.

The Florida constitution guarantees that a competent person has the constitutional right to choose or refuse medical treatment, and that right extends to all relevant decisions concerning one's health. The state has a duty to ensure that a person's wishes regarding medical treatment are respected. That obligation serves to protect the rights of the individual from intrusion by the state unless the state has a compelling interest great enough to override this constitutional right (e.g., protection of innocent third parties).

Harrell argued that the hospital should not have intervened in her private decision to refuse a blood transfusion. She claimed that the state had never been a party in this action, had not asserted any interest, and that the hospital had no authority to assume the state's responsibilities.

The Florida District Court of Appeal concluded that a health care provider must not be forced into the position of having to argue against the wishes of the facility's own patient. Patients do not lose their right to make decisions affecting their lives when they enter a health care facility. A health care provider's function is to provide medical treatment in accordance with the patient's wishes and best interests, not supervene the wishes of a competent adult. A health care provider must comply with the wishes of a patient to refuse medical treatment unless ordered to do otherwise by a court of competent jurisdiction. A health care provider cannot act on behalf of the state to assert state interests. When a health care provider, acting in good faith, follows the wishes of a competent and informed patient to refuse medical treatment, the health care provider is acting appropriately and cannot be subjected to civil or criminal liability. [20]

Ethical and Legal Issues

1. Is the Florida District Court of Appeal's conclusion binding in all states?
2. Do you think the hospital made the correct decisions in this case? Discuss your answer.

CASE: MOTHER REFUSES BLOOD, SPOUSE DISAGREES

What would you do if a patient, a Jehovah's Witness, signs a consent form refusing a blood transfusion and her husband, who is not a Jehovah's Witness, consents to a blood transfusion to save his wife's life?

The plaintiff, Bonita Perkins, in *Perkins v. Lavin*,[21] was a Jehovah's Witness. She gave birth to a baby at the defendant's hospital. After going home, she began hemorrhaging and returned to the hospital. She specifically informed the defendant's employees that she was not to be provided any blood or blood derivatives, and she signed a form to that effect:[22]

> I request that no blood or blood derivatives be administered to [plaintiff] during this hospitalization, notwithstanding that such treatment may be deemed necessary in the opinion of the attending physician or his assistants to preserve life or promote recovery. I release the attending physician, his assistants, the hospital, and its personnel from any responsibility whatever for any untoward results due to my refusal to permit the use of blood or its derivatives.

Because of the plaintiff's condition, it became necessary to perform an emergency dilation and curettage. She continued to bleed and her condition deteriorated dramatically. Her blood count dropped, necessitating administration of blood products as a lifesaving measure. Her husband, who was not a Jehovah's Witness, consented to a blood transfusion, which was administered. The plaintiff recovered and filed an action against the defendant for assault and battery. The plaintiff's claim as to assault and battery was sustained.

The plaintiff specifically informed the defendant that she would consider a blood transfusion an offensive contact. Although both parties have noted that the plaintiff's husband provided his consent for the transfusion, the defendant has not argued that his consent was sufficient to overcome plaintiff's direction that she was not to receive a transfusion. The plaintiff submitted sufficient evidence to the trial court to establish that there was, at least, a genuine issue as to whether the defendant intentionally invaded her right to be free from offensive contact. Because of the plaintiff's recognition that the defendant acted to save her life, a jury may find that she is entitled to only nominal damages.

Ethical and Legal Issues

1. Should the court be the ultimate decision maker when there is a dispute over whether or not a lifesaving measure should be administered to a nonconsenting patient?
2. Should a parent have the right to refuse a lifesaving treatment (e.g., transfusion) for a minor? Explain.

CASE: MOTHER REFUSES TREATMENT, SPOUSE AGREES

Vega, a Jehovah's Witness, executed a release requesting that no blood be administered to her during her hospitalization. Vega's husband also signed the release. She delivered a healthy baby. After the delivery, Vega bled heavily. Her obstetrician, Dr. Sood, recommended a dilation and curettage (D&C) to stop the bleeding. Although Vega agreed to permit Sood to perform the D&C, she refused to allow a blood transfusion. Before undergoing the procedure, she signed a second release refusing any transfusions and releasing the hospital from liability. Despite the D&C, Vega continued to hemorrhage.

Because Sood and the other physicians involved in Vega's care believed that it was essential that she receive blood in order to survive, the hospital requested that the court issue an injunction that would permit the hospital to administer blood transfusions. The trial court convened an emergency hearing at the hospital and appointed Vega's husband as her guardian. At the hearing testimony, Vega's husband testified that, on the basis of his religious beliefs as a Jehovah's Witness, he continued to support his wife's decision to refuse transfusions and believed that she would take the same position if she were able to participate in the hearing.

The court, relying on the state's interests in preserving life and protecting innocent third parties, granted the hospital's request for an injunction permitting it to administer blood transfusions. Vega was given blood transfusions. She recovered and was discharged from the hospital.

Vega sued, arguing that if her refusal of blood transfusions interfered with certain state interests, it should be the state itself, not a private hospital, that asserts state's interests. The hospital responded that because it was charged with Vega's care it had a direct stake in the outcome of the controversy and was a proper party to bring the action.

The hospital had a legitimate interest in receiving official guidance in resolving the "ethical dilemma" it faced: whether to practice medicine by trying to save a patient's life despite that patient's refusal to consent to treatment or to practice medicine in accordance with the patient's wishes and likely watch the patient die, knowing nonetheless that it had the power to save her life. The hospital had conflicting interests and was in the role not of opposing its patient but of a party seeking the court's guidance in determining its obligations under the circumstances.

Vega claimed that the state's interest in the welfare of her child is not sufficiently compelling as to outweigh her interest in refusing blood transfusions. Vega maintained that the trial court's injunction, issued at the behest of the hospital, violated her common-law right of self-determination, her federal constitutional right to bodily self-determination, her federal constitutional right to free exercise of religion, and her state constitutional right of religious liberty. The court concluded that, under the circumstances of this case, the issuance of the injunction, followed by the administration of blood transfusions, violated Vega's common-law right of bodily self-determination.

Although the hospital's interests are sufficient to confer standing in this case, they are not sufficient to take priority over Vega's common law right to bodily integrity, even when the assertion of that right threatens her own life. The hospital had no common-law right or obligation to thrust unwanted medical care on a patient who, having been sufficiently informed of the consequences, competently and clearly declined that care. The hospital's interests were sufficiently protected by Vega's informed choice, and neither it nor the trial court was entitled to override that choice. Vega's common-law right of bodily self-determination was entitled to respect and protection.[23]

Ethical and Legal Issues

1. What would you do if a patient refused a blood transfusion and the spouse agreed with her decision, knowing that a blood transfusion may be necessary to save her life?
2. Should a hospital challenge a patient's refusal of lifesaving blood transfusions?

Competent adolescents have the right to deny treatment according to Skagit County Superior Court Judge John Meyer when he had to decide if a 14-year-old patient with leukemia had the right to refuse a blood transfusion. The patient, Dennis Lindberg, a Jehovah's Witness had denied the transfusion based on his religious beliefs.

Ethics experts and Jehovah's Witness officials said such a court case is unusual these days. Most cases involving transfusions stem from surgical cases, and current policy at Children's is to inform parents that while the hospital will do everything it can to avoid transfusions, it will not let a child die for want of blood, said Dr. Doug Diekema, an ethics consultant there.[24]

Are Teens Old Enough for Life/Death Decisions?

When Skagit County Superior Court Judge John Meyer came to work he expected to be hearing a few small matters.

Instead, he made a decision in a case that he said has "perhaps more profound interest and implication than any matter I have ever heard on the bench."

Meyer decided Wednesday to allow 14-year-old Dennis Lindberg of Mount Vernon to refuse blood transfusions—based on his religious beliefs.

It's a case that brings into sharp relief the tensions in laws and ethics over whether adolescents should be able to make such serious health-care decisions for themselves.

Janet I. Tu, The Seattle Times, *November 30, 2007*

Judge John Meyer's decision should by no means be applied as a standard for all similar cases involving a minor patient's right to refuse treatment. The courts of various jurisdictions may have reached a different decision than that of Judge Meyer of the Skagit County Superior Court. In future cases of this sort, no court can use a customized cookie cutter approach to stamp out decisions because every case is composed of a different set of facts and circumstances to which the law must be applied. It seems to be an oxymoron to prohibit minors from obtaining treatment for most medical conditions without first obtaining parental consent on the one hand and on the other hand allowing the minor to deny lifesaving treatment. It is unclear how the courts will respond to the same or similar cases as they arise in other jurisdictions.

Interestingly, Dr. James L. Bernat wrote an article titled "Ask the Neurologist: What If Your Patient Refuses Blood Transfusions Due to Religious Beliefs? in *Neurology Today*, a publication of the American Academy of Neurology:

> One memorable experience in which I performed an ethics consultation on a minor patient whose Jehovah's Witness parents refused consent for blood transfusion yielded an unexpected outcome. After the bioethics committee requested and obtained a court order mandating treatment, rather than being angry or resentful with us for superseding their parental authority through the judiciary, the parents were relieved that their child would survive. It became clear to us in retrospect that they felt compelled to refuse blood transfusions on behalf of their child for them to remain true to their religious beliefs.[25]

CHAPTER REVIEW

1. *Consent*
   - Voluntary agreement by a person who possesses sufficient mental capacity to make an intelligent choice to allow something proposed by another to be performed on himself or herself.

- Forms of consent
  - *Express*
    - Verbal
    - Written
  - *Implied*
    - Presumption that consent has been authorized
2. *Informed consent*
   - Legal concept that provides that a patient has a right to know
     - Risks
     - Benefits
     - Alternatives of a proposed procedure
   - Informed consent is predicated on the duty of the physician to disclose to the patient sufficient information to enable the patient to evaluate a proposed medical or surgical procedure before submitting to it.
3. *Statutory consent*
   - Age of consent
   - Emergency consent
     - Generally presumed when immediate action is required to prevent death or permanent impairment of a patient's health
     - Documentation justifying the need for treatment
4. Capacity to consent
   - Individuals incompetent to give consent
   - No relatives or other parties from whom consent can be obtained
     - Application should be made for a court order that would allow a needed procedure.
5. Adequacy of consent
   - Requires that that consent be informed consent.
     - Varies depending on age, maturity, and mental status.
   - Competent patient
   - Spouse
   - Parental consent
   - Consent by minors
   - Incompetent patients
   - Guardian
6. Right to refuse treatment
   - Often based on religious beliefs.
   - Complexities occur when the consent for a minor's treatment is involved.
     - Generally because states interests are at issue, as in the case of a minor.
   - Patients refusing care should be requested to sign a release form.
     - Documentation should be placed in the patient's medical record as to their refusal of treatment.

consent	implied consent	statutory consent
express consent	informed consent	written consent
guardianship	oral consent	

REVIEW QUESTIONS

1. Discuss informed consent and how it applies the patient's right to self-determination.

2. Describe what information the patient should be provided prior to consenting to a recommended treatment.

3. Describe how various codes of professional ethics address a patient's right to informed consent and self-determination.

4. Explain and give examples of verbal, written, and implied consent.

5. Describe the purpose of statutory consent.

6. Describe under what circumstances statutory consent to treatment can be inferred.

7. Discuss why is it important to assess a patient's decision-making capacity.

8. Describe what factors the courts could take into consideration when determining the adequacy of consent.

9. Can a patient give consent and then withdraw it? Discuss your answer.

10. Explain why a patient has a right to refuse treatment.

NOTES

1. 141 U.S. 250, 251 (1891).
2. Wons v. Public Health Trust, 500 So. 2d 679, 687 (Fla. Dist. Ct. App. 1987), aff'd 541 So. 2d 96 (Fla. 1989).
3. In re Duran, 769 A.2d 497 (Pa. 2001).
4. Cruzan v. Director, Missouri Dep't of Health, 497 U.S. 261 (1990).
5. http://mobile.bloomberg.com/news/2013-12-30/unreported-robot-surgery-injuries-open-questions-for-fda.html
6. http://www.nursingworld.org/MainMenuCategories/EthicsStandards/CodeofEthicsforNurses/Code-of-Ethics.pdf.
7. 136 N.W. 1106 (Mich. 1912).
8. 28 N.E. 266 (Mass. 1891).
9. 611 A.2d 1148 (N.J. Super Ct. 1992).
10. 620 So. 2d 372 (La. Ct. App. 1993).

11. Id. at 380.

12. 390 N.Y.S.2d 523 (N.Y. Sup. Ct. 1976).

13. 632 N.E.2d 946 (Ohio Ct. App. 1993).

14. No. 38242 (Nev. 2004).

15. 534 A.2d 452 (Pa. 1987).

16. 500 So. 2d 679, 687 (Fla. Dist. Ct. App. 1987), aff'd 541 So. 2d 96 (Fla. 1989).

17. Public Law 101-508, November 5, 1990, sections 4206 and 4751 of the Omnibus Budget Reconciliation Act.

18. Cruzan v. Director, Missouri Dep't of Health, 497 U.S. 261, 269 (1990).

19. 689 N.E.2d 397 (Ill. App. Ct. 1997).

20. Harrell v. St. Mary's Hosp., Inc., 678 So. 2d 455 (Fla. Dist. Ct. App. 1996).

21. 648 N.E.2d 839 (Ohio App. 9 Dist. 1994).

22. Id. at 840.

23. Stamford Hosp. v. Vega, 674 A.2d 821 (Conn. Super. Ct. 1996).

24. *Carol M. Ostrom*, The Seattle Times, *November 29, 2007.* http://seattletimes.com/html/health/2004041765_transfusion29m.html.

25. *Neurology Today*, Vol. 11, Issue 10, May 19, 2011 pp. 27-8, 30-12.

PATIENT ABUSE

LEARNING OBJECTIVES

Upon completion of this chapter, the reader will be able to:

- Understand the pervasiveness of abuse
- Identify the signs of abuse
- Describe the reporting requirements for abuse

INTRODUCTION

Love and knowledge led upwards to the heavens, but always pity brought me back to earth; cries of pain reverberated in my heart of children in famine, of victims tortured, and of old people left helpless. I long to alleviate the evil, but I cannot, and I too suffer. This has been my life; I found it worth living.

—BERTRAND RUSSELL (ADAPTED)

Patient abuse refers to the mistreatment or neglect of individuals in the health care setting. Abuse often occurs to those who are most vulnerable and dependent on others for care (e.g., patients diagnosed with dementia and Alzheimer's disease, those who are physically weak). Abuse is not limited to an institutional setting and may occur in the patient's home. Abuse can take many forms—physical, psychological, medical, financial, and so forth. It is not always easy to identify because injuries can often be attributed to other causes. This chapter reviews child and senior abuse in a variety of settings.

CHILD ABUSE

An abused child is generally defined as a person younger than 18 years of age whose parent or other person legally responsible for his or her care inflicts, or allows to be inflicted, on that child physical injury by nonaccidental means that causes or creates a substantial risk of death, serious or protracted disfigurement, protracted impairment of physical or emotional health, or protracted loss or impairment of the function of any bodily organ; commits, or allows to be committed, a sex offense against that child; and/or allows, permits, or encourages the child to engage in an act considered unlawful. An abused child is one who may have suffered intentional serious mental, emotional, sexual, and/or physical injury inflicted by a parent or other person responsible for the child's care. The United States Code defines a *child abuse crime* as "a crime committed under any law of a State that involves the physical or mental injury, sexual abuse or exploitation, negligent treatment, or maltreatment of a child by any person."[1] Some states extend the definition to include a child suffering from starvation. Other states include moral neglect in the definition of abuse. Others mention immoral associations; endangering a child's morals; and the location of a child in a disreputable place or in association with vagrant, vicious, or immoral persons.

Child abuse continues to be of serious concern throughout the nation as noted by Joo Yeun Chang, the associate commissioner of the Children's Bureau, Department of Health and Human Services, in a report titled *Child Maltreatment 2012*.

- From 2008 to 2012, overall rates of victimization declined by 3.3%, from 9.5 to 9.2 per 1,000 children in the population. This results in an estimated 30,000 fewer victims in 2012 (686,000) compared with 2008 (716,000).
- Since 2008, overall rates of children who received a [Child Protective Services] CPS response increased by 4.7%, from 40.8 to 42.7 per 1,000 children in the population. This results in an estimated 107,000 additional children who received a CPS response in 2012 (3,184,000) compared to 2008 (3,077,000).
- Nationally, four-fifths (78.3%) of victims were neglected, 18.3% were physically abused, 9.3% were sexually abused, and 8.5% were psychologically maltreated.[2]

It is estimated that 1,640 children died of abuse and neglect at a rate of 2.20 children per 100,000 children in 2012.[3] The full document describing child maltreatment in 2012 is available from the Children's Bureau website at http://www.acf.hhs.gov/programs/cb/research-data- technology/statistics-research/child-maltreatment. The Children's Bureau in the Administration on Children, Youth and Families, the Administration for Children and Families within the U.S. Department of Health and Human Services (HHS), addresses this important issue in many ways. As noted in the following news clipping, the horrors of child abuse continue seemingly unabated.

NEWS

Mother gets 99 years for beating, gluing daughter: Has the US had it with bad parents?

Elizabeth Escalona, a 23-year-old mother of five, was sentenced to 99 years in prison after severely beating her daughter and gluing the girl's hands to a wall. The sentence is one sign that society—and the courts—are taking child abuse more seriously.

A 99-year prison sentence for a 23-year-old Dallas mother who admitted she had acted like a "monster" when gluing her daughter's hands and beating her into a coma last year suggests that society and the courts are taking a harsher view of neglectful, abusive, and violent parents, experts say.

Patrik Jonsson, The Christian Science Monitor, *October 13, 2012*

REPORTING ABUSE

The U.S. Code describes a state's reporting requirements for child abuse as follows:

> In each State, an authorized criminal justice agency of the State shall report child abuse crime information to, or index child abuse crime information in, the national criminal history background check system. A criminal justice agency may satisfy the requirement of this subsection by reporting or indexing all felony and serious misdemeanor arrests and dispositions.[4]

Child abuse statutes have been enacted by the states to protect abused children and provide civil immunity for those making or participating in good-faith reports of suspected child abuse. Most states also provide immunity from criminal liability. The New York State Social Services Law provides that "[a]ny person, official, or institution participating in good faith in the making of a report, the taking of photographs, or the removal or keeping of a child pursuant to this title shall have immunity from any liability, civil or criminal, that might otherwise result by reason of such actions."[5] Even in states that do not provide immunity, it is unlikely that anyone making a good-faith report of suspected child abuse would be subject to criminal liability. State laws generally specify what persons are required to report suspected child abuse that comes before them in their official capacities. In some states, failure to report a case of suspected child abuse carries criminal penalties as well as civil liability for the damages resulting from such failure.[6]

Child Abuse Fears Must Be Reported by Doctors, But Some Cases Pose Dilemmas

. . . As she turned her head on the way out the door, I noticed minor swelling around her eye. When I asked about it, she said, without hesitation, "Oh, my father hit me." Like all pediatricians, I am mandated by law to report any concern of child abuse . . .

Day after day, she begged me to rescind the report . . .

This spring, I received a message from her. She'd be home from college in the summer, she wrote. Could she shadow me at work as she explored a possible career in health care?

Her e-mail gave me hope.

Ilana Sherer, The Washington Post, August 15, 2011

Most states protect the persons required to report cases of child abuse. In a few states, certain identified individuals who are not required to report instances of child abuse, but who do so, are protected. Child abuse laws may or may not provide penalties for failure to report. Those in the health care setting who are required to report or cause a report to be made when they have reasonable cause to suspect that a child has been abused include the following: administrators, physicians, interns, registered nurses, chiropractors, social service workers, psychologists, dentists, osteopaths, optometrists, podiatrists, mental health professionals, and volunteers in residential facilities.

DETECTING ABUSE

What constitutes an abused child is difficult to determine because it is often impossible to ascertain whether a child was injured intentionally or accidentally. An individual who reports child abuse should be aware of the physical and behavioral indicators of abuse and maltreatment that appear to be part of a pattern (e.g., bruises, burns, broken bones). In reviewing the indicators of abuse and maltreatment, the reporter does not have to be absolutely certain that abuse or maltreatment exists before reporting. Rather, abuse and maltreatment should be reported whenever they are suspected, based on the existence of the signs of abuse and maltreatment and in light of the reporter's training and experience. Behavioral indicators include, but are not limited to, substantially diminished psychological or intellectual functioning, failure to thrive, no control of aggression, self-destructive impulses, decreased ability to think and reason, acting out and misbehavior, or habitual truancy. Such impairment must be clearly attributable to the unwillingness or inability of the person responsible for the child's care to exercise a minimum degree of care toward the child.

GOOD-FAITH REPORTING

Any report of suspected child abuse must be made with a good-faith belief that the facts reported are true. The definition of good faith as used in a child abuse statute may vary from state to state; however, when a health care practitioner's medical evaluation indicates reasonable cause to believe a child's injuries were not accidental and when the health care practitioner is not acting from his or her desire to harass, injure, or embarrass the child's parents, making the report will not result in liability.

Statutes generally require that when a person covered by a statute is attending a child and suspects child abuse, the staff member must report such concerns. Typical statutes provide that an oral report be made immediately, followed by a written report.

The criminal and civil risks for health care professionals lie not in *good-faith reporting* of suspected incidents of child abuse but in failing to report such incidents. Most states have legislated a variety of civil and criminal penalties for failure to report suspected child abuse incidents. New York, for example, provides:[7]

1. Any person, official, or institution required by this title to report a case of suspected child abuse or maltreatment who willfully fails to do so shall be guilty of a Class A misdemeanor.
2. Any person, official, or institution required by this title to report a case of suspected child abuse or maltreatment who knowingly and willfully fails to do so shall be civilly liable for the damages proximately caused by such failure.

IMMUNITY AND GOOD-FAITH REPORTING

A minor child and his mother brought an action for damages against physicians for failing to diagnose disease and filing erroneous child abuse reports in *Awkerman v. Tri-County Orthopedic Group*.[8] The Wayne County Circuit Court granted the physicians' motions for partial summary judgment, and the plaintiffs appealed. The Michigan Court of Appeals held that the child abuse reporting statute provides immunity to persons who file child abuse reports in good faith even if the reports were filed because of negligent diagnosis of the cause of the child's frequent bone fractures, which was eventually diagnosed as osteogenesis imperfecta. The court of appeals also held that damages for shame and humiliation were not recoverable pursuant to Michigan statute. Immunity from liability did not extend to damages for malpractice that may have resulted from the failure to diagnose the child's disease as long as all the elements of negligence were present.

Child Abuse Can Be Elusive

Child abuse is not always obvious to the caregiver and can unfortunately go undetected to the detriment of the child. I learned this early on in my training. I was a first-year resident at General Medical Center and was on tour in the hospital's pediatric unit with Peggy, the unit charge nurse. As we walked down the corridor I noticed a young child in room 106 in a full leg cast, which had been placed in traction. I asked Peggy what had happened to the patient. Peggy said, "Oh that's Gracie. Poor thing. She broke her femur tripping over a toy in her home." I thought to myself that was a major injury for tripping over a toy. I questioned Peggy further and she told me that she knew where I was leading by my questions and said, "Oh you can be assured that Gracie had not been abused. She has the sweetest mother and father. Although they are divorced one of her parents is here everyday. I even questioned the mother and she assures me it was an accident."

I had an uneasy feeling about the mother's story and decided to visit the radiology department to review Gracie's X-rays with the radiologist on duty. I walked into the imaging reading room where I found three radiologists reviewing various imaging studies. I introduced myself as a first-year resident to Dr. Patrick Williams, the medical director of radiology. I asked Dr. Williams, "Do you have time to review Gracie's X-rays with me." The radiologist replied, "No problem. What is Gracie's last name." I told him and he pulled up Gracie's X-rays electronically on a computer screen. As soon as he pulled up the X-rays he said, "Oh yes, Gracie has a compound fracture of the femur." He was very patient as he thoroughly reviewed with me Gracie's case. He pointed out the compound fracture of the femur with the computer cursor. I asked him, "Do you think the injury could have occurred from Gracie tripping over a toy at home on a plush carpet." He replied, "That would be highly unlikely." He called over one of his partners and said, "Does this patient's injury look like she tripped over a toy." Looking at me he said, "Is this what you were told you?" I said, "Well, yes, I was." He looked at me and said, "I have been reading imaging studies for over 20 years. It is highly unlikely that Gracie's compound fracture of her left femur is the result of her tripping over a toy." The third radiologist in the room commented, "Definitely not caused by a slip on a toy."

Following my review with the radiologists, I called Peggy and asked if she had time to review Gracie's medical record with me after lunch. Peggy replied, "Sure thing, I will see you after lunch."

After lunch I went to the pediatric unit. Upon arriving on the unit Peggy and Caroline, a hospital social service worker, greeted me. Caroline said, "I contacted child welfare in the county in which Gracie resides. They informed me that Gracie was an active child abuse case, which they have been following for the past 6 months. They thanked me for the information and will be in the hospital late this afternoon to follow up."

Discussion

1. Discuss what lessons the caregiver can learn from the resident's observations and persistence in learning more about the cause of Gracie's injury.
2. Assume you are the hospital's director of inservice education, explain what steps you might take to reeducate staff as how to identify and report suspicions of child abuse.

SENIOR ABUSE

People at their weakest are often treated the worst.

—Nina Santucci

Senior abuse is the harmful treatment of older people and includes abandonment; emotional, financial (e.g., theft or misuse of a senior individual's money or property by a person in a position of trust), verbal, mental, sexual, or physical abuse; corporal punishment; and involuntary restraint and seclusion. Neglect is the failure to provide the care necessary to prevent physical harm (e.g., the failure of staff to turn a patient periodically to prevent pressure sores) or mental anguish.

The American Psychological Association estimates that "4 million older Americans are victims of physical, psychological or other forms of abuse and neglect."[9]

Those statistics may not tell the whole story. For every case of elder abuse and neglect reported to authorities, experts estimate as many as 23 cases go undetected. The quality of life of older individuals who experience abuse is severely jeopardized, as they often experience worsened functional and financial status and progressive dependency, poor self-rated health, feelings of helplessness and loneliness and increased psychological distress. Research also suggests that older people who have been abused tend to die earlier than those who have not been abused, even in the absence of chronic conditions or life-threatening disease.[10]

A *USA Today* review of 2 years of inspection records (between 2000 and 2002) for more than 5,300 assisted-living facilities in seven states found that what should be havens for senior persons may in reality be exposing them to deadly risks. The study indicates that medication errors and poor staff training resulted in many of the injuries identified.[11]

The Centers for Medicare & Medicaid Services (CMS) is the federal agency responsible for reviewing the effectiveness of state surveys. CMS evaluates the performance of state surveyors by conducting federal surveys in which federal surveyors resurvey a nursing facility recently inspected by state surveyors. The results of the two surveys are compared as to the deficiencies identified between the two surveys.[12]

Federal comparative surveys can find two types of understatement: (1) missed deficiencies, which can occur when a state surveyor fails to cite a deficiency altogether, or (2) cases where state surveyors cite deficiencies at too low a level. In May 2008, we reported that a substantial proportion of federal comparative surveys conducted from fiscal years 2002 through 2007 identified missed deficiencies that either had the potential to or did result in harm, death, or serious injury to nursing home residents.[13]

There is no shortage of case stories as to the abuse of patients in nursing facilities. Both print and broadcast news are replete with stories of elder abuse. On Long Island nine nursing home employees were charged following investigation of a resident's death. "As CBS 2's Jennifer McLogan reported, of the nine employees charged, seven of them were arrested in connection with the October 2012 death of 72-year-old patient Aurelia Rios. Licensed professional Kethlie Joseph is charged with criminally negligent homicide and *administrator* David Fielding is accused of an alleged cover-up.[14]

On January 10, 2014 in an editorial titled *A Welcome Emphasis On Elder Abuse* the *News Tribune* writes, "Examples of elder abuse in the headlines range from baffling to horrifying: from the lonely old widower conned out of his life savings by a pretty young woman to the invalid grandmother found restrained to her bed, covered in bedsores and filth."[15] There is an endless stream of headlines and news stories as to how widespread and pervasive senior abuse is, as the following examples show:

- The California Attorney General has estimated that 200,000 elderly Californians are abused each year.[16]

- Financial Abuse Cost Elderly Billions[17]
- Like many Americans, Mary Kantorowski has been ordered to leave her home, but it's not a bank telling her to get out—it's her own son.[18]
- Jasmine Kassim, now serving 75 months in prison for bilking five seniors out of more than $1 million dollars.[19]
- Judge Timothy Lamb in addressing two defendants said, "In short, by your offending you have let down your colleagues, you have damaged patient trust and you have undermined the quality of care for the elderly and vulnerable at Whipps Cross (University Hospital)."[20]

REPORTING SENIOR ABUSE

Most states have enacted statutes mandating the reporting of senior abuse. In general, senior abuse is less likely to be reported than child abuse. Physical and emotional neglect, as well as verbal and financial abuse, are perceived as the most prevalent forms of senior abuse. Seniors often fail to report incidents of abuse because they fear retaliation and not being believed. Threats of placement in a nursing home or shame that a family member is involved often prevent senior citizens from seeking help.

Kansas statute 39-1402, for example, requires reporting of abuse, neglect or exploitation of its residents. The statute obligates the following persons to report elder abuse.

> (a) Any person who is licensed to practice any branch of the healing arts, a licensed psychologist, a licensed master level psychologist, a licensed clinical psychotherapist, a chief administrative officer of a medical care facility, an adult care home administrator or operator, a licensed social worker, a licensed professional nurse, a licensed practical nurse, a licensed marriage and family therapist, a licensed clinical marriage and family therapist, licensed professional counselor, licensed clinical professional counselor, registered alcohol and drug abuse counselor, a teacher, a bank trust officer and any other officers of financial institutions, a legal representative or a governmental assistance provider who has reasonable cause to believe that a resident is being or has been abused, neglected or exploited, or is in a condition which is the result of such abuse, neglect or exploitation or is in need of protective services, shall report immediately such information or cause a report of such information to be made in any reasonable manner to the department on aging . . .[21]

Kansas Governor Sam Brownback signed into law H.B. 2504 that imposes strict penalties against those who commit elder abuse. "Attorney General Derek Schmidt says elderly residents will have new protections against fraud and financial abuse under a new state law . . . The law is aimed at protecting people 70 and older who are victims of financial abuse. People convicted of large-scale abuse could be sentenced to more than 40 years in prison."[22]

Hidden Camera

Gale . . . wasn't prepared for the rough treatment and cruel taunts she says her ailing mother suffered at the nursing home. She cried as a nurse's aide chastised her mother for failing to straighten her arthritic-stricken legs. And she watched in disbelief as an assistant jerked her mother off her rubber bed pad and pushed her into the bed's metal rails. All of these images were caught . . . by a "granny cam"—a camera hidden in her mother's room.

Deborah Sharp, USA Today, *September 14, 1999*

Signs of senior abuse or neglect of a senior include the following:

- Physical Abuse
  - bruises, black eyes, welts, lacerations, and rope marks;
  - bone fractures, broken bones, and skull fractures;
  - open wounds, cuts, punctures, untreated injuries in various stages of healing;
  - sprains, dislocations, and internal injuries/bleeding;
  - broken eyeglasses/frames, physical signs of being subjected to punishment, and signs of being restrained;
  - laboratory findings of medication overdose or under utilization of prescribed drugs;
  - an elder's report of being hit, slapped, kicked, or mistreated;
  - an elder's sudden change in behavior; and
  - the caregiver's refusal to allow visitors to see an elder alone.
- Sexual Abuse
  - bruises around the breasts or genital area;
  - unexplained venereal disease or genital infections;
  - unexplained vaginal or anal bleeding;
  - torn, stained, or bloody underclothing; and
  - elder's report of being sexually assaulted or raped.
- Emotional or Psychological Abuse
  - being emotionally upset or agitated;
  - being extremely withdrawn and noncommunicative or nonresponsive;
  - unusual behavior usually attributed to dementia (e.g., sucking, biting, rocking); and
  - an elder's report of being verbally or emotionally mistreated.
- Neglect
  - dehydration, malnutrition, untreated bed sores, and poor personal hygiene;
  - unattended or untreated health problems;
  - hazardous or unsafe living condition/arrangements (e.g., improper wiring, no heat, or no running water);
  - unsanitary and unclean living conditions (e.g., dirt, fleas, lice on person, soiled bedding, fecal/urine smell, inadequate clothing); and
  - an elder's report of being mistreated.

- Abandonment
  - the desertion of an elder at a hospital, a nursing facility, or other similar institution;
  - the desertion of an elder at a shopping center or other public location; and
  - an elder's own report of being abandoned.
- Financial or Material Exploitation
  - sudden changes in bank account or banking practice, including an unexplained withdrawal of large sums of money by a person accompanying the elder;
  - the inclusion of additional names on an elder's bank signature card;
  - unauthorized withdrawal of the elder's funds using the elder's ATM card;
  - abrupt changes in a will or other financial documents;
  - unexplained disappearance of funds or valuable possessions;
  - substandard care being provided or bills unpaid despite the availability of adequate financial resources;
  - discovery of an elder's signature being forged for financial transactions or for the titles of his/her possessions;
  - sudden appearance of previously uninvolved relatives claiming their rights to an elder's affairs and possessions;
  - unexplained sudden transfer of assets to a family member or someone outside the family;
  - the provision of services that are not necessary; and
  - an elder's report of financial exploitation.
- Self-Neglect
  - dehydration, malnutrition, untreated or improperly attended medical conditions, and poor personal hygiene;
  - hazardous or unsafe living conditions/arrangements (e.g., improper wiring, no indoor plumbing, no heat, no running water);
  - unsanitary or unclean living quarters (e.g., animal/insect infestation, no functioning toilet, fecal/urine smell);
  - inappropriate and/or inadequate clothing, lack of the necessary medical aids (e.g., eyeglasses, hearing aids, dentures); and
  - grossly inadequate housing or homelessness.[23]

DOCUMENTATION

Caregivers who suspect abuse are expected to report their findings. Symptoms and conditions of suspected abuse should be defined clearly and objectively. The abuse of senior individuals is not a localized or isolated problem. Unfortunately, it permeates our society. *Behind Closed Doors,* a landmark book on family violence, stated that the first national study of violence in American homes estimated that one in two homes was the scene of family violence at least once a year.[24]

We have always known that America is a violent society. . . . What is new and surprising is that the American family and the American home are perhaps as much or more violent than any other single institution or setting (with the exception of the military, and only then in the time of war). Americans run the greatest risk of assault, physical injury and even murder in their own homes by members of their own families.[25]

It is difficult to determine the extent of senior abuse because the abused are reluctant to admit that their children or loved ones have assaulted them. Unfortunately, the abuse of senior persons remains hidden from the public, and the findings of the 1990 report are as current today as when they were first published in 1990 when the Senate Select Committee on Aging reported the following:[26]

- Senior abuse is less likely to be reported than child abuse.
- Physical violence, including negligence, and financial abuse appear to be the most common forms of abuse, followed by abrogation of basic constitutional rights and psychological abuse.
- Most instances of senior abuse are recurring events rather than one-time occurrences.
- Victims are often 75 years of age or senior, and women are more likely to be abused than men.
- Senior people are often ashamed to admit that their children or loved ones abuse them, or they may fear reprisals if they complain.
- Many middle-aged family members, finally ready to enjoy time to themselves, are resentful of a frail and dependent senior parent.
- Finally, the majority of the abusers are relatives.

The plaintiffs in *In re Estate of Smith v. O'Halloran*[27] instituted a lawsuit in an effort to improve deplorable conditions in many nursing homes. The court concluded that:[28]

The evidentiary record . . . supports a general finding that all is not well in the nation's nursing homes and that the enormous expenditures of public funds and the earnest efforts of public officials and public employees have not produced an equivalent return in benefits. That failure of expectations has produced frustration and anger among those who are aware of the realities of life in some nursing homes, which provide so little service that they could be characterized as orphanages for the aged.

Surveyors of health care organizations should look for signs of patient abuse by watching for the following:

- Physician's order for restraints
- Time-limited orders
- The number of patients that are physically restrained
- The types of restraints being used
- Whether or not the restraints are applied correctly
- How often restrained patients are observed by the staff
- Signs of overmedication
- Signs of mental and physical abuse of patients
- Signs of harassment, humiliation, or threats from staff or patients
- Whether patients are comfortable with the staff
- The numbers of patients with bruises or other injuries
- Evidence of patient neglect or patients left in urine or feces without cleaning

The defendant in *State v. Cunningham*,[29] the owner and administrator of a residential care facility, housed 30 to 37 mentally ill, mentally retarded, and senior residents. The Iowa Department of Inspections and Appeals conducted various surveys at the defendant's facility between October 1989 and May 1990. All of the surveys except for one resulted in a $50 daily fine assessed against the defendant for violations of the regulations.

On August 16, 1990, a grand jury filed an indictment charging the defendant with several counts of wanton neglect of a resident in violation of Iowa Code section 726.7 (1989), which provides, "A person commits wanton neglect of a resident of a health care facility when the person knowingly acts in a manner likely to be injurious to the physical, mental, or moral welfare of a resident of a health care facility. . . . Wanton neglect of a resident of a health care facility is a serious misdemeanor."

The district court held that the defendant had knowledge of the dangerous conditions that existed in the health care facility but willfully and consciously refused to provide or to exercise adequate supervision to remedy or attempt to remedy the dangerous conditions. The residents were exposed to physical dangers and unhealthy and unsanitary physical conditions and were grossly deprived of much-needed medical care and personal attention. The conditions were likely to and did cause injury to the physical and mental well-being of the facility's residents. The defendant was found guilty on five counts of wanton neglect. The district court sentenced the defendant to 1 year in jail for each of the five counts, to run concurrently. The district court suspended all but 2 days of the defendant's sentence and ordered him to pay $200 for each count, plus a surcharge and costs, and to perform community service. A motion for a new trial was denied, and the defendant appealed.

The Iowa Court of Appeals held that there was substantial evidence to support a finding that the defendant was responsible for not properly maintaining the nursing facility, which led to prosecution for wanton neglect of the facility's residents. The defendant was found guilty of knowingly acting in a manner likely to be injurious to the physical or mental welfare of the facility's residents by creating, directing, or maintaining hazardous conditions and unsafe practices; fire hazards and circumstances impeded safety from fire. The facility was not properly maintained (e.g., findings included broken glass in patients' rooms, excessive hot water in faucets, dried feces on public bathroom walls and grab bars, insufficient towels and linens, cockroaches and worms in the food preparation area, no soap available in the kitchen, at one point only one bar of soap and one container of shampoo found in the entire facility). Dietary facilities were unsanitary and inadequate to meet the dietary needs of the residents. There were inadequate staffing patterns and supervision in the facility, and improper dosages of medications were administered to the residents.[30]

The defendant argued that he did not "create" the unsafe conditions at the facility. The court of appeals disagreed. The statute does not require that the defendant create the conditions at the facility to sustain a conviction. The defendant was the administrator of the facility and responsible for the conditions that existed.

Ethical and Legal Issues

1. Do you agree with the court's finding? Discuss your answer.
2. Discuss how both ethics and the law are intertwined in this case.

CASE: ABUSE OF RESIDENTS

The operator of a nursing facility appealed an order by the Department of Public Welfare revoking his license because of resident abuse in *Nepa v. Commonwealth Department of Public Welfare*.[31] Substantial evidence supported the department's finding. Three former employees testified that the nursing facility operator had abused residents in the following incidents:[32]

He unbuckled the belt of one of the residents, causing his pants to drop, and then grabbed a second resident, forcing them to kiss. (Petitioner's excuse for this behavior was to shame the resident because of his masturbating in public.)

On two occasions he forced a resident to remove toilet paper from a commode after she had urinated and defecated in it. (Denying that there was fecal matter in the commode, the petitioner made the excuse that this would stop the resident from filling the commode with toilet paper.)

He verbally abused a resident who was experiencing difficulty in breathing and accused him of faking as he attempted to feed him liquids.

The nursing facility operator claimed that the findings of fact were not based on substantial evidence and that even if they were the incidents did not amount to abuse under the code. The defendant attempted to discredit the witnesses with allegations from a resident and another employee that one of his former employees got into bed with a resident and that another had taken a picture of a male resident while in the shower and had placed a baby bottle and a humiliating sign around the neck of another resident. The court was not impressed. Although these incidents, if true, were reprehensible, they were collateral matters that had no bearing on the witnesses' reputation for truthfulness and therefore could not be used for impeachment purposes. The court held that there was substantial evidence supporting the department's decision and that the activities committed by the operator were sufficient to support revocation of his license:[33]

> We believe Petitioner's treatment of these residents as found by the hearing examiner to be truly disturbing. These residents were elderly and/or mentally incapacitated and wholly dependent on Petitioner while residing in his home. As residents, they are entitled to maintain their dignity and be cared for with respect, concern, and compassion.

> Petitioner testified that he did not have adequate training to deal with the patients he received who suffered from mental problems. Petitioner's lack of training in this area is absolutely no excuse for the reprehensible manner in which he treated various residents. Accordingly, DPW's order revoking Petitioner's license to operate a personal care home is affirmed.

Ethical and Legal Issues

1. Do the facts of this case support the court's finding? Discuss your answer.
2. Discuss why senior citizens are often reluctant to report abuse.

CASE: ABUSIVE SEARCH

A nurse in *People v. Coe*[34] was charged with a willful violation of the public health law in connection with an allegedly abusive search of an 86-year-old resident at a geriatric center and with the falsification of business records in the first degree. The resident, Mr. Gersh, had heart disease and difficulty in expressing himself verbally. Another resident claimed that two $5 bills were missing. Nurse Coe assumed that Gersh had taken them because he had been known to take things in the past. The nurse proceeded to search Gersh, who resisted. A security guard was summoned, and another search was undertaken. When Gersh again resisted, the security guard slammed a chair down in front of him and pinned his arms while the defendant nurse searched his pockets, failing to retrieve the two $5 bills. Five minutes later, Gersh collapsed in a chair gasping for air. Coe administered cardiopulmonary resuscitation but was unsuccessful, and Gersh died.

Coe was charged with violation of the New York Penal Law for falsifying records because of the defendant's "omission" of the facts relating to the search of Gersh. These facts were considered relevant and should have been included in the nurse's notes regarding this incident. "The first sentence states, 'Observed resident was extremely confused and talks incoherently. Suddenly became unresponsive . . .' This statement is simply false. It could only be true if some reference to the search and the loud noise was included."[35] A motion was made to dismiss the indictment at the end of the trial.

The court held that the search became an act of physical abuse and mistreatment, that the evidence was sufficient to warrant a finding of guilt on both charges, and that the fact that searches took place frequently did not excuse an otherwise illegal procedure:[36]

> It may well be that this incident reached the attention of the criminal justice system only because, in the end, a man had died. In those instances which are equally violative of residents' rights and equally contrary to standards of common decency but which do not result in visible harm to a patient, the acts are nevertheless illegal and subject to prosecution. A criminal act is not legitimized by the fact that others have, with impunity, engaged in that act.

Ethical and Legal Issues

1. With the number of senior abuse cases occurring so frequently, discuss why society waits for extreme violence to occur before preventative actions are taken.
2. Having studied ethics and the moral breakdown that appears to have occurred in society, what steps do you believe can be taken to reverse the trend of violence faced by our seniors?

CASE: FORCIBLE ADMINISTRATION OF MEDICATIONS

The medical employee in *In re Axelrod*[37] sought review of a determination by the commissioner of health that she was guilty of resident abuse. Evidence showed that the employee, after a resident refused medication, "held the patient's chin and poured the medication down her throat."[38] There was no indication or convincing evidence that an emergency existed that would have required the forced administration of the medication. The court held that substantial evidence supported the commissioner's finding that the employee had been guilty of resident abuse.

Ethical and Legal Issues

1. Discuss the ethical and legal ramifications of this case.
2. What sentence should the employee receive? Why?
3. What message should the court be sending to other potential abusers of patients?

INTIMIDATION OF ABUSIVE RESIDENT/DISCIPLINARY OVERKILL

A difficult and abusive 80-year-old resident of a veteran's home in *Beasley v. State Personnel Board*[39] slapped the face of an aide who was assisting him. The resident, referring to his inability to have sex, said that he might as well have his penis cut off. The aide, Beasley, stated that she said to the resident if he did not behave, then she might accommodate him. A nursing supervisor who passed by at that moment noted that a nursing assistant and a hospital aide who were standing nearby laughed and did nothing to intervene. Beasley was fired and the other two employees were suspended for 10 days. After the state board upheld the punishments, the three employees went by mandate to the superior court, where Beasley's dismissal was ruled too severe. The trial court found that action against the nursing assistant and hospital aide, although harsh, was within discretion.

On appeal, the court held that Beasley's comments did not constitute misconduct, and the veterans' home nursing assistant and hospital aide did not commit actionable conduct by "sort of laughing." When this incident was viewed in its context and in light of the whole record, it did not support the state personnel board's finding that Beasley's attitude toward patients was poor.

CASE: DEFICIENT CARE

In *Montgomery Health Care Facility v. Ballard,*[40] three nurses testified that the facility was understaffed. "One nurse testified that she asked her supervisor for more help but that she did not get it."[41] A nursing home resident, Mrs. Stovall, expired as the result of multiple infected bedsores. The estate of the patient brought a malpractice action against the nursing home. First American Health Care, Inc., is the parent corporation of the Montgomery Health Care Facility, a nursing home. The trial court entered a judgment on a jury verdict against the home, and an appeal was taken. The Alabama Supreme Court held that reports compiled by the Alabama Department of Public Health concerning deficiencies found in the nursing home were admissible as evidence. Evidence showed that the care given to the deceased was deficient in the same ways as noted in the survey and complaint reports, which indicated that deficiencies in the home included:[42]

> Inadequate documentation of treatment given for decubitus ulcers; 23 patients found with decubitus ulcers, 10 of whom developed those ulcers in the facility; dressings on the sores were not changed as ordered; nursing progress notes did not describe

patients' ongoing conditions, particularly with respect to descriptions of decubitus ulcers; ineffective policies and procedures with respect to sterile dressing supplies; lack of nursing assessments; incomplete patient care plans; inadequate documentation of doctor's visits, orders, or progress notes; am care not consistently documented; inadequate documentation of turning of patients; incomplete "activities of daily living" sheets; "range of motion" exercises not documented; patients found wet and soiled with dried fecal matter; lack of bowel and bladder retaining programs; [and] incomplete documentation of ordered force fluids.

From a corporate standpoint, the parent corporation of the nursing facility could be held liable for the nursing facility's negligence, where the parent company controlled or retained the right to control the day-to-day operations of the home. The defendants had argued that the punitive damage award of $2 million against the home was greater than what was necessary to meet society's goal of punishing them. The Alabama Supreme Court, however, found the award not to be excessive. "The trial court also found that because of the large number of nursing home residents vulnerable to the type of neglect found in Mrs. Stovall's case, the verdict would further the goal of discouraging others from similar conduct in the future."[43]

Ethical and Legal Issues

1. Could any legislation be enacted or policies, procedures, rules, and regulations be implemented as proactive measures to prevent this type of widespread abuse? Describe your answer.

2. Do you agree with the court that the award will discourage others from similar behavior? Explain.

LOOK CLOSER, SEE ME

Donna Fannin read the poem "Look Closer, See ME" to every nursing assistant class she ever taught. This wonderful poem was found among the meager belongings of an 89-year-old nursing home patient in Scotland following her death. It has been widely published since then. It is a reminder to us all that our bodies and relationships continue to change, and someday many of us will experience what she has felt.[44]

Look Closer, See ME

What do you see, Nurses?/ What do you see?/ What are you thinking?/ When you're looking at me?

A crabbit old woman,/ Not very wise,/ Uncertain of habit/ With faraway eyes? Who dribbles her food/ And makes no reply/ When you say in a loud voice,/ "I do wish you'd try!"

Who seems not to notice/ The things that you do,/ And forever is losing/

A stocking or shoe? Who, resisting or not,/ Lets you do as you will,/ With bathing and feeding,/The long day to fill.

Is that what you're thinking?/ Is that what you see?/ Then open your eyes,

Nurse,/ You're not looking at ME. I'll tell you who I am/ As I sit here so still/ As I do at your bidding/ As I eat at your will.

I'm a small child of ten,/ With a Mother and Father,/ Brothers and sisters/

Who love one another. A young girl of sixteen,/ With wings on her feet,/ Dreaming that soon,/ A lover she'll meet.

A bride soon at twenty,/ My heart gives a leap./ Remembering the vows/

We have promised to keep. At twenty-five now,/ I have young of my own,/ Who need me to guide them,/And a secure happy home.

A woman of thirty/ My young they grow fast,/ Bound to each other/ With ties

that should last. At forty, my young sons/ Have grown and have gone,/ But my man's beside me/To see I don't mourn.

At fifty, once more/ Babies play round my knee,/ Again we know children,/

My husband and me. Dark days are upon me,/ My husband is dead./ I look to the future/ And shudder with dread.

For my young are all rearing/ Young of their own,/ And I think of the years/And the love I have known.

I'm an old woman now,/ And nature is cruel,/ 'Tis her jest to make old age/

Look like a fool. The body, it crumbles,/ Grace and vigor depart/ There is now a stone,/ Where I once had a heart.

But inside this old carcass,/ A young girl still dwells,/ And now and again,/

My battered heart swells. I remember the joys,/ I remember the pain,/ And I'm living and loving/ All over again.

I think of the years,/ All too few, gone too fast,/ And accept the stark fact/ That

nothing can last. So, open your eyes, people,/ Open and see,/ Not a crabbit old woman,/ Look closer, See ME.

CHAPTER REVIEW

1. Patient Abuse
   - Mistreatment or neglect of individuals who are under the care of a health care organization.
   - Abuse is not limited to an institutional setting and may occur in an individual's home as well as in an institution.
   - Signs of abuse include:
     - Physical (e.g., sexual), psychological, medical, financial
     - Difficult to identify because injuries can be attributed to other causes
2. Child Abuse
   - Defined as a child under the age of 18 one who has suffered intentional serious mental, emotional, sexual, and/or physical injury inflicted by a parent or other person responsible for the child's care.

- Reporting child abuse.
  - All states have enacted various child abuse statutes to provide civil immunity for those making or participating in good-faith reports of suspected child abuse.
- Detecting child abuse.
  - Individual who report child abuse should be aware of the physical and behavioral indicators of abuse and maltreatment that appear to be part of a pattern (e.g., bruises, burns, broken bones).
  - Caregivers must report the suspicion of child abuse with good faith motives.
  - Caregivers are immune from liability for good faith reporting.

3. Senior Abuse
- Seniors often fail to report incidents of abuse because they fear retaliation and not being believed.
- Most states have enacted statutes mandating the reporting of senior abuse.
- Signs of Elder Abuse:
  - Unexplained or unexpected death; broken bones; sudden and unexpected emotional outbursts, agitation, or withdrawal; bruises, welts, discoloration, or burns; absence of hair; dehydration and malnourishment without an illness-related cause; hesitation to talk openly; implausible stories; and unusual or inappropriate bank account activity.
- Reporting elder abuse
  - Caregivers who suspect abuse are expected to report their findings. Symptoms and conditions of suspected abuse should be defined clearly and objectively.
  - Signs of abuse should be accurately and thoroughly documented.
- Senior abuse is less likely to be reported than child abuse.
- Cases of elder abuse include:
  - Neglect
  - Physical abuse
  - Abusive search
  - Forcible administration of medications
  - Intimidation
  - Deficient care

4. *Look Closer, See ME*
- A poem close to many hearts and interpreted "don't see through the patient, see the patient you are treating."

TEST YOUR UNDERSTANDING

TERMINOLOGY

child abuse crime	patient abuse
good faith reporting	senior abuse

REVIEW QUESTIONS

1. What is patient abuse?

2. Discuss common signs of abuse for both children and seniors.

3. Describe what should a caregiver do when he or she suspects another unrelated person, caregiver or family member has been abusing a patient.

4. Discuss the importance of accurate and complete documentation of suspected abuse.

5. Describe what good-faith reporting means.

6. Discuss why patients are often reluctant to complain about their abusers and caregivers.

7. When a health care provider reports abuse, should the accuser's identity be revealed to the accused? Explain your answer.

8. Should caregivers be disciplined for reporting abuse if it proves to be false? Explain your answer.

9. Discuss the patient poem "Look Closer, See Me."

NOTES

1. Title 42 U.S. Code, Chapter 67 § 5119c (3).
2. http://www.acf.hhs.gov/sites/default/files/cb/cm2012.pdf
3. http://www.acf.hhs.gov/sites/default/files/cb/cm2012.pdf#page=11.
4. Title 42 U.S. Code, Chapter 67, Subchapter VI § 5119 (a).
5. N.Y. Soc. Serv. Law A4 419 (McKinney 1992).
6. N.Y. Soc. Serv. Law A4 420 (McKinney 1992).
7. N.Y. Soc. Serv. Law A4 420 (McKinney 1992).
8. 373 N.W.2d 204 (Mich. Ct. App. 1985).
9. http://www.apa.org/pi/aging/resources/guides/elder-abuse.aspx.
10. *Id.*
11. "Havens for elderly may expose them to deadly risks," *USA Today*, May 25, 2004, at 1.
12. http://www.gao.gov/new.items/d10434r.pdf.
13. *Id.*
14. *CBS New York/AP, February 11, 2014.* http://newyork.cbslocal.com/2014/02/11/9-arrested-in-l-i-nursing-home-probe-following-patients-death/.
15. http://www.thenewstribune.com/2014/01/10/2986582/a-welcome-emphasis-on-elder-abuse.html
16. Arthur Meirson, Prosecuting Elder Abuse: Setting the Gold Standard in the Golden State, 60 HASTINGS L.J. 431, 434 (2008).

17. http://www.nbcnews.com/id/41992299/ns/business-consumer_news/t/financial-abuse-costs-elderly-billions/#.U1eogcYgvG4.

18. http://www.newser.com/tag/18247/1/elder-abuse.html.

19. http://www.lawyersandsettlements.com/articles/financial-elder-abuse/interview-financial-elder-abuse-19203.html#.U1fuLcYgvG4.

20. *Suzannah Hills*, MailOnline, *August 23, 2013.* http://www.dailymail.co.uk/news/article-2400887/Jailed-Whipps-Cross-Hospital-carers-physically-verbally-abused-patients.html.

21. http://kansasstatutes.lesterama.org/Chapter_39/Article_14/.

22. *Greg Palmer*, WIBW.com, *April 22, 2014. The Associated Press*, The Kansas City Star, *April 22.* http://www.wibw.com/home/headlines/Kansas-Elder-Abuse-Measure-Becomes-Law-256157141.html.

23. http://ncea.aoa.gov/FAQ/Type_Abuse/#abandonment.

24. Richard J. Gelles, Murray A. Strauss, & Suzanne K. Steinmetz, *Behind Closed Doors: Violence in the American Family,* Anchor Press/Doubleday: Garden City, NY (1980).

25. *Id.*

26. Senate Subcommittee on Health and Long-Term Care, supra note 53.

27. 557 F. Supp. 289 (D. Colo. 1983).

28. *Id.* at 293.

29. *State v. Cunningham,* 493 N.W.2d 884 (Iowa Ct. App. 1992).

30. *Id.* at 887–888.

31. 551 A.2d 354 (Pa. Commw. Ct. 1988).

32. *Id.* at 355.

33. *Id.* at 357.

34. 501 N.Y.S.2d 997 (N.Y. Sup. Ct. 1986).

35. *Id.* at 1001.

36. *Id.*

37. 560 N.Y.S.2d 573 (N.Y. App. Div. 1990).

38. *Id.*

39. 178 Cal. Rptr. 564 (Cal. Ct. App. 1981).

40. 565 So. 2d 221, 224 (Ala. 1990).

41. *Id.* at 224.

42. *Id.* at 223–224.

43. *Id.* at 226.

44. Donna Fannin, "Your Granny's Nurses: Look Closer, See ME," Gather.com, May 16, 2006; http://www.gather.com/viewArticle.action?articleId=281474976752728.

Understanding the Role of and Conceptualizing Health Policy and Law

LEARNING OBJECTIVES

By the end of this chapter, you will be able to:

- Describe generally the important role played by policy and law in the health of individuals and populations
- Describe three ways to conceptualize health policy and law

INTRODUCTION

In this chapter, we introduce the role played by policy and law in the health of individuals and populations and describe three conceptual frameworks with which you can approach the study of health policy and law. Later, we narrow our focus, providing a measure of clarity in an area that is neither readily discernable—even to those who use and work in the health care and public health systems—nor easily redrawn by those who shape them through policy and law.

The goals of this chapter are to describe why it is important to include policy and law in the study of health care and public health and how you might conceptualize health policy and law when undertaking your studies. To achieve these goals, we first briefly discuss the vast influence of policy and law in health care and public health. You will have a much better feel for how far policy and law reach into these areas as you proceed, but we dedicate a few pages here to give you a sense of why it is critical to examine policy and lawmaking as part of your broader health studies. We then describe three ways to conceptualize health policy and law. As you will discover, the three conceptual frameworks are interwoven, with no one framework dominating the discussion.

ROLE OF POLICY AND LAW IN HEALTH CARE AND PUBLIC HEALTH

The forceful influence of policy and law on the health of individuals and populations is undeniable. Policy and law have always been fundamental in shaping the practice of individual health care in the United States and to achieving both everyday and landmark public health improvements.

Centuries-old legal principles have, since this country's inception, provided the bedrock on which healthcare quality laws are built, and today the healthcare industry is regulated in many different ways. Indeed, federal and state policy and law shape virtually all aspects of the healthcare system, from structure and organization, to service delivery, to financing, and to administrative and judicial oversight. Whether pertaining to the accreditation and certification of individual or institutional healthcare providers, requirements to provide care under certain circumstances, the creation of public insurance programs, the regulation of private insurance systems, or any other number of issues, policy and law drive the healthcare system to a degree unknown by most people.

In fact, professional digests that survey and report on the subjects of health policy and law typically include in their pages information on topics like the advertising and marketing of health services and products, the impact of health expenditures on federal and state budgets, antitrust concerns, healthcare contracting, employment issues, patents, taxation, healthcare discrimination and disparities, consumer protection, bioterrorism, health insurance, prescription drug regulation, physician-assisted suicide, biotechnology, human subject research, patient privacy and confidentiality, organ availability and donation, and more. Choices made by policymakers and decisions handed down through the legal system impact how we approach, experience, analyze, and research all of these and other specific aspects of the healthcare system.

Once you have read the next four preparatory chapters—one on policy and the policymaking process, one on law and the legal system, and one each covering the structure and organization of the healthcare and public health systems—and begin to digest the substantive chapters that follow them, the full force of policy and law in shaping the individual healthcare system will unfold. For now, simply keep in the back of your mind the fact that policy and law heavily influence the way in which health care is accessed, medicine is practiced, treatments are paid for, and much more.

The role of policy and law in public health is no less important than in individual health care, but the influence of policy and law in the field of public health is less frequently articulated. In fact, policy and law have long played a seminal role in everyday public health activities (think, for example, of food establishment inspections, occupational safety standards, policies related to health services for persons with chronic health conditions such as diabetes, and policies and laws affecting the extent to which public health agencies are able to gauge whether individuals in a community suffer from certain health conditions), as well as in many historic public health accomplishments such as water and air purification, reduction in the spread of communicable diseases through compulsory immunization laws, reduction in the number of automobile-related deaths through seatbelt and consumer safety laws, and several others.[a] Public health professionals and students quickly learn to appreciate that combating public health threats requires both vigorous policymaking and adequate legal powers. Additionally, in recent years, enhanced fears about bioterrorism and new and emerging infectious diseases have only increased the public's belief that policy and law are important tools in creating an environment in which people can achieve optimal health and safety.

Of course, policies and laws do not always cut in favor of what many people believe to be in the best interests of public health and welfare. A policy or law might, for example, favor the economic interests of a private, for-profit company over the residents of the community in which the company is located.[b] Why? Because one main focus of policy and law in the realm of public health is on locating the appropriate balance between public regulation of private individuals and corporations and the ability of those same parties to exercise rights that allow them to function free of overly intrusive government intervention. Achieving this balance is not easy for policymakers. Not all interested parties agree on things like the extent to which car makers should alter their operations to reduce environmentally harmful auto emissions, or the degree to which companies should be limited in advertising cigarettes, or whether gun manufacturers should be held liable in cases where injuries or killings result from the negligent use of their products.

How do policymakers and the legal system reach a (hopefully) satisfactory public health/private right balance? The competing interests at the heart of public health are mainly addressed through two types of policies and laws: those that define the functions and powers of public health agencies, and those that aim to directly protect and promote health.[c] State-level policymakers and public health officials create these types of policies and laws through what are known as their *police powers*. These powers represent the inherent authority of state and local governments to regulate individuals and private business in the name of public health promotion and protection. The importance of police powers cannot be overstated; it is fair to say that they are the most critical aspect of the sovereignty that states retained at the founding of the country, when the colonies agreed to a governmental structure consisting of a strong national government. Furthermore, the reach of police powers should not be underestimated, particularly since they permit public health authorities to coerce private interests to engage in (or refrain from) activities in the name of public health and welfare. However, states do not need to exercise their police powers in order to affect or engage in public health-related policymaking. Because the public's health is impacted by many social, economic, and environmental factors, public health agencies also conduct policy-relevant research, disseminate information aimed at helping people engage in healthy behaviors, and establish collaborative relationships with healthcare providers and purchasers and with other government policymaking agencies.

Federal policy and law also play a role in public health. Although the word "health" never appears in the U.S. Constitution, the document confers powers on the federal government—to tax and spend, for example—that allow it to engage in public health promotion and disease prevention activities. For example, the power to tax (or establish exemptions from taxation) allows Congress to incentivize healthy behaviors, as witnessed by the heavy taxes levied on packages of cigarettes; the power to spend enables Congress to establish executive branch public health agencies and to allocate public health-specific funds to states and localities.

CONCEPTUALIZING HEALTH POLICY AND LAW

You have just read about the importance of taking policy and law into account when studying health care and public health. The next step is to begin thinking about how you might conceptually approach the study of health policy and law.

There are multiple ways to conceptualize the many important topics that fall under the umbrella of health policy and law. We introduce three conceptual frameworks in this section: one premised on the broad topical domains of health policy and law, one based on prevailing historical factors, and one focused on the individuals and entities impacted by a particular policy or legal determination (see Box 1).

BOX 1 Three Conceptual Frameworks for Studying Health Policy and Law

Framework 1. Study based on the broad TOPICAL DOMAINS of:

a. Health care

b. Public health

c. Bioethics

Framework 2. Study based on HISTORICALLY DOMINANT SOCIAL, POLITICAL, AND ECONOMIC PERSPECTIVES:

a. Professional autonomy

b. Social contract

c. Free market

Framework 3. Study based on the perspectives of KEY STAKEHOLDERS:

a. Individuals

b. The public

c. Healthcare professionals

d. Federal and state governments

e. Managed care and traditional insurance companies

f. Employers

g. The pharmaceutical industry

h. The research community

i. Interest groups

j. Others

We draw on these frameworks to various degrees in this text. For example, the topical domain approach of Framework 1 is on display in the sections about individual rights in health care and public health and healthcare quality policy and law. Framework 2's focus on historical perspectives is highlighted in the health reform section and the government health insurance programs section. Finally, Framework 3, which approaches the study of health policy and law from the perspectives of key stakeholders, is discussed in the policy and the policymaking process section. We turn now to a description of each framework.

The Three Broad Topical Domains of Health Policy and Law

One way to conceptualize health policy and law is as consisting of three large topical domains. One domain is reserved for policy and law concerns in the area of *healthcare*, another for issues arising in the *public health* arena, and the last for controversies in the field of *bioethics*. As you contemplate these topical domains, bear in mind that they are not individual silos whose contents never spill over into the others. Indeed, this sort of spillage is common (and, as noted, is one reason why fixing health policy problems can be terribly complicated). We briefly touch on each domain below.

Health Care Policy and Law

In the most general sense, this domain is concerned with an individual's access to care (e.g., what policies and laws impact an individual's ability to access needed care?), the quality of the care the person received (e.g., was it appropriate, cost-effective, and non-negligent?), and how the person's care is going to be financed (e.g., is the person insured?). However, "access," "quality," and "financing" are themselves rather large sub-domains, with their own sets of complex policy and legal issues, and in fact it is common for students to take semester-long policy and/or law courses focused on just one of these sub-domains.

Public Health Policy and Law

The second large topical domain is that of public health policy and law. A central focus here is on why and how the government regulates private individuals and corporations in the name of protecting the health, safety, and welfare of the general public. Imagine, for example, that the federal government was considering a blanket policy decision to vaccinate individuals across the country against the deadly smallpox disease, believing that the decision was in the best interests of national security. Would this decision be desirable from a national policy perspective? Would it be legal? If the program's desirability and legality are not immediately clear, how would you go about analyzing and assessing them? These are the kinds of questions with which public health policy and law practitioners and scholars grapple.

Bioethics

Finally, there is the *bioethics* domain to health policy and law. Strictly speaking, the term "bioethics" is used to describe ethical issues raised in the context of medical practice or biomedical research. More comprehensively, bioethics can be thought of as the point at which public policy, law, individual morals, societal values, and medicine intersect. The bioethics domain houses some of the most explosive questions in health policy, including the morality and legality of abortion, conflicting values around the meaning of death and the rights of individuals nearing the end of life, and the policy and legal consequences of mapping the human genetic code.

Social, Political, and Economic Historical Context

Dividing the substance of health policy and law into broad topical categories is only one way to conceptualize them. A second way to consider health policy and law is in historical terms, based on the social, political, and economic views that dominate a particular era.[d] Considered this way, health policy and law have been influenced over time by three perspectives, all of which are technically active at any given time, but each of which has eclipsed the others during specific periods in terms of political, policy, and legal outcomes. These perspectives are termed *professional autonomy*, *social contract*, and *free market*.[e]

Professional Autonomy Perspective

The first perspective, grounded in the notion that the medical profession should have the authority to regulate itself, held sway from approximately 1880 to 1960, making it the most dominant of the three perspectives in terms of both the length of time it held favored status and its effect in the actual shaping of health policy and law. This model is premised on the idea that physicians' scientific expertise in medical matters should translate into legal authority to oversee essentially all aspects of delivering health care to individuals—in other words, according to proponents of the physician autonomy model, legal oversight of the practice of medicine should be delegated to the medical profession itself. While this perspective remained dominant, policy- and lawmakers were generally willing to allow physicians to control the terms and amount of payments

for rendered healthcare services, the standards under which medical licenses would be granted, the types of patients they would treat, the type and amount of information to disclose to patients, and the determination as to whether their colleagues in the medical profession were negligent in the treatment of their patients.

Social Contract Perspective

The second perspective that informs a historical conceptualization of health policy and law is that of the "modestly egalitarian social contract."[f] This paradigm overshadowed its competitors, and thus guided policy decision making, from roughly 1960 to 1980, a time notable in U.S. history for social progressiveness, civil rights, and racial inclusion. At the center of this perspective is the belief that complete physician autonomy over the delivery and financing of health care is potentially dangerous in terms of patient care and healthcare expenditures, and that public policy and law can and sometimes should enforce a "social contract" at the expense of physician control. Put differently, this perspective sees physicians as just one of several stakeholders (including but not limited to patients, employers, and society) that lay claim to important rights and interests in the operation of the healthcare system. Health policies and laws borne of the social contract era centered on enhancing access to health care (e.g., through the Examination and Treatment for Emergency Medical Conditions and Women in Labor Act), creating new health insurance programs (Medicare and Medicaid were established in 1965), and passing anti-discrimination laws (one of the specific purposes of Title VI of the federal 1964 Civil Rights Act was wiping out healthcare discrimination based on race).

Free Market Perspective

The final historical perspective—grounded in the twin notions of the freedom of the marketplace and of market competition—became dominant in the 1990s and continues with force today. It contends that the markets for healthcare services and for health insurance operate best in a deregulated environment, and that commercial competition and consumer empowerment will lead to the most efficient healthcare system. Regardless of the validity of this claim, this perspective argues that the physician autonomy model is falsely premised on the idea of scientific expertise, when in fact most healthcare services deemed "necessary" by physicians have never been subjected to rigorous scientific validation (think of the typical treatments for the common cold or a broken leg). It further argues that even the modest version of the social contract that heavily influenced health policy and law during the civil rights generation is overly regulatory. Furthermore, market competition proponents claim that both other models are potentially inflationary, since in the first case self-interest will lead autonomous physicians to drive up the cost of their services, and in the second instance public insurance programs like Medicare would lead individuals to seek unnecessary care.

To tie a couple of these historical perspectives together and examine (albeit in somewhat oversimplified fashion) how evolving social and economic mores have influenced health policy and law, consider the example of Medicaid, the joint federal–state health insurance program for low-income individuals. In 1965, Medicaid was borne out of the prevailing societal mood that it was an important role of government to expand legal expectations among the poor and needy. Its creation exemplified a social contract perspective, which in the context of health promotes the view that individuals and society as a whole are important stakeholders in the healthcare and public health systems. Medicaid entitled eligible individuals to a set of benefits which, according to courts during the era under consideration, was the type of legal entitlement that could be enforced by beneficiaries when they believed their rights under the program were infringed.

These societal expectations and legal rights and protections withstood early challenges during the 1970s, as the costs associated with providing services under Medicaid resulted in state efforts to roll back program benefits. Then, in the 1980s, Medicaid costs soared higher, as eligibility reforms nearly doubled the program's enrollment and some providers (e.g., community health centers) were given higher payments for the Medicaid services they provided. Still, the social contract perspective held firm, and the program retained its essential egalitarian features.

As noted above, however, the gravitational pull of the social contract theory weakened as the 1980s drew to a close. This, coupled with the fact that Medicaid spending continued to increase in the 1990s, led to an increase in the number of calls to terminate program members' legal entitlement to benefits.[g] Also in the 1990s, federal and state policymakers dramatically increased the role of private managed care companies in both Medicaid and Medicare, an example of the trend toward free market principles described above.

Key Stakeholders

A third way to conceptualize health policy and law issues is in terms of the stakeholders whose interests are impacted by certain policy choices or by the passage or interpretation of a law. For example, imagine that in the context of interpreting a state statute regulating physician licensing, your state's highest court ruled that it was permissible for a physician to not treat a patient even though the doctor had been serving as the patient's family physician. What stakeholders could be impacted by this result? Certainly the patient, and other patients whose treatment may be colored by the court's decision. Obviously the doctor, and other doctors practicing in the same state, could be impacted by the court's conclusion. What about the state legislature? Perhaps it unintentionally drafted the licensing statute in ambiguous fashion, which led the court to determine that the law conferred no legal responsibility on the physician to respond to a member of a family that was part of the doctor's patient load. Or maybe the legislature is implicated in another way—maybe it drafted the law with such clarity that no other outcome was likely to result, but the citizenry of the state was outraged because its elected officials have created public policy out of step with constituents' values. Note how this last example draws in the perspective of another key stakeholder—the broader public.

Of course, patients, healthcare providers, governments, and the public are not the only key stakeholders in important matters of health policy and law. Managed care and traditional insurance companies, employers, the pharmaceutical industry, the medical device industry, the research community, interest groups, and others all may have a strong interest in various policies or laws under debate.

CONCLUSION

The above descriptions of the roles played by policy and law in the health of individuals and populations, and of the ways to conceptualize health policy and law, were cursory by design. But what we hope is apparent to you at this early stage is the fact that the study of policy and law is essential to the study of both health care and public health. Consider the short list of major problems with the U.S. health system as described in a 2005 book edited and written by a group of leading scholars: the coverage and financing of health care, healthcare quality, health disparities, and threats to population health.[h] All of the responses and fixes to these problems—and to many other healthcare- and public health-related concerns—will invariably and necessarily involve creative policymaking and rigorous legal reform (and indeed, the 2010 Patient Protection and Affordable Care Act, about which you will read in various sections, addressed each of these topics to one degree or another). This fact is neither surprising nor undesirable: Policy and law have long been used to effectuate positive social change. Since the founding of this country, the fields of health care and public health have experienced this phenomenon, and given the many serious problems playing out in these arenas right now, there is little reason to expect that policy and law will not be two of the primary drivers of health-related reform in the years ahead.

Policy and legal considerations are not only relevant in the context of major healthcare and public health problems going forward, however—they are critical to the daily functioning of the health system, and to the health and safety of individuals and communities across a range of everyday life events. Consider pregnancy and childbirth, for example. There are approximately 11,000 births each day in this country, and society views pregnancy and childbirth as more or less normal and unremarkable events. In fact, the process of becoming pregnant, accessing and receiving high-quality prenatal health care, and experiencing a successful delivery is crucial not only to the physical, mental, and emotional health and well-being of individuals and families, but to the long-term economic and social health of the nation. It also implicates a dizzying number of interesting and important policy questions. Consider the following:

- Should there be a legal right to health care in the context of pregnancy and, if so, should that right begin at the point of planning to get pregnant, at the moment of conception, at the point of labor, or at some other point?
- Regardless of legal rights to care, how should the nation finance the cost of pregnancy care? Should individuals and families be expected to save enough money to pay out-of-pocket for what is a predictable event? Should the government help subsidize the cost of prenatal care? If so, in what way? Should care be subsidized at the same rate for everyone, or should subsidy levels be based on financial need?
- Regarding the quality of care, what is known about the type of obstetrical care women should receive, and how do we know they are getting that care? Given the importance of this type of care, what policy steps are taken to assure that the care is sound? What should the law's response be when a newborn or pregnant woman is harmed through an act of negligence? When should clinician errors be considered preventable and their commission thus tied to a public policy response? And what should the response be?
- What should the legal and social response be to prospective parents who act in ways risky to the health of a fetus? Should there be no societal response because the prospective parents' actions are purely a matter of

individual right? Does it depend on what the actions are?
- Is it important to track pregnancy and birth rates through public health surveillance systems? Why or why not? If it is an important function, should the data tracking be made compulsory or voluntary?
- How well does the public health system control known risks to pregnancies, both in communities and in the workplace?
- Finally, who should answer these questions? The federal government? States? Individuals? Should courts play a role in answering some or all of them and, if so, which ones? Whose interests are implicated in each question, and how do these stakeholders affect the policymaking process?

There are scores of topics—pregnancy and childbirth among them—that implicate a range of complex health policy questions, and these are the types of questions this text prepares you to ask and address. Before you turn your attention to the essential principles, components, and issues of health policy and law, however, you must understand something about policy and law generally, and about the organization and purposes of the healthcare and public health systems. The next two chapters provide a grounding in policy and law and supply the basic information needed to study policy and law in a health context. There, we define policy and law; discuss the political and legal systems; introduce the administrative agencies and functions at the heart of the government's role in health care and public health; and more. With this information at your disposal, you will be better equipped to think through some of the threshold questions common to many policy debates, including: which sector—public, private, or not-for-profit (or some combination of them)—should respond to the policy problem?; if government responds, at what level—federal or state—should the problem be addressed?; what branch of government is best-suited to address—or more attuned to—the policy issue?; when the government takes the lead in responding to a policy concern, what is the appropriate role of the private and not-for-profit sectors in also attacking the problem?; and what legal barriers might there be to the type of policy change being contemplated? Once you have the knowledge to be able to critically assess these types of questions, you will be able to focus more specifically on how the healthcare and public health systems operate in the United States, and on the application of policy and law to critical issues in health care and public health.

ENDNOTES

a. See, e.g., Wendy E. Parmet, "Introduction: The Interdependency of Law and Public Health," in *Law in Public Health Practice*, eds. Richard A. Goodman et al. (Oxford, England: Oxford University Press, 2003).

b. For a non-fictional and utterly engrossing example of the ways in which law and legal process might stand in the way of effective public health regulation, we recommend Jonathan Harr, *A Civil Action* (New York, NY: Vintage Books, 1995).

c. See, e.g., Larry O. Gostin, Jeffrey P. Koplan, and Frank P. Grad, "The Law and the Public's Health: The Foundations," in *Law in Public Health Practice*, eds. Richard A. Goodman et al. (Oxford, England: Oxford University Press, 2003).

d. The particular historical framework described here was developed to apply to health care, rather than public health. We do not mean to imply, however, that it is impossible to consider public health from an historical, or evolutionary, vantage point. In fact, it is fair to say that public health practice may have just entered its third historical phase. Throughout the 1800s and most of the 1900s, protection of the public's health occurred mainly through direct regulation of private behavior. In the latter stages of the 20th century, strict reliance on regulation gave way to an approach that combined regulation with chronic disease management and public health promotion, an approach that necessitated a more active collaboration between public health agencies and healthcare providers and purchasers. Now, it appears that public health professionals are adding to this revised practice model another strategic initiative: building collaborative relationships with policymaking agencies whose responsibilities are not directly related to public health—for example, agencies whose primary fields are transportation or agriculture.

e. The discussion of these perspectives is guided by Rand E. Rosenblatt, Sylvia A. Law, and Sara Rosenbaum, *Law and the American Health Care System* (Westbury, CT: The Foundation Press, Inc., 1997), 24–35; and Rand E. Rosenblatt, "The Four Ages of Health Law," *Health Matrix: Journal of Law-Medicine*. 2004;14:15.

f. Rand E. Rosenblatt, Sylvia A. Law, and Sara Rosenbaum, *Law and the American Health Care System*, 2. The authors write that the American social contract lags behind those of other developed countries, and thus use the phrase "modestly egalitarian" in describing it.

g. By 2005, proponents of weakening Medicaid-enrolled persons' entitlement to program benefits had made significant strides: Congress passed a law called the Deficit Reduction Act that, among other things, granted states the ability to redefine the benefits and services to which Medicaid beneficiaries are entitled.

h. David Mechanic, Lynn B. Rogut, David C. Colby, and James R. Knickman, eds., *Policy Challenges in Modern Health Care* (New Brunswick, NY: Rutgers University Press, 2005), 10.

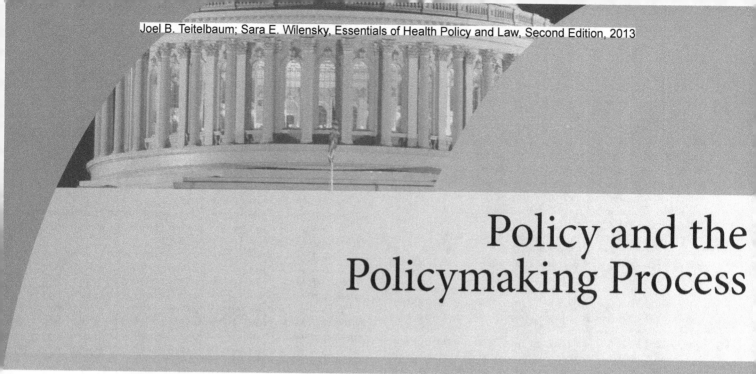

Policy and the Policymaking Process

LEARNING OBJECTIVES

By the end of this chapter, you will be able to:

- Describe the concepts of policy and policymaking
- Describe the basic function, structure, and powers of the legislative branch of government
- Describe the basic function, structure, and powers of the executive branch of government
- Explain the role of federal and state governments in the policymaking process
- Explain the role of interest groups in the policymaking process

INTRODUCTION

The first steps for any student of health policy are to understand what policy is generally and to learn about the policymaking process. It is vital to consider policy questions in the particular context in which they arise, both in terms of the general politics of the issue and the values and powers of the policymaker. As you will discover, there is no single definition of policy. Even so, this chapter arms you with the information needed to know what issues to consider when thinking about a public policy problem, how to account for a variety of competing policy views, and what policy options are possible given the political process in the United States.

The chapter first defines what policy is and then moves to a discussion of the policymaking process by examining the roles and powers of two of the political branches of government—the legislative and executive branches. As part of this discussion, we introduce you to federal and state agencies

that make up the healthcare and public health bureaucracy. We conclude with a discussion about the roles of interest groups in policymaking and the influence they wield in the policymaking process.

DEFINING POLICY

In this section we consider various aspects of what we mean by the term *policy*. Before delving into the policymaking process, we identify which issues fall within the realm of a public policy decision and, generally, what kinds of decisions might be made by policymakers.

Identifying Public Problems

Scholars have defined policy in many different ways. Consider a few of them:

> Authoritative decisions made in the legislative, executive, or judicial branches of government that are intended to direct or influence the actions, behaviors, and decisions of others.[1(p243)]

> A course of action adopted and pursued by a government, party, statesman, or other individual or organization.[2(p124)]

> Authoritative decisions and guidelines that direct human behavior toward specific goals either in the private or the public sector.[3(p125)]

The differences in these definitions raise several important issues. The first question to consider is whether private actors make policy or whether policymaking is an activity for the government only. The first definition refers only to governmental policymakers, the second definition allows for both public and private policymakers, and the third definition is unclear on this issue. Of course, the government is a key player in any policy field, and it is certainly true that decisions by government entities represent public policy. However, in this text we also focus on private actors who make policy, such as commercial insurance companies, private employers, influential individuals, and others who can all be part of health policy. For example, when a major health insurance company decides to cover obesity prevention measures, or when the Bill and Melinda Gates Foundation provides grants to develop crops that are high in essential vitamins and minerals to improve the nutrition of people in developing countries, they are making health policy decisions.

Regardless of whether the policymaker is a public or private figure, it is necessary that the decision being made is an *authoritative* decision. These are decisions made by an individual or group with the power to implement the decision, and there are a variety of levels where these kinds of decisions can take place. For example, within government, authoritative decisions may be made by the president, cabinet officials, agency heads, members of Congress, governors, state legislatures, public health commissioners, and many others.

But all decisions by public and private individuals or entities are not necessarily policy decisions. The key issue to determining whether a "decision" represents a "policy" is whether the question at hand is an individual concern or a public policy problem. A public policy problem goes beyond the individual sphere and affects the greater community. Whereas an individual might decide to take advantage of employer-sponsored health insurance, a public policy question is whether all employers should be required to offer health insurance to their employees. Whereas an individual might decide to purchase a generic (as opposed to a brand name) drug to save money, a public policy question is whether patients should be induced to buy less expensive generic drugs. When deciding whether something is a public policy decision, the focus is not only on who is making a decision, but also on what kind of decision is being made.

Furthermore, just because a problem is identified as a public policy problem does not necessarily mean the only solution involves government intervention. For example, consider the problem of an influenza vaccine shortage. Although there are government-oriented solutions to this problem, such as expanding public research and development or creating production incentives (through tax cuts or subsidies) to encourage private manufacturers to produce more vaccine, other solutions may rely solely on private actors. Private companies may decide to invest in the research and development of new ways to produce vaccines, or to build new plants to increase production capacity, because they believe they can make a profit in the long run. Just as private individuals and entities can make policy decisions for their own benefit, they can also play a central role in solving public policy problems. A lengthier discussion about options for solving public policy problems and arguments for and against government intervention is found in a review of health economics.

Structuring Policy Options

Considered broadly, there are different ways to approach public policy problems. For example, some policy options are voluntary, whereas others are mandatory. It is important to recognize that authoritative decisions do not always *require* others to act or refrain from acting in a certain way. Some of the most important and effective policies are those that provide incentives to others to change their behavior. Indeed, the power of persuasion is very important to public officials, particularly at the federal level, which is limited in its ability to force states and individuals to take certain actions. This stems from the fact that the 10th Amendment of the U.S. Constitution limits Congress and the executive branch to specific powers and reserves all other powers for the states. However, members of the federal government may use their enumerated powers, such as those to tax and spend, to persuade states and others to act in desired ways.

For example, the Constitution does not give the legislative or executive branches the power to protect the public's health, meaning that the area is primarily within the purview of states to regulate. As a result, Congress and the president cannot require states to create emergency preparedness plans. Yet, Congress may provide incentives to states to do so by offering them federal money in return for state preparedness plans that meet certain criteria established by the federal government.

In addition, it is important to remember that inaction can also be a policy decision. Deciding to do nothing may be a decision to keep a prior decision in place or not to engage in a new issue. For example, a governor could decide against trying to change a restrictive abortion law or a state legislature could choose not to pass a law expanding the allowable scope of practice for nurse practitioners. Both of these inactions result in important policy decisions that will affect the choices and opportunities available to individuals, advocacy organizations, and others.

This brief discussion about policy has raised several important issues to consider when identifying policy options. The next section provides a detailed discussion of the policymaking process, providing you with the background knowledge necessary to identify and understand the roles and powers of various policymakers.

PUBLIC POLICYMAKING STRUCTURE AND PROCESS

The public policymaking structure refers to the various branches of government and the individuals and entities within each branch that play a role in making and implementing policy decisions. In this section, we review the structure, powers, and constituency of these branches, with a focus on the U.S. House of Representatives, the U.S. Senate, and various commissions and agencies that assist Congress, the president, White House staff, and federal executive branch administrative agencies. In addition to reviewing the policymaking structure, we discuss the processes used by these various individuals and entities for making public policy decisions.

State-Level Policymaking

The federal government does not have a monopoly on policymaking. Indeed, important policy decisions are regularly made at the state level as well, especially in the healthcare arena. However, because state governments are similar to the federal government in many ways, the policymaking duties and powers that we discuss below can often be applied to a state-level analysis. At the same time, there is a significant amount of variation in how states structure their legislative and executive branches, agencies, and offices, and it is not possible to review the differences that exist among all 50 states. Accordingly, after a brief discussion of state-level policymaking, this chapter focuses primarily on the federal policymaking structure and process.

Like the federal government, each state has three branches of government. State legislatures pass laws, appropriate money within the state, and conduct oversight of state programs and agencies. States also have their own judiciary with trial and appellate courts. The governor is the head of the state executive branch and can set policy, appoint cabinet members, and use state administrative agencies to issue regulations that implement state laws. Although there are limits to a state's power to regulate healthcare issues, state regulation is an extremely important aspect of health policy. Just a few examples of the healthcare matters states can regulate include provider licensing, accreditation, some aspects of health insurance, and most public health concerns.

At the same time, it is also important to realize that all state governments are not exactly alike. The governor has more power in some states than others, agencies are combined in different ways among the states, state legislatures may meet annually or biannually, state legislators may be full-time or part-time employees, and so on. Because these differences exist, it is essential for policy analysts to understand the specific structure of the state in which their client resides.

Furthermore, there are important differences between the federal government and the states. Unlike the federal government, almost all states are required to have a balanced budget, and most states cannot borrow money for operating expenses. These rules mean that states must act to raise revenue or cut programs if they project that their budget will be in deficit by the end of the fiscal year. In addition, in 2008, 30 states had at least one tax and expenditure limit rule that restricts the growth of government revenues or spending to a fixed numerical target, sometimes using changes in population level or the inflation rate as guideposts. In addition, 16 states require a legislative supermajority or voter approval to raise taxes (a supermajority means that more than a simple majority—over 50%—is required; for example, a two-thirds majority vote could be required).[4] As a result, state officials may be more likely than federal officials to make the difficult choice to either limit programs or cut resources from one program to fund another.

As is evident from this brief discussion, state level policymaking is both a rich area for discussion and a difficult area to make generalizations about because each state is unique. Having highlighted some of the key differences and similarities among the states and between the states and the federal government, we now turn to the legislative and executive branches of the federal government.

The Federal Legislative Branch

Article 1 of the U.S. Constitution makes Congress the lawmaking body of the federal government by granting it "All legislative Powers" and the right to enact "necessary and proper laws" to effectuate its prerogatives.[5] Congressional responsibilities are fulfilled by the two chambers of Congress, the Senate and the House of Representatives ("the House"). The Constitution grants specific powers to Congress, including but not limited to the power to levy taxes, collect revenue, pay debts, provide for the general welfare, regulate interstate and foreign commerce, establish federal courts inferior to the Supreme Court, and declare war.[6] The Senate has the specific power to ratify treaties and confirm nominations of public officials.

The Senate consists of two elected officials from each state, for a total of 100 senators.[a] Each senator is elected in a statewide vote for a six-year term, whereas representatives in the House sit for two-year terms. Due to the lengthy term of its members, the Senate is considered less volatile and more concerned with long-term issues than the House. A senator must be at least 30 years old, a U.S. citizen for at least nine years, and a resident of the state he or she is seeking to represent.[7]

The House includes 435 members allocated proportionally based on the population of the 50 states, with each state guaranteed at least one representative.[b] For example, in 2010, California was allotted 53 representatives, while Vermont had only 1. Due to the proportionality rule, members from larger states dominate the House and often hold leadership positions.[8] Members of the House are elected by voters in congressional districts and serve two-year terms. They must be at least 25 years old, a U.S. citizen for at least seven years, and a resident of the state where the election takes place.[9]

Leadership Positions

Leadership roles in Congress are determined by political party affiliation, with the party in the majority gaining many advantages. The vice president of the United States is also the president of the Senate and presides over its proceedings. In the vice president's absence, which is common given the other obligations of the office, the president pro tempore, a mostly ceremonial position, presides over the Senate. In most cases the vice president is not a major player in Senate voting, but with the power to break a tie vote, the vice president wields an important power. The Speaker of the House ("Speaker") presides over that chamber and has the authority to prioritize and schedule bills, refer bills to committees, and name members of joint and conference committees. Other than the vice president's senatorial role, leadership positions in Congress are not elected by the voters, but determined by the members from the party who have been elected to Congress. Other key Congressional leadership positions include:

Senate majority leader—Speaks on behalf of the majority party, schedules floor action and bills, works on committees, directs strategy, and tries to keep the party united.

House majority leader—Works with the Speaker to direct party strategy and set the legislative schedule.

House and senate minority leaders—Speak on behalf of the minority party, direct strategy, and try to maintain party unity; as members of the minority, they do not have the legislative duties of the majority leader/Speaker.

House and senate majority and minority whips—Track important legislation, mobilize members to support leadership positions, keep a count of how party members are planning to vote, and generally assist their leaders in managing their party's legislative priorities.

Committees

Committees have been referred to as the "workhorses" of Congress; they are where many key decisions are made and legislative drafting takes place. Given the vast array of issues that Congress contends with in any given legislative session, it is impossible for every member to develop expertise on every issue. Although members vote on bills that cover a wide range of issues, members often concentrate on the areas relevant to the committees on which they serve.

Committees have a variety of important roles, including drafting and amending legislation; educating members on key issues; shepherding the committee's legislation on the floor when it goes before a vote by all the members of one chamber; working with the president, his administration, and lobbyists to gain support for a bill; holding hearings; and conducting oversight of executive branch departments, agencies, commissions, and programs within their purview. Committee members often gain expertise in the areas covered by their committees, and other members often rely on their advice when making voting decisions.

Standing committees are generally permanent committees with specified duties and powers. There are 20 standing committees in the House and 17 in the Senate. House committees tend to be larger than those in the Senate, with about 40 members per committee. Some committees have *authorization* jurisdiction, allowing them to create programs and agencies. Other committees have *appropriation* authority, meaning they are responsible for funding various programs and agencies. Standing committees also have *oversight* authority, meaning they monitor how programs are run and funds are spent. Each chamber of Congress has established specific oversight committees for some programs and issues that cut across committee jurisdiction, as well as committees that review the efficiency and economy of government actions.[10(pp2–3)]

Not surprisingly, some of the most powerful and popular committees are those that deal with appropriating money. These include:

House Ways and Means and Senate Finance committees—These committees have jurisdiction over legislation concerning taxes, tariffs, and other revenue-generating measures, and over entitlement programs such as Medicare and Social Security. The Constitution requires all taxation and appropriations bills to originate in the House, and House rules require all tax bills to go through the Ways and Means committee.

House and Senate Appropriations committees—These committees have responsibility for writing federal spending bills.

House and Senate Budget committees—These committees are tasked with creating the overall budget plan that helps guide tax and appropriation committee work.

House Rules committee—This committee has jurisdiction over the rules and order of business in the House, including rules for the floor debates, amendments, and voting procedures. Unlike in the Senate, all House bills must go to the House Rules committee before reaching the House floor for a vote by all representatives.

Table 1 identifies the key health committees and subcommittees and their health-related jurisdictions.

Congressional Commissions and Staff Agencies

Although the committee system helps members of Congress focus on particular areas, members often need assistance with in-depth research and policy analysis. Commissions and staff agencies provide members with information they might not otherwise have the time to gather and analyze. There are too

TABLE 1 Key Health Committees and Subcommittees

Senate Committee	Health-Related Jurisdiction
Finance Committee: Subcommittee on Health Care	Department of Health and Human Services • Centers for Medicare and Medicaid Services (Medicare, Medicaid, State Children's Health Insurance Program) • Administration for Children and Families Department of the Treasury • Group health plans under the Employee Retirement Income Security Act
Appropriations Committee: Subcommittee on Labor, Health and Human Services, Education and Related Agencies	Department of Health and Human Services • Office of Public Health Service • National Institutes of Health • Centers for Disease Control and Prevention • Health Resources and Services Administration • Substance Abuse and Mental Health Services Administration • Agency for Healthcare Research and Quality Occupational Safety and Health Review Commission Social Security Administration
Appropriations Committee: Subcommittee on Agriculture, Rural Development and Related Services	Department of Health and Human Services Food and Drug Administration
Appropriations Committee: Subcommittee on Interior, Environment and Related Agencies	Department of Health and Human Services • Indian Health Services • Agency for Toxic Substances and Disease Registry
Health, Education, Labor, and Pensions Committee: Subcommittee on Public Health	Bioterrorism and Public Health Preparedness Department of Health and Human Services • Food and Drug Administration • Centers for Disease Control and Prevention • National Institutes of Health • Administration on Aging • Substance Abuse and Mental Health Services Administration • Agency for Healthcare Research and Quality
Committee on Agriculture, Nutrition and Forestry: Subcommittee on Research, Nutrition and General Legislation	• Food stamps • National school lunch program • School breakfast program • Special milk program for children • Special supplemental nutrition program for women, infants and children (WIC)

(Continues)

TABLE 1 Key Health Committees and Subcommittees *(Continued)*

House Committee	Health-Related Jurisdiction
Committee on Ways and Means: Subcommittee on Health	Social Security Act • Maternal and Child Health block grant • Medicare • Medicaid • Peer review of utilization and quality control of health care organizations
Appropriations Committee: Subcommittee on Labor, Health and Human Services, Education and Related Agencies	Department of Health and Human Services • Office of Public Health Service • National Institutes of Health • Centers for Disease Control and Prevention • Health Resources and Services Administration • Substance Abuse and Mental Health Services Administration • Agency for Healthcare Research and Quality Occupational Safety and Health Review Commission Social Security Administration
Appropriations Committee: Subcommittee on Agriculture, Rural Development and Related Services	Department of Health and Human Services • Food and Drug Administration
Appropriations Committee: Subcommittee on Interior, Environment and Related Agencies	Department of Health and Human Service • Indian Health Services • Agency for Toxic Substances and Disease Registry
Energy and Commerce Committee: Subcommittee on Health	Department of Health and Human Services • Medicaid

many commissions and agencies to list here, but a few key ones include:

Congressional Budget Office—Provides Congress with cost estimates of bills and federal mandates to state and local governments, as well as forecasts economic trends and spending levels.

Government Accountability Office—An independent, nonpartisan agency that studies how federal tax dollars are spent and advises Congress and executive agencies about more efficient and effective ways to use federal resources.

Congressional Research Service—The public policy research service that conducts nonpartisan, objective research on legislative issues.

Medicare Payment Advisory Commission—An independent federal commission that gives Congress advice on issues relating to the Medicare program, including payment, access to care, and quality of care.

How Laws Are Made

One way that members of Congress indicate their policy preferences is by passing laws that embody their values and the values of their constituents. This is a lengthy process, with many steps along the way that could derail a bill (see Figure 1).

Before a committee considers a bill, it must be introduced by a member of Congress. Once this occurs, the Speaker refers the bill to one or more committees in the House, and the majority leader does the same in the Senate. The bill may die in committee if there is not sufficient support for it, although there are rarely invoked procedures that allow a bill to be reported to the full chamber even without committee approval. While the bill is in committee, members may hold hearings on it or "mark up" the bill by changing or deleting language in the proposed bill or by adding amendments to it. If a majority of the committee members approves a bill, it goes to the full chamber (House or Senate, depending on where the bill originated).

The full House or Senate then debates the merits of the bill and puts it to a vote. If a majority does not support the bill, it dies on the chamber floor. If a majority supports the bill, it is sent to the other chamber for consideration. The second chamber may pass the exact same bill or a different version of the bill. If the second chamber does not pass any version of the bill, it dies on the chamber floor and no version of the bill moves forward. If the second chamber passes an identical bill, it goes directly to the president for consideration.

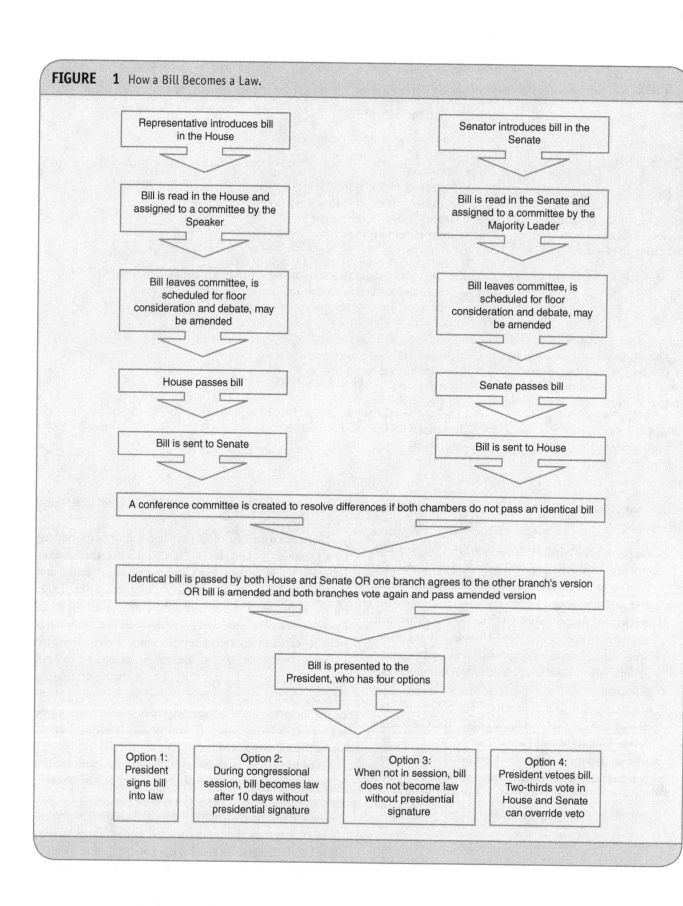

FIGURE 1 How a Bill Becomes a Law.

Representative introduces bill in the House

Bill is read in the House and assigned to a committee by the Speaker

Bill leaves committee, is scheduled for floor consideration and debate, may be amended

House passes bill

Bill is sent to Senate

Senator introduces bill in the Senate

Bill is read in the Senate and assigned to a committee by the Majority Leader

Bill leaves committee, is scheduled for floor consideration and debate, may be amended

Senate passes bill

Bill is sent to House

A conference committee is created to resolve differences if both chambers do not pass an identical bill

Identical bill is passed by both House and Senate OR one branch agrees to the other branch's version OR bill is amended and both branches vote again and pass amended version

Bill is presented to the President, who has four options

Option 1:
President signs bill into law

Option 2:
During congressional session, bill becomes law after 10 days without presidential signature

Option 3:
When not in session, bill does not become law without presidential signature

Option 4:
President vetoes bill. Two-thirds vote in House and Senate can override veto

If there are differences in the bills passed by the House and Senate, the two chambers must reach a consensus through an exchange of amendments for the bill to have a chance of becoming law. Consensus building is facilitated by a "conference committee" made up of members from both chambers. If the committee cannot reach a consensus, the bill dies. If the committee reaches a consensus, the bill is sent back to each chamber for a vote on the new version of the bill. If either chamber does not approve of it, the bill dies at that point. If both the House and the Senate pass the new version, it is sent to the president for consideration.

The president may choose to sign the bill into law, or the president may choose to veto the bill. If the president chooses not to sign the bill while Congress is in session, the bill becomes law after 10 days; if Congress is not in session and the bill goes unsigned, the bill dies (this is referred to as a "pocket veto"). If the president vetoes the bill, Congress may override the veto with approval of a two-thirds majority in each chamber.

Congressional Budget and Appropriations Process[11,12]

Although the budget and appropriation processes may sound dry, it is about much more than numbers and charts. If you take a close look at budget documents, they include narratives that discuss why certain programs are being funded and what the government hopes to achieve by doing so. In many ways, this process is a key policy tool for members of Congress and the president; they are able to show which programs and issues have their support through their funding decisions.

Given both the amount of money involved in running the United States (over $3 trillion in 2011) and the various jurisdictions of congressional committees, it is not surprising that the federal budget process is fairly complex. The Congressional Budget and Impoundment Control Act of 1974 ("Budget Act") and subsequent amendments were passed by Congress to create a process that brings together the numerous committees involved in crafting an overall budget plan. The budget process works in concert with the appropriations process, which involves congressional passage of bills from each of the appropriations committees to distribute the funds provided for in the overall budget.

The president is required to submit a budget proposal to Congress by the first Monday in February. This proposal is the administration's request; it is not binding on Congress. Each chamber then passes a *budget resolution*, identifying how the chamber would spend federal money delineated by different categories of spending (e.g., defense, agriculture,

transportation). Members from each chamber then meet to develop a single *conference report* reflecting a consensus agreement on the overall budget. Congress then passes a *concurrent budget resolution*, which is binding upon the House and Senate as a blueprint for revenue collection and spending. However, it is not a law and the president is not bound by the budget resolution.

Over the six weeks subsequent to the passage of the concurrent budget resolution, the House and Senate budget committees hold hearings to discuss the budget, and other committees review the budget as it pertains to their jurisdiction. The latter committees provide the budget committees with their "views and estimates" of appropriate spending and/or revenue levels for the upcoming year. In addition, the Congressional Budget Office provides the budget committees with its budget and economic outlook reports and provides the budget and appropriations committees with its analysis of the president's proposal.

In March, the House and Senate budget committees each craft a budget plan during public meetings known as "markups." When the markups are complete, each committee sends a budget resolution to its respective chamber. The budget resolution contains a budget total, spending breakdown, reconciliation instructions, budget enforcement mechanisms, and statements of budget policy. Budget totals are provided as aggregates and as committee allocations.

The federal budget includes two types of spending: *discretionary* and *mandatory*. Discretionary spending refers to money that is set aside for programs that must be funded annually in order to continue—if the programs are not funded by Congress, they will not receive federal dollars to continue their operations. For example, the Head Start program, which provides early childhood education services, is a discretionary program that relies on annual appropriations. Mandatory spending refers to spending on entitlement and other programs that must be funded as a matter of law. For example, the Medicaid program is an entitlement that provides health insurance to eligible low-income individuals. The *authorizing legislation* (the law that created the program) for Medicaid includes eligibility rules and benefits. Because Medicaid is an entitlement program, Congress must provide enough money so the Medicaid agency can meet the obligations found in the authorizing legislation.

The appropriations committees write bills to cover discretionary spending. These committees make their decisions based on the amount of funds available and any *reconciliation instructions*, which direct the appropriate authorizing committee to make changes in the law for mandatory spending programs to meet budgetary goals. Appropriations bills and reconciliation instructions must be signed by the president to become law.

Members of the House and Senate have the opportunity to make changes to the work of the budget committees. Once the House and Senate pass their own versions of the budget resolution, they establish a conference committee to resolve any differences. Once the differences are resolved, each full chamber votes on the compromise budget.

Congress often does not meet Budget Act deadlines (shown in Table 2). If the appropriations bills are not passed by every October 1—the beginning of the fiscal year—Congress may pass a *continuing resolution* that allows the government to continue to spend money. If Congress does not pass a continuing resolution or if the president vetoes it, all nonessential activities of federal agencies must stop until additional funds are provided.

Constituents

With the wide array of issues they take on, members of Congress may have an equally wide array of constituents to be concerned about when making policy decisions. Clearly, members are concerned about pleasing the voters who elect them. Even though there may be a variety of policy views to consider, members often prioritize their home constituents. In addition to courting their home-state voters, members often try to court independents or voters from the opposing party in their home state to strengthen their appeal. High approval

ratings deter challengers from trying to take an incumbent's congressional seat and allow members of Congress more leeway to pursue their goals and policies.

Although concern for their home-state base may be their first priority, representatives and senators often need to be concerned about supporting their party's position on issues. Today, elected federal politicians are usually affiliated with the Democratic or Republican Party, and voters may be influenced by the party's stance on issues. Also, if the balance of power between the two parties is close in Congress, the parties usually cannot afford to have members defect from their party's positions. Members' concern regarding keeping their party strong is magnified if they hold leadership positions in Congress or are considering running for national office.

Finally, the views of the president may be important for members to consider, depending on whether the member and the president share the same party, the particular issue involved, and the president's popularity. Members who are in the same party as the sitting president have incentive to help the president remain popular because they will likely advance many of the same policies. In addition, presidents are often prodigious fundraisers and campaigners who may be able to assist members during election season. Even when members disagree with the president, the president's power to affect their influence in Congress may be a deterrent to opposing the president. Of course, if the president is exceedingly popular, it is difficult for members of either party to oppose presidential policy goals.

TABLE 2 Federal Budget Process Timeline	
First Monday in February	President submits budget proposal to Congress.
March	House completes its budget resolution.
April	Senate completes its budget resolution.
April 15	House and Senate complete concurrent budget resolution.
May	Authorizing committees develop reconciliation language when necessary and report legislation to budget committees. House and Senate develop conference report on reconciliation, which is voted on by each chamber.
June 10	House concludes reporting annual House appropriations bills.
June 15	If necessary, Congress completes reconciliation legislation.
June 30	House completes its appropriations bills.
September 30	Senate completes its appropriations bills. House and Senate complete appropriations conference reports and vote separately on the final bills.
October 1	Fiscal year begins.

Source: Adapted from House Committee on the Budget Majority Caucus, Basics of the Budget Process. 107th Cong. Briefing Paper. 2001.

The Federal Executive Branch

Article 2 of the U.S. Constitution establishes the executive branch and vests executive power in the most well-known member of the branch, the president.[13] Of course, the president does not act alone in running the executive branch. Presidents rely on Executive Office agencies and staff such as the Council of Economic Advisors and Office of Management and Budget, as well as policy development offices such as the National Security Council and Domestic Policy Council (see Box 1 for a description of one such office). In addition, there are 15 cabinet departments led by individuals selected by the president (subject to Senate confirmation) and additional non cabinet-level agencies, all of which are responsible for, among other duties, interpreting and implementing the laws passed by Congress. All of these advisors identify issues to be addressed and formulate policy options for the president to consider. In theory, all of these parts of the executive branch work in furtherance of the goals set by the president.

The Presidency

The president is the head of the federal executive branch. As powerful as that may sound, the country's founders created three distinct branches of government and limited the president's power in order to ensure that no single individual gained too much control over the nation. As you will see, in some ways the president is very powerful, and in other ways his power is quite limited.

Although there have been third-party candidates for president in the past, generally speaking our country now operates on a two-party system, with the Democratic and Republican Parties as the major parties. Each party selects a candidate for president who represents the party in the election. Presidents (and their vice presidents) are elected through a nationwide vote to serve a four-year term. An individual is limited to serving two four-year terms as president, which may or may not be consecutive.[14,c] To be eligible for election, candidates must be at least 35 years old, a natural-born citizen of the United States, and a resident of the country for at least 14 years.

Presidents have many roles. As the unofficial *Chief of State*, the president is seen as the symbol of the country and its citizens.[15(p40)] As the official *Chief Executive Officer*, the president manages the cabinet and executive branch. The president also holds the position of *Commander in Chief of the Armed Forces*, and as such is the top ranking military official in the country. The U.S. Constitution vests the president with other powers, such as the ability to appoint judges to the federal courts, sign treaties with foreign nations, and appoint ambassadors as liaisons to other countries. These powers are all subject to the advice and consent of the Senate.[15(p41)]

Agenda Setting   A key tool of the presidency is the ability to put issues on the national agenda and offer a recommended course of action: "[F]raming agendas is what the presidency is all about."[16(p371)] Presidents help set the national agenda because of the role of the president as the country's leader and the amount of media attention given to presidential actions, decisions, and policy recommendations. Unlike many other politicians or interest groups, the president does not have to work hard to receive media coverage. Whether it is the annual State of the Union address, release of the president's budget proposal, a major speech, a press conference, a photo shoot with a foreign leader, or the release of a report, the president's message is continually publicized. In addition, the president's message can be delivered by the vice president, cabinet officers, and party leaders in Congress.

The notion of appealing directly to the country's citizens to focus on a particular issue and to influence legislative debates is referred to as "going public." In going public, presidents try to use support from the American people to gain the attention of Congress and sway votes on policy decisions. Because members of Congress are highly concerned about pleasing their constituency to improve their chance for re-election, "the president seeks the aid of a third party—the public—to force other politicians to accept his preferences."[17(p3)]

BOX 1   Office of Management and Budget (OMB)

The Office of Management and Budget (OMB) reports directly to the president and plays an important role in policy decisions. OMB is responsible for preparing the presidential budget proposal, which includes reviewing agency requests, coordinating agency requests with presidential priorities, working with Congress to draft appropriation and authorization bills, and working with agencies to make budget cuts when needed. In addition to these budgetary functions, OMB provides an estimate of the cost of regulations, approves agency requests to collect information, plays a role in coordinating domestic policy, and may act as a political intermediary on behalf of the president. OMB also has an oversight and evaluation function over select federal agencies as a result of the Government Performance and Results Act, which requires agencies to set performance goals and have their performance evaluated.

Sometimes it may be advantageous for the president to place an item on the policy agenda in a less public manner. For example, if a policy is controversial with the general public or if members of the president's party disagree with a proposal, it may be more effective to promote a policy behind the scenes. The president, either directly or through intermediaries, can carefully let members of Congress know which policies are favored. Using combinations of promises of favors and threats to members' interests, the president may be able to influence the outcome of policy debates in Congress even without going public.

In addition to deciding whether to approach Congress publicly or behind the scenes, the president must choose whether to present a preferred policy decision with more or less detail. A policy can be presented broadly through principles or general guidelines, or specifically through proposed legislation that is presented to Congress. Each method for conveying the president's goals has pros and cons. If a policy choice is presented in a broad manner, Congress may interpret the policy in a way that the president dislikes. However, if the president presents Congress with a specific proposal or draft legislation, Congressional members may view the president as infringing upon their role as the legislative body and resist working with him.

Whether presidents are successful in placing policy issues on the national agenda and having them resolved in accordance with their preferences depends in part on how much "political capital" a president has available. Political capital is defined as the strength of the president's popularity and of his party, in Congress and in other contexts. Members of Congress are more likely to support a popular president who has the ability to mobilize the public's support, improve members' standing by association with the president and the president's party, and raise money for their campaigns.

Even the most popular president cannot always dictate what issues are on the national agenda, however. Events and decisions outside the president's control often influence what topics most concern the nation. The terrorist attacks of September 11, 2001, the subsequent anthrax scare, and the subway and bus bombings in London and Madrid all served to place combating terrorism at the top of the policy and political agenda during the George W. Bush Administration. Concerns about an avian flu epidemic and numerous food recalls put public health and food safety issues on the national agenda. The devastation wrought by the BP oil spill in the Gulf of Mexico made improved responses to environmental disasters a high priority for a short time. Recently, however, all other issues have been dwarfed by concerns about the federal deficit, high unemployment, and a lagging economy. Thus, even the most popular presidents must be responsive to national and international events that may be beyond their control.

Presidential Powers   As noted earlier, if Congress passes legislation the president dislikes, he has the power to veto it, thereby rejecting the bill. However, the president does not have to actually use the veto to shape policy. The president may be able to persuade Congress to change a piece of legislation simply by threatening to veto it, especially if it is a law that is only expected to pass by a slim majority. In general, vetoes are used infrequently, with presidents vetoing only 3% of all legislation since George Washington was president.[15(p43)]

Presidents also have the power to issue executive orders. These are legally binding orders that the president gives to federal administrative agencies under the control of the Executive Office. In general, these orders are used to direct federal agencies and their officials in how they implement specific laws. Executive orders are controversial because under our system of government, Congress, not the executive, is tasked with making laws. In addition, significant policy decisions can be accomplished by using executive orders. For example, an executive order was used by President Truman to integrate the armed forces, by President Eisenhower to desegregate schools, by President Clinton to designate 1.7 million acres in southern Utah as a national monument, and by President George W. Bush to create the federal Office of Homeland Security (which subsequently became a cabinet-level department when Congress established it through legislation).

If Congress believes an executive order is contrary to congressional intent, it has two avenues of recourse. It can amend the law at issue to clarify its intent and effectively stamp out the executive order that is now clearly contrary to the law. (Bear in mind that because the president may veto any bill, in effect it takes a two-thirds majority of Congress to override an executive order.) As an alternative, Congress may challenge the executive order in court, claiming that the president's actions exceed his constitutional powers.

Constituents   From this description of the presidency, it is evident that presidents have several layers of constituents to consider when making policy choices. Certainly, the president represents every citizen and the country as a whole as the only nationally elected official (along with the vice president) in the nation. However, the president is also a representative of a particular political party and therefore must consider the views of that party when making policies. The party's views may be evident from the party platform, policies supported by party leadership in Congress, and voters who identify themselves as party members. In addition, the president must keep in mind the foreign policy duties of the office. Depending on the issue, it may be important for the president to take into account the views of other nations or international organizations, such as the United Nations or the World Health Organization.

How does the president decide which policies to pursue? Presidents are driven by multiple goals. They want "their policies to be adopted, they want the policies they put in place to last, and they want to feel they helped solve the problems facing the country."[4(p82)] In addition, presidents often speak of wanting to leave a legacy or ensure their place in history when they leave office.

Given the vast array of constituents that presidents must consider, the president's policy decision-making process involves several layers. As shown in Figure 2, presidents consult their agency staff to identify problems, decide which problems are priorities, determine what solutions are available to address those problems, and choose the policy option that is the preferred course of action. In addition, the president's staff interacts with members of Congress and other political players to gauge their support for or opposition to various policies. Of course, how the media portrays both problems and potential solutions can be an important ingredient in whether politicians and the general public support the president's initiatives.

In addition, which policies presidents choose to promote may depend in part on when policy decisions are made. First-term presidents must satisfy their constituents if they hope to be re-elected. Although all presidents want to see their favored policies implemented throughout their time in office, second-term presidents may be more willing to support more controversial goals because they cannot run for re-election. Yet, second-term presidents may also be constrained by the desire to keep their party in power, even though another individual will hold the presidential office.

Administrative Agencies

When studying the structure of our government, it is common to review Congress, the presidency, and the court system. Administrative agencies, however, are often overlooked despite the power they wield over the way our country is run.

Structurally, almost all administrative agencies are part of the executive branch, and thus under the power and control of the president. Practically, administrative agencies often work out of the public's eye to implement the laws passed by Congress and the executive orders signed by the president.

Federal agencies fall into two main categories: executive department agencies and independent agencies. Executive department agencies are under the direct control of the

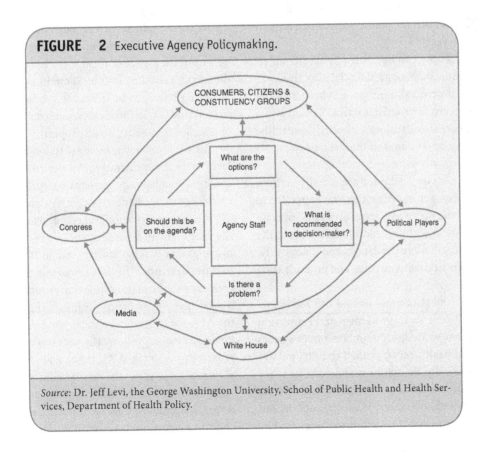

FIGURE 2 Executive Agency Policymaking.

Source: Dr. Jeff Levi, the George Washington University, School of Public Health and Health Services, Department of Health Policy.

president, and department heads serve at the pleasure of the president. These departments include the 15 cabinet-level departments and their subunits; some of the more well-known executive departments are the Department of Health and Human Services, the Department of Education, the Treasury Department, the Department of State, the Department of Defense, and the Department of Homeland Security. Independent agency heads are appointed by the president and confirmed by the Senate. They serve a fixed term and may only be removed "for cause," meaning there must be a legitimate reason to fire them. Examples of independent agencies include the Securities and Exchange Commission, the U.S. Postal Service, and the National Labor Relations Board.

Overall, the president fills approximately 2,400 federal jobs.[4(p160)] In general, these political appointees have short tenures, lasting an average of two years.[4(p161)] When the administration changes hands after an election, new appointees are usually selected to run the agencies. The daily operations of agencies are run by career civil servants, public employees who do not necessarily come and go with each administration but who often remain at an agency for years, gaining expertise and institutional knowledge about the agencies in which they work. Frequently, there may be tension between the goals of the political appointee and those of the career bureaucrat, who may have the advantage of familiarity with members of Congress and who knows that the political appointee is likely to be replaced in a few years.

Administrative agencies can be created by statute, internal department reorganization, or presidential directive.[15(p50)] However they are initially created, agencies must have statutory authority in order to receive appropriations from Congress and act with the force of law. This statutory authority, or enabling statute, outlines the agency's responsibilities and powers.

Agency Powers　By necessity, statutes are usually written broadly. Congress does not have the time or expertise to include every detail about how a new program should operate or how a new department will be structured. It is up to the executive branch agency to fill in the details, and it does so by issuing policy statements, developing rules, and promulgating regulations.

For example, in 2001, Congress passed the Medicare, Medicaid, and SCHIP Benefits Improvement and Protection Act, which included a new Medicaid reimbursement system for federally qualified health centers called the Prospective Payment System.[18] Basically, the statute mandated that every health center calculate a baseline per-visit cost that was the average of their 1999 and 2000 costs. Under the act, health center reimbursement rates would be determined each year by the baseline rate plus an inflationary factor called the Medicare Economic Index, adjusted to account for any increase or decrease in a health center's change in scope of service. That was all the statute said. It was up to the Center for Medicare and Medicaid Services (CMS), the federal agency in charge of the Medicaid program, to work out the details. CMS had the choice of issuing regulations, policy notices, information sheets, or the like to flesh out the broadly worded statute.

Many questions were left unresolved by the statute. For example, if the center opened in 2000, how would its baseline be calculated? What if there was an extraordinary event in 1999 or 2000, like a hurricane, that severely damaged a health center—would that affect the baseline calculation? What does a change of scope of service mean? Does it count as a change in scope of service if the health center adds a few dentists to its current dental practice, or would it have to add a new service in order to trigger the statutory definition? Who determines whether a change in scope of service occurred? The health center? The state Medicaid agency? The regional Medicaid office? CMS? As you can imagine, the list of questions that results from broadly written statutes is almost endless. Agencies are usually the ones that provide the answers.

Promulgating regulations is the most important and powerful role of agencies. Agency regulations have the force of law and must be obeyed, just as one obeys a law passed by the legislative branch. Yet, an agency's power to create rules and regulations is not unlimited. The thing being regulated must be within the power of the agency to regulate, as defined by the agency's enabling statute. Sometimes it is not clear whether an agency has acted in an area that is beyond the scope of its authorizing law. In those cases, a court may be the final arbiter of whether the agency acted properly.

In addition, agencies must follow the requirements set forth in the Administrative Procedure Act (APA).[19] The APA contains detailed requirements compelling agencies to issue a notice of their intent to issue a new rule or change an existing rule, and provide for and respond to public comments on the proposed rule. Some agencies are also required to hold hearings and develop rules based on the evidence presented in those hearings.[4(p172)] It is important to know that the APA creates procedural standards that require an agency to follow a particular *process* when promulgating regulations, but that the APA does not relate to the *substance* of the regulations. As long as an agency follows the necessary notice and comment requirements of the APA, it has wide latitude to issue rules within its scope of power, even if many of the public comments opposed the proposed rules. If an agency does not follow the APA requirements, interested parties may sue the agency in court to force compliance with the law.

Constituents Agency heads, since they are not elected, do not have constituents in the same way that the president and members of Congress do. In theory, as members of the executive branch, agency heads should only be concerned with the wishes of the president. In reality, however, that is not always the case. Some presidents have firmer control of their departments than others. If the president gives the departments and agencies broad discretion to make policy decisions, the agencies may have few policy constraints. Practically, however, agency heads want their operation to run smoothly, which includes having a good working relationship with the individuals or entities regulated by that agency. If an agency antagonizes the people or groups being regulated, they might reach out to their congressional representatives to try to change or limit the agency's personnel or authority. In addition, because Congress appropriates funds to and maintains oversight of many agencies, agency heads are well served by taking Congress' interests into account.

Table 3 summarizes the general public policymaking machinery. We next turn our attention to the specific parts of the government bureaucracy that operate in the health arena.

THE HEALTH BUREAUCRACY

The Federal Government

Although several federal agencies have health-related responsibilities, the three most significant health agencies are the Department of Health and Human Services (HHS), the Department of Defense (DOD), and the Department of Veterans Affairs (VA). HHS houses many of the major public health insurance programs and health services that provide care, information, and more to millions of U.S. residents; the DoD and VA operate health insurance programs specifically for military personnel and their families.

Department of Health and Human Services

HHS includes hundreds of programs that cover activities as varied as medical and social science research, preschool education services, substance abuse and prevention services, and health insurance programs, just to name a few. As shown in Figure 3, the department has 11 operating divisions. The main purpose of each agency is described in Table 4.

Each operating division has numerous bureaus or divisions that operate health programs. For example, the HIV/AIDS Bureau (HAB) is one of six bureaus in HRSA. The HIV/AIDs Bureau implements the Ryan White CARE Act,[20] which provides health care to individuals with HIV and AIDS. Similarly, the FDA has eight offices or centers; the one whose job is perhaps most well-known to the general public is the Center for Drug Evaluation and Research, which is responsible for testing and approving new drugs before they can be sold to the public. These are just two examples of the many sub-agency units that perform vital functions in our federal health care bureaucracy.

HHS also includes numerous offices that assist the Secretary of HHS in running the department. The Assistant Secretary of Health is the principal advisor to the HHS secretary on public health matters. This individual oversees the U.S. Public Health Service (PHS), the Commissioned Corps (health professionals used for both emergency responses and as health promoters), and the Office of Public Health and Sciences (OPHS). PHS employs both commissioned corps members and civilians to run its public health programs.

TABLE 3 Summary of Public Policymaking Entities

	Congress	President	Administrative Agencies
Main Function	Legislative body	Chief executive of the country	Implement statutes through rulemaking
Main Tools/Powers	Support/oppose legislation Appropriations Oversight	Agenda setting Persuasion Propose solutions Budget proposals Executive orders	Create regulations Provide information
Constituents	Voters in state or district Voters in nation if in leadership role or have national aspirations Party President	Nation (all voters) Public who voted for the president Party Other nations International organizations	President Congress Individuals and entities regulated or served by the agency

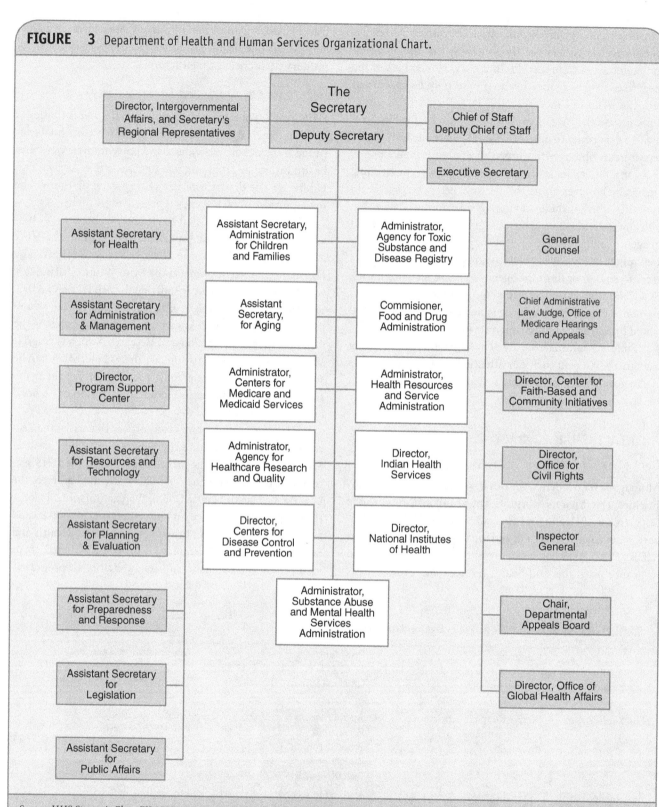

FIGURE 3 Department of Health and Human Services Organizational Chart.

Source: HHS Strategic Plan, FY 2007–2012. Appendix F: Operating and staff divisions and their functions. U.S. Department of Health and Human Services website. Available at http://aspe.hhs.gov/hhsplan/2007/hhasplanpdf/hhsplanappE.pdf. Accessed July 25, 2011.

TABLE 4 Department of Health and Human Services Agencies

Agency	Main Purpose of Agency
Administration for Children and Families (ACF)	To promote economic and social well-being of families, children, individuals, and communities.
Administration on Aging (AoA)	To promote the dignity and independence of older people, and to help society prepare for an aging population.
Agency for Healthcare Research and Quality (AHRQ)	To support, conduct, and disseminate research that improves access to care and the outcomes, quality, cost, and utilization of healthcare services.
Agency for Toxic Substances and Disease Registry (ATSDR)	To serve the public by using the best science, taking responsive public health actions, and providing trusted health information to prevent harmful exposure and diseases related to toxic substances.
Centers for Disease Control and Prevention (CDC)	To promote health and quality of life, by preventing and controlling disease, injury, and disability.
Center for Medicare and Medicaid Services (CMS)	To ensure effective, up-to-date healthcare coverage and to promote quality of care for beneficiaries.
Food and Drug Administration (FDA)	To rigorously assure the safety, efficacy, and security of human and veterinary drugs, biological products, and medical devices, and assure the safety and security of the Nation's food supply, cosmetics, and products that emit radiation.
Health Resources and Services Administration (HRSA)	To provide the national leadership, program resources, and services needed to improve access to culturally competent, quality health care.
Indian Health Service (IHS)	To raise the physical, mental, social, and spiritual health of American Indians and Alaska Natives to the highest level.
National Institutes of Health (NIH)	To employ science in pursuit of fundamental knowledge about the nature and behavior of living systems and the application of that knowledge to extend healthy life and reduce the burdens of illness and disability.
Substance Abuse and Mental Health Services Administration (SAMHSA)	To build resilience and facilitate recovery for people with or at risk for substance abuse and mental illness.

Source: HHS Strategic Plan, FY 2007–2012. Appendix F: Operating and staff divisions and their functions. U.S. Department of Health and Human Services website. Available at http://aspe.hhs.gov/hhsplan/2007/hhsplanpdf/hhsplanappE.pdf. Accessed July 25, 2011.

PHS employees also work in the Bureau of Prisons, U.S. Coast Guard, National Oceanic and Atmospheric Administration, Environmental Protection Agency, Division of Immigration Health Services, and U.S. Marshal Services. OPHS consists of 11 offices, including the Office of the Surgeon General, Office of Population Affairs, and Office of Minority Health.

HHS also has divisions concerned with planning and evaluation, legislation, administration and management, budget and finance, program support, public affairs, and global health affairs. In 2001, President George W. Bush created the Center for Faith-Based and Community Initiatives, which strives to increase participation by faith-based community organizations in providing health and human services.[21] Offices concerned with the legality and efficiency of the department's activities include those of the General Counsel and Inspector General, and the Office of Civil Rights.

As a result of the recent focus on preventing terrorism, HHS includes an Assistant Secretary for Preparedness and Response. This individual is the principal advisor to the Secretary of HHS on matters relating to bioterrorism and other public health emergencies, and helps coordinate efforts in these areas at all levels of government. Other federal departments also have a role in public health emergency preparedness. The Department of Homeland Security (DHS), which includes the Federal Emergency Management Agency (FEMA), is tasked with preparing for and coordinating the federal response to emergencies, whether due to natural or man-made disasters. The CDC houses the Strategic National

Stockpile of emergency pharmaceutical supplies. Other agencies, such as the Environmental Protection Agency (EPA), DoD, and VA, play significant roles in emergency preparedness and response.

Department of Veterans Affairs and Department of Defense

Any veteran who does not receive a dishonorable discharge is potentially eligible for healthcare services through the Veterans Health Administration (VHA). The VHA is the largest healthcare delivery system in the country, with hundreds of medical centers, nursing homes, and outpatient clinics that serve over 1 million patients each year.[22(p357)]

VHA-sponsored health plans offer a wide array of preventive, ambulatory, and hospital services as well as medications and medical and surgical supplies. VHA providers are organized into integrated networks aimed at providing cost-effective services based on local need. There are no premiums (monthly payments) for the plan, but veterans have to make co-payments (a charge per visit) unless they are exempt based on disability or income level. Unlike most healthcare plans, the VHA system is completely portable, meaning that veterans can access VHA facilities anywhere in the country.

Veterans who wish to receive care through the VHA must enroll in the program. Because the VHA receives an annual appropriation from Congress, it may not have sufficient funds to pay for all of the care demanded by eligible veterans. For that reason, the VHA uses a priority system to ensure that veterans who are low-income or have service-related disabilities can be enrolled into a plan. Other veterans may have to wait to be enrolled if there are insufficient funds. In addition, priority in accessing care is given to enrolled veterans who need care for service-related disabilities or have a sufficiently severe service-related disability and need care for any health concern. Veterans not in a priority group may have to wait to see an appropriate provider once they are enrolled.

Although veterans may receive care through VHA, they are not required to do so. If eligible, they may choose to obtain services through other public or private healthcare programs or health insurance plans. They may also choose to receive some services through VHA and others from non-VHA programs or plans.

The VHA does not provide coverage to veterans' family members, but the DoD does through its TRICARE program. TRICARE provides healthcare services to current and retired military personnel and their families. TRICARE offers a variety of plans with various eligibility requirements and costs to the patient.

State and Local Governments

As discussed earlier, the Constitution gives states primary responsibility for protecting the public's health. States have health-related agencies that deal with health financing, aging, behavioral health, environmental health, children and family services, veterans, facility licensing and standards, provider credentialing, and more. Although all states have agencies that generally cover the same functions, their structure, responsibilities, and lines of authority vary greatly.

With the variation among state agencies, it is not surprising that there are significant differences across the states in terms of their approach to public health and health services needs. All states have agencies to run their Medicaid and SCHIP programs, as well as other state-specific health services programs. Although a review of enabling statutes and mission statements found that only one-fifth of states address most of the concepts identified by PHS as essential public health functions, most states cover the traditional public health tasks such as surveillance, investigation, and education.[23(p154)]

Local public health agencies (LPHA) carry out the public health functions of the state. Most commonly, LPHAs are formed, managed by, and report to a local government, such as a county commission or local board of health. This structure provides LPHAs with significant latitude to interpret and implement state statutes. In some states, the state and local governments jointly oversee the LPHA.

LPHAs may provide services directly or, as is increasingly common, may contract or provide support to others who perform the services. The services provided by LPHAs vary considerably, though there is an emphasis on addressing communicable diseases, environmental health, and children's health issues. LPHAs often provide services such as immunizations, community assessments, epidemiology and surveillance, food safety and inspections, and tuberculosis testing. Some, but not all, also provide diabetes care, glaucoma screening, substance abuse treatment, mental health services, and more.[23(pp160–161)]

INTEREST GROUPS

Before leaving the discussion of policy, the policymaking process, and the health bureaucracy, we must say a few words about interest groups. *Interest group* is a general term used for a wide variety of organizations that are created around a particular issue or population and have the goal of influencing policy and educating others about their views and concerns.[4(p117)] Interest groups are different from most of the other stakeholders that have been discussed because interest groups do not have the power to make policy. Although members of the executive and legislative branches of government have a key role in determining which policies are adopted, interest groups have the limited, but still significant, role of trying to influence the decisions of policymakers.

There are many types of interest groups, including trade associations, think tanks, advocacy groups, and lobbying firms. A few examples include the Pharmaceutical Research and Manufacturers of America, whose mission is to "conduct effective advocacy for public policies that encourage discovery of important new medicines for patients by pharmaceutical/biotechnology research companies"[24]; the National Association of Public Hospitals, which has as its goal to "provide national, regional and local advocacy on behalf of public and other hospitals and health systems, conduct research and analysis, and provide a host of related services needed by our members"[25]; the Center for Budget and Policy Priorities, which "conducts research and analysis to help shape public debates over proposed budget and tax policies and to help ensure that policymakers consider the needs of low-income families and individuals . . . in these debates"[26]; the AARP, which is "dedicated to enhancing quality of life for all as we age . . . through information, advocacy and service"[27]; and the Heritage Foundation, which has as its goal to "formulate and promote conservative public policies based on the principles of free enterprise, limited government, individual freedom, traditional American values, and a strong national defense."[28]

Just as members of Congress do not have the time or ability to become experts in every issue that comes before them, the same is true for the average citizen. Many people do not have the time and ability to learn about all of the issues that are important to them, develop proposals, rally public support for their positions, monitor current activity, lobby to add or remove issues from the agenda, and reach out to politicians who make policy decisions. Instead, interest groups take on those duties: "Their job is to make the case for their constituents before government, plying the halls of Congress, the executive branch, the courts, and the offices of other interest groups to provide a linkage between citizens and government."[4(p119)]

Interest Group Powers

Interest groups do not have the power to pass laws. However, they can influence policy in a variety of ways throughout the policymaking process. For example, recall all the steps it takes for a bill to become a law. Anywhere along that continuum is an opportunity for interest groups to make their case. The first step for interest groups is often to commission research that they use to support their position. This can be most important in the early stages of policy development, when politicians might have an open mind about various proposals.[4(p131)] However, it does not matter how much information a group has if it is not able to gain access to the decision makers. Even a few minutes with a politician may be a few more minutes than the opposition has to make its case directly to a decision maker.[4(p131)] Finally, interest groups need to develop a persuasive argument, a way to frame the issue that convinces politicians to agree with their view of a policy matter.

Interest groups have a variety of tools at their disposal when developing strategies for lobbying. They may initiate a *grassroots* campaign, asking their members to contact their representatives with a particular message. Because interest group members are the voters with the power to re-elect public officials, strong grassroots campaigns can be quite effective. Or, they may try a *grasstops* strategy and harness the influence of community leaders and other prominent individuals,[4(p139)] or, they may join with other interest groups to create coalitions and strengthen their influence through numbers. Interest groups may start a media campaign to align public sentiment with their goals. Of course, providing candidates with money, often through political action committees, is a time-honored way to try to influence the outcome of policy debates.

Whatever methodology they use, interest groups are an important part of the policymaking process. One researcher has called interest groups an "indispensable" part of making policy decisions.[29(p85)] They provide a way to give a voice to their members, who may not otherwise feel able to participate effectively in the policymaking process.

CONCLUSION

This journey through the policymaking process in the United States was intended to provide you with an understanding of policy and a context for your discussions and analysis of health policy issues. It is vital that you become familiar with both the nature of policy and the institutions that make and influence policy. As you have seen, the definition of policy is subject to much debate, yet it is necessary to define what policy means before attempting to engage in policy analysis. We have also walked through the specific duties and powers of the executive and legislative branches of the federal government and included key points about state-level policymaking as well. Finally, all policy students must be aware of and understand the influence of interest groups. They have and use numerous opportunities to influence the policymaking process, and their strength and concerns must be accounted for when analyzing policy issues. As you move further into health policy study, use the information provided in this overview to help you think about and frame your own policy positions.

REFERENCES

1. Longest BB Jr. *Health Policy Making in the United States.* 2nd ed. Chicago, IL: Health Administration Press; 1998.

2. Subcommittee on Health and Environment of the Committee on Interstate Commerce, U.S. House of Representatives. *A Discursive Dictionary of Health Care.* Washington, DC: GPO; 1976.

3. Hanley BE. Policy development and analysis. In: Leavitt JK, Mason DJ, Chaffee MW, eds. *Policy and Politics in Nursing and Health Care.* 3rd ed. Philadelphia, PA: WB Saunders; 1998:125–138.

4. Weissert CS, Weissert WG. *Governing Health: The Politics of Health Policy.* 2nd ed. Baltimore, MD: Johns Hopkins University Press; 2002.

5. U.S. Const. art. 1, § 1; U.S. Const. art. 1, § 8.

6. U.S. Const. art. 1, § 1.

7. U.S. Const. art. 1, § 3.

8. U.S. Const. art. 1, § 3.

9. U.S. Const. art. 1, § 2.

10. Schneider J. The committee system in the U.S. Congress. *Congressional Research Service.* Washington, DC: Library of Congress; 2003.

11. Senate Committee on the Budget. *The Congressional Budget Process: An Explanation.* 105th Cong., 2nd sess. Committee Print 67; 1998.

12. House Committee on the Budget Majority Caucus. *Basics of the Budget Process.* 107th Cong. Briefing Paper; 2001.

13. U.S. Const., art. 2, § 1.

14. U.S. Const., amend. XXII, §1.

15. Committee on House Administration. *Our American Government.* House Concurrent Res. 221. 106th Cong., 2nd sess.; 2000. H. Doc. 216.

16. Davidson RH. The presidency and the Congress. In: Nelson M, ed. *The Presidency and the Political System.* Washington, DC: Congressional Quarterly Press; 1984.

17. Kernell S. *Going Public: New Strategies of Presidential Leadership.* 3rd ed. Washington, DC: CQ Press; 1997.

18. Publ L No. 106-554, relevant sections codified at 42 U.S.C. § 1396a(a).

19. 5 U.S.C. §500.

20. Ryan White Comprehensive AIDS Resources Emergency Act of 1990, amended in 1996 and 2000, 42 U.S.C 300ff.

21. Executive Order No. 13198, *Code of Federal Regulations*, title 3, sec. 750–752 (2002).

22. Sultz HA, Young KM. *Health Care USA: Understanding Its Organization and Delivery.* 3rd ed. Gaithersburg, MD: Aspen; 2001.

23. Turnock BJ. *Public Health: What It Is and How It Works.* 3rd ed. Sudbury, MA: Jones and Bartlett; 2004.

24. Pharmaceutical Research and Manufacturing Association. *About pharma.* Available at http://www.phrma.org/about/about-phrma. Accessed July 25, 2011.

25. National Association of Public Hospitals. *About NAPH.* Available at http://www.naph.org/Main-Menu-Category/About-NAPH/NAPH-Mission.aspx. Accessed July 25, 2011.

26. Center for Budget and Policy Priorities. *About us.* Available at http://www.cbpp.org/about/. Accessed July 25, 2011.

27. American Association of Retired Persons. *Overview.* Available at http://www.aarp.org. Accessed July 25, 2011.

28. The Heritage Foundation. *About Heritage.* Available at http://www.heritage.org/about. Accessed July 25, 2011.

29. Lindbloom C. *The Policy-Making Process.* Englewood Cliffs, NJ: Prentice-Hall; 1980.

ENDNOTES

a. Under Article 1 of the Constitution, Congress has jurisdiction over the District of Columbia. Both the Senate and the House have committees that oversee some governmental functions of the District. The District elects two "shadow senators" who are allowed to lobby Congress on issues but who do not have voting rights. In terms of representation, this places the District in a position similar to other political bodies administered by the United States, such as Puerto Rico, the U.S. Virgin Islands, and American Samoa. The District's shadow senators (and a shadow representative in the House) were created by the citizens of the District in anticipation of the passage of the 1978 District of Columbia Voting Rights amendment to the U.S. Constitution, which would have granted the District the same voting rights as the states. The amendment never passed, but the District government has maintained the shadow positions nonetheless.

b. In addition to the 435 representatives, Puerto Rico has a resident commissioner, and the District of Columbia, Guam, the U.S. Virgin Islands, and American Samoa each has a delegate who is allowed to sponsor legislation and vote in committees, but may not vote on the House floor. The citizens of the District of Columbia also elect a nonvoting shadow representative.

c. In circumstances where the president serves two years or less of the term of another president, an individual may hold office for 10 years.

Understanding Health Insurance

LEARNING OBJECTIVES

By the end of this chapter, you will be able to:

- Understand the role of risk and uncertainty in insurance
- Define the basic elements of health insurance
- Differentiate various insurance products
- Discuss incentives created for providers and patients in various types of insurance arrangements
- Discuss health policy issues relating to health insurance

INTRODUCTION

Unlike many other countries, the United States does not have a national healthcare delivery system; whether individuals have access to healthcare services—and whether they receive health care of appropriate quantity and quality—often depends on whether they are insured. Even if an individual is insured, the kind of coverage she has can affect her ability to obtain care. Understanding health insurance, however, requires more than understanding its importance to healthcare access.

Policymakers must also know how providers, suppliers, employers, states, and others respond to changes in the health insurance market. For example, if policymakers decide to reduce the number of uninsured by creating a new government-sponsored health insurance program, they must know whether providers will participate in the program and what features will make it more or less attractive to providers. Or, if policymakers want to reduce the number of uninsured by increasing access to employer-sponsored health insurance plans, they must know which policy changes will make it more

or less likely that employers will offer (or expand) insurance coverage to their employees. In either case, policymakers might also want to know whether an initiative will affect the financial viability of public hospitals or health centers.

Several themes emerge when considering these types of health insurance-related policy questions. First, insurance is rooted in the concepts of uncertainty and risk; reducing uncertainty and risk by, for example, offering a health insurance product, participating as a provider in a health insurance plan, or purchasing health insurance coverage as a consumer creates various incentives for insurers, the insured, providers, and governments to act or refrain from acting in certain ways. As noted in the vignette, one goal of the Patient Protection and Affordable Care Act (ACA) is to reduce the risk of insuring small businesses and individuals by creating a large purchasing pool through state health insurance exchanges.[1] Second, to a large extent, insurance carriers choose the design of their health insurance products, and employers and individuals choose whether to (and what type of) health insurance to purchase. Indeed, insurance carriers have had wide latitude to determine the individuals or groups that may join a plan, employers have had broad discretion to determine whether to offer coverage and what type to offer, and individuals have had the choice whether to purchase health insurance coverage, although this choice was often illusory due to the high cost of health care. Once again, the ACA attempts to change these choices and incentives. For example, many insurance plans will have to meet new requirements, such as offering a package of "essential health benefits"; most employers will have to provide health insurance coverage or pay a penalty;

aged care, a particular form of health insurance dominant in today's market.

A BRIEF HISTORY OF THE RISE OF HEALTH INSURANCE IN THE UNITED STATES

Although 83% of people in this country are insured today, health insurance was not always an integral part of our society.[2(p22)] The initial movement to bring health insurance to the United States was modeled after activities in Europe. In the late 1800s and early 1900s, the European social insurance movement resulted in the creation of "sickness" insurance throughout many countries: Germany in 1883, Austria in 1888, Hungary in 1891, Britain in 1911, and Russia in 1912, to name just a few examples. These programs varied in scope and structure, from a compulsory national system in Germany, to industry-based requirements in France and Italy, to extensive state aid in Sweden and Switzerland. Although the Socialist and Progressive parties advocated for the adoption of similar social insurance systems in the United States in the early 1900s, their efforts were unsuccessful.[3]

In the absence of government-sponsored health insurance plans, the private sector insurance industry flourished with the growth of Blue Cross, Blue Shield, and commercial insurance carriers. Blue Cross established its first hospital insurance plan at Baylor University in 1929 by agreeing to provide 1,500 teachers with 21 days of hospital care per year for the price of $6 per person.[3(p295)] The hospital industry supported the growth of private insurance as a way to secure payment for services during the Depression. Blue Shield, the physician-based insurance plan, began in 1939 as a way to forestall renewed efforts to enact compulsory national health insurance and to avoid growth in consumer-controlled prepaid health plans, both of which would have reduced the type of physician autonomy endemic at that time.[3(p307)]

World War II led to rapid growth in employer-sponsored health insurance. With employees scarce and a general wage freeze in effect, a 1942 War Labor Board ruling that employee fringe benefits of up to 5% of wages did not violate the wage freeze created a strong incentive for employers to provide health benefits to attract new workers and keep their current ones. After the war, labor unions gained the right to bargain collectively, leading to another expansion of employee health plans. In 1954, the Internal Revenue Service declared that employers could pay health insurance premiums for their employees with pre-tax dollars, further increasing the value of the fringe benefit to employers.[a] By 1949, 28 million people had commercial hospital insurance, 22 million had commercial

and most individuals will have to purchase health insurance or pay a penalty. For each choice, the question is: What policy goal (e.g., equity, universal coverage, fiscal restraint, market efficiency) should drive the design and regulation of health insurance?

This chapter begins with a short history of health insurance in this country and then reviews the health insurance concepts key to understanding the structure and operation of health insurance. It concludes with an overview of man-physician insurance, and 4 million had independent hospital plans. At that time, over 31 million had Blue Cross hospital coverage and 12 million had Blue Shield coverage.[3(p327)] Employer-sponsored health insurance, not national health insurance, was well on its way to becoming entrenched as the primary form of health insurance.

The federal government first became a major player in health insurance with the passage of Medicaid and Medicare in 1965. These programs were created, in part, to fill in coverage gaps left by the private insurance market—namely, coverage for the elderly, disabled, and low-income populations who had too little income and too high health risks to be viable candidates for insurance coverage from the insurance carriers' point of view. Like many major policy changes, the passage of these programs was a multi-layered compromise. Before the final design of these programs was established, several proposals were considered. The American Medical Association (AMA) supported a combination federal–state program to subsidize private insurance policies for the elderly to cover hospital care, physician care, and prescription drugs; Representative John Byrnes (R-WI), ranking Republican on the House Ways and Means Committee, endorsed an AMA-like proposal but with federal, instead of federal–state, administration; the Johnson Administration supported hospital insurance for the elderly through Social Security; and Senator Jacob Javitz (R-NY) supported federal payments to state programs to provide health care to poor, elderly individuals.[4(pp46–48)] In the end, the Medicare and Medicaid programs were passed in one bill with features from all of these proposals. For example, Medicare was established as a federally funded program with

two parts, one for hospital insurance and one for physician insurance, and Medicaid as a state–federal program for the poor.

By the 1970s a number of factors converged to place rising healthcare costs on the national agenda: advances had been made in medical technology, hospitals expanded and became more involved in high-tech care, physician specialties became more common, hospitals and physicians had a large new pool of paying patients due to Medicaid and Medicare, wages for medical staff increased, and an aging population required an increasing amount of services.[3(pp383–384)] In addition, the prevailing fee-for-service (FFS) insurance system rewarded healthcare professionals for providing a high quantity of services. As the name suggests, fee-for-service reimbursement means the providers are paid for each service they provide—the more services (and more expensive services) rendered, the more reimbursement the provider receives. From 1960 to 1970, hospital care expenditures tripled from $9.3 billion to $28 billion and physician service expenditures almost matched that growth rate, increasing from $5.3 billion to $13.6 billion.[6(pp257–258)] Federal and state governments were also feeling the burden of high healthcare costs. From 1965 to 1970, federal and state governments collectively experienced a 21% annual rate of increase in their healthcare expenditures.[3(p384)]

As is discussed in more detail later in this chapter, managed care moves away from the FFS system by integrating the payment for services and the delivery of services into one place in an attempt to rein in healthcare costs and utilization. The federal Health Maintenance Organization Act of 1973 was intended to spur the growth of managed care by providing incentives to increase the use of health maintenance organizations (HMOs). The act relied on federal loans and grants and a mandate that employers with 25 or more employees offer an HMO option if one was available in their area.[6(pp262–263)] Even so, managed care did not flourish due to opposition by patients who did not want their provider and service choices restricted, and by providers who did not want to lose control over their practices.

As healthcare cost and quality concerns remained a national priority, the managed care industry eventually found a foothold in the health insurance market. Indeed, enrollment in managed care doubled during the 1990s, with almost 80 million enrollees by 1998. In 2010, only 1% of workers were in conventional, non-managed care arrangements.[7] Although only about 24% of Medicare enrollees choose managed care arrangements, some 70% of Medicaid beneficiaries receive some or all of their services through managed care, though for many of them it is mandatory that they receive services through a managed care arrangement.[8,9]

HOW HEALTH INSURANCE OPERATES

This section provides an overview of the purpose and structure of health insurance. It begins with a review of basic health insurance terminology, considers the role of uncertainty and risk in insurance, and concludes with a discussion of how insurance companies set their premium rates.

Basic Terminology

As you read earlier, the health insurance industry first developed when the FFS system was standard. Under this system, not only do providers have incentive to conduct more and more expensive services, but patients are unbridled in their use of the healthcare system because FFS does not limit the use of services or accessibility to providers. As we will discuss later in this chapter, managed care developed as a response to the incentives created by the FFS system. However, even though there are numerous differences between FFS and managed care, many of the fundamental principles of how insurance operates are applicable to any type of health insurance contract. The following discussion reviews how health insurance works generally, regardless of the type of insurance arrangement.

The health insurance consumer (also known as the *beneficiary* or *insured*) buys health insurance in advance for an annual fee, usually paid in monthly installments, called a *premium*. In return, the health insurance carrier (or company) pays for all or part of the beneficiary's healthcare costs if she or he becomes ill or injured and has a covered medical need. (A covered need is a medical good or service that the insurer is obligated to pay for because it is covered based on the terms of the insurance contract or policy. As discussed in detail elsewhere, the ACA requires many plans to cover all "essential health benefits," which at the time of this writing have not yet been defined by the Obama Administration through the regulatory process.) Insurance contracts cannot identify every conceivable healthcare need of beneficiaries, so they are generally structured to include categories of care (outpatient, inpatient, vision, maternity, etc.) to be provided if deemed medically necessary. Definitions of the term *medically necessary* vary by contract and are important when determining whether a procedure is covered.

Even if the beneficiary never needs healthcare services covered by the insurance policy, she still pays for the policy through premiums. The consumer benefits by having financial security in case of illness or injury, and the insurance company benefits by making money selling health insurance.

In addition to premiums, the beneficiary typically pays other costs under most health insurance policies. Many policies have *deductibles*, which is the amount of money the beneficiary must pay on her own for her healthcare needs each year before the insurance carrier starts to help with the costs. For example, if a policyholder has a $500 deductible, the beneficiary must pay 100% of the first $500 of healthcare costs each year. The insurance carrier is not liable to cover any costs until the individual's healthcare bill reaches $501 in a given year. If the individual does not need more than $500 worth of health care in a specific year, the insurance carrier generally will not help that individual pay her healthcare costs.

Furthermore, a beneficiary generally continues to incur some costs in addition to the premiums even after the deductible has been met. Insurance carriers often impose cost sharing on the beneficiary through *co-payment* or *co-insurance* requirements. A co-payment is a set dollar amount the beneficiary pays when receiving a service from a provider. For example, many HMOs charge their beneficiaries $10 every time

> ## BOX 3 Discussion Questions
>
> As a general matter, all types of insurance under traditional economic models cover expensive and unforeseen events, not events that have small financial risk or little uncertainty.[5(p195)] For example, auto insurance does not cover regular maintenance such as an oil change, and home insurance does not protect against normal wear and tear, such as the need to replace an old carpet. Accordingly, many economists argue that health insurance should not cover regular, foreseeable events such as physical exams or low-cost occurrences such as vaccinations. Other economists support a different school of thought. An alternative economic view is that health insurance should insure one's health, not just offer protection against the financial consequences of major adverse health events. Because people without health insurance are less likely to obtain preventive care such as physical exams or vaccinations, these economists believe it is in everyone's best interest, ethically and financially, to promote preventive care. Therefore, it is appropriate for insurance to cover both unpredictable and expensive events as well as predictable and less expensive events. Which theory do you support? What do you think is the best use of insurance? If insurance does not cover low-cost and predictable events, should another resource be available to assist individuals, or should people pay out of their own pockets for these healthcare needs?

a beneficiary sees a primary care provider. Co-insurance refers to a percentage of the healthcare cost the individual must cover. For example, 20% is a common co-insurance amount. This means the beneficiary pays 20% of all healthcare costs after the deductible has been met, with the insurance carrier paying the other 80%.

Uncertainty

From a traditional economic perspective, insurance exists because of two basic concepts—risk and uncertainty. The world is full of risks—auto theft, house fires, physical disabilities—and uncertainty about whether any such events might affect a particular individual. As a result, people buy a variety of forms of insurance (e.g., automobile insurance, home insurance, life or disability insurance) to protect themselves and their families against the financial consequences of these unfortunate and unforeseen events.

Although genetic predisposition or behavioral choices such as smoking or working a high-risk job may increase the chances that an individual will suffer from a health-related problem, in general there is a high level of uncertainty as to whether a particular person will become sick or injured and need medical assistance. Health insurance protects the consumer from medical costs associated with both expensive and unforeseen events. Even if the consumer does not experience a negative event, a benefit exists from the peace of mind and reduced uncertainty of financial exposure that insurance provides.

In terms of health status and wise use of resources, when insurance allows consumers to purchase necessary services they would not otherwise be able to afford, it functions in a positive manner. Conversely, when insurance leads consumers to purchase unnecessary healthcare goods or services of low value because the consumer is not paying full cost, it works in a negative manner. The difficult task is trying to figure out how to set the consumer's share of the burden at just the right point to encourage and make available the proper use of health care, while discouraging improper usage.

Risk

Risk is a central concern in insurance. Consumers buy insurance to protect themselves against the risk of unforeseen and costly events. But health insurers are also concerned about risk—the risk that their beneficiaries will experience a covered medical event.

Individuals purchase health insurance to protect themselves against the risk of financial consequences of healthcare needs. Because of differences in risk level, individuals who are generally healthy or otherwise do not anticipate having health expenses may place a lower value on insurance than individuals who are unhealthy or those who are healthy but expect to have medical expenses, such as pregnant women. Therefore, healthy individuals tend to seek out lower-cost insurance plans or refrain from obtaining insurance altogether if it is not, in their view, cost effective. Unhealthy individuals or healthy individuals who often use the healthcare system would obviously prefer a low-cost insurance plan (with comprehensive benefits) but are generally more willing to pay higher premiums because of the value they place on having insurance.

Health insurance carriers are businesses that need to cover their expenditures, including the cost of accessing capital needed to run their company, to stay in the market.[b] They earn money by collecting premiums from their beneficiaries, and they pay out money to cover their beneficiaries' healthcare costs above the deductible amount and to cover the costs of running a business (overhead, marketing, taxes, etc.). One way health insurance companies survive is to make sure the premiums charged to beneficiaries cover these costs. From the insurance carrier's perspective, it would be ideal to be

---

BOX 4 Discussion Questions

As discussed earlier, risk and uncertainty are important concepts in health insurance. Individuals purchase health insurance policies to protect themselves financially against healthcare costs, and insurance carriers try to set premiums that will cover the cost of the services used by their beneficiaries. Currently (when allowed by law), insurance carriers may consider factors such as medical history, demographics, type of occupation, size of the beneficiary pool, and similar criteria when setting the terms of an insurance policy. Should health insurance carriers also have access to and be able to use genetic testing results when carriers decide whether to insure an individual, what premiums to charge, or which services to cover? If you think the answer to that question should be "no," why is genetic information different from all of the other kinds of information insurance carriers may take into account when making those decisions? Conversely, what is the strongest argument you can make in favor of allowing insurance carriers to consider an applicant's genetic information? How would allowing genetic testing alter an individual's or a provider's diagnosis and treatment decisions? What is the primary policy goal that affects your view?

---

able to charge lower premiums to attract healthy individuals who are less likely to use their benefits, and higher premiums to unhealthy individuals who are more likely to need medical care.

However, insurance companies have difficulty matching healthy people with low-cost plans and unhealthy people with high-cost plans because of the problem of *asymmetric information*. This is the term used by economists when one party to a transaction has more information than the other party. In the case of insurance, the imbalance often favors the consumer because insurance carriers generally do not know as much as the individual does about the individual's healthcare needs and personal habits. Although relatively healthy low-cost individuals want to make their status known because insurance carriers might be willing to sell them an insurance product for a lower price, relatively unhealthy individuals do not want their status known because insurance companies might charge them higher premiums. For this reason, when an insurance carrier lacks complete information, it is more beneficial to unhealthy beneficiaries than to healthy ones.

Together, uncertainty about risk and the presence of asymmetric information lead to the problem of *adverse selection*. In terms of health insurance, adverse selection is when unhealthy people over-select (that is, select beyond a random distribution) a particular plan. This occurs because people at risk for having high healthcare costs choose a particular plan because of that plan's attractive coverage rules.[10(pp12–13)] The consumer who knows he is a high risk for needing services will be more likely to choose a more comprehensive plan because it covers more services, even though it is probably a more expensive option. This leaves the insurer that offers the comprehensive plan with a disproportionate number of high-risk beneficiaries. As a result of the relatively high-risk pool, beneficiaries will have high service utilization rates and, in turn, the insurance carrier would need to raise premiums to be able to pay for the increased cost of covering services for beneficiaries. In turn, some of the healthier individuals might choose to leave the plan because of the higher premiums, resulting in an even riskier beneficiary pool and even higher premiums, and the cycle continues. The healthier consumers may find a lower-cost plan or may choose to go without health insurance and pay the penalty under the ACA, while the insurance plan is left with an increasingly higher percentage of relatively unhealthy people. This is the problem of adverse selection.

One instance where adverse selection is a key concern is with an increasingly popular type of health plan, the high deductible health plan (HDHP). As the name suggests, these plans have very high deductibles (usually defined as at least

$1,000 for an individual or $2,000 for a family). In 2010, annual premiums for the average HDHP were $4,702 for individuals and $11,683 for families.[7(p141)] As with other insurance plans, consumers pay most of their healthcare expenses out-of-pocket until they reach the deductible.[8] HDHPs are often used in conjunction with health reimbursement arrangements (HRAs) or health savings accounts (HSAs), which allow individuals to set aside money for future healthcare needs. Health reimbursement arrangements are funded solely by employers, who usually commit to making a specified amount of money available for healthcare expenses incurred by employees or their dependents, while HSAs are created by individuals, but employers may also contribute to HSAs if the employers offer a qualified HDHP. Individual contributions to HSAs are made with pre-income tax dollars, and withdrawals to pay for qualified healthcare expenses are also not taxed. As shown in Figures 1 and 2, high-deductible plans are increasingly popular with employers and employees.

Those who support HDHPs assert that high deductible plans promote personal responsibility because enrollees have a financial incentive to avoid overutilizing the healthcare system and to choose cost-effective treatment options. As a result, HDHPs are favored by employers and others as a cost-cutting strategy. Others are concerned that HDHPs will result in adverse selection, harming low-income and unhealthy individuals. Critics argue that enrollees of high deductible plans are more likely to be wealthier and healthier individuals who can afford high out-of-pocket expenses and are less likely to use the healthcare system.[11] As a result, relatively poorer and sicker individuals will choose a comprehensive group health insurance plan (assuming one is available and affordable), resulting in plans facing the possibility of adverse selection due to having a relatively high-risk insurance pool. In addition, there are concerns that employers will replace their more expensive comprehensive plan options with HDHPs, potentially resulting in less affordable health care for poorer and sicker individuals. Finally, critics also contend that the lower service utilization associated with HDHP enrollees is due to their better health status, not price sensitivity, undermining one of the main arguments in support of these plans.[11]

Setting Premiums

Assuming that insurance companies make their decisions in the context of asymmetric information, they cannot determine with certainty the appropriate amount of premium to charge each individual. Instead, insurance companies rely on making educated guesses about the risk each individual or group of individuals has of needing healthcare services. The

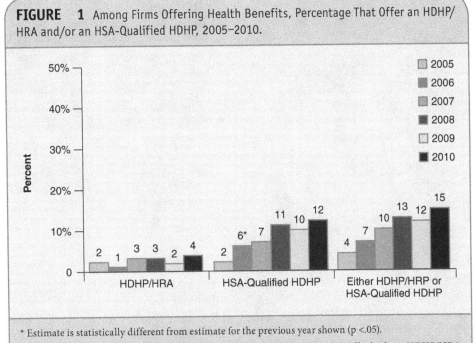

FIGURE 1 Among Firms Offering Health Benefits, Percentage That Offer an HDHP/HRA and/or an HSA-Qualified HDHP, 2005–2010.

* Estimate is statistically different from estimate for the previous year shown (p <.05).

‡ The 2010 estimate includes 0.3% of all firms offering health benefits that offer both an HDHP/HRA and an HSA-qualified HDHP. The comparable percentages for 2005, 2006, 2007, 2008 and 2009 are 0.3%, 0.4%, 0.2%, 0.3% and 0.1%, respectively.

Source: Kaiser/HRET Survey of Employer-Sponsored Health Benefits, 2005–2010.

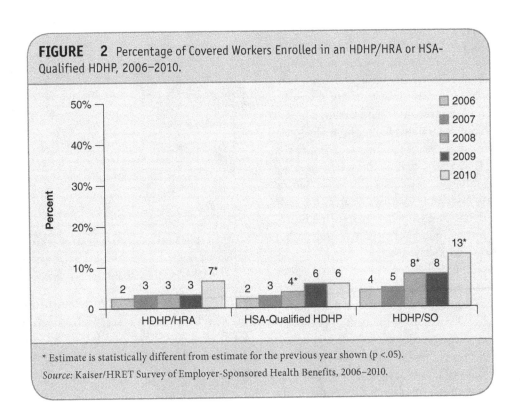

FIGURE 2 Percentage of Covered Workers Enrolled in an HDHP/HRA or HSA-Qualified HDHP, 2006–2010.

* Estimate is statistically different from estimate for the previous year shown (p <.05).

Source: Kaiser/HRET Survey of Employer-Sponsored Health Benefits, 2006–2010.

two main methods of setting premiums are *experience rating* and *community rating*.

When insurance companies use experience rating to make an educated guess about the risk of someone's needing healthcare services, they are relying on how much a beneficiary or group of beneficiaries spent on medical services previously to determine the amount of the premium for each member or group. Thus, if an individual or group had very high medical costs in a given year, premiums are likely to rise the following year. Conversely, community rating does not take into account health status or claims history when setting premiums. In "pure" community rating, insurers use only geography and family composition to set rates; in "modified" community rating, insurers may be allowed to consider other characteristics, such as age and gender.

Which rating system makes more sense from a policy perspective as a basis for setting premiums may depend on whether you evaluate the insurance market based on efficiency or equity (think back to discussions of competing conceptual frameworks). If the market is judged based on efficiency, then the key issue is whether the optimal amount of risk has shifted from consumers to insurers. If there are individuals willing to pay a higher amount for greater coverage and insurers willing

to provide greater coverage for the higher amount, but something in the market prevents this transaction from occurring, then the optimal amount of risk shifting has not occurred. Or, if individuals value a certain level of insurance coverage at a price that is less than the price at which insurers are willing to provide that coverage, but individuals buy coverage anyway at the higher price, the market is not optimally efficient (due to excess coverage).

Conversely, the market may be judged based on equity or fairness. Even the most efficient market may result in some inequities. Some individuals may be uninsured, some may have to pay more than other individuals for the same level of insurance, some may not be able to purchase the level of coverage they desire, and some individuals may not be able to join a particular plan. These inequities are often a concern in the context of the uninsured, especially as uninsurance relates to low-income individuals or those with high health needs due to random events, such as an accident or genetic condition.

Regardless of the underwriting methodology used, premiums are cheaper for people purchasing insurance as part of a large group rather than buying health insurance individually or as part of a small group. Due to the law of averages, larger groups of people are more likely to have an average risk rate. When people join a group for reasons unrelated to health status, such as working for the same company, it is also more likely that the group will have an average risk rate. Groups with average risk rates are attractive to insurers because the cost of insuring a few unhealthy people will probably be offset by savings from insuring many healthy ones. Conversely, in smaller groups it is more likely that the group will have a relatively high risk rate and less likely that the cost of insuring an unhealthy person can be offset by the savings of insuring a few other healthy people. This is the problem faced by Bob, the small business owner described at the outset of the chapter who has one high-cost employee. Even though he would like to offer health insurance coverage to his employees, Bob and other small business owners like him often are able to offer only expensive or limited coverage, if they can offer any health insurance benefit at all. In order to help individuals and small business owners like Bob, some states require insurers to use a community rating system to set premiums for these groups and in the state health insurance exchanges that were created by the ACA.

Carriers also prefer to insure large groups because most of the administrative costs associated with insurance are the same whether the carrier is covering a few people or a few thousand.[12(pp342–344)] In fact, group coverage has traditionally required fewer marketing resources than individual coverage, which targets customers one at a time. However, the proliferation of information on the Internet may change this equation.

Medical Underwriting

The prior discussion about rate setting assumed asymmetric information (i.e., where the insurer has little information about the consumer's health status and the consumer has substantial information about his or her own healthcare needs). Of course, there are ways for insurers to gain information about the medical needs of a consumer looking to join a health plan: Physical exams, questionnaires, medical records, occupation, and demographics all provide clues about the health status of the consumer. Although it is much more difficult to accomplish, insurers may also try to predict an individual's future costs through questionnaires that ask, for example, whether an individual engages in risky activities (e.g., riding a motorcycle) or through genetic testing (which is itself an emerging health policy and law issue).

Whether companies are allowed to consider an applicant's medical history or other personal information to help assess risk of healthcare needs in the future—a practice referred to as medical underwriting—is a somewhat complicated legal question that involves both federal and state law. The Health Insurance Portability and Accountability Act of 1996 (HIPAA)[13] includes an important protection for consumers by prohibiting group health plans from excluding or limiting otherwise qualified individuals due to pre-existing conditions (a pre-existing condition is a medical condition, such as cancer or diabetes, that is present at the time an individual applies to enroll in an insurance plan). The ACA expands this protection by requiring all health insurers to sell policies to all applicants, regardless of pre-existing conditions, This requirement is already in effect for children and will take effect for adults in 2014.

Prior to HIPAA, many individuals with pre-existing conditions were denied insurance altogether, denied coverage for particular medical care, or charged very high premiums if they sought to purchase a policy. These practices led to a problem referred to as "job lock." Because most Americans receive insurance coverage through their employers, many employees with pre-existing conditions could not switch jobs for fear that their new company's insurance policy would be denied to them on account of their pre-existing condition. One study estimated that job lock resulted in a 4% reduction in voluntary turnover.[12(p341)]

Although HIPAA and the ACA do not regulate the amount of premiums that may be charged, all members of a group generally pay the same premium due to the laws' nondiscrimination provisions. In HIPAA, these provisions prohibit plans or insurance carriers from requiring any individual to pay a higher premium or contribution than another "similarly situated" individual[14] in the plan based on eight health factors: health status, physical or mental medical conditions, claims experience (i.e., the individual has a history of high health claims), receipt of health care, medical history, genetic information, evidence of insurability, and disability.[15] However, because those who purchase individual health insurance plans are not covered by HIPAA's protections, the ACA protections were needed as well. The ACA also prohibits plans from charging individuals higher premiums due to their pre-existing conditions.

MANAGED CARE

The prior sections reviewed the history, basic structure, and purpose of health insurance generally. In this section, we discuss a specific kind of health insurance structure that has come to dominate the American market: managed care. We will describe why managed care emerged, some of the frequent cost-containment strategies used by managed care organizations, and the most common managed care structures in the market today.

Managed care became the predominant healthcare financing and delivery arrangement in the United States because healthcare costs had risen to alarming levels and there were few mechanisms for containing costs under the FFS system. As mentioned earlier, FFS does not create incentives for providers or patients to utilize healthcare services sparingly. Providers have an incentive under FFS to provide more services and more expensive services (but not necessarily higher-quality services) because their income rises with each procedure or office visit and fees are higher for more expensive services. As long as providers are accessible, insured patients can request services and assume their insurance company will pay most or all of the costs to the extent that the services are covered by the health plan and medically necessary.

In addition, the FFS system does not create incentives for providers or patients to use the lowest-cost quality care available. Many people believe specialists provide higher quality care and turn to them even for minor needs that do not truly require expensive specialty services, and the FFS system does not discourage this behavior. Furthermore, because traditional insurance coverage requires a specific diagnosis for reimbursement, patients are discouraged from seeking preventative services when they are symptom-free under FFS.[16(p332)] At the same time, traditional insurance companies do not have the ability to control costs or quality of care under FFS—their job is limited to determining whether a service is covered and medically necessary and providing the agreed-upon reimbursement. They have little ability to measure or improve the quality of care provided by healthcare professionals and cannot control costs by limiting the amount or type of services received; instead, they can only raise premiums and other rates in the future to cover increasing costs.

To alter the inherent incentives under FFS and to grant insurers some ability to control the quality and utilization of services, managed care integrates the provision of and payment for healthcare services. Through various strategies discussed in the following sections, managed care organizations (MCOs) and managed care plans create incentives to provide fewer services and less expensive care, while still maintaining the appropriate level of healthcare quality. Managed care organizations also attempt to alter patients' decision making through cost-sharing requirements, cost containment tools, utilization restrictions, and free or low-cost coverage for preventive care.

Managed care organizations take various forms, but certain general features apply to all of them to varying degrees. All MCOs provide a comprehensive, defined package of benefits to the purchaser/member for a pre-set fee (including both monthly premium and cost-sharing requirements). Services are offered to members through a network of providers, all of whom have a contractual relationship with the MCO. The MCOs choose which providers to include in their networks and what services are rendered by network providers. Most notably, they also use financial incentives and other mechanisms to control the delivery, use, quality, and cost of services in ways that are not present in FFS insurance systems.[6(p260)]

Cost Containment and Utilization Tools

Managed care introduced a variety of tools in its attempt to contain costs and control healthcare service utilization. The cost containment strategies of *performance-based salary bonuses or withholdings*, *discounted fee schedules*, and *capitated payments* shift financial risk or limit payments to providers who, in turn, have an incentive to choose the least costly, but still effective, treatment option. The utilization control strategies of *gatekeeping* and *utilization review* focus on making sure that only appropriate and necessary care is provided to patients. Another type of strategy, *case management*, is designed to make sure that necessary care is provided in the most coordinated and cost-effective way possible.

Provider Payment Tools

Depending on the structure of the MCO, providers are paid by salary, discounted fee schedule, or capitation rate. Providers in what are called staff-model MCOs are employees of the MCO and are paid an annual salary. The salary structure often includes bonuses or salary withholdings that are paid (or withheld) upon meeting (or not meeting) utilization or performance goals, thus shifting some financial risk from the MCO to the provider. A discounted fee schedule is a service-specific fee system as is used in FFS. However, an MCO-style fee schedule pays lower reimbursement rates than is true in FFS systems; providers agree to accept less than their usual fee in return for the large volume of patients available to them by being a part of the MCO provider network. The MCO retains the financial risk in a discounted fee system, but the costs are lower for the company due to the discounted rate paid to providers. Finally, a capitated payment rate is a fixed monthly sum per member that the provider receives regardless of the number or type of services provided to patients. The physician receiving the capitated rate is responsible for providing all of the care needed by his or her MCO patients, within the provider's scope of practice. As a result, the financial risk in the case of capitated arrangements is shifted entirely from the MCO to the provider. Depending on the contract between the provider and MCO, the insurance company may or may not guarantee the provider a minimum number of patients in exchange for accepting a capitated rate. These provider-focused cost containment strategies are summarized in Table 1.

Both the salaried and capitation payment methods have very different incentives for providers than is the case under the FFS system. Instead of being paid more for doing more, MCO providers are paid the same amount regardless of the number or type of services they provide. Given the use of bonuses and withholdings, salaried providers may be paid more if they make treatment decisions deemed favorable by an MCO. By using these incentives, MCOs encourage providers to render the fewest and most cost-effective services necessary.

Critics of managed care payment methodologies argue that MCO plan members will not receive all necessary care if providers are incentivized to provide fewer services and less-costly care. Instead of treating patients using both the most cost-efficient and medically necessary services, critics claim MCOs encourage providers to save money by providing fewer services and less specialized care than necessary; MCOs counter that their own incentive is to keep their members healthy so they do not need expensive services in the future. In addition, MCOs point to their ability to impose quality control measures on providers as a way to ensure that patients are properly treated. In response, critics argue that because members switch health plans relatively frequently, MCOs do not have an incentive to keep their members healthy because the MCOs will not realize the long-term savings as members come and go.

Which side has the better argument? There is no definitive answer. On the one hand, studies have found that treatment decisions under MCO arrangements are mostly influenced by clinical factors (not economic ones), that there is little or no measurable difference in the health outcomes of patients in FFS versus managed care plans, that the quality of care provided under FFS and managed care plans is basically equal, and that most Americans are satisfied with their health plan, whether it is FFS or through an MCO.[16(pp351–352)] On the other hand, studies have also shown that mental health patients do not fare as well in MCOs as in FFS plans; that nonprofit HMOs (a type of MCO) score better on quality measures than for-profit ones; and that managed care enrollees are less likely than FFS patients to give excellent ratings to their plan overall, the quality of services they receive, access to specialty care, and time spent with physicians.[16(pp351–352)]

Utilization Control Tools

Managed care organizations also employ other techniques, not related to provider payment methods, to control use of healthcare services. Once again, the goal in using these tools is to reduce the use of unnecessary and costly services. We review three common utilization control tools: gatekeeping, utilization review, and case management.

Gatekeepers monitor and control the services a patient receives. Members of managed care plans are often required to select a primary care provider from the MCO network upon enrollment. This provider acts as the member's "gatekeeper" and is responsible for providing primary care, referring patients for additional care, and generally coordinating the patient's care. Having a gatekeeper allows the MCO, not the patient or specialty provider, to determine when a patient needs additional or specialty services, diagnostic tests,

TABLE 1 Provider Payment Cost Containment Strategies			
Strategy	**Provider Payment Method**	**How Costs Are Controlled**	**Who Assumes Financial Risk**
Salary and bonuses/ withholds	Provider receives a salary as an employee of an MCO	Incentive for provider to perform fewer and/or less costly services	MCO and provider
Discounted fee schedule	Provider receives a lower fee than under FFS for each service to members	Pays provider less per service rendered than under FFS	MCO (but also has lower costs)
Capitation	Provider receives a set payment per month for each member regardless of services provided	Incentive for provider to perform fewer and/or less costly services	Provider

hospital admissions, and the like. As with the cost containment strategies discussed earlier, there are critics who contend that utilization-based bonuses or salary withholdings give gatekeepers financial incentive not to provide specialty referrals even when it is in the best interest of the patient.

Utilization review (UR) allows an MCO to evaluate the appropriateness of the services provided and to deny payment for unnecessary services. Managed care organization personnel review and approve or deny the services performed or recommended by network providers. Utilization review specialists are often healthcare professionals, and MCOs generally use existing clinical care guidelines to determine whether services are appropriate.

Utilization review may occur prospectively, concurrently, or retrospectively. Prospective UR means that an MCO reviews the appropriateness of treatment before a service is rendered. A request for a recommended service is sent to a UR panel for approval or denial. A denial does not mean a patient cannot move forward with his preferred treatment plan; however, it does mean that the patient will have to pay for the treatment out of his own pocket. Prospective UR is distinguished from concurrent UR, which is when the MCO review of the appropriateness of treatment occurs while treatment is being rendered. For example, a patient may need a procedure that requires hospitalization. Even though the procedure is performed and covered, a UR specialist might still determine the number of days the patient may remain in the hospital or whether certain services, such as home care or physical therapy, will be covered upon discharge from the hospital. Finally, retrospective review means the MCO reviews the appropriateness of treatment (and therefore its coverage) after a service is rendered. In this case, a patient's medical records are reviewed to determine whether the care provided was appropriate and billed accurately; MCOs will not provide reimbursement for services deemed inappropriate

or unnecessary. This latter type of review may also be used to uncover provider practice patterns and determine incentive compensation.[16(p339)] Regardless of when the review occurs, the use of UR is controversial because it may interfere with the patient–provider relationship and allow for second-guessing of provider treatment decisions by a third party who is not part of the diagnosis and treatment discussions.

Case management is a service utilization approach that uses trained personnel to manage and coordinate patient care. Although gatekeeping serves as a basic form of case management for all members, many patients with complex or chronic conditions, such as HIV/AIDS or spinal cord injuries, may benefit from more intensive case management. These patients may have frequent need for care from various specialists and thus benefit from assistance by personnel who are familiar with the many resources available to care for the patient and who are able to provide information and assistance to patients and their families. A case manager works with providers to determine what care is necessary and to help arrange for patients to receive that care in the most appropriate and cost-effective settings.[16(pp336–337)] Although the general idea of case management is not controversial, some people believe it can be implemented in a manner that acts more as a barrier than an asset to care because additional approval is needed before a patient receives care and because another layer of bureaucracy is placed between the patient and the provider. Table 2 summarizes the three service utilization control strategies just discussed.

As you might imagine, managed care's use of service utilization control mechanisms frequently leads to disputes between patients and their managed care company over whether the company is improperly affecting the provider–patient relationship (and negatively impacting the quality of care provided) by making decisions as to the type or quantity of care a patient should receive. This is both a highly charged

TABLE 2 Service Utilization Control Strategies

Strategy	Description	Potential Concerns
Gatekeeper	Uses a primary care provider to make sure only necessary and appropriate care is provided.	Gatekeepers may have financial incentive to approve fewer services or less costly care.
Utilization review	Uses MCO personnel to review and approve or deny services requested by a provider to make sure only necessary and appropriate care is provided.	Interferes with patient–provider relationship; someone other than the patient's provider decides whether treatment is appropriate.
Case management	Uses MCO personnel to manage and coordinate patient care to make sure care is provided in the most cost-effective manner.	May act as a barrier to receiving care if the case manager does not approve a desired service or service provider.

health policy issue and a complicated legal issue, and one that is discussed in more detail in a review of individual rights in health care. For purposes of this chapter, it is enough to note that MCOs must have a grievance and appeal process to at least initially handle these sorts of disputes. Although companies' processes differ in their specifics, they generally allow members to appeal a coverage decision, provide evidence to support the appeal, and receive an expedited resolution when medically necessary. The ACA included a number of provisions relating to the appeals process required of insurance plans; these provisions establish a federal standard for state external appeals laws governing products in the individual and group markets and create a new federal appeals process for self-insured plans (the provisions do not affect Medicaid and Medicare, which have their own appeals processes).[17] The need for adequate grievance and appeal procedures can be particularly acute for patients with special healthcare needs, such as those with physical or mental disabilities, and patients who otherwise use the healthcare system more frequently than most.

Common Managed Care Structures

There are three managed care structures common in the market today: health maintenance organizations (HMOs), preferred provider organizations (PPOs), and point-of-service plans (POS). All three provide preventive and specialty care, but the rules relating to accessing care differ for each. In general, HMOs have the most restrictive rules pertaining to patients and providers, PPOs have the least restrictive rules, and POSs fall in the middle.

BOX 8 Discussion Questions

Cost containment strategies embraced by MCOs were a direct result of the FFS experience with ever-increasing utilization and healthcare costs. However, many consumers and providers chafe at the restrictions imposed by MCOs and are concerned that someone other than the provider is making treatment decisions. Are these restrictions appropriate and necessary? Do you favor some of the restrictions over others? Is it appropriate for one entity to be responsible for both paying for and providing care? Should someone other than an MCO—say the federal or state governments—have primary responsibility for making determinations about service utilization?

As shown in Figure 3, PPOs are the most popular type of managed care plan, while very few people are still insured by a conventional FFS plan. In general, the more control an MCO has over its providers and members, the easier it is to control utilization of services and, therefore, healthcare costs and quality. Conversely, providers and patients prefer to have as much autonomy as possible, so the more restrictive MCO structures may be less desirable in that respect. However, the distinctions among managed care structures have become blurred recently because of the consumer and provider backlash against MCO restrictions.

Health Maintenance Organizations

When managed care first became prominent in the 1970s, HMOs were the most common type of MCO. There are several characteristics shared by all HMOs:

- They pay providers a salary to cover the cost of any and all services that beneficiaries need within a provider's scope of practice;
- They negotiate a capitated rate with plan purchasers (e.g., employers) which prices the plan based on a per member per month amount for each type of provider;
- They coordinate and control receipt of services;
- They arrange for care using only their network providers, and
- They are responsible for providing care according to established quality standards.

Despite these commonalities, HMOs may be structured through a variety of models, including staff-model/closed panel, group model, network model, individual practice associations (IPAs), and direct contract model.[16(pp340–344)] Each model has advantages and disadvantages from the perspective of the HMO, its providers, and its members, as shown in Table 3.

Preferred Provider Organizations

As is evident from Table 3, every form of HMO is fairly restrictive. In all models, the HMO provides coverage only if members seek care from network providers and providers may or may not be limited to serving only HMO members. As both patients and providers began rebelling over these restrictions, new forms of MCOs emerged, often formed by providers and hospitals themselves.

Like HMOs, PPOs have a provider network, referred to as preferred providers. Unlike HMOs, however, PPOs provide coverage to patients seeking care from any provider, regardless of whether the provider is part of the member's PPO preferred

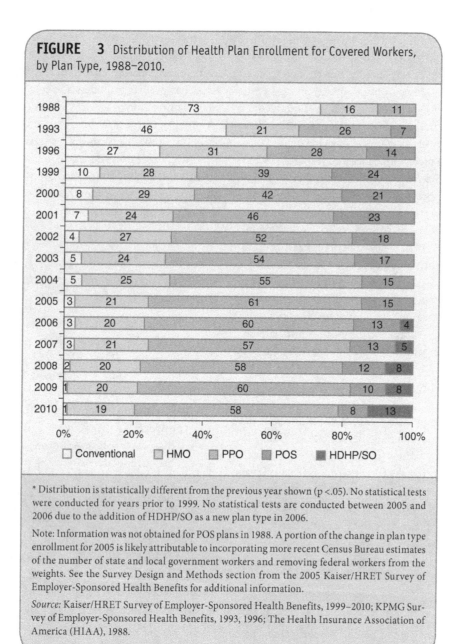

FIGURE 3 Distribution of Health Plan Enrollment for Covered Workers, by Plan Type, 1988–2010.

* Distribution is statistically different from the previous year shown (p <.05). No statistical tests were conducted for years prior to 1999. No statistical tests are conducted between 2005 and 2006 due to the addition of HDHP/SO as a new plan type in 2006.

Note: Information was not obtained for POS plans in 1988. A portion of the change in plan type enrollment for 2005 is likely attributable to incorporating more recent Census Bureau estimates of the number of state and local government workers and removing federal workers from the weights. See the Survey Design and Methods section from the 2005 Kaiser/HRET Survey of Employer-Sponsored Health Benefits for additional information.

Source: Kaiser/HRET Survey of Employer-Sponsored Health Benefits, 1999–2010; KPMG Survey of Employer-Sponsored Health Benefits, 1993, 1996; The Health Insurance Association of America (HIAA), 1988.

provider network. However, the amount of the service price that the PPO will cover is greater for an in-network provider than an out-of-network provider. For example, a PPO may agree to cover 80% of the cost for an in-network physician visit, but only 70% of the cost for a similar, but out-of-network, physician visit. PPO patients thus have the option of paying more but choosing among a greater number of providers or paying less but choosing among a more limited number of (in-network) providers. In addition, a PPO member's cost-sharing responsibilities are often higher than is the case for HMO members.

In exchange for being in the network, providers agree to accept a discounted rate for their services, often 25–35% below their usual rates.[16(p345)] Because PPO members have a financial incentive to seek providers who are in-network, these healthcare professionals find it worthwhile to accept a reduced rate from the PPO in exchange for the higher likelihood that PPO members will select them over non-network

			Must		
	HMO–Provider	**Provider**	**Members Seek**	**May Providers**	
	Relationship and	**Employment**	**Care from**	**Care for**	
HMO Model	**Payment Type**	**Arrangement**	**Network?**	**Nonmembers?**	**General Comments**
Staff-model/ closed panel	HMO employs providers, pays a salary, often includes bonuses or withholds.	Employed by HMO.	Yes	No	Provides services only in HMO's office and affiliated hospitals. Relatively speaking, HMO has the most control over providers and service utilization, but has fixed costs of building and staff. HMO may contract with outside providers if necessary. Providers and consumers often do not like restrictions imposed by HMO. Providers do not need to solicit patients. Consumers may find it most cost-effective option.
Group	HMO contracts with one multi-specialty group for a capitated rate.	Employed by own provider group.	Yes	Depends on terms of contract	HMO has less control over utilization. HMO contracts for hospital care on a prepaid or FFS basis. Providers may prefer this model because they remain independent as opposed to becoming an employee of the HMO and because they may serve nonmembers if their contract permits.
Network	HMO contracts with several group practices (often primary care practices) for a capitated rate.	Employed by own provider group.	Yes	Depends on terms of contract	The group practices may make referrals, but are financially responsible for reimbursing outside providers. HMO has less control over utilization due to greater number of contracts and ability of providers to subcontract. Providers may prefer additional autonomy, but also take on financial risk of providing primary and specialty care. Members may have a relatively greater choice of providers.
IPA	HMO contracts with IPA for a capitated rate.	IPA is intermediary between HMO and solo practitioners and groups. IPA pays providers a capitated rate.	Yes	Depends on terms of contract	HMO has reduced control over providers but may have less malpractice liability because IPA is an intermediary.[1] HMO may contract with specialty physicians as needed and for hospital care on a prepaid or FFS basis. Providers may prefer contracting with IPA instead of HMO to retain more autonomy. Members may have greater choice of providers.
Direct contract	HMO contracts directly with individual providers for a capitated rate.	Self-employed.	Yes	Depends on terms of contract	HMO has more leverage over providers because it contracts with them as individuals, but its administrative costs are much higher than having one contract or a few contracts with groups. Providers have less leverage regarding practice restrictions when contracting on an individual basis.

TABLE 3 Key Characteristics of Common HMO Models

BOX 9 Discussion Questions

In terms of containing healthcare costs and improving healthcare quality, do you think healthcare consumers and professionals need even more restrictions than are currently used in managed care? Are there any reasons to revert back to the FFS system, even knowing its inflationary qualities? If you think that managed care is not the answer to our still-rising healthcare costs and quality concerns, what other tools might help lower costs and improve the quality of care? Should any tools be imposed by government regulation or agreed to voluntarily by insurers and the insured?

providers. Furthermore, unlike the capitation system found in HMOs, PPO providers do not assume financial risk for providing services. Depending on the terms of their contract with the PPO, preferred providers may or may not agree to limit their practice to PPO members. Although it is rare, PPOs may choose to guarantee preferred providers a minimum number of patients.

Even though an MCO has much less control over service utilization in the PPO model than the HMO model, PPOs still provide more incentives to use care judiciously than is the case in an FFS system. For example, in-network PPO providers are paid less than their customary rate by the company when they provide care to PPO members and often agree to abide by quality control and utilization review strategies used by the PPO. In addition, PPO patients have an incentive to use certain providers who will cost them less and have cost-sharing requirements unlike anything found under FFS. The PPO model attempts to locate a middle ground between the very restrictive HMO models and the FFS structure that resulted in very high health care utilization and costs.

Point-of-Service Plans

In another effort to contain costs while still providing patients the freedom to choose their provider, POS plans combine features of HMOs and PPOs. Like an HMO, POS plans have a provider network, use a capitated or other payment system that shares financial risk with providers, and requires members to use a gatekeeper to help control service utilization. However, designated services may be obtained from out-of-network providers who are paid on an FFS basis, but use of these providers costs the member more money, as with the PPO model. A POS gatekeeper must approve all in-network care and may also have some control over out-of-network

care, depending on the terms of the plan. The call by many consumers for increased choice in providers has become forceful enough that some HMOs are now offering POS plans, which they may refer to as open-ended (as opposed to closed panel) models.

The Future of Managed Care

Managed care is likely to remain an integral part of the health system despite its drawbacks. Patients chafe at utilization restrictions, as is evident by the increase in PPO popularity and the emergence of the hybrid HMO/POS. Accurate or not, there is a widespread perception that managed care plans deny necessary care and provide lower quality care.[16(p352)] Providers also complain that managed care interferes with their ability to practice medicine in a manner of their choosing, placing them in ethical dilemmas due to the use of financial incentives and possibly lowering the quality of care they provide due to limits on tests and procedures they order. Yet, the key circumstance that led to the creation of managed care—high healthcare expenditures—has not abated. While the country struggles with ever-growing healthcare costs, even under managed care, the willingness to experiment with various cost and utilization containment strategies is likely to remain in place.

CONCLUSION

This introduction to health insurance serves as a building block for additional study, which expands upon many of the key health policy and law themes mentioned here. It should be clear to readers that health policy analysts and decision makers must be particularly attuned to health insurance issues; without knowing both the basic structure of health insurance and how various incentives impact the actions of healthcare consumers, professionals, and insurance carriers, they cannot make informed recommendations and policies addressing the key health issues of the day.

REFERENCES

1. Pub L No. 111-148, The Patient Protection and Affordable Care Act.

2. U.S. Bureau of the Census. *Income, Poverty, and Health Insurance Coverage in the United States: 2009*. Washington, D.C.: Bureau of the U.S. Census; 2010.

3. Starr P. *The Social Transformation of American Medicine: The Rise of a Sovereign Profession and the Making of a Vast Industry*. New York, NY: Basic Books, Inc.; 1982.

4. Stevens R, Stevens R. *Welfare Medicine in America: A Case Study of Medicaid*. New Brunswick, NJ: Transaction Publishers; 2003.

5. Council of Economic Advisors. Health care and insurance. In: *Economic Report of the President*. Washington, D.C.: GPO; 2004.

6. Sultz HA, Young KM. *Health Care USA: Understanding Its Organization and Delivery*. 3rd ed. Gaithersburg, MD: Aspen Publishers; 2001.

7. Kaiser Family Foundation and Health Research and Educational Trust. *Employer health benefits. 2010.* Available at http://ehbs.kff.org /pdf/2010/8085.pdf. Accessed February 1, 2011.

8. Kaiser Family Foundation. *Medicare Advantage—fact sheet. 2010.* Available at http://www.kff.org/medicare/upload/2052-14.pdf. Accessed July 20, 2011.

9. Kaiser Family Foundation. *Medicaid and managed care: key data, trends, and issues. 2010.* Available at http://www.kff.org/medicaid /upload/8046.pdf. Accessed July 20, 2011.

10. Penner S. *Introduction to Health Care Economics and Financial Management: Fundamental Concepts with Practical Application.* Philadelphia, PA: Lippincott Williams and Wilkins; 2004.

11. Davis K. Consumer-directed health care: will it improve system performance? *Health Serv Res.* 2004;39:1219–1233.

12. Phelps CE. *Health Economics.* 3rd ed. Boston, MA: Addison-Wesley; 2003.

13. Pub. L. No. 104-191, 110 Stat. 1936 *codified* in sections 18, 26, 29, and 42 U.S.C.

14. Nondiscrimination in Health Coverage in the Group Market; Interim Final Rules and Proposed Rules, 66 Fed. Reg. 1378, 1382 (January 2001) *codified* in 29 CFR 2590.702.

15. 42 U.S.C. § 300gg-1; Nondiscrimination in Health Coverage in the Group Market; Interim Final Rules and Proposed Rules, 1378–1384, 1396–1403.

16. Shi L, Singh DA. *Delivering Health Care in America: A Systems Approach.* 3rd ed. Gaithersburg, MD: Aspen Publishers; 2004.

17. Rosenbaum S. *Appeals of claims for benefits. 2010.* HealthReformGPS. Available at http://www.healthreformgps.org/resources/appeals-of-claims-for-benefits/. Accessed July 20, 2011.

ENDNOTES

a. Section 106 of the IRS Code of 1954 states that employers who pay a share of premiums for employees' hospital and medical insurance may exclude that amount from the gross income of employees.

b. There are both for-profit and not-for-profit insurance companies. Both types of companies seek to earn enough revenues to cover expenses and the cost of accessing capital. However, for-profit companies return excess revenue to their investors whereas not-for-profit companies put excess revenue back into the company.

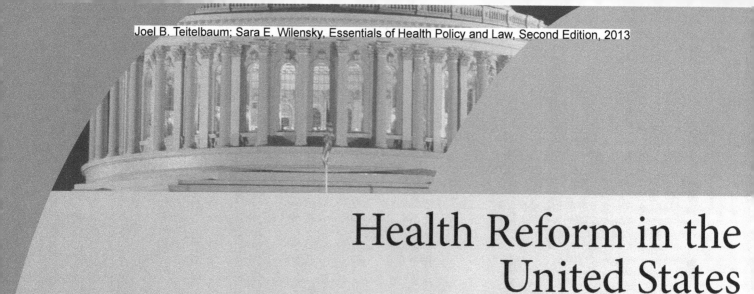

Health Reform in the United States

VIGNETTE

Casey is a recent college graduate with a degree in fine arts. She works in retail to pay the bills until her career as an artist takes off. It is 2011 and her employer does not offer health insurance coverage as an employee benefit; however, even if her employer did offer coverage, Casey would rather spend her limited funds on art supplies than on her portion of the coverage. Despite her low income, Casey makes too much money to qualify for any of the public health insurance programs in her state.

One evening when Casey was up late working on an art project, she cut a tendon in her hand with a sharp knife. She rushed to the emergency room, where she waited for 7 hours before being treated because of the high volume of patients that night. Doctors stitched up her hand, provided her with pain killers, and told her she would need physical therapy to ensure she regained full function in her hand. Casey looked into private physical therapy programs but found them unaffordable. The public clinics in her area that provided free or reduced-cost care did not offer physical therapy services. Casey decided to forgo the physical therapy and rehabilitate

her hand on her own. In addition, she received a $1,500 bill from the hospital, an amount equal to her savings.

If the above scenario took place in 2014, the result may have been very different. By then, it is very likely Casey would have health insurance because most individuals will be required to obtain insurance starting that year (or pay a penalty). Although she would not have had the choice to purchase art supplies instead of health insurance, she would be much more likely to receive the care she needs. There would be a better chance her employer would offer affordable coverage, but even if health coverage wasn't offered, Casey would have better public and private options available to her.

INTRODUCTION

In the United States the persistent rate of uninsurance, concerns about the quality of health care services, and the rising cost of health care have led to numerous attempts to implement national health reform that provides comprehensive and universal health insurance coverage. Most people in the United States have health insurance through a patchwork collection of private plans and public programs. Unfortunately, like Casey, there are also many people who are uninsured. As discussed in Chapter 4, over the last several decades the rate of uninsurance has consistently hovered between 12% and 16% of the population.[1](p. 24) In 2009, 50.7 million people in this country (16.7% of the population) did not have health insurance,[1](p. 22) and most of them were without coverage for at least 2 years.[2](p. 7) U.S. spending on health care has been perpetually high, accounting for 17.6% of the gross domestic product in 2009.[3] Despite the high level of spending on health care, the United States ranks poorly on a variety of quality measures, such as infant mortality rates and life expectancy (see Chapters 4 and 11 for a more detailed discussion of quality).

Although there has been general agreement about the problems facing the U.S. health care system, politicians and voters have disagreed about the best solutions. As a result, numerous attempts to pass national health reform legislation did not succeed. What was different in 2010? Why was the Obama administration successful when so many had failed before? This chapter begins with a discussion of why it has been so difficult to achieve broad health reform in this country. It continues by examining the numerous failed attempts at national health reform over the last century. The chapter then analyzes why health reform was enacted in 2010 and ends with an overview of the health reform law. Throughout this chapter we revisit themes highlighted in previous chapters: choosing between state flexibility and national uniformity; determining the appropriate role for government, the private sector, and individuals in health care financing and delivery; defining a primary decision-making goal (e.g., fiscal restraint, equity/social justice, improved health outcomes, uniformity, etc.); and settling on the appropriate scope of coverage to offer beneficiaries.

DIFFICULTY OF HEALTH REFORM IN THE UNITED STATES

The array of problems facing the health care system has led to numerous health reform proposals and implemented policies. The concept of health reform can have several different meanings. Given the patchwork health care system, health reform often refers to changes that seek to reduce the number of uninsured. Due to the high and increasing cost of health care services, health reform might also include changes that seek to contain costs and control utilization. The notion of health reform could also address other shortcomings, such as trying to reduce medical errors, strengthen patient rights, build the public health infrastructure, or confront the rising cost of medical malpractice insurance. The Patient Protection and Affordable Care Act (ACA), the health reform law passed in 2010, touches on many of these issues.[4]

We begin with a discussion about why health reform is difficult to achieve in the United States and then introduce some of the reforms that have been attempted on a national level with varying degrees of success. Numerous authors have addressed the main factors that deter significant social reform in this country, including health reform.[5-7] Factors that are prominently discussed include the country's culture, the nature of U.S. political institutions, the power of interest groups, and path dependency (i.e., the notion that people are generally opposed to change).

Culture

This country's culture and lack of consensus about health reform have impeded attempts to create universal coverage health plans. The twin concepts of entrepreneurialism and individualism have had a real impact on health policy decisions: Americans generally oppose government solutions to social welfare problems.[7(p. 438)] Opposition is high to health reforms that rely either on a direct government-run program or public funding through tax increases.[7(p. 438)] Far less than half of Americans (24%) strongly favor a single-payer health plan, and even the notion of a "public option," a government health plan to compete with private insurers, was soundly rejected in the 2010 health care debate.[8]

At the same time the country also believes the government has some role to play in health reform. Large majorities favor tax credits to assist the uninsured with purchasing health insurance, expanding government programs for low-income individuals, and government mandates that employers provide insurance.[9] In 2010 almost half of Americans (47%) believed it was the federal government's responsibility to ensure that all Americans have health coverage, down from a high of 69% in 2007.[8] In addition to having different views about how to reduce the number of uninsured, there is no agreement about the overall scope of the health care problems we face.[10] Going into the 2010 presidential election, most Americans believed the extant health system needed major changes, yet 22% believed only minor changes were required and another 17% thought the system should basically stay the same.[11]

U.S. Political System

The country's system of government has also made it difficult to achieve universal coverage. Traditionally, social welfare programs—including the provision of health care—have been the responsibility of the states. Initially, there was almost no federal involvement in the provision of health care, and when the federal government became more heavily involved in 1965, Medicaid continued to keep the locus of decision making on the state level. Of course, there are select populations, such as the elderly (Medicare) and veterans (Veterans Health Administration), who have a federalized health insurance system. However, the country appears to support a Medicaid-type expansion over a new federalized program.[8]

Although states are generally home to social welfare changes, it is very difficult to provide universal health care on a state-by-state basis. If state health reform efforts lead the way, the country could have a patchwork of programs and policies that vary from state to state, with the potential to make health coverage even more complex and inefficient than it currently is. In addition, states must consider whether they are making policy decisions that will give employers an incentive to choose to locate in another state with fewer or less onerous legal requirements. If employers leave the state, it could result in loss of jobs and have downstream effects on the state's economy.

The federal government also has resource advantages over states, making it easier for the federal level to be the engine for health reform. Each state has a much smaller tax and revenue base than the federal government to draw from to implement health reform plans. In addition, once the federal government decides to tax a good or service, a state's ability to tax that same good or service is constrained by the individual's willingness and ability to pay a higher price. Unlike the federal government, all states (except Vermont) have some type of balanced budget requirement.[9] Without the ability to deficit spend, states must make difficult choices about resource allocation that federal policymakers often avoid (and thus generate enormous deficits). These restrictions, however, may also help with reform efforts by forcing states to a crisis point where a decision must be made to avoid an untenable situation. The federal government rarely reaches such a crisis point, meaning tough decisions are often left for the next Congress or administration.

In addition, state reform efforts are also constrained by the Employee Retirement Income Security Act of 1974 (ERISA).[a] As discussed in Chapter 11, ERISA is a federal law that regulates "welfare benefit programs," including health plans, operated by private employers. ERISA limits states' ability to reform because it broadly preempts state laws that "relate to" employer-sponsored plans and because it applies to nearly all individuals who receive health benefits through a private employer.[b] One effect of the law, for example, is that states have little regulatory control over the benefits covered in employer-sponsored health plans because ERISA accords employers near-total discretion over the design of their benefit packages.[12(p. 237)]

Despite these hurdles, it is also important to recognize that a health reform strategy focusing on states has benefits as well. At its best, state-level reform can be accomplished more rapidly and with more innovation than at the federal level. State legislatures may have an easier time convincing a narrower band of constituents important to the state than Congress has in accommodating the varied needs of stakeholders nationwide. Along the same lines, states are able to target reforms to meet the particular needs of their population instead of covering more diverse needs across the entire country. Additionally, through the use of "direct democracy" (referenda, ballot initiatives, etc.), citizens can more easily have an impact on decisions by state-level policymakers than

by federal legislators. Finally, because the health care delivery system is run primarily on the state level, states have the expertise and ability to implement many planks of health care reform.

Other aspects of the U.S. political system also make it difficult to institute sweeping reform. For example, although presidents have significant influence on policy agenda setting and proposing budgets, they have very limited power to make changes without the assistance of Congress (as discussed in detail in Chapter 2). The federal government is often politically divided, with different parties holding power in the executive and legislative branches. This division often results in partisanship and policy inaction due to different policy priorities and views.

Furthermore, although members of Congress may ride the coattails of a popular president from their own party, they are not reliant on the president to keep their jobs. The issues and views their constituents care about most may not align with the president's priorities. In those cases, members of Congress have a strong incentive to adhere to the wishes of those who vote for them instead of simply following the president's lead. Barring an overwhelming wave of discontent, as occurred in the 2010 midterm elections when Democrats suffered historic losses in Congress, it is usually difficult to unseat incumbents. For example, 98% of incumbents successfully defended their seats in 2004.[13] As a result, legislators in Congress may have confidence in focusing on their district's or state's needs before those of the entire nation.

Federal legislative rules also support inaction or incremental reform over sweeping changes. In the Senate 60 (of 100) votes are needed to break a filibuster in most cases. Thus, even the political party in the majority can have difficulty effectuating change. Also, because both the House and Senate have to pass bills containing the same policies and language to have any chance at becoming law, a large political majority in one chamber or the other does not guarantee the ability to enact a policy. As a result, in many cases, members of Congress have to work together, at least to some degree, to devise a consensus policy that satisfies enough members to pass a bill. This need to build consensus makes radical change unlikely.

Interest Groups

As discussed in more detail in Chapter 2, decisions by politicians are often influenced by interest groups. The role of interest groups is to represent their members' interests in policy decisions. These groups can be corporate for-profit entities or nonprofit consumer-oriented organizations. They lobby politicians and the general public about the virtues or vices of specific proposals, work to improve proposals on the policy agenda, and attempt to defeat proposals they believe are not in the best interest of their group. By contributing to political campaigns or by helping to draw supportive voters out on election day, interest groups gain the ear, and often the influence, of politicians who vote on issues important to the group.

In terms of health reform, interest groups representing various providers, businesses, employer groups, insurance companies, and managed care organizations have often been opposed to comprehensive health reform.[7(pp. 438–439)] There are numerous points along the path from developing a policy idea to voting for or against a bill when interest groups can attempt to affect politicians' views. The more radical the policy proposal, the more interest groups are likely to become engaged in the political decision-making process, making it difficult to pass a bill that includes comprehensive reform.

In general, it is easier to oppose a proposal than develop one and pass a bill. Opponents of proposals are not required to show a better alternative to whatever is on the table. Instead, they can simply point to aspects of the policy idea that are unpopular and call for the proposal to be rejected. This was the tactic used by the Health Insurance Association of America in their well-known "Harry and Louise" television ads that opposed the Clinton administration's comprehensive health reform bill in 1993, the Health Security Act. In the ad, Harry and Louise, two "average" Americans, are seen discussing the health care system over breakfast. Although they both agree the system needs to be improved, they highlight certain aspects of the Clinton plan that were particularly controversial, such as an overall cap on funds for health care needs and restrictions on provider choice. The punch line for the ad was "There's got to be a better way."[14] Similarly, before the 2010 midterm elections, many Republicans promised to "repeal and replace" the health reform bill without specifying their favored replacement option. To be effective in opposing health reform, opponents did not have to propose an alternative that was scrutinized and compared with the existing proposal. Simply saying "the country can do better" was enough to help create significant opposition to the plan.

Path Dependency

Finally, the concept of "path dependency" has been a hindrance to major health reform. "The notion of path dependency emphasizes the power of inertia within political institutions."[7(p. 439)] That is, once a certain way of doing things becomes the norm, it is hard to change course. Yet, this theory does not mean that health reform is impossible. Inertia may be overcome at "critical moments or junctures" that open a window for change.[7(p. 439)] For example, the passage of Medicaid and Medicare in 1965 was a radical change from the

past pattern of limited federal government involvement in health care. The catalysts for this change were the growing social pressure for improving the health care system and the landslide victory of Democrat Lyndon Johnson as president and of liberal and moderate Democrats in Congress. The 1992 election of Democrat Bill Clinton, who ran on a platform emphasizing broad health reform, coupled with the Democratic majority in Congress (until 1994), also presented a window of opportunity. Although Clinton's plan was not ultimately successful, it appeared the American public and politicians were open to changing the course of the health care "path" that had been taken to date. In 2010 another "critical moment" appeared, and President Obama took advantage of the circumstances to push through the health reform bill. Although path dependency suggests that inertia and fear of change have made broad reform difficult to achieve, it is not impossible to succeed.

Path dependency is also evident on the individual level; that is, once individuals are accustomed to having things a certain way, it is difficult for them to accept change. Currently, about 85% of Americans have health insurance, most through employer-sponsored coverage. Comprehensive health reform would likely change the condition of the insured population to some degree by changing either their source of coverage, the benefits included in coverage, the cost of coverage, or some other factor. During the debate over the ACA, about one-third of people surveyed reported that the bill would probably make them worse off, and another third thought it would not make any difference to them.[10] Professor Judith Feder refers to this problem as the "crowd-out" politics of health reform.[15] "[T]he fundamental barrier to universal coverage is that our success in insuring most of the nation's population has 'crowded out' our political capacity to insure the rest."[15(p. 461)] In other words, many of the insured do not want a change in the health care system that will leave them worse off to make the uninsured better off.

According to Professor Feder, the way to solve the political crowd-out dilemma is by changing the very nature of American culture. The focus on individualism must be replaced with a concern for the community and recognition that all Americans are part of a single community. "[T]he challenge to improving or achieving universal coverage is to decide whether we are a society in which it is every man, woman or child for him/herself or one in which we are all in it together."[15(p. 464)] Even with the passage of the ACA, the country remains divided about the extent that "we are all in it together." Shortly before the ACA passed, over half of people surveyed (54%) said they would not be willing to pay more so others could have access to health insurance.[16]

411

UNSUCCESSFUL ATTEMPTS TO PASS NATIONAL HEALTH REFORM

Since the early 1900s, when medical knowledge became advanced enough to make health care and health insurance a desirable commodity, there have been periodic attempts to implement universal coverage through national health reform. The Socialist Party was the first U.S. political party to support health insurance in 1904, but the main engine behind early efforts for national reform was the American Association for Labor Legislation (AALL), a "social progressive" group that hoped to reform capitalism, not overthrow it.[17(p. 243)] In 1912 Progressive Party candidate Theodore Roosevelt supported a social insurance platform modeled on the European social insurance tradition that included health insurance, workers' compensation, old-age pensions, and unemployment. With his loss to Woodrow Wilson, the national health insurance movement was without a strong national leader for three decades.

The AALL continued to support a form of health insurance after Roosevelt's defeat and drafted a model bill in 1915. This bill followed the European model, limiting participation to working class employees and their dependents. Benefits included medical aid, sick pay, maternity benefits, and a death benefit. These costs were to be financed by employers, employees, and the state. The AALL believed that health insurance for the working population would reduce poverty and increase society's productivity and well-being through healthier workers and citizens.

Opposition to AALL's bill came from several sources.[17(pp. 247–249)] Although some members of the American Medical Association (AMA) approved of the bill conceptually, physician support rapidly evaporated when details emerged about aspects of the plan that would negatively impact their income and autonomy. The American Federation of Labor (a labor union) opposed compulsory health insurance because it wanted workers to rely on their own economic strength, not the state, to obtain better wages and benefits. In addition, the federation was concerned that it would lose power if the government, not the union, secured benefits for workers. Employers were generally opposed to the bill, contending that supporting public health was a better way to ensure productivity. In addition, they feared that providing health insurance to employees might promote malingering instead of reducing lost workdays. After experiencing the high cost associated with workers' compensation, employers were also not eager to take on an additional expensive benefit. Of course, the part of the insurance industry that had already established a profitable niche in the death benefit business was strongly opposed to a bill that included a death benefit provision.

Employers, providers, and insurers have, in general, remained staunch opponents of national health reform over the years, whereas unions have supported national reform efforts. However, this dynamic has recently changed with more provider groups, employers, and even some insurers calling for a national solution to the problems of rising health care costs and the uninsured.

The country's entry into World War I in 1917 also changed the health reform debate. Many physicians who supported the AALL bill entered the military, shifting their focus away from the domestic health policy debate. Anti-German sentiment was high, so opponents of the bill gained traction by denouncing compulsory health insurance as anti-American. One pamphlet read as follows: "What is Compulsory Social Health Insurance? It is a dangerous device, invented in Germany, announced by the German Emperor from the throne the same year he started plotting and preparing to conquer the world."[17(p. 253)]

The next time national health insurance might have taken hold was from the mid-1930s through the early 1940s because the country was coping with the difficulties of the Depression. During this time, there was a significant increase in government programs, including the creation of Social Security in 1935, which provided old-age assistance, unemployment compensation, and public assistance. Yet, the fourth prong of the social insurance package, health insurance, remained elusive. President Franklin Roosevelt heeded his staff's advice to leave health insurance out of Social Security because of the strong opposition it would create.[17(p. 267)]

Even so, members of Roosevelt's administration continued to push for national health insurance. The Interdepartmental Committee to Coordinate Health and Welfare Activities was created in 1935 and took on the task of studying the nation's health care needs. This job fell to its Technical Committee on Medical Care. Instead of supporting a federal program, the committee proposed subsidies to the states for operating health programs. Components of the proposal included expanding maternal and child health and public health programs under Social Security, expanding hospital construction, increasing aid for medical care for the indigent, studying a general medical care program, and creating a compensation program for those who lost wages due to disability.

Although President Roosevelt established a National Health Conference to discuss the recommendation, he never fully supported the medical care committee's proposal. With the success of conservatives in the 1938 election and the administration's concerns about fighting the powerful physician and state medical society lobbies, national health reform did not have a place on Roosevelt's priority list. Senator Robert

Wagner (D-NY) introduced a bill that followed the committee's recommendations in 1939, and although it passed in the Senate, it did not garner support from the president or in the House.

World War II provided another opportunity for the opposition to label national health insurance as socialized medicine. But once the war ended, President Roosevelt finally called for an "economic bill of rights," which included medical care. President Truman picked up where Roosevelt left off, strongly advocating for national health insurance. President Truman's proposal included expanding hospitals, increasing public health and maternal and child health services, providing federal aid for medical research and education, and, for the first time, a single health insurance program for all.[17(p. 281)] Heeding lessons from earlier reform failures, Truman emphasized that his plan was not socialized medicine and that the delivery system for medical and hospital care would not change.

Again, there was strong opposition to the proposal. The AMA vehemently rejected the proposal, and most other health care groups opposed it as well. Although the public initially approved of it, there was no consensus about how national health insurance should be structured, and more people preferred modest voluntary plans over a national, compulsory, comprehensive health insurance program.[17(p. 282)] Additional opposition came from the American Bar Association, the Chamber of Commerce, and even some federal agencies concerned about losing control over their existing programs. In the end, only the hospital construction portion of the proposal was enacted.

When Truman won reelection on a national health insurance platform in 1948, it appeared the tide had turned. However, the AMA continued its strong opposition and its attempts to link national health insurance to socialism. Congress considered various compromises but never reached a consensus. The public remained uncertain about what kind of plan to favor. Employers maintained their opposition to compulsory insurance. In addition, one large group of potential supporters—veterans—was disinterested in the debate because they had already secured extensive medical coverage through the Veterans Administration. As the Korean War moved forward, Truman's focus shifted away from national health insurance and toward the war effort and other priorities.

National health insurance did not return to the national policy agenda until the 1970s. The landscape was quite different from that during Truman's era. Medicaid and Medicare had been created, health care costs had begun to rise exponentially, and the economy was deteriorating. In 1969 President Nixon declared that a "massive crisis" existed in health care and that unless it was fixed immediately, the country's medical system would collapse.[17(p. 381)] The general public seemed to agree, with 75% of respondents in one survey concurring that the health care system was in crisis.[17(p. 381)] Democrats still controlled Congress by a significant margin, and Senator Edward Kennedy (D-MA) and Representative Martha Griffiths (D-MI), the first woman to serve on the powerful House Ways and Means Committee, proposed a comprehensive, federally operated health insurance system.

At the same time a movement supporting health care and patient rights was gaining momentum. These included rights to informed consent, to refuse treatment, to due process for involuntary commitment, and to equal access to health care.[17(p. 389)] The public was both anxious to obtain care and willing to challenge the authority of health care providers.

The Nixon administration's first attempt at health reform focused on the need to change the financing of the health care system from one dominated by a fee-for-service system, which created incentives to provide more and more expensive services, to one that promoted restraint, efficiency, and the health of the patient. The result was a "health maintenance strategy" intended to stimulate the private industry to create health maintenance organizations (HMOs) through federal planning grants and loan guarantees, with the goal of enrolling 90% of the population in an HMO by the end of the 1970s.[17(pp. 395–396)] Ironically, group health plans, often labeled socialized medicine, had become the centerpiece of a Republican reform strategy.

Nixon's proposal included an employer mandate to provide a minimum package of benefits under a National Health Insurance Standards Act, a federally administered Family Health Insurance Program for low-income families. The program had a less generous benefit package than the one required by the National Health Insurance Standards Act, reductions in Medicare spending to help defray the costs, a call for an increase in the supply of physicians, and a change in how medical schools were subsidized. Opponents were plentiful, and this plan did not come to fruition. Some believed the plan was a gift to private insurance companies. Advocates for the poor were outraged at the second tier of benefits for low-income families. The AMA was concerned about HMOs interfering with physician practices and supported an alternative that provided tax credits for buying private insurance.

After the 1972 election, Nixon proposed a second, more comprehensive plan that covered everyone and offered more comprehensive coverage. Private insurance companies would cover the employed and a government-run program would cover the rest of the population, with both groups receiving the same benefit package. Senator Kennedy and Representative Wilbur Mills (D-AR) supported a similar plan, and it appeared a compromise was close at hand. However, labor unions and liberal organizations preferred the original Kennedy plan and resisted compromising with the hope of gaining power in the 1974 post-Watergate elections. Fearing the same political shift, insurance companies actually supported a catastrophic insurance plan proposed by Senator Russell Long (D-LA), believing it was better than any plan that would come out of a more liberal Congress after the elections. Once again, there was no majority support for any of the bills, and a national health insurance plan was not enacted.

Although President Jimmy Carter gave lip service to national health reform, he never fully supported a proposal. It was not until the election of Bill Clinton in 1992 that the next real attempt at national health insurance was made. The Clinton administration plan, dubbed the Health Security Act, was designed to create national health insurance without spending new federal funds or shifting coverage from private to public insurance. It relied on the concept of "managed competition," which combined elements of managed care and market competition.

Under the Health Security Act, a National Health Board would have established national and regional spending limits and regulated premium increases. "Health alliances" would have included a variety of plans that were competing for the business of employees and unemployed citizens in each geographic area. All plans were to have a guaranteed scope of benefits and uniform cost sharing. Employers were required to provide coverage for their workers at a defined high level of benefits, and those with 5,000 employees or fewer had to purchase plans through the health alliance. Subsidies were provided for low-income individuals and small businesses. Funding was to be provided from cost-containment measures that were reinvested. Forced by the Congressional Budget Office (CBO) to provide an alternative funding strategy should the cost containment not create enough funds, the plan also included the option of capping insurance premium growth and reducing provider payments.

Like the national health insurance plans before it, the Health Security Act had opponents from many directions. The health alliances were attacked as big government, employers resisted mandates and interference with their fringe benefits, some advocates feared that cost containment would lead to care rationing, the insured were concerned about losing some of their existing benefits or cost-sharing arrangements, the elderly feared losing Medicare, and academic health centers were concerned about losing funds based on new graduate medical education provisions.[17(p. 463)] In addition, the usually strong support from unions was missing because of an earlier disagreement with the president on trade matters. It is also generally accepted that the Clinton administration made several political mistakes that made a difficult political chore nearly impossible. The Health Security Act never made it to a vote.

WHY THE PATIENT PROTECTION AND AFFORDABLE CARE ACT PASSED

In many ways, 2010 was a very unlikely year to pass a national health reform plan. The country had been bitterly divided ideologically in recent years. Both the popular and electoral votes were almost evenly split in the 2000 and 2004 presidential elections. George W. Bush beat Al Gore despite losing the popular vote in 2000, and Bush beat John Kerry in 2004 with only 51% of the popular vote.[18] Even though Barack Obama won the electoral vote in a landslide over John McCain (365 to 173), only 53% of the population voted for Obama in 2010.[19]

In addition to the ideological divide, a financial crisis erupted toward the end of the 2008 presidential election. In October 2008, President Bush signed into law the Emergency Economic Stabilization Act, which included the $700 billion Troubled Asset Relief Program (TARP), which allowed the federal government to take over distressed assets, primarily bad mortgage loans, from private financial institutions.[20] It was argued that TARP was necessary to save the financial industry from collapsing, which could have led to another Great Depression. Even with TARP, the United States (and many other countries) entered into a recessionary period. Many individuals lived in homes they could no longer afford, banks limited lending opportunities, and employers laid off millions of workers due to the drop in consumer spending. In an effort to improve the economy, Obama signed into law the American Recovery and Reinvestment Act of 2009, also known as the stimulus bill.[21] This almost $800 billion effort was intended to save existing jobs, create new jobs, and spur long-term growth of the U.S. economy.[22] Although TARP was not popular with politicians or the general public, it was seen as necessary by members of both political parties and signed into law by a Republican president. Unlike TARP, however, the stimulus bill was not a bipartisan effort. Republicans in the House unanimously opposed the stimulus bill and only three Republicans voted for the bill in the Senate.

Not surprising, health care was not the only issue on voters' minds during the election campaign. Shortly before the election, 43% of registered voters ranked the economy as their number one priority. Economic concerns trumped health care, which ranked second, by an almost 2-to-1 margin.[23] Although voters from both political parties ranked the economy as their top priority, differences emerged along party lines regarding the next most important issue. Democratic voters ranked health care second, whereas both Republican and Independent voters were more concerned about the size and power of the federal government. These results were not surprising; Democrats have ranked health care as a higher priority than Republican and Independent voters did in every presidential election from 1988 to 2008.[24(p. 2053)]

Against this backdrop of a faltering economy, partisan differences, and the recent passage of two massive government spending bills, President Obama pursued a national health reform plan. Given the history of failed reform efforts, it would have been an accomplishment to pass health reform in the best of times, and clearly this was not the best of times. How did Obama and the 111th Congress succeed? It was a combination of having commitment, exhibiting leadership, applying lessons from past failures, and being pragmatic that lead to the passage of health reform.

Commitment and Leadership

It is highly unlikely that the 2010 health reform effort would have succeeded without a passionate and committed president willing to make health reform a priority. Health care has long been a priority for Democrats, and President Obama was no exception. Perhaps Obama's dedication to pass health reform stemmed in part from his personal experience. Obama's mother was uninsured when she died of ovarian cancer. As he said in one of his campaign ads: "My mother died of cancer at 53. In those last, painful months she was more worried about paying her medical bills than getting well. I hear stories like hers every day."[25]

Some of Obama's political advisors suggested waiting to tackle health reform until after taking action to address the poor economy and rising unemployment. Even voters who supported Obama were split over what his priorities should be during his first days in office.[26] Just days before the election, Obama suggested that the economy and energy independence were higher priorities than health reform. To Obama, that meant he should tackle several major issues at once, not put health reform on the back burner. "Priority number 3 would be health reform. I think the time is right to do it."[27]

Health reform efforts did not begin smoothly. President Obama initially wanted former Senator Tom Daschle to run both the Department of Health and Human Services (DHHS) and the White House Office on Health Reform. It was thought that his experience with the Senate, relationships with legislators, and confidence of the president were the right combination to take the lead on health reform. When his nomination was derailed due to tax problems, it was not a good omen. As deliberations in Congress lagged, Democrats were not able to present a bill to President Obama before recessing for the summer. During the summer of 2009, members of Congress went home to their constituents and held town hall meetings to discuss health reform. Some of the meetings erupted in vocal opposition to health reform, and the media focused on these town hall meetings throughout the summer. Obama and the Democrats were criticized for losing the momentum for reform by letting the debate linger.

At the same time, there were several instances during the political process when the health reform effort appeared doomed and President Obama's leadership made a difference. Obama attempted to reclaim the upper hand on health reform with a speech to a joint session of Congress in September 2009. He memorably proclaimed, "I am not the first president to take up health reform, but I intend to be the last."[28] Though support for health reform had been on the decline for several months, September 2009 polls showed that 62% still thought it was important to address health reform at that time, and 53% thought the country as a whole would be better off if health reform passed.[29] Less support existed for the Democrats' specific reform proposal, however, with 46% in support of the proposed change and 48% opposed to it.[30]

In January 2010, an event occurred that some assumed was the death knell of health reform. In the 2008 elections, Democrats made significant gains in Congress, earning a 59–41 majority in the Senate and a 257–178 majority in the House. Furthermore, Senator Arlen Specter of Pennsylvania switched parties, giving Democrats the crucial 60th vote needed for a filibuster-proof majority. President Obama, Senate Majority Leader Harry Reid (D-NV), and House Speaker Nancy Pelosi (D-CA) would have to balance the competing interests of conservative Democrats who were concerned with having too much government intervention, progressive Democrats who sought a public insurance option to compete with private companies, Blue Dog Democrats who were most concerned with fiscal discipline, and prolife and prochoice factions who would battle over whether and how abortion services would be included in any health reform bill. Then, in August 2009, Senator Ted Kennedy (D-MA) died. In office for 47 years, Kennedy was not only a lifelong supporter of health reform but also an expert negotiator who could work with Republicans and possibly achieve a bipartisan consensus. The January 2010 special election to fill his seat was won by Republican Scott Brown, who campaigned against the Democrats' health reform plan. In a postelection poll, 42% of voters said they voted for Brown to stop the health reform bill.[31]

Despite this setback and concerns by some that health reform efforts should be abandoned, Obama, along with Reid and Pelosi, remained strong in his conviction to pursue reform. President Obama's senior advisors said it would be a "terrible mistake" to walk away from the process based on Brown's victory, and Pelosi reminded her caucus how detrimental it was when Democrats abandoned the health reform effort during the Clinton administration.[32] In his State of the Union address, just a week after the special election, President Obama tied his health reform efforts to fixing the economy and reiterated his commitment to the issue[33]:

> And it is precisely to relieve the burden on middle class families that we still need health reform. Now let's be clear, I did not choose to tackle this issue to get some legislative victory under my belt. And by now it should be fairly obvious that I didn't take on health reform because it was good politics. . . . Here is what I ask of Congress though: Do not walk away from reform. Not now. Not when we are so close. Let us find a way to come together and finish the job for the American people.

Obama was not alone in providing leadership on health reform. Reid's and Pelosi's determination to see health reform succeed and their skill in mobilizing and controlling their caucuses were essential to the passage of the ACA. It is likely that health reform would not have passed without the skillful efforts of all three leaders working together. Even so, it is clear that the health reform effort would not even have begun without a president who put health reform at the top of the agenda and stuck with it throughout all the pitfalls.

Lessons from Failed Health Reform Efforts

The Obama administration tried to avoid the pitfalls that doomed health reform efforts in the past. Although the most recent failed effort from the Clinton administration probably provided the most relevant lessons, Obama confronted some of the same obstacles that reformers had faced decades earlier. At times, President Obama was accused of learning some of the lessons too well, swinging the pendulum too far to the other side. Although that debate may continue, clearly the way in which the Obama administration applied those lessons brought him success where others before him had failed.

President Clinton was criticized for not moving quickly enough to try to enact health reform after he was elected in 1992. He did not present a plan to Congress until a year into his presidency, having been sidetracked by other issues, such as the economy, including a budget showdown with Republicans, and whether gays should be allowed to serve in the military. Even after he finally sent his health care proposal to Congress, Clinton was preoccupied with other issues that sapped his political capital, such as passing the North American Free Trade Agreement and the fallout from the deaths of 18 American soldiers in Somalia.

President Obama, over the objection of some aides, chose to address health reform as quickly as possible despite also having to tackle the poor economy and possible collapse of the financial sector. Obama was elected into office with a 70% approval rating, and he moved to capitalize on his popularity.[34] It was almost inevitable that his approval rating would decline as he tried to turn the promise of a campaign into the reality of running the country. As Lyndon Johnson said after winning the 1964 election in a landslide, "Everyday while I'm in office, I'm gonna lose votes."[35(p. 172)] In addition, it is almost universally expected that the president's party will lose seats in the midterm elections. In the past 10 midterm elections, the incumbent party lost an average of 18.5 seats in the House and 2.5 seats in the Senate.[36(p. 1097)] Obama was correct to assume his Democratic majorities in Congress would not last long. After the 2010 midterm elections, the Democrats lost control of the House and several seats in the Senate.

President Obama also dealt with interest groups in a different way than his predecessors had done. Previous failed efforts of health reform have shown that those vested interests can be important players in the debate. In general, though not in all instances, provider groups, insurers, and employers have opposed health reform, whereas unions have supported health reform efforts. All these stakeholders have been known to devote significant resources and to lean on their representatives to support their point of view. During their reform effort, the Clinton administration warred with many stakeholder groups, with insurance companies and small businesses taking a leading role.[14]

Obama took a different tact from Clinton's by making deals with various stakeholders at the outset of the health reform debate. The lure of millions of newly insured customers helped convince the Pharmaceutical Research and Manufacturers of America and the American Hospital Association to contribute to health reform financing through reduced Medicare and Medicaid payments. In addition, the health insurance industry supported universal coverage under health reform. After being credited for helping derail the Clinton health plan, the Health Insurance Association of America favored the general idea of health reform though it differed with Obama and the Democrats' plan on some of the specifics. To be fair, Clinton may not have been able to broker deals with these stakeholders in the 1990s no matter how hard he tried. A combination of a changing health care environment, the likelihood that some type of health reform was likely to pass, and the uncertain future of employer-sponsored insurance made it more palatable for interest groups to try to influence instead of oppose the 2010 legislation.[37]

Clinton was also criticized for not mastering the legislative process. The Clinton administration chose to design the health reform plan itself and developed a complicated and secretive process, headlined by the Health Care Task Force, run by Hillary Clinton, to do it. While naming Hillary Clinton as the leader of the task force signaled the administration's commitment to the issue, she became a lightning rod for criticism, and questions about the appropriateness of the First Lady taking on such a significant policy role detracted from the substance of the health reform debate. Instead of negotiating with Congress, the administration debated the specifics of health reform among its own advisors and then asked Congress to pass the bill they had developed. Shutting out members of Congress instead of negotiating with them and taking over Congress' role in developing legislation was not, it turned out, a formula for success.

President Obama learned from Clinton's mistakes, as well as other presidents' legislative achievements. Instead of presenting a detailed plan or written legislation to Congress, success has often been found in outlining ideas and principles and letting Congress work through the details. When President Johnson was trying to get a Medicare bill passed, he told key members of Congress that he would not delve into the details of the bill, but he generally pushed for a larger package. When President George W. Bush was pursuing a new Medicare prescription drug benefit, he outlined his desire for an approach that worked with the private sector and encouraged competition but let Congress find the exact formula that would pass.[36(p. 1097)]

Similarly, Obama set out his principles but left the work of drafting a bill and fleshing out the details to Congress. On June 2, 2009, President Obama sent a letter to Senators Kennedy and Baucus, two leaders in the health reform effort, outlining his "core belief" that Americans deserved better and more affordable health insurance choices and that a health reform bill must not add to the federal deficit.[38] Although he let the negotiators know what his priorities were, Obama stayed above the fray during the legislative process. Whereas he preferred a public option to compete with private insurers, he did not insist on it. Although Obama campaigned against an individual mandate as a presidential candidate, he was open to including it in the bill. The president refused to be drawn into the debate over taxing generous health plans or creating a Medicare cost-containment commission. Instead, he focused his efforts on persuading Congress not to give up on the effort, bringing together various factions of the Democratic caucus and reaching out to the public to garner support for health reform.

The legislative process for completing the bill was long, rocky, and ultimately partisan. The House of Representatives moved more quickly and with less fractious debate than did the Senate. Instead of having multiple House committees work on competing bills, as occurred during the Clinton administration, House Democratic leaders created a "Tri-Committee" bill, jointly sponsored by Charles Rangel (D-NY), Henry Waxman (D-CA), and George Miller (D-CA), the chairmen of the House Ways and Means, Energy and Commerce, and Education and Labor (later renamed the Education and Workforce committee) committees, respectively. On November 7, 2009, the House passed its health reform bill with only two votes to spare, 220–215.[39] Only one Republican voted for it, and 39 conservative Democrats voted against it. The bill from the more liberal House contained several provisions that were likely to be rejected by the Senate: a public health insurance option to compete with private plans, a national health insurance exchange instead of state-based exchanges, more generous subsidies for low-income individuals, a broader expansion of Medicaid, and higher taxes on wealthier Americans.

Finance Committee Chairman Max Baucus (D-MT) led the effort in the Senate. The legislative process he established was lengthy, and some observers believed he compromised on too many issues in an attempt to forge a bipartisan bill. For a time, Senator Charles Grassley (R-IA) actively participated in the health reform deliberations, and a few other Republican senators appeared willing to consider a bipartisan measure. Ultimately, however, a bipartisan agreement could not be reached. In a 2009 Christmas Eve vote, the Baucus bill passed 60–39, with all Democrats and two Independents voting for the measure and all Republicans voting against it.[40]

Shortly after the New Year, members of the House and Senate began meeting to resolve differences between the House- and Senate-passed bills. Before those differences were resolved, however, Scott Brown was elected to fill Kennedy's seat in the Senate, and the Democrats no longer had a filibuster-proof majority. Before the special election that led to Brown's victory, it was assumed that after the Senate passed a health reform measure, House and Senate negotiators would work out their differences in a conference committee, with each chamber then voting to pass the compromise bill. With Brown's election and his opposition to health reform, however, this plan became unworkable. Democratic congressional leaders were left with few options, all of them unpalatable: the House could pass the Senate version of the bill; Democrats could try to use the reconciliation process to pass a new comprehensive bill; the House and Senate could compromise on a much smaller, more incremental health reform bill that focused on areas where a bipartisan agreement could be reached; or Democrats could abandon their efforts to pass a health reform bill. The day after Brown's election, House

Speaker Pelosi appeared to eliminate the easiest (legislatively speaking) of these paths by declaring that the House would not pass the Senate version of the bill: "I don't think it's possible to pass the Senate bill in the House. I don't see the votes for it at this time."[41]

In the end, a compromise was reached. House and Senate leaders agreed to use the budget reconciliation process to amend the Senate bill. The House then passed the Senate version of the bill, along with a companion reconciliation bill that amended certain aspects of the Senate bill. The reconciliation bill included more generous subsidies for individuals to purchase insurance than existed in the stand-alone Senate bill, the closure of the Medicare Part D doughnut hole, a tax on more generous insurance plans, changes to the penalties on individuals who would not buy insurance and for employers who would not offer insurance, and an increase in Medicare and investment taxes for higher earners. The Senate then passed the reconciliation bill, which could not be filibustered and only required a simple majority vote to pass. Once again, the vote to approve the bills was along party lines. The House approved the Senate bill by a vote of 219–212, with all Republicans and 34 Democrats voting against it.[42] President Obama signed the bill into law on March 23, 2010.[4]

Some observers argue that Obama may have "overlearned" the lesson about working with Congress and that in doing so he did not provide enough guidance to legislators and allowed the debate over health reform to linger too long.[36(p. 1097)] On one hand, it is difficult to criticize Obama's approach, because he was ultimately successful. On the other hand, could the problems stemming from the 2009 town halls and Scott Brown's election have been avoided, and would public opinion of the health reform effort be higher if the process had been better managed? Only time will tell whether Obama was successful over the long term (e.g., Is the law effective? Will the public support it over time? Will it be repealed?) and whether the political cost of the lengthy battle hurt the Democrats more than passing the bill helped them.

Political Pragmatism

President Obama is both credited and criticized for being as pragmatic as necessary to help ensure that health reform passed. He was comfortable making deals with industry stakeholders even though those agreements limited the savings and other changes that could have been achieved in the health reform bill. Obama ultimately signed a bill that did not include a public option even though he preferred that one was included, and his liberal base thought health reform without such an option was not true reform. An argument over abortion nearly derailed the bill in its final days, and Obama supported a compromise on abortion language to keep enough Democrats in the fold. Even his goal of universal coverage was not met in the name of passing health reform. Obama's willingness to be pragmatic instead of staunchly principled, taking some victories instead of an all-or-nothing approach, allowed him to succeed in passing a health reform bill where others had failed.[37(p. 1116)] Some people argued it was worse to pass a flawed bill than not pass a bill at all, but Obama believed the promise of reducing the uninsured rate and gaining numerous health insurance market reforms were worth the compromises he made.

PATIENT PROTECTION AND AFFORDABLE CARE ACT

The ACA's reforms are expected to reduce the number of uninsured by 32 million people, including 16 million new Medicaid enrollees. This would leave approximately 23 million nonelderly residents uninsured. Although the ACA is estimated to cost $940 billion over 10 years, the CBO projects that the health care and revenue provisions in the law will reduce the federal deficit by $124 billion during that span.[43]

Although the ACA does not completely alter the way health insurance is provided by establishing a single-payer system or even a large government-run insurance plan to compete with private insurers, it makes significant philosophical and practical changes in how health insurance is regulated, structured, and administered in this country. The ACA is wide ranging and includes new requirements affecting individuals, employers, and states. Key provisions of the law are discussed in more depth below although most provisions relating to Medicaid and Medicare are detailed in Chapter 10. **Figure 1** provides a timeline for when major provisions of the ACA will be implemented.

Many people contend that the ACA falls short in its reform of the health care delivery system. And in many cases, they are correct. The ACA is most notable for the transformation changes it makes to health insurance—both access to it and its content—rather than for structural reforms made to the delivery system. Many provisions that focus on improving the health care delivery system, increasing the quality of care received by patients, reducing health care costs, and incentivizing providers to reconsider traditional methods of delivering care are often in the form of temporary pilot programs that may never be enacted permanently even if they prove to be valuable. Other analysts contend that these provisions were written as strongly as they could be at the time given the political environment and data available to policy makers. According to this view, the ACA provides the secretary of DHHS with unprecedented authority to make the pilot programs permanent, and it would have been irresponsible to implement more permanent wholesale changes without more evidence. In any case, as sweeping as the ACA is, it is far from being the last step that needs to be taken to improve how health care is provided in this country.

Individual Mandate

An individual mandate is a requirement that individuals purchase health insurance. This is not a new idea. President Clinton proposed an individual mandate in 1993 as part of his Health Security Act, and other competing proposals at the time, including those supported by Republicans, also included an individual mandate. Massachusetts, the only state in the country to require that everyone over age 18 have insurance, included an individual mandate as one way to achieve that goal. Switzerland and the Netherlands also included an individual mandate in their health reform plans.[44] During the 2008 election, Obama supported a mandate for children to be covered but suggested waiting to see if a mandate was necessary for adults after implementing other major health reform changes.

Individual mandates can be set up in a variety of ways, but usually individuals who do not comply will be required to pay some sort of penalty. The penalty is intended to both provide an incentive to comply with the law and to raise funds to cover the cost of health care for those individuals who choose not to carry health insurance. Individual mandates are considered to be a cornerstone of health reform efforts because they ensure that everyone covered by the mandate will be in an insurance pool to help cover costs and share risk.

The mandate is considered essential because without it, people who are in poor health or otherwise expect to use more health care services will be more likely to purchase health insurance, whereas healthier people will be more likely to opt out of insurance coverage. This would lead to an insurance pool that is sicker and more expensive, a problem referred to as adverse selection (discussed in more detail in Chapter 8). In addition, healthy individuals who choose not to purchase health insurance but then later need health care will likely receive some care even though they are uninsured. This is especially true if the individuals have the resources to pay for health care services. These individuals are referred to as free riders because they avoid paying premiums for health insurance during their healthy years but then enjoy the benefits of health care services when they are sick (free riders are discussed in more detail in Chapter 8). In 2007, more than 9 million people who earned at least $75,000 were uninsured. Because it is likely that many of these individuals could have afforded to purchase health insurance, some analysts consider

this evidence of the free rider problem.[44] In addition, the individual mandate is essential because it was the carrot that enticed health insurers to support health reform.

Starting in 2014, the ACA's individual mandate requires that almost everyone purchase health insurance or pay a penalty. This penalty is phased in over time, beginning at the greatest of $95 or 1% of taxable income per person in 2014 and growing to the greatest of $695 or 2.5% of taxable income per person in 2016. After 2016, the penalty amount increases through cost of living adjustments. Individuals are exempt from this requirement if their income is below the tax filing threshold (in 2010 this was $9,350 for singles and $18,700 for couples), the lowest-cost plan option exceeds 8% of their income, they qualify for a religious exemption, they are incarcerated, they are undocumented immigrants, they were without coverage for less than 3 months, or they are Native Americans.

The individual mandate is controversial. In addition to believing that the individual mandate represents unwanted government intrusion into private decision making, opponents of the individual mandate argue that Congress does not have the legal authority to impose such a requirement. This argument is grounded in jurisprudence relating to the federal Constitution's Commerce Clause, which gives Congress the power to "regulate commerce with foreign nations, and among the several states, and with the Indian tribes."[45] Since the 1940s, the Supreme Court has interpreted the Commerce Clause to permit Congress to regulate economic activity that carries across state lines or are local concerns that substantially affect interstate commerce. Several Commerce Clause cases have allowed the regulation of individual conduct. For example, the Court has upheld laws that prohibit an individual from refusing to interact with a minority and those that regulate an individual's ability to grow wheat or marijuana for home consumption.[46] In addition, regulating health insurance has also been deemed to be within the scope of the Commerce Clause.[47]

The crux of the argument against the individual mandate is that the Commerce Clause does not permit Congress to require an individual to purchase a good or service, such as health insurance. In other words, the argument goes, an individual's decision not to purchase health insurance cannot be considered "economic activity" that Congress may regulate. Instead, it is argued, Congress is trying to regulate economic *in*activity—the decision not to purchase health insurance— and that this is not covered by the Commerce Clause.[48]

Those who contend the Commerce Clause permits Congress to establish an individual mandate to purchase health insurance argue that everyone uses health care services at some point in their lives. Decisions regarding health insurance are an economic activity because no one can opt out of the health care market—the decision individuals make is not whether to participate but how to participate in it. People will participate by purchasing health insurance now to cover the cost of future services or by paying out of pocket later at the time services are needed. Furthermore, it is argued that the decision to purchase health insurance affects everyone's economic activity because of the nature of pricing health insurance. To date, the Supreme Court has not ruled on a case where Congress compels an individual to buy a good or service, and the lower courts that have considered challenges have split on the issue. As of June 2011, 26 cases have been filed in the courts seeking to overturn the ACA. With so many challenges making their way through the judicial system, this legal question will ultimately be decided by the Supreme Court.

State Health Insurance Exchanges

The ACA establishes a new entity called health insurance exchanges, which are intended to create a more organized and competitive market for purchasing health insurance. These exchanges are state-based and geared toward those who purchase health insurance as individuals (through American Health Benefit Exchanges) or through small businesses (through the Small Business Health Options Program). Starting in 2014, these exchanges will offer a variety of health insurance plans that meet ACA criteria regarding plan benefits, payments, and consumer information. CBO projects that by 2019, 24 million individuals will purchase their own health insurance through an exchange and another 5 million individuals with access to employer-sponsored insurance will pick an exchange option.[49]

The exchanges are a critical component of health reform because it would be untenable to require individuals to purchase health insurance without also making comprehensive and affordable health insurance options available.

> ### BOX 1 Discussion Questions
>
> What will happen to ACA if the individual mandate is found to be unconstitutional? Will the whole reform bill unravel? Will it work but not as well? Are there alternatives to the individual mandate that accomplish the same goals without potentially running afoul of the Constitution?

As discussed in Chapter 8, individuals and small businesses often face expensive and less comprehensive health insurance choices because their insurance pools are not so large that the premiums paid by healthy individuals offset the costs associated with sicker ones. The exchanges are intended to create a new market by bringing together large numbers of individuals or small businesses to create bigger insurance pools. Individuals are eligible to purchase health insurance through an exchange if they are U.S. citizens or legal immigrants, are not incarcerated, and do not have access to affordable employer-sponsored insurance.

States are required to establish exchanges for individuals and small businesses by January 1, 2014 (although the federal government will provide a fallback option if any state fails, or chooses not, to offer one). States may choose to establish one exchange for both groups or create separate exchanges. Although the ACA defines a small business as one with fewer than 100 employees, states may choose to limit the small business exchange to organizations with fewer than 50 employees for the first 2 years. As of 2017, states may also choose to allow companies with more than 100 employees to enroll in an exchange. States may form a regional exchange with other states or allow multiple exchanges within one state as long as each exchange covers a distinct geographic area. In addition, the Office of Personnel Management is required to offer at least two multistate plans within each exchange.

All plans that participate in the exchange must offer a standard benefits package called "essential health benefits" (Table 1).[50] This represents the first time private health insurance plans are subject to a federal standard regarding which benefits must be offered. The ACA outlines the categories of services that must be provided in the essential health benefits package, but important questions about how the scope of services is defined will be decided through the regulatory process. As part of this process, the ACA requires the secretary of DHHS to ensure the scope of benefits is equal to the benefit level found in a "typical employer plan." If a state requires plans to offer any services beyond the essential health benefits package, the state must defray the cost of the additional service through a payment to the enrollee or the plan. Plans may not design their benefit or reimbursement packages in ways that discriminate based on age, disability, or expected length of life.[51]

One exception to the essential health benefits requirement is the option for plans to offer catastrophic coverage with limited benefits and low premiums. A catastrophic plan may be offered only to individuals under the age of 30 who would be exempt from the individual mandate requirement

TABLE 1 Essential Health Benefits

All plans in the state exchanges must offer the following benefits:

- Ambulatory patient services
- Emergency services
- Hospitalization
- Maternity and newborn care
- Mental health services
- Substance abuse services
- Prescription drugs
- Rehabilitative services, habilitative services and devices
- Laboratory services
- Prevention and wellness services
- Chronic disease management services
- Pediatric services, including vision and dental services

because the cost of the lowest priced plan available to them exceeds 8% of their income. The coverage level would be set at the current health savings account coverage level but with preventive benefits and three primary care visits exempt from the deductible.

There was significant debate about whether to allow or require plans in the exchange to offer abortion services. In fact, the debate was so divisive, it almost doomed the entire health reform bill at the 11th hour. A compromise was reached with the intent of keeping the status quo regarding federal funding for abortion services (i.e., limit federal funding for abortion services to cases where the life of the pregnant woman is in danger or the pregnancy is a result of rape or incest). Under the compromise, states may enact a law that prohibits plans that participate in their state exchanges from providing abortion services. If a state does not enact such a law and a plan chooses to offer abortion services in other circumstances, the plan must create separate financial accounts to ensure that federal premium and cost-sharing subsidies are not used toward those abortion services. In addition, at least one of the multistate plans is required not to provide abortion services beyond those that are currently allowed with federal funding. As with most compromises, neither side was entirely pleased with the outcome. Those who want more restrictive abortion policies found the separate accounting process to be a meaningless exercise, whereas those who want more permissive abortion policies were disturbed by the ability of states to prohibit plans from offering abortion services.

Because all exchange plans must offer the same essential health benefits package, one key difference among the plans is the cost to the enrollee. Four levels of plans may be offered, and they are distinguished by their actuarial value. Actuarial value is the share of covered benefits generally paid by the insurer based on the cost-sharing provisions in the plan. The higher the actuarial value, the more the plan pays for a given set of services. For example, in a plan with 70% actuarial value, the plan pays 70% of the cost of services on average across all enrollees, and enrollees pay 30%. Actuarial value is set by average cost, but any single enrollee in that plan may pay more or less than 30% of the cost of services. In general, plans with a higher actuarial value will also have higher premiums to cover the cost of providing services to enrollees. The four ACA-approved plan levels by actuarial value are bronze (60% actuarial value), silver (70% actuarial value), gold (80% actuarial value), and platinum (90% actuarial value). Plans must offer at least one silver- and one gold-level option in each exchange in which they participate.

The ACA also requires the exchanges to ensure that plans are meeting other requirements of participating in the exchange. These requirements relate to marketing practices, provider networks, outreach and enrollment, following insurance market regulations, and providing information in plain language. In addition, the entity running the exchange must provide a call center for customers, maintain a website, rate plans in the exchange, develop uniform applications, provide information regarding eligibility for public programs, assist individuals in calculating their tax credits, and certify individuals who are exempt from the individual mandate requirement.

Premium and Cost-Sharing Subsidies

The ACA includes a host of premium tax credits and cost-sharing subsidies to help make it affordable for people to purchase health insurance in a state exchange. Given the mandate to purchase insurance, it was necessary to include some assistance to make it possible for low-income individuals to comply with the new requirement. The tax credits and subsidies will be available starting in 2014, the same year the individual mandate and the state health insurance exchanges go into effect.

Premium tax credits are available to individuals who purchase health insurance in state exchanges and have incomes between 133% and 400% of the federal poverty level. In 2010, 400% of poverty was $43,200 for an individual and $88,200 for a family of four.[52] The tax credits are advanceable and refundable, meaning they will be available when health insurance is purchased and regardless of whether the individual

TABLE 2 Premium Tax Credit Schedule

Income Level by Federal Poverty Level (FPL)	Premium as a Percent of Income
Up to 133% FPL	2% of income
133–150% FPL	3–4% of income
150–200% FPL	4–6.3% of income
200–250% FPL	6.3–8.05% of income
250–300% FPL	8.05–9.5% of income
300–400% FPL	9.5% of income

owes any taxes. Cost-sharing subsidies are available to people who earn up to 250% of poverty. Under the ACA, individuals with income less than 133% of poverty will be eligible for Medicaid in 2014.

To qualify for assistance, an individual must be a U.S. citizen or legal resident, must not be eligible for any public health insurance program (including military coverage), and must not have access to employer-sponsored health insurance. Exceptions exist if an available employer plan does not cover at least 60% of covered benefits or if the employee's share of premium contributions exceeds 9.5% of the employee's income.

The amount of the premium tax credit is tiered based on income and set so individuals will not have to pay more than a certain percentage of their income on premiums (Table 2). The tax credit amount is based on the cost of the second-lowest-cost silver plan in the exchange and location where the individual is eligible to purchase insurance. Individuals who want to purchase a more expensive plan have to pay the difference in cost between the second-lowest-cost silver plan and the plan they prefer to purchase. Under the ACA, DHHS will adjust the premium people are expected to pay to reflect that premium costs typically grow faster than income levels. For example, assume Bob's income is 250% of poverty (about $27,000) and the cost of the second-lowest-cost silver plan in Bob's area is $5,700. Under the premium tax credit schedule, Bob will pay no more than 8.05% of his income, or $2,173. Bob's tax credit is $3,527, which is $5,700 minus $2,173.[53]

Cost-sharing subsidies are available to help low-income people reduce the amount of out-of-pocket spending on health

insurance (Table 3). The subsidies are tiered by income level and set so plans pay a higher percentage of service costs. In other words, they are set to increase the actuarial value of the plan for low-income individuals.

In addition to the premium tax credits and cost-sharing subsidies, the ACA limits the overall amount of out-of-pocket costs paid by individuals with incomes up to 400% of poverty (Table 4). The limits are based on the maximum out-of-pocket costs for health savings accounts ($5,950 for single coverage, $11,900 for family coverage in 2009) and will be indexed annually.

Employer Mandate

Beginning in 2014, employers with 50 or more employees and at least 1 employee who qualifies for a tax credit are required to offer affordable health insurance or pay a penalty. As a result, covered employers have three options: (1) provide affordable health insurance and not pay a penalty, (2) provide health insurance not considered affordable and pay a penalty, or (3) do not provide health insurance and pay a penalty. The penalties are based on whether an employer offers health insurance and whether any full-time employees take a premium tax credit. The amount of the penalty increases over time based on the

TABLE 3 Cost-Sharing Subsidy Schedule

Income Level by Federal Poverty Level (FPL)	Actuarial Value
100–150% FPL	94%
150–200% FPL	87%
200–250% FPL	73%

TABLE 4 Out-of-Pocket Spending Limits	
Income Level by Federal Poverty Level (FPL)	**Out-of-Pocket Limit**
100–200% FPL	⅔ of maximum
200–300% FPL	½ of maximum
300–400% FPL	⅓ of maximum

national increase in premium costs. The employer mandate was put in place to encourage employers to continue offering or start offering health insurance. Without such a mandate, employers may have found it profitable not to offer health insurance and let their employees purchase health care through state exchanges, shifting more of the costs of health reform to the public sector and taxpayers.

For employers who do not offer health insurance and have at least one full-time employee who takes the premium tax credit, the penalty is $2,000 per employee after the first 30 employees. In other words, if such an employer has 50 employees, the employer would pay a $40,000 penalty ($2,000 × 20 employees).

Employers who offer health insurance do not pay a penalty if the insurance is considered affordable. Insurance is affordable if the plan has an actuarial value of at least 60% or if the premiums do not cost more than 9.5% of an employee's income. Employees who would have to pay more than 9.5% of their income on premiums have the option to purchase insurance through an exchange and receive a premium tax credit.

Employers who provide unaffordable insurance have to pay a penalty for each employee who takes a tax credit, not counting the first 30 employees. The penalty is $3,000 per employee who takes a tax credit but may not exceed more than $2,000 times the number of employees over 30. For example, if the employer has 50 employees and offers unaffordable coverage, the employer would pay a maximum penalty of

$40,000 ($2,000 × 20). If only 10 employees take a tax credit, the penalty would be $30,000 ($3,000 × 10). If all 50 employees take a tax credit, the penalty would be $40,000, which is the maximum penalty allowed, not $150,000 ($3,000 × 50).

Employers must offer vouchers to employees who earn up to 400% of poverty, would have to pay premiums between 8% and 9.8% of their income, and choose to enroll in a state exchange. The voucher is equal to the amount the employer would have paid for the employee in the employer's plan and is used to offset premium costs in the exchange plan. Employees who receive vouchers are not eligible for subsidies.

Congress was concerned about the impact of the employer mandate on small businesses. Given their smaller pool of employees, small businesses have often found it quite expensive to offer health insurance to their employees. In addition to exempting businesses with fewer than 50 employees from the employer mandate and creating a health insurance exchange for small businesses, Congress also included a small business tax credit to encourage these employers to provide coverage. Employers are eligible for the tax credit if they have fewer than 25 full-time equivalent employees, average annual wages under $50,000, and pay for at least half of the cost of health insurance coverage for their employees. The tax credit covers a portion of the cost of the employer's contribution toward employees' premiums. The credit is capped based on the average premium costs in the employer's geographic area and phases out as firm size and annual wages increase.

Changes to the Private Insurance Market

In addition to creating a new marketplace for private insurance through state exchanges, the ACA includes a variety of changes to private health insurance rules and requirements. These requirements cover everything from rate setting to benefits to who must be covered. Although the overall health reform law is controversial, many of these private market reforms have overwhelming support. Together, these changes filled in gaps left by the private market that many people believed were unfair to consumers.

The following coverage changes took effect in 2010:

- **Preexisting conditions:** Individual and group plans may not exclude children due to their health status or based on preexisting conditions.
- **Dependent coverage:** Individual and group plans must provide dependent coverage up to age 26.
- **Preventive services:** New health plans may not impose cost sharing for certain preventive services, including
  - Preventive services with an A or B rating from the U.S. Preventive Services Task Force

BOX 3 Discussion Questions

Premium and cost-sharing subsidies are estimated to cost $350 billion over 10 years. Is this a good use of resources? Are these subsidies well designed? Are they sufficient to make health insurance affordable? Do they cover people with incomes that are too high? Should they cover more people?

- Immunizations recommended by the Centers for Disease Control and Prevention's Advisory Committee on Immunization Practices.
- Preventive care and screening for women based on guidelines to be issued by the Health Resources and Services Administration.

- **Coverage limits:** Individual and group plans may not impose lifetime dollar limits on coverage (and ability to impose annual limits on the dollar value of coverage is prohibited as of 2014).
- **Rescission:** Individual and group plans may not rescind coverage except in the case of fraud.
- **Appeals:** New health insurance plans must have an effective appeals process that includes an external review option.

Congress also focused on the issue of how insurers determine premium rates and what they spend those resources on within their plans. The ACA charges DHHS with establishing an annual process to review "unreasonable" increases in premiums.[4(§1003)] In 2010, 43 states had some type of rate review law, and the federal process is intended to work with, not preempt, those state laws.[54] As of January 2011, DHHS was in the notice and review process for its proposed rule on this subject. In addition, the ACA requires that plans spend at least 85% (large group plans) or 80% (small group or individual plans) of their premium dollars on medical care and quality improvement services, not administrative or other expenses (e.g., profits). Regulations clarifying this medical loss ratio, as it is called, took effect on January 1, 2011.[55] Insurers must provide enrollees with a rebate if they do not spend the requisite percentage on clinical and quality improvement services.

A number of significant changes will also take place in 2014, when the individual mandate, employer mandate, and state health insurance exchanges begin:

- **Guaranteed issue and renewability:** Individual and group plans may not exclude or charge more to individuals based on preexisting conditions or health status in the individual market, small group market, and exchanges.
- **Rate variation limits:** Premium rates may vary based on only age, geographic area, family composition, and tobacco use in the individual market, small group market, and exchanges.
- **Coverage limits:** Individual and group plans may not place annual dollar limits on coverage.
- **Essential health benefits:** Insurers providing coverage to small businesses, individuals, and in the exchanges have to provide essential health benefits through one of

four categories of plans (bronze, silver, gold, platinum) and adhere to annual cost-sharing limits.
- **Wellness plans:** Employers may offer rewards that reduce the cost of coverage to employees for participating in a wellness plan.

These private market changes do not affect all plans equally. Plans in small group or nongroup markets must follow these rules whether or not they are offered in an exchange. On the other hand, the ACA included two significant exceptions to these reforms. First, insurance plans that were in existence when the ACA was signed into law are referred to as "grandfathered plans" and are subject to some, but not all, of the new rules. The grandfathered plans must follow new requirements relating to preexisting conditions, lifetime and annual limits, waiting period limits, and dependent coverage rules. These plans are exempt, however, from having to provide essential health benefits, preventive services without copays, and limited cost sharing, although many of the large employer plans already have some of these features. A plan may retain its grandfathered status as long as it does not make significant changes to plan benefits or cost-sharing rules. If it loses its grandfathered status, the plan will have to meet all applicable requirements.

It is estimated that over the next several years, most people who obtain health insurance through a large employer will remain in a plan that is grandfathered under the ACA. Because small businesses are more likely to make significant changes to their health plans, it is estimated that only about one-third of these plans will remain grandfathered over the next several years. It is likely that most people in the individual health care market will receive care in an ACA-covered plan, not a grandfathered plan, sooner rather than later because these individuals switch plans frequently.[56]

The second major exception is for self-funded plans. These are plans where an employer does not buy insurance from a company but instead takes on the insurance risk itself. Self-funded plans are exempt from state law and subject to federal rules under ERISA (see Chapter 11 for more details on ERISA). Self-funded plans must adhere to ACA rules regarding dependent coverage, cost sharing for preventive services, annual and lifetime limits, and waiting period limits but do not need to comply with essential health benefit requirements.[57]

Financing Health Reform

Congress financed health reform primarily through Medicare and Medicaid savings, excise taxes and fees on the health care industry, changes to the income tax code, and a tax on some health insurance plans. (The provisions that alter Medicaid and Medicare are discussed in more detail in Chapter 10.) In addition, it is estimated that individuals ($17 billion) and employers ($52 billion) will pay $69 billion in penalties over a 10-year period for violating the insurance mandates.[58] Several of these financing changes were made as part of the deals the Obama administration struck with various stakeholders.

The ACA's main financing features are as follows:

- **Medicare provider reimbursement:** Reduces "market basket" or cost updates for inpatient and outpatient hospital reimbursement. Reduces payments for preventable hospital readmissions and hospital-acquired infections. Includes productivity adjustments for certain providers that will result in lower reimbursement rates. Estimated savings: $196 billion.
- **Medicare Advantage payments:** Reduces reimbursement rates and imposes cost-sharing limits for Medicare's managed care plans. Estimated savings: $136 billion.
- **Medicare Part A (Hospital Insurance):** Increases Medicare Part A tax rate for high-income earners. Estimated revenue: $210 billion.
- **Medicare premiums:** Reduces Medicare Part D (prescription drug) premium subsidy for high-income beneficiaries. Estimated savings: $36 billion.
- **Medicare employer subsidy:** Eliminates tax deduction for employers who receive a Medicare Part D (prescription drug coverage) subsidy. Estimated revenue: $4.5 billion.
- **Disproportionate share hospital (DSH) payments:** Reduces Medicare payments to DSH hospitals. Payments may increase over time based on percentage of uninsured served and uncompensated care provided. Reduces Medicaid DSH payments and requires DHHS to develop new funding formula. Estimated savings: $36 billion.
- **Medicaid prescription drugs:** Increases rebates drug manufacturers give to state Medicaid programs. Estimated savings: $38 billion.
- **Income tax code provisions:** Increases the threshold from 7.5% to 10% of adjusted gross income to claim deduction for unreimbursed medical expenses. Prohibits purchasing over-the-counter drugs with tax free savings accounts, increases tax burden on distributions not used for qualified medical expenses, and limits amount individuals may put in to accounts toward medical expenses. Estimated revenue: $29 billion.
- **Health industry fees:** Imposes a 10% tax on indoor tanning services, 2.3% tax on all taxable medical devices, annual fees on the pharmaceutical manufacturing sector, and fees on the health insurance sector. Estimated revenue: $107 billion.
- **Health insurance plans:** Imposes a tax on employer-sponsored health insurance plans with aggregate expenses that exceed $10,200 for individual coverage or $27,500 for family coverage. Estimated revenue: $32 billion.

Although it is the responsibility of the CBO to estimate the cost of legislation as it is written, time-bound cost estimates have their limitations. First, the CBO must assume that all the provisions in the bill will be implemented as written. With Republican gains in Congress in the 2010 midterm elections and the possibility of a new administration after the 2012 presidential election, it is not guaranteed that all these taxes, fees, and other features will remain in place. One of the

---

BOX 4 Discussion Questions

The ACA includes a tax on insurers for more generous health plans. Because it is likely insurers will pass on the cost of the tax to consumers, the idea behind the tax is to provide incentives for people to choose lower-cost plans. In theory, the less money employers spend on health care costs (and other fringe benefits), the more they will spend on wages. The income tax paid for by workers on their higher wages will provide revenue that can be used to pay for health reform. In addition, people may be less likely to obtain unnecessary care if fewer services are covered by their plan or if cost sharing is higher.

Is it likely that employers will trade lower benefits for higher wages? Are there times or industries where this trade-off is more or less likely to occur?

In 2010, the average cost of an employer plan was $5,079 for single coverage and $13,770 for family coverage. Beginning in 2018, plans that exceed $10,200 for individual coverage and $27,500 for family coverage are taxed. Congress rejected lower thresholds for the tax ($8,500/$23,000) that would have raised an estimated $149 billion. Did Congress pick the right thresholds for the tax? Should they be higher or lower?

Why did Congress delay implementation of the tax until 2018? What are the pros and cons to having the tax start well after the main provisions of health reform are in place?

most unpopular cost-saving tools—a tax on more generous health insurance plans—is not slated to take effect until 2018. Second, because the 10-year estimate, by design, does not consider costs beyond the first decade, some expected costs are not included in the estimate. For example, the CBO concluded that the new Community Living Assistance Services Supports program to help the elderly remain in their homes will save $70 billion over 10 years. It is also expected, however, that the program will cost more than the premiums bring in after the first decade, meaning the program will add to the federal deficit in the long run if it is not altered. In response to congressional inquiries, the CBO also offered a "rough estimate" for the decade beginning in 2020 and found that the ACA would continue to provide a slight reduction in the federal deficit as compared to the pre-ACA law.[59] Third, cost estimates cannot account for provisions that are left out of a bill. For example, Congress has passed several annual "fixes" to the Medicare physician fee schedule formula to avoid significant reimbursement cuts to doctors. Even though this problem is expected to cost the federal government billions of dollars over the next decade, the health reform bill did not include the cost of a permanent fix to the formula. For these reasons, cost estimates should not be taken as the final word on the cost of any bill, as changes in political will can undermine the best projections.

Public Health, Workforce, Prevention, and Quality

The ACA also includes a variety of programs and pilot projects that focus on improving quality of care and increasing access to preventive care. (The provisions related to Medicaid or Medicare are discussed in Chapter 10.) These provisions show both a commitment to these issues and the limitations of that commitment. Although task forces and pilot programs can be useful tools to try new ideas and gather data to inform future changes, their temporary nature can also mean that progress ends once the experiment is over especially in tight budget times. Whether these steps lead to lasting reform and needed change in the delivery of health care and in public health practice remains to be seen.

The ACA's quality improvement efforts are highlighted by the new National Quality Improvement Strategy and the new comparative effectiveness institute. The priorities of the National Quality Improvement Strategy include improving delivery of health care services, patient outcomes, and population health. A process will be created to develop quality measures, and a community-based collaborative care network will be established to integrate and coordinate services for low-income and uninsured populations. The new comparative effectiveness institute, the Patient Centered Outcomes Research Institute, is designed to consider the clinical effectiveness of medical treatments. The idea behind comparative effectiveness is to determine which procedures, devices, and pharmaceuticals provide the best value for a given outcome. The institute is designed to provide information to help others make decisions, but Congress stipulated that findings from the institute may not be construed as mandates or recommendations for payment, coverage, or treatment decisions.

The health reform law also provides funds to promote public health, wellness, and a stable and high-quality health care workforce. The ACA calls for the creation of a national prevention, health promotion, and public health council to develop a national strategy to improve the nation's health. A new regular corps and ready reserve corps will be established to assist when public health emergencies occur. In addition, a variety of programs and incentives are in place to promote employer wellness programs. Finally, the workforce shortage is addressed through graduate medical education reforms that promote primary care training, increases in scholarships and

---

BOX 5 Discussion Questions

As of 2009, the U.S. Preventive Services Task Force no longer recommends routine screening mammograms for women ages 40 to 49, although they said the decision should be made by the patient and her physician. The U.S. Preventive Services Task Force found that physicians would need to screen 1,000 women to save 1 woman's life and concluded that it was not worth the risks associated with false positives (anxiety, unnecessary biopsies, overtreatment). Others, such as the American Cancer Society, disagree with the U.S. Preventive Services Task Force and conclude that the lifesaving effects of routine mammogram screening outweigh the potential harm.

The idea of comparative effectiveness research is to provide information about the value of different tools. Once that information is available, who should make the decisions about whether to provide coverage and reimbursement for a particular good or service? Can one objectively assess the risks and benefits associated with mammograms or other services or medications? Should decisions be made solely by the patient and treating provider? Does it matter if decisions affect taxpayers (for example, if a patient is covered by a government program such as Medicare or the Veterans Administration)?

FIGURE 1

Early retirees: A temporary reinsurance program will help offset the costs of expensive premiums for employers providing retiree health benefits.

Access to care: Funding will be increased by $11 billion over five years for community health centers and the National Health Services Corps to serve more low-income and uninsured people.

Small-business tax credits: Small businesses (25 or fewer employees and average wages under $50,000) that offer health care benefits will be eligible for tax credits of up to 35 percent of their premium costs for two years.

Coverage for young adults: Parents will be able to keep their children on their health policies until they turn 26.

"Doughnut hole" rebates: Medicare will provide $250 rebates to beneficiaries who hit the Part D prescription drug coverage gap known as the "doughnut hole."

Benefit disclosure: Employers will be required to disclose the value of benefits provided for each employee's health insurance coverage on the employee's W-2 forms.

New payment and delivery approaches: A new Center for Medicare and Medicaid Innovation will test reforms that reward providers for quality of care rather than volume of services. Medicare will increase payment for primary care physicians by 10 percent for primary care services.

CLASS Act: A national, voluntary insurance program for purchasing community living assistance services and support (CLASS) will be established. All working adults will automatically enrolled—unless they opt out—though payroll deductions that, after five years, will qualify them for monthly payments toward services to help them stay at home should they become disabled.

2010 →

2011 →

High-risk pool: People with preexisting conditions who have been uninsured for at least six months will have access to affordable insurance through a temporary, subsidized high-risk pool. Premiums will be based on the average heath status of a standard population. Annual out-of-pocket costs will be capped at $5,950 for individuals and $11,900 for families.

Protection for children: Insurers can no longer deny health coverage to children with preexisting conditions or exclude their conditions from coverage.

Preventive care: All new group and individual health plans will be required to provide free preventive care for proven preventive services. In 2011, Medicare also will provide free preventive care.

Annual review of premium increases: Health insurers will be required to submit justification for unreasonable premium increases to the federal and relevant state governments before they take effect, and to report the share of premiums spent on nonmedical costs.

New insurance rules: Insurance companies will be banned from rescinding people's coverage when they get sick, and from imposing lifetime caps on coverage. Restrictions will be placed on annual limits.

Pharmaceutical manufacturer fee: An annual, nondeductible fee will be imposed on pharmaceuticals and importers' branded drugs, based on market share.

OTC drug reimbursement restrictions: Over-the-counter drugs not prescribed by a doctor will no longer be reimbursable through flexible spending accounts or health reimbursement arrangements, or on a tax-free basis in health savings accounts.

Physician quality reporting: Medicare will launch a Physician Compare Web site where beneficiaries can compare measures of physician quality and patient experience.

"Doughnut hole" discounts: Medicare beneficiaries in the Part D prescription drug coverage "doughnut hole" will receive 50 percent discounts on all brand-name drugs. By 2020, the "doughnut hole" coverage gap will be closed.

Premium share spending: Health plans in the large-group market that spend less than 85 percent of their premiums on medical care, and plans in the small-group and individual markets that spend less than 80 percent on medical care, will be required to offer rebates to enrollees.

Source: Courtesy of the Commonwealth Fund.

Medicare value-based purchasing: Medicare will reward hospitals that provide higher quality or better patient outcomes.

Administrative simplification: Health insurers must follow administrative simplification standards for electronic exchange of health information to reduce paperwork and administrative costs.

Flexible spending limits: Contributions to flexible spending accounts (FSAs) will be limited to $2,500 a year, indexed to the Consumer Price Index (CPI).

Shared responsibility for coverage: Individuals will be required to carry health insurance, and employers with 50 or more workers will be required to offer health benefits or be subject to a fine of $2,000 per employee (not counting the first 30 employees) if any worker receives governmental assistance with premiums through the insurance exchanges.

Insurance industry fee: Insurers will pay an annual fee, based on market share, to help pay for reform.

New rules for insurers: Insurers will be banned from restricting coverage or basing premiums on health status. Annual, in addition to lifetime, limits on benefits are banned.

Premium subsidies: Premium and cost-sharing assistance on a sliding scale will make coverage affordable for families with annual incomes between $30,000 and $88,000 that buy plans through the exchanges.

Medicare managed care plans: Four- and five-star Medicare private plans will receive 5 percent bonuses as a reward for providing better clinical quality and patient experiences.

High-cost insurance plans: Insurers will face a 40 percent excise tax on policies with premiums over $10,2000 for individuals or $27,500 for family coverage.

2012	2013	2014	2018

Insurance exchanges: New state-based market-places will offer small businesses and people without employer coverage a choice of affordable health plans that meet new essentials benefit standards.

Essential benefits package: The Department of Health and Human Services will establish an essential standard benefits package for policies sold in the exchanges and individual and small-group markets with a choice among tiers of plans (bronze, silver, gold, and platinum) that have different levels of cost-sharing.

Independent payment advisory board: A new independent payment advisory board within the executive branch will work to identify areas of waste and federal budget savings in Medicare. The board's recommendations must not ration care, raise taxes, or change Medicare benefits, eligibility, or cost-sharing.

Medicaid expansion: Medicaid eligibility will be expanded to all legal residents with incomes up to 133 percent of the federal poverty level. Currently, states have different—an in many cases very low—eligibility thresholds, and most states do not cover adults without children.

Source: Courtesy of the Commonwealth Fund.

oans to support primary care providers and workforce diversity, and education, training, and loan repayment programs o address the primary care nursing shortage.

States and Health Reform

Before the ACA and in the wake of numerous failed attempts at national health reform, states had been an active player in health reform. Filling the gap left by the lack of federal action, states took steps to experiment with individual mandates, employer mandates, small business pools, and programs to reduce the number of uninsured. Although the ACA is a federal law, it is full of state obligations and opportunities for state innovation. Even though governors in many states have expressed opposition to health reform, it is likely that states will expend significant efforts toward implementing the ACA over the next several years. The reform implementation challenges facing the states are compounded by the poor economy, which has forced many states to cut government agency personnel and budgets. States will have their hands full developing and running health insurance exchanges, regulating the private health insurance market, and implementing Medicaid changes.

CONCLUSION

After decades of trying and against the predictions of numerous experts, the United States passed a national health reform law that provides near-universal coverage, includes protections for individuals who have been historically excluded from the insurance market, and shows a concern for improving health care quality and access to preventive care. From a philosophical perspective, the ACA moves America toward a society where (almost) everyone is expected to have insurance. In this way, health insurance is considered both an obligation and a right: individuals are required to obtain insurance, and the government is obligated to make it affordable and accessible.

Yet, this is not the end of the story. The ACA remains a controversial bill with almost half of those polled expressing opposition to it, a number of states pursuing legal challenges to the bill, and newly elected Republicans pushing to repeal it. Implementation challenges will be great, from the need for numerous regulations to be created on the federal and state level in a short amount of time, to the ability of the states' health care delivery systems to handle an influx of newly insured individuals, to the ability of the American people to understand their new responsibilities and rights. As complex as the ACA is, gaps remain. Not everyone will be insured under the new system. The law's cost-containment and health care delivery reform measures are often in the form of temporary programs

whose future is unknown. Questions remain whether the subsidies are enough to make insurance affordable for all and whether Congress will implement the unpopular financing measures needed to fund the law when they take effect several years down the line. Although the ACA is a significant step in reforming the U.S. health care system, it is not the last step that needs to be taken.

REFERENCES

1. U.S. Bureau of the Census. *Income, Poverty, and Health Insurance Coverage in the United States: 2009.* Washington, D.C.: Bureau of the United States Census; 2010.

2. Kaiser Family Foundation. *The Uninsured: A Primer—Key Facts About Americans Without Health Insurance.* 2010. Available at: http://www.kff.org/uninsured/upload/7451-06.pdf. Accessed January 6, 2011.

3. Goldstein A. Health-care spending rose less in 2009. *Washington Post.* January 6, 2011: A15.

4. Pub. L. No. 111-148, the Patient Protection and Affordable Care Act.

5. Gordon C. *Dead on Arrival: The Politics of Health Care in Twentieth-Century America.* Princeton, N.J.: Princeton University Press; 2003.

6. Blake CH, Adolino JR. The enactment of national health insurance: A boolean analysis of twenty advanced industrial countries. *J Health Politics Policy Law.* 2001;26:670–708.

7. Jost TS. Why can't we do what they do? National health reform abroad. *J Law Med Ethics.* 2004;32:433–441.

8. Newport F. US still split on whether gov't should ensure health care. Gallup. Nov. 18, 2010. Available at: http://www.gallup.com/poll/144839/Split-Whether-Gov-Ensure-Healthcare.aspx. Accessed January 6, 2011.

9. National Conference of State Legislatures. *NCSL Fiscal Brief: State Balanced Budget Provisions.* Washington, DC; 2010. Available at http://www.ncsl.org/documents/fiscal/StateBalancedBudgetProvisions2010.pdf. Accessed January 7, 2011.

10. Kaiser Family Foundation. *Kaiser Health Tracking Poll: August 2009.* Available at: http://www.kff.org/kaiserpolls/upload/7965.pdf. Accessed January 6, 2011.

11. Kaiser Family Foundation. *Kaiser Health Tracking Poll: Election 2008.* Available at: http://www.kff.org/kaiserpolls/upload/7832.pdf. Accessed January 6, 2011.

12. Weissert CS, Weissert WG. *Governing Health: The Politics of Health Policy,* 2nd ed. Baltimore: Johns Hopkins University Press; 2002.

13. Friedman J, Holden R. The gerrymandering myth. *The New Republic Online;* 2006. Available at: https://ssl.tnr.com/p/docsub.mhtml?i=w060529&s= friedmanholden060106. Accessed on October 25, 2006.

14. West DM, Heith D, Goodwin C. Harry and Louise go to Washington: Political advertising and health care reform. *J Health Politics Policy Law.* 1996;21:35–68.

15. Feder J. Crowd-out and the politics of health reform. *J Law Med Ethics.* 2004;32:461–464.

16. Kaiser Family Foundation. *Kaiser Health Tracking Poll: November 2009.* Available at: http://www.kff.org/kaiserpolls/upload/8019.pdf. Accessed January 6, 2011.

17. Starr P. *The Social Transformation of American Medicine: The Rise of a Sovereign Profession and the Making of a Vast Industry.* New York: Basic Books; 1982.

18. Federal Election Commission. *2000 Presidential Popular Vote Summary for All Candidates Listed on at Least One State Ballot.* 2000. Available at: http://www.fec.gov/pubrec/fe2000/prespop.htm. Accessed on October 29, 2010; CNN. *Election results—US president.* 2010. Available at: http://www.cnn.com/ELECTION/2004/pages/results/president/. Accessed October 29, 2010.

19. CNN. *Election Center 2008*. 2008. Available at: http://www.cnn.com/ELECTION/2008/results/president/. Accessed October 29, 2010.

20. Pub. L. No. 110–343.

21. Pub. L. No. 111-5.

22. Recovery.gov. *The Recovery Act*. Available at: http://www.recovery.gov/About/Pages/The_Act.aspx. Accessed October 29, 2010.

23. Jones JM. Economy top issue for voters; size of government may be more pivotal. Gallup. October 26, 2010. Available at: http://www.gallup.com/poll/144029/Economy-Top-Issue-Voters-Size-Gov-May-Pivotal.aspx. Accessed October 29, 2010.

24. Blendon RJ, Altman DE, Benson JM, et al. Voters and health reform in the 2008 presidential election. *New Engl J of Med*. 2008;359(19):2050–2061.

25. CNN. Obama talks about mother's cancer battle in ad. September 21, 2007. Available at: http://politicalticker.blogs.cnn.com/2007/09/21/obama-talks-about-mothers-cancer-battle-in-ad/. Accessed November 2, 2010.

26. Appleby J. Health reform up in the air as the economy sinks. *USA Today*. December 20, 2008. Available at: http://www.usatoday.com/news/health/2008-12-18-health_N.htm. Accessed November 2, 2010.

27. Pear R. Senator takes initiative on health reform. *New York Times*. November 11, 2008. Available at: http://www.nytimes.com/2008/11/12/washington/12health.html. Accessed November 2, 2010.

28. Obama's health care speech to Congress. *New York Times*. September 9, 2009. Available at: http://www.nytimes.com/2009/09/10/us/politics/10obama.text.html. Accessed November 2, 2010.

29. Kaiser Family Foundation. *Kaiser Health Tracking Poll: September 2009*. Available at: http://www.kff.org/kaiserpolls/upload/7990.pdf. Accessed November 2, 2010.

30. Cohen J, Balz D. Opposition to Obama's health care plan is high, but easing. *Washington Post*. September 14, 2009. Available at: http://www.washingtonpost.com/wp-dyn/content/article/2009/09/13/AR2009091302962.html. Accessed November 2, 2010.

31. Condon S. Scott Brown win shakes up health care fight. *CBS News*. January 20, 2010. Available at: http://www.cbsnews.com/8301-503544_162-6119035-503544.html. Accessed November 2, 2010.

32. Brown CB, O'Connor P. The fallout: Democrats rethinking health care bill. *Politico*. January 21, 2010. Available at: http://www.politico.com/news/stories/0110/31693.html. Accessed November 2, 2010.

33. State of the Union: President Obama's speech. *ABC News*. January 27, 2010. Available at: http://abcnews.go.com/Politics/State_of_the_Union/state-of-the-union-2010-president-obama-speech-transcript/story?id=9678572&page=1. Accessed November 2, 2010.

34. Saad L. Obama and Bush: A contrast in popularity. *Gallup*. November 10, 2008. Available at: http://www.gallup.com/poll/111838/obama-bush-contrast-popularity.aspx. Accessed November 4, 2010.

35. Blumenthal D, Morone JA. *The Heart of Power: Health and Politics in the Oval Office*. Berkeley: University of California Press; 2009.

36. Morone J. Presidents and health reform: From Franklin D. Roosevelt to Barack Obama. *Health Affairs*. 2010; 29(6):1096–1100.

37. Oberlander J. Long time coming: Why health reform finally passed. *Health Affairs*. 2010;29(6):1112–1116.

38. Text of a letter from the president to Senator Edward M. Kennedy and Senator Max Baucus. Washington, DC: The White House Office of the Press Secretary; June 2, 2009. Available at: http://www.whitehouse.gov/the_press_office/Letter-from-President-Obama-to-Chairmen-Edward-M-Kennedy-and-Max-Baucus. Accessed November 5, 2010.

39. Affordable Health Care for America Act, H.R. 3962.

40. Patient Protection and Affordable Care Act, H.R. 3590.

41. Murray S, Kane P. House won't pass Senate bill to save health care reform. *Washington Post*. January 22, 2010. Available at: http://www.washingtonpost.com/wp-dyn/content/article/2010/01/21/AR2010012101604.html?sid=ST2010012005092. Accessed November 5, 2010.

42. Murray S, Montgomery L. House passes health care reform bill without Republican votes. *Washington Post*. March 22, 2010. Available at: http://www.washingtonpost.com/wp-dyn/content/article/2010/03/21/AR2010032100943.html?sid=ST2010032201830. Accessed November 5, 2010.

43. Congressional Budget Office. *Cost Estimate for H.R. 4872, Reconciliation Act of 2010*. Washington, DC: Congressional Budget Office; 2010. Available at: http://www.cbo.gov/ftpdocs/113xx/doc11379/AmendReconProp.pdf. Accessed December 23, 2010.

44. Health Affairs. *Health Policy Brief—Individual Mandate*. Washington, DC: Project Hope; 2010. Available at: http://www.healthaffairs.org/healthpolicybriefs/brief.php?brief_id=14. Accessed December 22, 2010.

45. United States Const. Art. 1, §8.

46. *Heart of Atlanta Motel, Inc. v. United States*, 379 U.S. 241 (1964); *Wickard v. Filburn*, 317 U.S. 111 (1942); *Gonzalez v. Raich*, 545 U.S. (2005).

47. Jost TS. State lawsuits won't succeed in overturning the individual mandate. *Health Affairs*. 2010; 29(6):1225–1228.

48. Shapiro I. State suits against health reform are well grounded in law—and pose serious challenges. *Health Affairs*. 2010;29(6):1229–1233.

49. Kaiser Family Foundation. *Explaining Health Care Reform: Questions About State Health Insurance Exchanges*. 2010. Available at: http://www.kff.org/healthreform/upload/7908-02.pdf. Accessed December 23, 2010.

50. Rosenbaum S, Teitelbaum J, Hayes K. The essential health benefit provisions of the Affordable Care Act: Implications for people with disabilities. *Commonwealth Fund*. Pub. 1485, Vol. 3. Available at: http://www.commonwealthfund.org/~/media/Files/Publications/Issue%20Brief/2011/Mar/1485_Rosenbaum_essential_hlt_benefits_provisions_ACA_disabilities_reform_brief_v2.pdf. Accessed June 24, 2011.

51. Rosenbaum S, Teitelbaum J, Hayes K. Crossing the Rubicon: The impact of the Affordable Care Act on the content of insurance coverage for persons with disabilities. *Notre Dame J of Law, Ethics, and Public Policy*. 2011; 25(2):527–562.

52. Center for Medicare and Medicaid Services. *2010 Federal Poverty Guidelines*. Washington, DC: Center for Medicare and Medicaid Services; 2010. Available at: https://www.cms.gov/MedicaidEligibility/downloads/POV10Combo.pdf. Accessed December 23, 2010.

53. Kaiser Family Foundation. *Explaining Health Reform: Questions About Health Insurance Subsidies*. Available at: http://www.kff.org/healthreform/upload/7962-02.pdf. Accessed December 23, 2010.

54. Proposed Rule for Rate Increase Disclosure and Review, 75 *Federal Register* 81004 (2010).

55. Interim Final Rule, Health Insurance Issuers Implementing Medical Loss Ratio Requirements Under the Patient Protection and Affordable Care Act, 75 *Federal Register* 74864 (2010).

56. HealthReform.gov. *Fact Sheet: Keeping the Health Plan You Have: The Affordable Care Act and "Grandfathered" Plans*. Available at: http://www.healthreform.gov/newsroom/keeping_the_health_plan_you_have.html. Accessed January 3, 2011.

57. Kaiser Family Foundation. *Health Reform Resource. FAQ—How Does the New Law Apply to Companies with Self-Funded Plans*. Menlo, CA: Kaiser Family Foundation. Available at: http://healthreform.kff.org/faq/how-does-new-law-apply-to-companies-with-self-funded-plans.aspx. Accessed January 3, 2011.

58. Water PN. *How Health Reform Helps Reduce the Deficit*. Washington, DC: Center for Budget and Policy Priorities; 2010. Available at: http://www.cbpp.org/cms/index.cfm?fa=view&id=3178. Accessed January 4, 2011.

59. Congressional Budget Office. *Cost Estimate for H.R. 4872, Reconciliation Act of 2010*. Washington, DC: Congressional Budget Office; 2010. Available at: http://www.cbo.gov/ftpdocs/113xx/doc11379/AmendReconProp.pdf. Accessed December 23, 2010.

ENDNOTES

a. 88 Stat. 832.

b. ERISA § 514, 29 USC. § 1144.

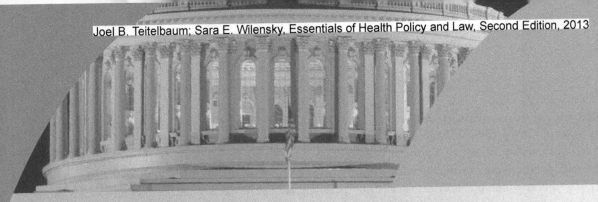

Government Health Insurance Programs: Medicaid, CHIP, and Medicare

LEARNING OBJECTIVES

By the end of this chapter, you will be able to:

- Describe the basic structure, administration, financing, and eligibility rules for:
  - Medicaid
  - State Children's Health Insurance Program (CHIP)
  - Medicare
- Understand how the Patient Protection and Affordable Care Act alters Medicaid, CHIP, and Medicare
- Discuss key health policy questions and themes relating to each of these public programs

INTRODUCTION

Elsewhere, the significant role of employer-sponsored health insurance in financing health care, the flexibility that private insurers have in designing health insurance coverage and selecting who they will cover, why private insurers do not have incentive to cover high-risk populations, and how the Patient Protection and Affordable Care Act (ACA) has changed the health insurance and healthcare delivery landscape have been discussed in detail. Medicaid, the State Children's Health Insurance Program (CHIP), and Medicare were established in part because the private health insurance market was not developing affordable, comprehensive health insurance products for society's low-income, elderly, and disabled populations. Federal and state governments chose to fill some of those gaps through Medicaid, CHIP, and Medicare. The gaps were substantial, as shown by the over 100 million beneficiaries served by these three programs today.[1] Due to the needs of vulnerable populations and the requirements necessary to make health

insurance coverage for them viable, these programs are quite different from standard private health insurance plans.

There are numerous other important health insurance and direct service programs funded by federal, state, and local governments. Just a few examples include the Ryan White Care Act, which provides HIV/AIDS services to infected individuals and their families; the Women, Infants and Children Supplemental Nutrition Program, which provides nutritional

BOX 1 Vignette

Governor Manha is in a quandary. She believes everyone should have access to health care and would like to support state policies that make care accessible and affordable. While she supported President Obama's goal of reducing the number of uninsured, she is concerned that some of the provisions in the Patient Protection and Affordable Care Act are too burdensome on the states, particularly in a fragile economy. The Governor wonders how her state can afford the mandated Medicaid expansion when the recent trend has been to cut services across the board. How will state agencies cope with their new responsibilities when positions are being defunded and employees are being furloughed? Should she spend her state's time and resources to establish a health insurance exchange when the federal government will step in if she does not act? At the same time, does she want to leave decisions about how the exchange will be operated in her state to bureaucrats in Washington, D.C.?

supplements and education to poor women and their children; and the Indian Health Service, which provides federal health services to American Indians and Alaska Natives. Although these and many other health programs are vital to the health of our population, this chapter focuses only on the three major government health insurance programs in this country, because in addition to providing health insurance to millions, these programs are also influential in terms of setting healthcare policy. For example, when Medicare, a program serving over 47 million people, makes a decision to cover a certain treatment, private insurance companies often follow suit, establishing a new standard for generally accepted practice in the insurance industry.[2] Conversely, states may decide to try healthcare innovations with their Medicaid programs that, if successful, may become commonplace across the country. Thus, understanding these three major programs is essential in terms of both how this country finances and delivers health care and how it makes health policy decisions.

The ACA made wide-ranging changes to Medicaid, CHIP, and Medicare. In general, the ACA included a significant Medicaid eligibility expansion, altered which children are eligible for Medicaid and CHIP, added new benefits to Medicare, and included a host of changes intended to produce savings in the Medicare program. Since many of these provisions do not take place until 2014, this chapter describes these programs as they currently exist and highlights how the new health reform law will change them.

As you learn about specific rules for each program, keep in mind the numerous tensions that are present throughout the healthcare system as policymakers decide how to design and implement public insurance programs. This chapter touches on several recurring themes relating to these tensions, which were evident during the debate that led to passage of the ACA: choosing between state flexibility and national uniformity; determining the appropriate role for government, the private sector, and individuals in healthcare financing and delivery; defining a primary decision-making goal (fiscal restraint, equity/social justice, improved health outcomes, uniformity, etc.); and settling on the appropriate scope of coverage to offer beneficiaries.

Before delving into the details of each program, it is necessary to explain the difference between entitlement and block grant programs. Medicaid and Medicare are *entitlement* programs, whereas CHIP is a *block grant* program. Some of the themes listed earlier, such as the appropriate role of government and primary decision-making goals, are implicated in the decision of whether to establish a program as an entitlement or a block grant.

In an *entitlement* program, everyone who is eligible for and enrolled in the program is legally entitled to receive benefits from the program. In other words, the federal or state governments cannot refuse to provide program beneficiaries all medically necessary and covered services due to lack of funds or for other reasons. Because everyone who is enrolled has a legal right to receive services, there cannot be a cap on spending. The absence of a spending cap has the advantage of allowing funds to be available to meet rising healthcare costs and unexpected needs, such as increased enrollment and use of services during recessions or natural or man-made disasters.

Opponents of entitlement programs focus on the open-ended budget obligation entitlements create. With healthcare costs straining federal and state budgets, critics would prefer to establish a cap on the funds spent on entitlement programs such as Medicaid. It is impossible to determine how many people will enroll in the program or how many and what kind of healthcare services they will use in any given year, so governments cannot establish exact budgets for their Medicaid program. In addition to these fiscal objections, many opponents reject the notion that government should play a large role in providing health insurance, preferring to leave that function to the private market.

Entitlement programs are often contrasted with *block grant* programs such as CHIP. A block grant is a defined sum of money that is allocated for a particular program (often, but not always, from the federal government to the states) over a certain amount of time. If program costs exceed available funds, additional money will not be made available and program changes have to be made. Such changes could include

BOX 2 Discussion Questions

Do you think it makes more sense to structure government healthcare programs as entitlements or block grants? What are the economic and healthcare risks and benefits of each approach? Does your answer depend on who is paying for the program? Who the program serves? What kinds of benefits the program provides? Do you think various stakeholders would answer these questions differently? How might the answers change if you ask a member of the federal government, a governor, a state legislator, an advocate, or a tax-paying citizen who is not eligible for benefits under the program?

terminating the program, capping enrollment in the program, reducing program benefits, or finding additional resources. Unlike entitlement programs, individuals who qualify for block grant programs may be denied services or receive reduced services due to lack of funds.

The arguments for and against block grant programs are similar to those found with entitlement programs. Proponents of block grant programs laud the limited and certain fiscal obligation and reduced role of government in providing health insurance. Opponents of block grant programs object to the lack of legal entitlement to services and the finite amount of funds available to provide health insurance.

MEDICAID

Medicaid is the country's federal–state public health insurance program for the indigent. In this section, we discuss fundamental aspects of the Medicaid program, including its structure, eligibility, benefits, and financing, as well as changes to Medicaid made by the ACA. Unlike private health insurance plans, which are based on actuarial risk, the Medicaid program is designed to ensure that funds are available to provide healthcare services to a poorer and generally less-healthy group of beneficiaries; in order to do so, Medicaid has several features not found in private health insurance plans.

Program Administration

Medicaid is jointly designed and operated by the federal and state governments. The Centers for Medicare and Medicaid Services is the federal agency in charge of administering the Medicaid program. Each state, the District of Columbia, and certain U.S. Territories,[a] as defined in the statute,[3] have the option to participate in the Medicaid program, and all have chosen to do so. The federal government sets certain requirements and policies for the Medicaid program though statute,[4] regulations,[5] a *State Medicaid Manual*,[6] and policy guidance such as letters to state Medicaid directors.[7] Each state has its own Medicaid agency that is responsible for implementing the program in the state. States file a Medicaid State Plan with the federal government outlining the state's own eligibility rules, benefits, and other program requirements; this plan is effectively a contract between states and the federal government and between states and program beneficiaries.

The federal and state governments jointly set rules concerning who is covered and which services are provided by Medicaid. The federal government outlines which populations must be covered (*mandatory populations*) and which ones may be covered (*optional populations*), as well as which benefits must be covered (*mandatory benefits*) and which ones may be

BOX 3 Discussion Questions

What are the benefits and drawbacks of having a health program that varies by state versus having one that is uniform across the country? Do you find that the positives of state flexibility outweigh the negatives, or vice versa? Does your analysis change depending on what populations are served? Does your analysis change depending on whose point of view you consider? Is it fair that similarly situated individuals may be treated differently in different states? Does this occur in other aspects of society?

covered (*optional benefits*). Between these floors and ceilings, states have significant flexibility to determine how Medicaid will operate in their particular state. In general, states must cover mandatory populations and benefits, and they may choose to cover any combination of optional populations or benefits, including the choice not to offer any optional coverage at all. In addition, states may seek a waiver from federal rules, allowing states to experiment with coverage and benefit design while still drawing down federal funds to operate their program. Given all of these possible permutations, it is often said that "if you have seen one Medicaid program, you have seen one Medicaid program"; in other words, within the broad federal parameters, every state (and territory) has a unique Medicaid structure—no two programs are exactly alike. As a result, similarly situated individuals in different states may have very different experiences in terms of the generosity of benefits they are entitled to or even if they are eligible for the program at all.

Eligibility

Traditionally, Medicaid has covered low-income pregnant women, children, adults in families with dependent children, individuals with disabilities, and the elderly. About one-half of all Medicaid beneficiaries are children, while adults account for another 25% of enrollees and the disabled and elderly make up the remaining one-quarter.[8] Approximately 9 million people are called *dual enrollee* or *dual eligible* elderly, meaning they qualify for both Medicaid and Medicare.[9] Although most dual enrollees are eligible for full Medicaid benefits, a small portion of them receives only premium and/or cost-sharing assistance to help them pay for Medicare, not full Medicaid benefits.

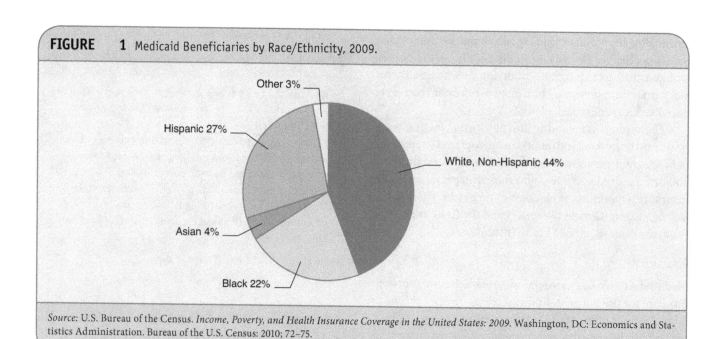

FIGURE   **1**   Medicaid Beneficiaries by Race/Ethnicity, 2009.

Other 3%

Hispanic 27%

White, Non-Hispanic 44%

Asian 4%

Black 22%

Source: U.S. Bureau of the Census. *Income, Poverty, and Health Insurance Coverage in the United States: 2009.* Washington, DC: Economics and Statistics Administration. Bureau of the U.S. Census: 2010; 72–75.

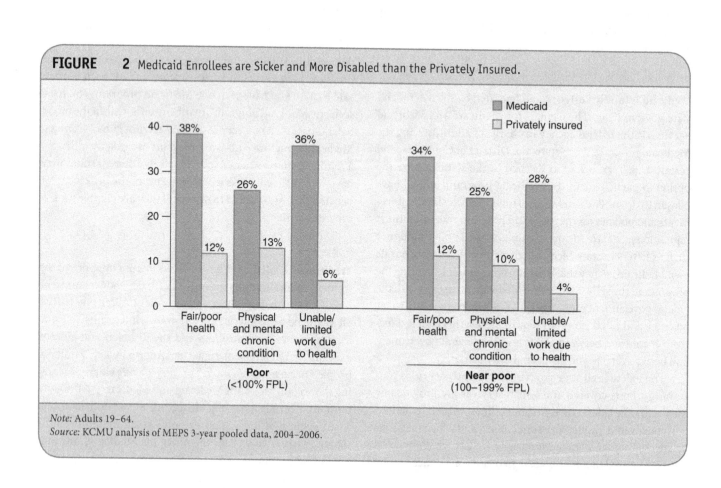

FIGURE   **2**   Medicaid Enrollees are Sicker and More Disabled than the Privately Insured.

■ Medicaid
□ Privately insured

40

38%

36%

34%

30

28%

26%

25%

20

13%

12%

12%

10%

10

6%

4%

0

Fair/poor health | Physical and mental chronic condition | Unable/ limited work due to health | Fair/poor health | Physical and mental chronic condition | Unable/ limited work due to health

Poor
(<100% FPL)

Near poor
(100–199% FPL)

Note: Adults 19–64.
Source: KCMU analysis of MEPS 3-year pooled data, 2004–2006.

BOX 4 Federal Poverty Level

Federal poverty guidelines are determined annually and calculated based on the number of individuals in a family. The guidelines are commonly referred to as the Federal Poverty Level (FPL), but U.S. Department of Health and Human Services (HHS) discourages the use of this term because the Census Bureau also calculates, using different methods, a figure referred to as the federal poverty thresholds. However, because the term Federal Poverty Level is still commonly used when discussing eligibility for federal and state programs, we use it here. The poverty guidelines are somewhat higher for Alaska and Hawaii due to administrative procedures adopted by the Office of Economic Opportunity.

Among all people with health insurance, members of ethnic or minority groups are more likely than Caucasians to have coverage through Medicaid. As shown in Figure 1, however, Medicaid beneficiaries are split almost evenly between white, non-Hispanic beneficiaries and beneficiaries who are members of ethnic or minority groups. Figure 2 indicates that overall, Medicaid beneficiaries are more likely to be in poorer health than privately insured individuals.

Overall, 89% of nonelderly Medicaid enrollees are either poor (meaning they earn less than 100% of the Federal Poverty Level [FPL]) or near-poor (meaning they earn between 100% and 250% of the FPL).[10] Yet, not all low-income individuals have been covered by the program, and over 28 million low-income Americans remain uninsured.[11] Traditionally left out of the program have been low-income adults without disabilities, women who are not pregnant, and the near-poor who earn too much money to qualify for Medicaid. However, the ACA included a significant eligibility expansion that is expected to add 16 million individuals to the program by 2019.[12] As discussed below in more detail, the expansion is designed to include the low-income groups that have been traditionally excluded from Medicaid.

Eligibility Requirements

Under current Medicaid rules, everyone must meet *all five* of the following requirements in order to be eligible:

Categorical: An individual must fit within a category (e.g., pregnant women) covered by the program.
Income: An individual/family must earn no more than the relevant income limits, which are expressed as an FPL percentage (e.g., 133% of the FPL).

Resources: An individual/family must not have nonwage assets (e.g., car, household goods) that exceed eligibility limits.
Residency: An individual must be a U.S. resident and a resident of the state in which they are seeking benefits.
Immigration status: Immigrants must meet certain requirements, including having been in the country for at least five years (for most immigrants).

As shown in Table 1, under current rules it is necessary to consider both categorical eligibility and income limits for all populations to understand who is covered by Medicaid and which populations are mandatory and which are optional. The groups in Table 1 represent some of the larger and more frequently mentioned categories of Medicaid beneficiaries, but it is not an exhaustive list. There are approximately 50 categories of mandatory and optional populations in the Medicaid program, with each state picking and choosing which optional populations to include and at what income level.

Medically Needy

Medicaid's *medically needy* category is an option that has been picked up by 32 states and the District of Columbia as of 2009.[13] As its name implies, this category is intended to cover individuals who have extremely high medical expenses. These individuals fit within a covered category, but earn too much money to be otherwise eligible for Medicaid. Medically needy programs have both income and asset requirements. In terms of income requirements, states subtract the costs of individuals' medical expenses from their income level. States have the choice of deducting the medical expenses as they are incurred each month, every six months, or any time in between. As soon as otherwise qualified individuals "spend down" enough money on medical expenses, they are eligible for Medicaid through the medically needy option based on their reduced income level for the remainder of the period.

The following is a simplified example of how the "spend down" process works. Let's say a state calculates incurred medical expenses every three months to determine eligibility for the medically needy option, and in this state an individual (who we'll call Peter) must earn no more than $8,500 a year to qualify as medically needy. Peter earns $11,000 per year and has $6,000 each year in medical expenses, incurred at a rate of $500 per month. After 3 months, Peter has spent $1,500 on medical expenses. Instead of considering the income level to be the annual amount earned ($11,000), the state subtracts Peter's medical expenses as they occur. So, after three months the state considers Peter to earn $9,500 annually ($11,000 − $1,500). Because this amount is still over the $8,500 limit,

TABLE 1 Select Medicaid Mandatory and Optional Eligibility Groups and Income Requirements Prior to ACA.

Eligibility Category	Mandatory Coverage	Optional Coverage
Infants under 1	≤133% FPL	≤185% FPL
Children 1–5	≤133% FPL	>133% FPL
Children 6–19	≤100% FPL	>100% FPL
Pregnant women	≤133% FPL	≤185% FPL
Parents	Below state's 1996 AFDC[a] limit	May use income level above state's 1996 AFDC limit
Parents in welfare-to-work families	≤185% FPL	
Elderly and disabled SSI[b] beneficiaries	SSI limits	Above SSI limits, below 100% FPL
Certain working disabled	May not exceed specified amount	Variable, SSI level to 250% FPL
Elderly—Medicare assistance only[c]	Variable, up to 175% FPL	Variable up to 175% FPL
Nursing Home Residents		Above SSI limits, below 300% SSI
Medically Needy		"Spend down" medical expenses to state set income level

AFDC = Aid to Families with Dependent Children.

SSI = Supplemental Security Income, a federal program that provides cash assistance to the aged, blind, and disabled who meet certain income and resource requirements.

Medicare Assistance only = payment for Medicare cost-sharing requirements.

Peter is not eligible under the medically needy option. In another three months, Peter will have spent $3,000 in medical expenses over the past 6 months. At that time, the state considers Peter to earn $8,000 annually ($11,000 – $3,000), making him eligible because he earns less than the $8,500 limit. For the rest of this period (i.e., three months), Peter is eligible for Medicaid. After another three months, the state recalculates his earnings and medical expenses. Each year, this entire calculation starts over. In the end, Peter will not be eligible for Medicaid for the first six months of the year, but will be eligible for Medicaid for the second six months of the year.

Immigrants

There are also special Medicaid eligibility rules relating to immigrants. The Personal Responsibility and Work Opportunity Reconciliation Act of 1996 (PRWORA) severely restricted immigrant eligibility for Medicaid (and most of the same rules in PRWORA were later applied to CHIP eligibility in 1997).[14] Prior to PRWORA, legal immigrants followed the same Medicaid eligibility rules as everyone else, but undocumented immigrants were not eligible at all. PRWORA instituted a five-year bar, meaning that most immigrants who come to

> **BOX 5 Discussion Questions**
>
> Does the medically needy category make sense to you? Do you think it is a good idea to discount medical expenses of high-need individuals so they can access the healthcare services they need through Medicaid? If so, is the process described above cumbersome and likely to result in people being on and off Medicaid (and therefore likely on and off treatment) because their eligibility is based on their spending patterns? Why should individuals with high medical needs have an avenue to Medicaid eligibility that is not available to other low-income people who have other high expenses, such as child care or transportation costs? Would it make more sense to simply raise the eligibility level for Medicaid so more low-income people are eligible for the program? Politically, which option would likely have more support? Does your view about the medically needy category vary depending on your primary decision-making goal (fiscal restraint, equity, improved health outcomes, etc.)?

the United States after August 22, 1996, are not eligible for Medicaid (or CHIP) for the first five years after their arrival. After five years, legal immigrants are eligible on the same basis as U.S. citizens, while undocumented immigrants remain ineligible for full Medicaid (or CHIP) benefits. However, both legal and undocumented immigrants who are otherwise eligible for Medicaid may receive emergency Medicaid benefits without any temporal restrictions. Immigrant eligibility eased slightly when CHIP was reauthorized in 2009.[15] States now have the option to cover legal immigrant children and/or pregnant women through Medicaid and CHIP in the first five years that they are in the United States.

Proponents of the immigrant restrictions believe they discourage people who cannot support themselves from coming to the United States and prevent immigrants from taking advantage of publicly funded programs they did not support through taxes before their arrival. In addition, some proponents believe that healthcare resources should go first to U.S. citizens, not non-citizens.

Opponents of the restrictions assert that most immigrants pay taxes once they arrive in this country and therefore deserve to receive the full benefits of those taxes.[16(p15)] They also find the restriction ill-suited as a deterrent because immigrants often come to the United States for economic opportunities, not social benefits.[17] Furthermore, restricting immigrants' access to health care may be a public health hazard for all members of the community because contagious diseases do not discriminate by immigration status. Finally, opponents contend that having higher numbers of uninsured individuals in the United States will further strain the ability of providers to care for all vulnerable populations in a community and lead to rising healthcare costs because uninsured immigrants are much less likely to obtain preventive care or early treatment for illnesses or injuries.[16(p15)] As a result, 27 states have decided to use state-only funds to provide Medicaid or CHIP services to some or all individuals who are otherwise ineligible due to their immigration status, and 20 states have implemented the new coverage option available after CHIP reauthorization.[18] Even so, immigrants are still less likely to be insured or have access to care than native citizens.

Medicaid Eligibility Expansion Under the Affordable Care Act

As mentioned earlier, the ACA significantly expanded Medicaid eligibility. Beginning in 2014, all non-Medicare-eligible individuals under age 65, with incomes up to 133% FPL,[b] will be eligible for Medicaid in every state. In addition, children ages 6–19 must be covered up to 133% FPL, instead of at 100% FPL as under current rules. Since 2010, states have had the option of covering low-income childless adults without a waiver. Undocumented immigrants, as well as legal immigrants who have resided in the United States for fewer than five years, will not be eligible for Medicaid under the expansion, although states have the option to cover legal immigrant pregnant women and children who have been in the country fewer than five years (matching the new rules put in place under CHIP).

The eligibility expansion for all non-Medicare-eligible individuals under 65 years of age with incomes up to 133% FPL marks a drastic departure from how Medicaid has generally been structured. Unlike Medicaid's traditional eligibility structure, newly eligible individuals only have to satisfy an income threshold and do not have to meet a resource test or fit within a pre-approved category. In addition, states usually have significant flexibility in determining how individual income and other personal resources are calculated. Under the ACA expansion, however, all states are required to accept newly eligible individuals using the federal income level calculation and without accounting for other assets. As discussed in more detail below, Medicaid has a generous benefit package that must be provided equally to all categorically eligible beneficiaries. While states may choose to offer a variety of benefits, they are only required to offer a benefit package that

---

BOX 6 Discussion Questions

Looking at Medicaid's traditional eligibility rules, you notice numerous value/policy judgments—pregnant women and children are favored over childless adults, the medically needy are favored over other low-income individuals with high costs, non-immigrants are favored over immigrants. Under the ACA expansion, these distinctions mostly disappear and eligibility depends purely on income level in the case of the biggest expansion group. Which approach do you prefer? If the ACA approach were expanded beyond 133% of FPL, the costs of the Medicaid program would soar. Given limited resources, do you think it would be better to cover more people at a higher poverty level across the board or continue to favor some groups over others through the categorical requirement? Should we decide that, for some populations, the government should step in and provide coverage regardless of the cost? In other words, is there a point where equity trumps financial constraints?

is at least as generous as the essential health benefit package offered in the state exchanges. Finally, while Medicaid financing is usually based on a federal–state matching system, the federal government will cover the cost of almost all of the described expansions through 2019. Overall, the ACA expansion has created a two-tier Medicaid program, with newly eligible individuals falling under one set of eligibility, financing, and benefit rules, and the rest of Medicaid beneficiaries adhering to different standards.

Benefits

Medicaid benefits are structured in the same way as Medicaid eligibility—some are mandatory and some are optional, and the newly eligible individuals under the ACA expansion have their own set of rules. Again, this means that no two Medicaid programs are alike, as each state picks its own menu of optional benefits to provide.

Historically, Medicaid programs have offered a rich array of benefits, including preventive services, behavioral health services, long-term care services, supportive services that allow people with disabilities to work, institutional services, family planning services, and more. In fact, the coverage provided by Medicaid generally has been more generous than the typical private insurance plan, particularly in the case of children. While federal Medicaid regulations exclude very few services, there are prohibitions. Since 1977, Congress has prohibited the use of federal funds to pay for the costs of an abortion or Mifepristone (commonly known as RU-486), a drug that induces medical abortions. Also, drug addiction or alcohol dependency may not be used as reasons to qualify an individual as disabled under SSI (and therefore, under Medicaid), though if an individual is eligible for Medicaid for another reason, Medicaid programs may pay for substance abuse treatment.

All states provide the mandatory services listed on the left side of Table   2, and may provide the optional services listed on the right side. In addition to requiring a wide array of services, Medicaid also defines many service categories quite broadly. For example, under the category of medical or remedial services, a state may pay for diagnostic, screening, or preventive services provided in any settings that are recommended by a licensed practitioner "for the maximum reduction of physical or mental disability and restoration of an individual to the best possible functional level."[19]

One of the broadest service categories is the early and periodic screening, diagnosis, and treatment (EPSDT) package of services for beneficiaries under age 21. As the *E* in EPSDT indicates, this package of benefits provides preventive care to children to catch problems before they advance, and offers early treatment to promote healthy growth and development. EPSDT benefits include periodic and as-needed screening services, comprehensive health exams (to detect both physical and mental health conditions), immunizations, lab tests, health education, vision services, hearing services, dental services, *and* any other measure to "correct or ameliorate" physical or mental defects found during a screening, *whether or not those services are covered under a state plan*. In addition to these benefits, EPSDT also requires states to inform families about the importance of preventive care, seek out children in need of comprehensive care, and offer families assistance in securing care.

The "correct or ameliorate" standard is very different from the "medical necessity" standard that is used for adults in Medicaid and is commonly found in private health insurance plans. Typically, medically necessary services are those that restore "normal" function after an illness or injury. Not only does this standard generally preclude care before a diagnosis is made, but if recovery is not possible (for example, as a result of blindness), services that improve the quality of life or prevent deterioration of a condition may be denied. By contrast, the EPSDT correct or ameliorate standard means a state must provide coverage for preventive and developmental treatment, as well as for services needed to treat a specific diagnosis. Combined with the requirement to provide services regardless of state plan limitations, the correct or ameliorate standard means that almost any accepted treatment should be covered under EPSDT.

Although Medicaid benefits are quite generous, in 2006 Congress passed, and President Bush signed into law, the Deficit Reduction Act of 2005 (DRA),[20] which contains, among other things, state options for significant changes to Medicaid benefit and cost-sharing rules. As shown in Box   8, the DRA gives states the option to choose a "benchmark" or "benchmark-equivalent" package of services for certain population groups instead of following the mandatory and

TABLE 2 Medicaid Benefits (Non-Deficit Reduction Act Option)	
Mandatory	**Optional**
Acute Care Benefits	*Acute Care Benefits*
Physician services	Prescription drugs
Laboratory and X-ray services	Medical care or remedial care furnished by non-physician
Inpatient hospital services	licensed practitioners
Outpatient hospital services	Rehabilitation and other therapies
Early and periodic screening, diagnostic, and treatment	Clinic services
services (EPSDT) for beneficiaries under 21	Dental services, including dentures
Family planning services and supplies	Prosthetic devices, eyeglasses, and durable medical equipment
Federally qualified health center (FQHC) services	Primary care case management
Rural health clinic services	Tuberculosis-related services
Nurse midwife services	Other specified medical or remedial care
Certified pediatric and family nurse practitioner services	*Long-Term Care Benefits*
Long-Term Care Benefits	Intermediate care facility services for the mentally retarded (ICF/
Nursing facility services for individuals 21 and over	MR)
Home healthcare services for individuals entitled to nursing	Inpatient/nursing facility services for individuals age 65 years and
facility care	over in an institution for mental disease
New benefits in ACA	Inpatient psychiatric hospital services for individuals under 21
Tobacco cessation program for pregnant women	Home- and community-based waiver services
	Other home health care
	Targeted case management
	Respiratory care services for ventilator-dependent individuals
	Personal care services
	Hospice services
	Services furnished under a Program of All-inclusive Care for the
	Elderly (PACE program)
	New benefits in ACA
	New state option for community-based care
	New state option for home health care
	New state option for family planning services

Source: 42 U.S.C. § 1396d; 42 CFR Parts 430–498.

optional list of services identified in Table 2.[21] There are three benchmark packages: (1) the Federal Employee Health Benefits Plan (FEHBP), (2) a state's health plan for its own employees, and (3) the state's largest commercial non-Medicaid health maintenance organization (HMO) plan. In addition, the DRA allows the secretary of HHS to approve a plan as a benchmark.

Benchmarks provide a state with a standard to follow when designing its Medicaid package of benefits—it does not mean that Medicaid beneficiaries are enrolled in the plans identified as benchmarks. Furthermore, a state may instead choose to offer "benchmark-equivalent" coverage that includes certain basic services as shown in Box 8. These services must have the same actuarial value as the services provided by one of the three benchmarks listed above (i.e., the value of the services must be similar). States may choose to

supplement their benchmark-equivalent plans with additional services, as listed in Box 8. These additional services are required to be worth only 75% of the actuarial value of the same service provided in a benchmark plan. Finally, while the DRA still guarantees the same set of EPSDT services for children under 19, these services may be more difficult to access if they are provided through wrap-around benefits that supplements the benchmark package instead of within the package itself.[22]

The benefit changes allowed by the DRA may only be applied to certain populations, and these groups had to be part of a state plan prior to the law's enactment to receive the new benefits package. DRA-eligible populations include most categorically needy children, as well as parents and caretakers who receive Medicaid but not Temporary Assistance to Needy Families (the new welfare program created by

BOX 8 DRA Benefit Options

Benchmark Plans
Federal Employee Health Benefits Plan
State employee health plan
Largest commercial non-Medicaid HMO in the state
HHS secretary-approved plan

Benchmark-Equivalent Plan
Full actuarial value for the following services:
- Inpatient and outpatient hospital
- Physician (surgical and medical)
- Laboratory and X-ray
- Well-baby and well-child
- Other appropriate preventive services (defined by HHS secretary)

Additional Optional Benchmark-Equivalent Services
75% actuarial value for the following services:
- Prescription drugs
- Mental heath
- Vision
- Hearing

Note: States must wrap around EPSDT coverage as necessary.

BOX 9 Idaho Implementation of DRA[25]

Idaho took advantage of DRA options to modernize its Medicaid program in response to increasing costs and concerns about the value of its mental health services. The state hoped to reform Medicaid to improve its performance and efficiency, but did not expect to achieve significant cost savings. Idaho made a variety of changes, including separating beneficiaries into basic and enhanced benefit packages based on health needs, increasing assistance to help individuals access preventive services, expanding its premium assistance program, and changing eligibility and co-payments under Medicaid and CHIP. Early indications show improved access to preventive services, a shift to a focus on quality improvement through a pay-for-performance disease management program, and better use of the medical home model. Given the limited time since implementation, the ramifications of the tiered benefit package model are not clear. Furthermore, the state has had less success in changing beneficiary behavior (e.g., in making healthier lifestyle choices), has struggled to translate the pay-for-performance program into cost savings, and has had limited participation in the premium assistance program.

PRWORA). The list of populations excluded from the DRA is quite lengthy and includes beneficiary groups with high expenditures, such as the disabled, dual eligibles, and terminally ill hospice patients.[23]

In states that choose to utilize the options provided in the DRA, the potential exists for Medicaid benefits to be severely curtailed. As of 2008, seven states (Idaho, Kansas, Kentucky, South Carolina, Washington, West Virginia, and Wisconsin) have taken the DRA option to reduce benefits and increase cost-sharing, while 24 states have used the DRA to increase the role of private long-term care insurance.[24]

Amount, Duration, and Scope, and Reasonableness Requirements

Although states have a great deal of flexibility in designing their Medicaid benefit packages, states had to follow several federal requirements prior to the DRA. These rules, collectively referred to as "amount, duration, and scope" and "reasonableness" requirements, were intended to ensure that all Medicaid beneficiaries in a state received adequate, comparable, and nondiscriminatory coverage. As discussed below, some of these rules have changed under the DRA.

Private insurers typically are not drawn to Medicaid's population because of the likelihood that these individuals would have relatively high healthcare needs. In addition, private insurers use a variety of tools (such as limited open-enrollment periods, experience rating, medical condition-based limitations, and narrow medical necessity standards) to limit their financial exposure. Medicaid, on the other hand, was designed as a healthcare entitlement program, with the goal to provide services to a needy population that would otherwise be uninsurable through commercial plans.[26] Table 3 identifies some of the requirements that help the Medicaid program achieve this goal, as well as any changes to them found in the DRA.

Medicaid Spending

Health policymakers are concerned with not only how much money Medicaid costs, but also the distribution of program spending. In 2009, Medicaid spent $366 billion, accounting for approximately 16% of total personal healthcare spending in the United States.[27] Understanding which populations utilize the most services, which services are utilized most frequently, and which services and populations are most costly helps policymakers decide if they need to change the Medicaid program and, if so, what changes should be made.

As you can see from Figure 3, not all populations and services are equal when it comes to cost. Generally, children

and adults are fairly inexpensive to cover, whereas elderly and disabled beneficiaries use more, as well as more expensive, services. One of the biggest reasons the elderly and disabled account for a high proportion of Medicaid expenditures is their use of long-term care services, such as nursing homes and home- and community-based services. In addition, they are heavy users of prescription drugs and are relatively more likely to be hospitalized. As is the case with private insurance and Medicare, a relatively small group of individuals account for a large proportion of Medicaid spending. In calendar year 2004, 5% of beneficiaries accounted for over half of all Medicaid spending.[28] Figure 4 shows that over one-half

TABLE 3 "Reasonableness" and "Amount, Duration, and Scope" Requirements in Medicaid

Requirement	Requirement Purpose	DRA Changes to the Requirement
Reasonableness	State must provide all services to categorically-needy beneficiaries in sufficient amount, duration, and scope to achieve its purpose	States only have to meet amount, duration, and scope requirements found in the named benchmark or benchmark-equivalent plan
Comparability	All categorically needy beneficiaries in the state are entitled to receive the same benefit package in content, amount, duration, and scope	States may apply benchmark or benchmark-equivalent packages to some, but not all, populations
Statewideness	In most cases, states must provide same benefit package in all parts of the state	States may apply benchmark or benchmark-equivalent packages to some, but not all, populations
Non-discrimination	States may not discriminate against a beneficiary based on diagnosis, illness, or type of condition by limiting or denying a mandatory service	DRA does not include language changing Medicaid non-discrimination rules

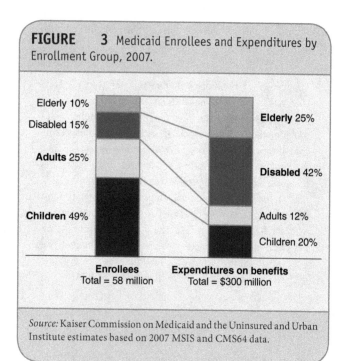

FIGURE 3 Medicaid Enrollees and Expenditures by Enrollment Group, 2007.

Elderly 10%

Disabled 15%

Adults 25%

Children 49%

Elderly 25%

Disabled 42%

Adults 12%

Children 20%

Enrollees
Total = 58 million

Expenditures on benefits
Total = $300 million

Source: Kaiser Commission on Medicaid and the Uninsured and Urban Institute estimates based on 2007 MSIS and CMS64 data.

of all Medicaid spending is for acute care services, and long-term care services account for over one-third of Medicaid expenditures.

In addition to expanding eligibility, the ACA also included a few changes to Medicaid benefits. States will have new options relating to community-based care, home health care, and family planning. In addition, all states will have to cover tobacco cessation programs for pregnant women. The ACA also includes a variety of demonstration programs that target key health issues such as obesity, high cholesterol, high blood pressure, diabetes, and tobacco use.

Medicaid Financing

The Medicaid program is jointly financed by the federal and state governments, with about 57% of the total program costs paid for by the federal government and the rest by the states. Even with the federal government picking up over half the tab, states have found their share of Medicaid costs to be increasingly burdensome, accounting for 16% of state budgets nationally.[29]

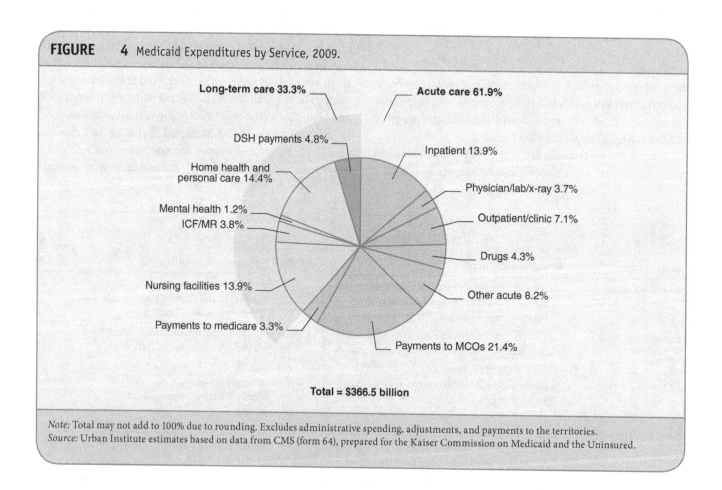

FIGURE 4 Medicaid Expenditures by Service, 2009.

Long-term care 33.3%

DSH payments 4.8%

Home health and personal care 14.4%

Mental health 1.2%

ICF/MR 3.8%

Nursing facilities 13.9%

Payments to medicare 3.3%

Payments to MCOs 21.4%

Acute care 61.9%

Inpatient 13.9%

Physician/lab/x-ray 3.7%

Outpatient/clinic 7.1%

Drugs 4.3%

Other acute 8.2%

Total = $366.5 billion

Note: Total may not add to 100% due to rounding. Excludes administrative spending, adjustments, and payments to the territories.
Source: Urban Institute estimates based on data from CMS (form 64), prepared for the Kaiser Commission on Medicaid and the Uninsured.

Program financing occurs through a matching payment system that divides the amount paid by the federal and state governments. The matching rate for most medical services, called the Federal Medical Assistance Percentage (FMAP), is determined by a formula that is tied to each state's per capita income. Poorer states—those with lower per capita incomes—receive more federal money for every state dollar spent on Medicaid, while the wealthier states receive less. In addition, the ACA allows for a 1% increase in FMAP for states that cover certain preventive services and immunizations without any cost-sharing requirements. The FMAP rate may not be lower than 50% for any state, meaning that the costliest scenario for a state government is that it splits program costs evenly with the federal government. FMAP rates range from 50% to 76%, although the 2009 stimulus bill included a temporary FMAP increase that expired in 2010.[29(p.27)] Given the variation in matching rates and state programs' size, federal funds are not distributed evenly among the states. In fact, five states (California, New York, Ohio, Pennsylvania, and Texas) account for almost one-third of all federal Medicaid spending.[30]

Medicaid is also partially financed through beneficiary co-payments, co-insurance, and premiums. Prior to the DRA, Medicaid cost-sharing was extremely limited, but the DRA included drastic changes to Medicaid's cost-sharing rules. In most cases, states historically could only charge "nominal" cost sharing, such as $2 per month per family, $.50 to $3.00 per service, or 5% of the state's payment rate.[31] In addition, pre-DRA, states were prohibited from charging any cost-sharing to some beneficiaries and for some services. Furthermore, cost-sharing requirements were "unenforceable," meaning health professionals could not refuse to provide services if a beneficiary did not pay a required cost-share amount.

Under the DRA, however, states have options to impose much higher cost-sharing requirements and to make these requirements enforceable, meaning a provider may refuse service or beneficiaries may be disenrolled from Medicaid if they do not pay the requisite amount. States may now charge Medicaid families earning between 100% and 150% FPL up to 10% of the cost of services, and may charge families earning above 150% FPL both premiums and up to 20% of the cost of services,[32] and the aggregate of these cost-sharing requirements may not exceed 5% of a family's income. Furthermore, the DRA permits higher cost sharing for prescription drugs and the use of emergency departments for nonemergency services. Some beneficiaries are protected from these increased costs. Cost-sharing is generally prohibited for children covered by a mandatory category and is limited to nominal levels for adults with incomes up to 100% FPL. In addition, premium requirements are not enforceable for these groups.[29(p.17)] As with the DRA benefit changes, many groups and services are excluded from the new cost-sharing options.

As noted earlier, the federal government is picking up the bulk of the cost of the ACA Medicaid expansions. From 2014–2016, the federal government will pay 100% of the cost of financing newly eligible enrollees. While the federal government's share will lessen over time, it will still cover 90% of the cost in 2020 and beyond. It is also expected that the Medicaid expansion will reduce the uncompensated care burden of states, since fewer individuals will be uninsured. Even so, many states are concerned about the financial burden of the Medicaid expansion and it is estimated that ACA changes to Medicaid and CHIP will cost states $20 billion over 10 years.[33] While the federal government will provide significant financial help through 2019, the eligibility expansion is intended to be permanent. In addition, the ACA included a maintenance-of-effort (MOE) rule forbidding states from reducing their own eligibility rules. States must keep the eligibility rules they had in place as of March 2010 (when the law was enacted) for adults until 2014, and for children until 2019. This requirement was included to prevent states from rolling back coverage expansions and from simply replacing state dollars with federal dollars without actually expanding coverage. There is, however, a significant exception to the MOE rule: States with a documented budget deficit may reduce eligibility for non-pregnant, non-disabled adults earning over 133% FPL.

Medicaid Provider Reimbursement

Medicaid's complex design also extends to its provider reimbursement methodology. States have broad discretion in setting provider rates. Not only do reimbursement rates vary by state, but they also vary by whether services are provided in a fee-for-service or managed care setting and by which type of provider (e.g., physicians, hospitals) renders a service.[c]

Fee-for-Service Reimbursement

When reimbursing fee-for-service (FFS) care under Medicaid, states are required to set their payment rates to physicians at levels that are "sufficient" to ensure Medicaid patients have "equal access" to providers compared to the general population.[34] Despite this language, Medicaid reimbursement is much lower than both Medicare and private practice rates. Low reimbursement is one reason that many providers are wary of treating Medicaid patients. In 2008, one study found that approximately 28% of physicians were not accepting *any* new Medicaid patients compared to the 74% of physicians who were accepting *all or most* new Medicare and privately insured patients.[35] The ACA includes a temporary bump in primary care payment rates for services provided in both FFS and managed care settings. For 2013 and 2014, primary care payment rates will equal 100% of Medicare payment rates, with the federal government covering the cost of the increased reimbursement. While this measure is intended to support primary care providers and boost access to primary care services, its temporary nature means it is unlikely to have a lasting effect.

Hospital FFS services are reimbursed at a rate that is "consistent with efficiency, economy, and quality of care."[36] However, there is no specified minimum reimbursement level that states are required to meet, resulting in rates that are lower than what hospitals receive from Medicare and private insurance. Hospitals that serve a high number of low-income patients may receive additional Medicaid payments called dis-proportionate share hospital (DSH) payments. Under the ACA, however, these payments will be reduced significantly.

Managed Care Reimbursement

As with the rest of the healthcare system, managed care has become an increasingly important part of the Medicaid program. About 36 million patients—71% of all Medicaid patients—were in Medicaid managed care plans in 2009.[37] All states except Alaska and Wyoming enroll some Medicaid beneficiaries in managed care, with 22 states enrolling over 80% of their beneficiaries in managed care plans.[37] States may require managed care enrollment for all beneficiaries except children with special healthcare needs, Native Americans, and Medicare recipients.[38]

Managed care organizations (MCOs) that enroll Medicaid beneficiaries receive a monthly capitated rate per member and assume financial risk for providing services. States and MCOs agree upon a set of services the MCOs will provide for the capitated rate. If there are any Medicaid-covered services that are not included in a state's managed care contract with MCOs, states reimburse them an amount in addition to the capitated rate or reimburse non-MCO providers on a fee-for-service basis to provide those services. In other words, beneficiaries are still entitled to all Medicaid services, even when they are enrolled in a managed care plan.

States are required to pay MCOs on an "actuarially sound basis," a term that is not defined in the Medicaid statute.[39] As with other types of provider rates, capitation rates vary widely among states. However, it is difficult to compare capitation rates across states because of the variation in Medicaid programs generally and in the types of services and populations covered by the managed care contracts.

BOX 14 Discussion Questions

Is higher Medicaid cost-sharing a good idea? What are the strongest arguments you can make for and against higher cost-sharing? Should Medicaid beneficiaries have the same cost-sharing responsibilities as privately insured individuals, or should the government bear more of the cost because Medicaid beneficiaries are low-income individuals? What is the primary decision-making goal that led to the exclusion of so many populations and services from the new cost-sharing options?

Medicaid Waivers

Much of the previous discussion about Medicaid highlighted both the numerous requirements placed on states and the enormous amount of flexibility states have in operating their program. Medicaid *waivers* provide still another level of flexibility for states. There are several different types of waivers under Medicaid; here, we focus only on the broadest one—the "section 1115" waiver. Under section 1115 of the Social Security Act, states may apply to the secretary of HHS to waive requirements of health and welfare programs under the Social Security Act, including both Medicaid and CHIP. The secretary may grant section 1115 waivers, also called demonstration projects, as long as the proposal "assists in promoting the objectives" of the federal program.[d] This broad standard has not been defined and leaves the secretary with enormous discretion to approve or reject waiver applications. One of the most important aspects of a waiver is the "budget neutrality" requirement. A state must show that the waiver project will not cost the federal government more money over a five-year period than if the waiver had not been granted. The MOE rule under the ACA also applies to waivers. Although the amount of money spent remains the same, by seeking a waiver, a state is agreeing to use itself as a "policy laboratory" in exchange for being able to operate its Medicaid program with fewer requirements. Ideally, other states and the federal government will learn from these demonstration projects and incorporate their positive aspects, while avoiding negative ones.

In 2001, the Bush administration created a specific type of section 1115 waiver called the Health Insurance Flexibility and Accountability (HIFA) demonstration. These waivers differ from traditional 1115 waivers in that they encourage integration of Medicaid and CHIP with private insurance through premium assistance programs and other means. HIFA waivers also allow states to achieve budget neutrality by reducing the amount, duration, and scope of optional benefits and increasing cost-sharing requirements for optional eligibility groups (changes that may now be possible under the DRA without the need for a formal waiver). Although states may reduce optional benefits and populations under HIFA, mandatory populations must remain covered and mandatory benefits may not be reduced. Given these rules, HIFA waivers often involve a trade-off between covering more people with fewer services or fewer people with more services.

As of June 2011, HHS approved section 1115 waivers in 30 states and the District of Columbia, some of which were HIFA-1115 waivers.[40] States have taken a variety of approaches to changing their Medicaid programs through these waivers. For example, several states have implemented managed care programs, created tiered benefit systems (meaning that not all beneficiaries are entitled to the same benefits) in exchange for covering new populations, altered federal financing, or expanded coverage to low-income adults.

The Future of Medicaid

Due to the high cost of the Medicaid program, the large federal deficit, other pressures on federal and state budgets, and ideological differences among policymakers, Medicaid reform has been a hot topic in recent years. Although the ACA included a significant Medicaid expansion, the battle over Medicaid and other entitlement programs continues. Opponents of the ACA are seeking to overturn the law, and reform of entitlement programs is a central part of the debate about how to reduce the federal deficit. Furthermore, with the newly eligible Medicaid population operating under different rules than traditional Medicaid enrollees, it appears that many policymakers are moving away from viewing Medicaid as a social insurance program that provides a certain set of healthcare benefits and specific legal protections to vulnerable populations. Instead, they are fashioning Medicaid as a program that more closely mirrors private insurance plans in terms of their use of risk, cost-sharing, limited benefits, and lack of extra protections that ensure fairness and access to care. On an ever-larger scale, some policymakers are advocating for ending Medicaid as an entitlement program and transforming it into a block grant program in which the federal government will give states a set amount of funds for a specified period of time to run their Medicaid program as they see fit.

What type of Medicaid reform or waivers, if any, do you support? Should Medicaid beneficiaries be treated like privately insured individuals, meaning increased cost-sharing requirements, fewer legal protections, and fewer guaranteed benefits than in the current Medicaid program? Is it fair to provide a more generous package of benefits to publicly insured individuals than most privately insured people receive? Can the country afford a more generous Medicaid program? Can it afford not to provide adequate health insurance and access to care to the poor and near poor? Is it best to let states experiment with new ideas? If you could design a new Medicaid program, what would be your primary decision-making goal?

STATE CHILDREN'S HEALTH INSURANCE PROGRAM

Congress created the State Children's Health Insurance Program (CHIP) in 1997 as a $40 billion, 10-year block grant program, codified as Title XXI of the Social Security Act.[41] When the program expired in 2007, Congress tried to extend it by passing two versions of the Children's Health Insurance Program Reauthorization Act (CHIPRA). Despite the bi-partisan support for these bills, then-President George W. Bush vetoed both versions and instead signed a temporary extension of the program. In 2009, Congress again passed CHIPRA and newly elected President Obama signed it into law as one of his first acts in office.[15] CHIPRA included $33 billion in federal funds for children's coverage and extended the program and its funding through 2013.[42] The ACA further extended the program until 2019, but only included funding through fiscal year 2015.

CHIP is designed to provide health insurance to low-income children whose family income is above the eligibility level for Medicaid in their state. The funding and eligibility expansions in CHIPRA are estimated to cover 6.5 million additional children in either Medicaid or CHIP.[42] Overall, CHIP has been successful at insuring low-income children, enrolling more than 7.7 million children by the end of 2010.[43] Nonetheless, over 8 million children remain uninsured as of 2009, and many of them live in low-income families.[44]

CHIP Structure and Financing

CHIP is an optional program for the states, but all 50 have chosen to participate. States have three options regarding how their CHIP program is structured:

States may incorporate CHIP into their existing Medicaid program by using CHIP children as an expansion population.

States may create an entirely separate CHIP program.

States may create a hybrid program with lower-income children part of Medicaid and higher-income children in a separate CHIP program.

In 2010, 17 states had a separate program, 12 states had a Medicaid expansion program, and 21 states had a hybrid program.[45]

As with Medicaid, federal CHIP funds are disbursed on a matching basis, although the federal match is higher for CHIP than for Medicaid; CHIP matching rates range from 65% to 85%, compared to 50% to 76% for Medicaid.[46] The ACA includes a significant increase in the CHIP match for states beginning in 2015, but did not fund the program past 2015.

The matching formula is set by law and was changed when CHIPRA was enacted. Originally, allotments were for three years and were based on state-specific estimates of the number of low-income uninsured children, the number of low-income children generally, and healthcare costs relative to other states. Under CHIPRA, allotments are for two years and fiscal year 2009 allotments were based on prior CHIP spending levels. State allotments will increase annually to account for growth in healthcare spending, increases in the number of children in the state, and state program expansions. Every two years, state allotments will be rebased to reflect actual use of CHIP funds.[47]

The changes to the CHIP allotment formula were intended to allow for more predictable budgeting and to account for state program expansions. In addition, it addresses a recurring problem under the old formula. Previously, if states did not use their full allotment, the unused money reverted to the federal treasury and could be used by the federal government for any purpose. This lead to frequent fights to keep the money in the CHIP and over how the unused funds would be redistributed. Many states became dependent on receiving redistributed funds to keep their CHIP afloat. The new formula and process should help avoid this problem through better budgeting predictability and shorter allotment timeframes. In addition, under CHIPRA, all unused funds are designated to go to Medicaid performance bonuses for increased enrollment and outreach, instead of reverting to the federal treasury.[47]

Table 4 highlights a number of differences between Medicaid and CHIP. One very important difference is that whereas Medicaid is an entitlement program, CHIP is a block grant. As mentioned earlier, as a block grant, the federal matching funds are capped (through the allotments). Thus, a state is not entitled to limitless federal money under CHIP, and children, even if eligible, are not legally entitled to services once the allotted money has been spent. If a state runs out of funds and operates its CHIP separate from Medicaid, it will have to cut back its CHIP program by eliminating benefits, lowering provider reimbursement rates, disenrolling beneficiaries, or wait-listing children who want to enroll in the program. A state with a Medicaid expansion CHIP or a hybrid structure would not receive new CHIP money, but would continue to receive federal funds for Medicaid-eligible children as allowed under the Medicaid rules and at the Medicaid matching rate.

CHIP Eligibility

CHIP originally allowed states to cover children up to 200% FPL, but CHIPRA expanded coverage to 300% FPL.[42] All but four states have chosen to cover children up to 200% FPL and 25 states cover children at or above 250% FPL.[48,e]

Since CHIP coverage is built on a state's Medicaid eligibility rules, when CHIP eligibility begins depends on when Medicaid eligibility ends. For example, if a state covers a child up to 150% FPL, CHIP eligibility in that state would start at over 150% FPL. If another state Medicaid program covers children

at 200% FPL, CHIP eligibility would start at over 200% FPL. Under the ACA, states must cover all children aged 6–19 up to 133% FPL in their Medicaid program, and children in families with incomes up to 133% who are currently in CHIP programs must be moved to the state's Medicaid program.[b] Even so, variations may still exist above that level. As a result, children in families with the same income levels could be in CHIP in one state and in Medicaid in another state.

Under the original CHIP, pregnant women were not eligible for coverage without a waiver, although an option to cover unborn children indirectly allowed pregnant women to access the program. CHIPRA explicitly allows for coverage of pregnant women and 6 states have utilized that option as of January 2011. CHIPRA also expanded eligibility by allowing states to cover lawfully residing immigrant pregnant women and children, even if they have not been in the U.S. for five

Feature	Medicaid	CHIP
Structure	Entitlement	Block grant
Financing	Federal–State match	Federal–State match at higher rate than Medicaid
Funds may be used for premium assistance	No (without a waiver)	Yes
Benefits	Federally defined, with option to use benchmark or benchmark-equivalent benefits package; broad EPSDT services for children	Benefits undefined; use benchmark package; limited "basic" services required
Cost-sharing	Limited or prohibited for some populations and services, higher amounts allowed for some populations and services	Cost-sharing permitted within limits, but prohibited for well-baby and well-child exams
Anti-discrimination provision	Yes	No

TABLE   4 Comparing Key Features of Medicaid and CHIP

years. Prior to CHIPRA, states could only cover these populations with state dollars. As of January 2011, 25 states have picked up this option for immigrant children and 17 states have done so for immigrant pregnant women.[48]

CHIPRA included a number of provisions to streamline enrollment and improve outreach. While states must verify the citizenship status of CHIP enrollees, just as they must for Medicaid enrollees, states may do so through an electronic data match with the Social Security Administration. This option eases the administrative burden of the citizenship verification requirement and makes it much less likely that eligible individuals will be dropped from the program. In addition, CHIPRA allows states to use "express lane eligibility," which permits states to take information provided when individuals apply for other public programs and use that information to assess eligibility for CHIP. Finally, CHIP includes performance bonuses and other financial incentives to states that adopt various enrollment simplification and outreach policies.[48]

CHIP Benefits and Beneficiary Safeguards

States must provide "basic" benefits in their CHIP programs, including inpatient and outpatient hospital care, physician services (surgical and medical), laboratory and X-ray services, well-baby and well-child care, and age-appropriate immunizations. Under CHIPRA, states must now provide dental coverage and may provide dental-only supplemental coverage for otherwise eligible children who have health insurance without dental coverage. States may also choose to provide additional benefits such as prescription drug coverage, mental health services, vision services, hearing services, and other services needed by children. CHIPRA requires that states that choose to provide mental health or substance abuse services to offer the same level of coverage as they do for medical and surgical benefits.[42]

Various standards may be used for a benefit package. The law outlines the following benchmarks that states may use when designing their programs:

- The health insurance plan that is offered by the HMO that has the largest commercial, non-Medicaid enrollment in the state.
- The standard Blue Cross Blue Shield preferred provider plan for federal employees.
- A health plan that is available to state employees.
- A package that is actuarially equivalent to one of the above plans.
- A coverage package that is approved by the HHS secretary.[49]

(Do these benchmark plans sound familiar? Clearly, the DRA revisions to Medicaid were modeled on the existing CHIP program.) Under a stand-alone CHIP program, the benefit package may be the same as the state's Medicaid package or equal to one of these benchmarks. States with separate CHIP programs commonly create benefit packages that are less generous than the ones available in their Medicaid programs.[47]

In addition to the benefit package options, there are other areas where CHIP provides states with more program flexibility and beneficiaries with less protection than is the case under Medicaid. CHIP does not have the same standards regarding reasonableness, benefit definitions, medical necessity, or nondiscrimination coverage on the basis of illness (though, as noted earlier, states may opt out of or alter some of these protections in Medicaid under the DRA). States, however, may not exclude children based on preexisting conditions. Also, like the new DRA cost-sharing option, states with separate CHIP programs may impose cost-sharing requirements up to 5% of a family's annual income for families with incomes at or above 150% FPL.[47]

CHIP and Private Insurance Coverage

In devising CHIP, Congress was concerned that Medicaid-eligible children would enroll in CHIP instead of Medicaid without reducing the overall number of uninsured children in a state. To avoid this outcome, CHIP requires that all children be assessed for Medicaid eligibility and, if eligible, enrolled in Medicaid instead of CHIP.[50] In addition, Congress wanted to make sure that the government did not start funding health insurance coverage that was previously being paid for in the private sector. In other words, it did not want to give individuals or employers an incentive to move privately insured children to the new public program. To avoid private insurance crowd out, Congress allowed states to institute enrollment-waiting periods and impose cost-sharing requirements as a disincentive to switch to CHIP.

CHIP Waivers

States may apply to the secretary of HHS to waive CHIP program requirements in exchange for experimenting with new ways to increase program eligibility or benefits. Initially, the most common use of CHIP waivers was to expand eligibility for uncovered populations, such as childless adults and parents and pregnant women who are not eligible under a state's Medicaid program. Using CHIP funds to provide coverage for adult populations was controversial because the program was designed to provide health insurance to children. While CHIPRA expands eligibility options for pregnant women, it also prohibits states from obtaining new waivers to cover adults with CHIP funds.[47]

In addition, a few states have used CHIP waivers to create premium assistance programs. Premium assistance means that public subsidies (in this case, CHIP funds) are available to help beneficiaries cover the cost of private health insurance premiums for employer-sponsored coverage or other health insurance plans that are available to them. States favor premium assistance programs as a way to reduce the state's cost of providing a child with health insurance. Premium assistance programs may also reduce crowd out by providing an incentive for people to keep their children in private coverage instead of enrolling them in CHIP. States must abide by numerous rules when creating a premium assistance program and the combination of these rules and the high cost of private insurance has led to low enrollment in CHIP premium assistance programs in the few states that have initiated them. The use of premium assistance programs may increase in the future, as CHIPRA includes provisions to help reduce these barriers.[42]

The Future of CHIP

The future of CHIP is clouded by the ACA. While CHIP has been a very successful (and bi-partisan) program, it is possible that some states will drop the program due to fiscal pressures and the availability of newer insurance options.[51] States will bear increased costs due to the ACA's Medicaid expansion and if CHIP's enhanced match is not extended past 2015, many states may choose to spend their state dollars elsewhere. Given the ACA's individual insurance mandate, most children who are dropped from CHIP would be required to obtain coverage through another source. While other insurance options should be available—employer coverage, Medicaid, or through state health exchanges—many children may be moved to less generous and more expensive coverage if CHIP is not available.

MEDICARE

Medicare is the federally funded health insurance program for the elderly and some persons with disabilities. As a completely federally funded program with uniform national guidelines, Medicare's administration and financing is quite different from that found in Medicaid and CHIP. This section reviews who Medicare serves, what benefits the program provides, how Medicare is financed, and how Medicare providers are reimbursed. As with Medicaid and CHIP, the ACA included several provisions relating to Medicare. These changes include new coverage for preventive services, bonus payments for primary care services, and assistance in paying for prescription drugs. At the same time, a number of changes will result in reduced reimbursement for providers. Taken together, the ACA's Medicare-related provisions are expected to result in $533 billion in savings and $105 billion in new Medicare spending, for a net reduction of $428 billion in Medicare spending over 10 years.[52]

BOX 19 Discussion Questions

Although many Medicare beneficiaries are poor, there is no means test (income- or resource-specific eligibility level) to determine eligibility as there is with Medicaid and CHIP. Is there a good public policy reason for this difference? What would be the basis for making this distinction? Does the government have a different role to play in providing health care based on the population involved?

Medicare Eligibility

Medicare covers two main groups of people—the elderly and the disabled. In 2010, there were 39 million elderly and 8 million persons with disabilities or end-stage renal disease[ii] enrolled in Medicare.[2] To qualify for Medicare under the elderly category, individuals must be at least 65 years old and be eligible for Social Security payments by having worked and contributed to Social Security for at least 10 years. Individuals who are 65 but do not meet the work requirements may become eligible for Medicare on the basis of their spouse's eligibility. To qualify for Medicare as a person with disabilities, individuals must be totally and permanently disabled and receive Social Security Disability Insurance (SSDI) for at least 24 months, or have a diagnosis of either end-stage renal disease or amyotrophic lateral sclerosis. The disability categories do not have an age requirement, so these Medicare beneficiaries may be under age 65. Unlike Medicaid and CHIP, Medicare eligibility is not based on an income or asset test—in other words, individuals of any income level are eligible for Medicare if they meet the eligibility requirements.

Even though Medicare does not target low-income elderly and disabled, a significant portion of Medicare beneficiaries are indigent and in poor health. Almost 25% of Medicare beneficiaries are in families with annual incomes of $10,000 or less and just over half have incomes under 200% FPL.[2] These low-income beneficiaries are more likely to be female, in fair or poor health, part of a racial or ethnic minority group, and disabled than other beneficiaries. As shown in Figure 5, among all Medicare beneficiaries, many have three or more chronic conditions, are in poor or fair health, or have a cognitive impairment. Even though approximately 78% of Medicare beneficiaries identify as non-Hispanic white, almost twice as many African-American and Hispanic beneficiaries report being in fair or poor health compared to non-Hispanic white beneficiaries.[2(p3)]

Medicare Benefits

Medicare is split into several parts, each covering a specified set of services. Beneficiaries are automatically entitled to Part A, also known as Hospital Insurance (HI). Part B services, also known as Supplemental Medical Insurance (SMI), covers physician, outpatient, and preventive services. (The ACA added coverage for certain preventive services without cost-sharing, including an annual comprehensive risk assessment, provided without cost-sharing when delivered in an outpatient setting.) Part B is voluntary for enrollees, but 95% of Part A beneficiaries also opt to have Part B. Beneficiaries may choose to receive their benefits through Part C, Medicare Advantage, which includes the Medicare managed care program and a few other types of plans. Part D is the new prescription drug benefit. Table 5 lists Medicare benefits by part and Figure 6 illustrates current and projected spending on Medicare benefits. Significant growth is expected in spending on outpatient prescription drugs over the next 10 years. Although Medicare benefits are quite extensive, the list excludes services that one might expect to be covered in health insurance

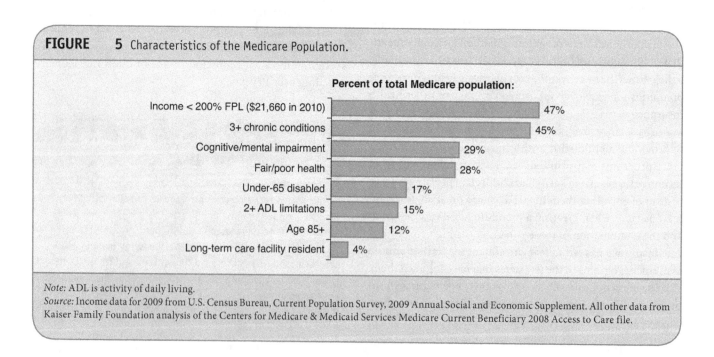

FIGURE 5 Characteristics of the Medicare Population.

Percent of total Medicare population:

Income < 200% FPL ($21,660 in 2010)	47%
3+ chronic conditions	45%
Cognitive/mental impairment	29%
Fair/poor health	28%
Under-65 disabled	17%
2+ ADL limitations	15%
Age 85+	12%
Long-term care facility resident	4%

Note: ADL is activity of daily living.
Source: Income data for 2009 from U.S. Census Bureau, Current Population Survey, 2009 Annual Social and Economic Supplement. All other data from Kaiser Family Foundation analysis of the Centers for Medicare & Medicaid Services Medicare Current Beneficiary 2008 Access to Care file.

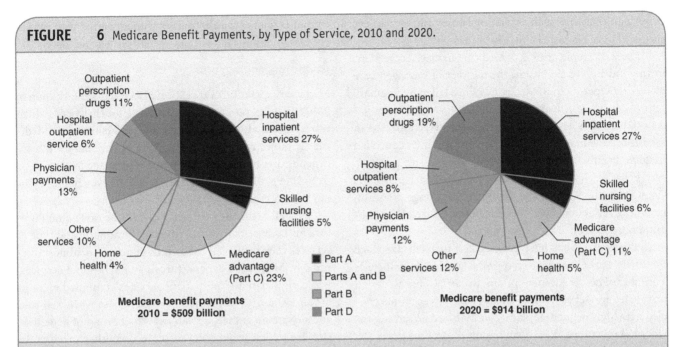

Notes: Totals do not include administrative expenses and are net of recoveries. Other Services include hospice services; durable medical equipment; ambulance services, independent, physician in-office, and hospital outpatient department laboratory services; hospital outpatient services that are not paid for using the prospective payment system (PPS); Part B prescription drugs; rural health clinic services; outpatient dialysis; and benefit payments not allocated to specific services, including adjustments to reflect year-to-date spending (2010), and savings from the Independent Payment Advisory Board (2020).
Source: Congressional Budget Office, Medicare Baseline, August 2010.

TABLE 5 Medicare Benefits

Part	Services Covered
A	Inpatient hospital, 100 days at skilled nursing facility (SNF), limited home health following hospital or SNF stay, and hospice care.
B	Physician, outpatient hospital, X-ray, laboratory, emergency room, and other ambulatory services; medical equipment; limited preventive services, including: one preventive physical exam, mammography, pelvic exam, prostrate exam, colorectal cancer screening, glaucoma screening for high-risk patients, prostrate cancer screening, and cardiovascular screening blood test; diabetes screening and outpatient self-management; bone-mass measurement for high-risk patients; hepatitis-B vaccine for high risk patients; pap smear; and pneumococcal and flu vaccinations. New ACA benefits: In 2010, cost-sharing eliminated for select preventive services; coverage for personalized prevention plan, including comprehensive health assessment.
C	Managed care plans, private fee-for-service plans, special needs plans, and medical savings accounts. The plans provide all services in Part A and Part B and generally must offer additional benefits or services as well.
D	Prescription drug benefit.

targeting the elderly, such as nursing home care, routine eye care, and hearing exams and hearing aids.[2(p6)]

There was rapid growth of Medicare managed care plans in the mid-to-late 1990s, but the number of managed care plans participating in Medicare has since fallen by one-half. Future Medicare Advantage enrollment projections vary.[29] As of 2010, over 11 million beneficiaries were enrolled in Medicare Advantage plans, over double the number enrolled in 2005. Even with this growth, only one-quarter of Medicare beneficiaries opt to enroll in managed care plans.[2(p9)] Changes in the ACA to the Medicare Advantage program, including reimbursement cuts, mean the future of the program is uncertain.

Although HMOs have participated in Medicare since the 1970s, Part C has evolved over the last decade to include a number of new insurance options. In 1997, Congress added private fee-for-service plans,[f] medical savings accounts coupled with high-deductible plans, county-based preferred provider organizations (PPOs), and point-of-services plans.[2(p9)] As part of the Medicare Prescription Drug Improvement and Modernization Act of 2003 (MMA),[54] Congress added regional PPOs and "special needs plans" for the institutionalized and for beneficiaries with severe and disabling conditions.[2(p9)]

The MMA also created Part D, Medicare's prescription drug benefit. The drug benefit was made available to recipients beginning in 2006. Medicare contracts with private drug insurance plans in each of 34 regions. If at least two plans are not available in a region, the government contracts with a fallback plan (a private plan that is not an insurer) to serve that area. All plans must cover at least two drugs in each therapeutic class or category of Part D drugs. Dual enrollees (individuals enrolled in both Medicaid and Medicare) are no longer eligible for prescription drug coverage under Medicaid; they must receive their prescription drug benefit through Medicare.

To obtain prescription drugs through Medicare, beneficiaries have the choice of remaining in traditional fee-for-service Medicare under Parts A and B and enrolling in a separate private prescription drug plan, or enrolling in a Part C plan through Medicare Advantage that includes prescription drug coverage. Medicare Advantage plans are required to offer basic prescription drug benefits and may offer supplemental prescription drug benefits for an additional premium. Some beneficiaries may also have access to employer-sponsored health insurance that includes prescription drug benefits. These beneficiaries may keep their employer coverage only, keep their employer coverage and enroll in Part D, or drop their employer coverage. Finally, beneficiaries may also choose not to obtain any prescription drug coverage. However, in certain circumstances, a beneficiary who declines to enroll in Part D during the allotted enrollment period may pay increased premiums if he decides to enroll at a later date.

Medicare Spending

Medicare expenditures are expected to reach $504.3 billion in 2010 (final figures are not yet available for that year), which would account for 12% of the total federal budget.[2(p15)] Medicare is projected to constitute 20.8% of national healthcare expenditures by 2014 and spending is expected to grow 6.2% from 2009–2019. Spending levels would be even higher without savings created by the ACA.[55]

Not all Medicare beneficiaries cost the same amount to care for because of the disparities in the amount and type of services they require. As shown in Figure 6, almost one-third of Medicare's expenditures pay for hospital services, while physician and outpatient services combined account for almost a fifth of Medicare payments. As with Medicaid and private insurance, a relatively small group of beneficiaries use a high proportion of these and other services. In 2006, 10% of all beneficiaries accounted for 58% of Medicare expenditures.[2(p16)]

The ACA established an Independent Payment Advisory Board, which has the task of submitting proposals to reduce the rate of Medicare spending if Medicare exceeds specified targets. The Secretary of Health and Human Services is

---

BOX 20 Discussion Questions

Lawmakers were concerned that adding a prescription drug benefit to Medicare would encourage employers to drop prescription drug coverage to the beneficiaries who receive prescription drugs through retiree health plans. In an effort to avoid a shift in elderly people who rely on public insurance instead of private insurance for their prescription drug coverage, Congress included in the MMA a tax-free subsidy to encourage employers to maintain prescription drug coverage. While the ACA eliminates the tax deduction, the subsidy remains in place. The amount of the subsidy is based on the prescription drug costs of individuals who remain with the employer's plan and do not enroll in Part D.

Is this subsidy a good idea? Is the proper role of government to pay private companies to maintain insurance coverage? If so, should it occur for other benefits? Do you have a preference between giving incentives for private entities to provide insurance coverage versus the government financing the coverage directly?

required to implement proposals submitted by the board unless Congress enacts alternative proposals that achieve the same level of savings. Congress limited the board's options by prohibiting consideration of proposals that ration care, increase revenue, change benefits, change eligibility, or change cost-sharing. In addition, hospitals and physicians are exempt from board proposals until 2020.[52]

Medicare Financing

Medicare is a federally funded program. Unlike Medicaid and CHIP, state governments do not generally contribute to Medicare spending, and therefore a matching system is not required. Although Medicare financing is simpler than Medicaid financing in many respects, each Medicare part has its own financing rules, adding some complexity to the program (see Figure 7). In addition, beneficiary contributions in the form of premiums, deductibles, and co-payments contribute to financing Medicare expenditures.

Part A (HI) benefits are paid from the HI Trust Fund, funded through a mandatory payroll tax. Employers and employees each pay a tax of 1.45% of a worker's earnings (self-employed persons pay both shares, for a total tax of 2.9%), which is set aside for the Trust Fund. The ACA increases this rate for higher income tax payers. Beginning in 2013, individuals will have to pay a tax of 2.35% on earnings over $200,000 for individuals or $250,000 for couples.[52] In addition, beneficiaries pay a deductible for each inpatient hospital episode, and co-insurance for hospital care beyond 60 days, skilled nursing care beyond 20 days, outpatient drugs, and inpatient respite care.

By relying on payroll taxes, Medicare Part A uses current workers and employers to pay for health benefits for the disabled and those over 65 years old, many of whom are already retired. This formula is problematic in the face of the looming retirement of those from the Baby Boom generation; between 2010 and 2030, it is projected that a 10-million-person increase in the working population will have to support an increase of 30 million new elderly Medicare beneficiaries. To put it another way, in 2003, payroll taxes from almost four workers supported each Medicare beneficiary, but in 2030, it is expected that taxes on only 2.4 workers will be available to support each Medicare beneficiary.[56] Because of this and for other reasons, the 2010 Medicare Board of Trustees estimated that the Part A HI Trust Fund would be exhausted by 2029.[2(p20)]

Part B (SMI) is financed through general federal tax revenues and monthly premiums, deductibles, and cost-sharing paid by beneficiaries. Beneficiaries with incomes over $85,000 (or $170,000 for a couple) will pay a higher income-related monthly premium than other beneficiaries. Instead of increasing each year, this income threshold was frozen from 2009 to 2019 as part of the ACA, meaning more beneficiaries will be subject to the higher premium during those years. In addition to the monthly premium, beneficiaries pay an annual deductible for physician and medical services and have co-insurance requirements for outpatient hospital care, ambulatory surgical care, clinical diagnostic services, outpatient mental health services, and most preventive services.

Despite the federal government's and beneficiaries' investment in Medicare benefits, the program covers less than half of beneficiaries' actual healthcare expenses.[56] As a result, many beneficiaries have some type of supplemental insurance. Figure 8 illustrates the most common type of supplemental options: employer-sponsored insurance; Medicare Advantage plans, which offer extra benefits; Medicaid; and Medigap polices. Medigap policies are sold by private insurers and are intended to cover the cost of payments required by Medicare, such as premiums and co-payments. In addition, some Medigap policies offer benefits that are not covered by Medicare.

Part C Medicare Advantage plans provide services from Parts A and B and receive their funding from the sources described above. The federal government contracts with private plans and pays them a capitated rate to provide Medicare

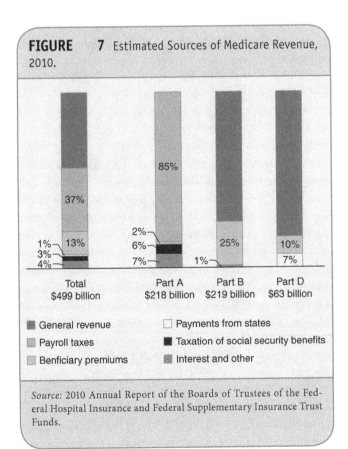

FIGURE 7 Estimated Sources of Medicare Revenue, 2010.

Total $499 billion — 37%, 13%, 1%, 3%, 4%
Part A $218 billion — 85%, 2%, 6%, 7%
Part B $219 billion — 25%, 1%
Part D $63 billion — 10%, 7%

- General revenue
- Payroll taxes
- Benficiary premiums
- Payments from states
- Taxation of social security benefits
- Interest and other

Source: 2010 Annual Report of the Boards of Trustees of the Federal Hospital Insurance and Federal Supplementary Insurance Trust Funds.

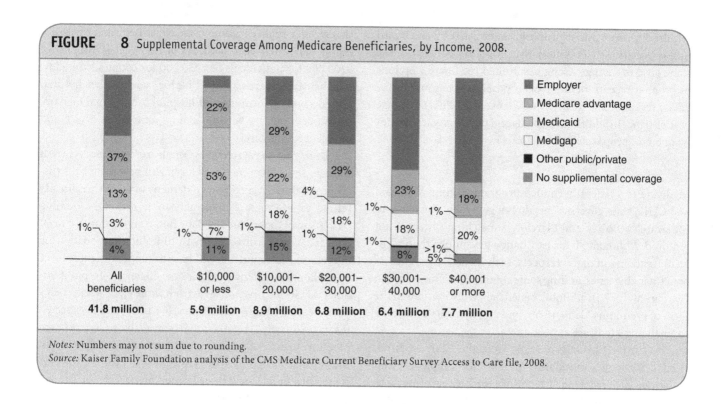

FIGURE 8 Supplemental Coverage Among Medicare Beneficiaries, by Income, 2008.

Legend:
- Employer
- Medicare advantage
- Medicaid
- Medigap
- Other public/private
- No supplemental coverage

	All beneficiaries	$10,000 or less	$10,001–20,000	$20,001–30,000	$30,001–40,000	$40,001 or more
	41.8 million	5.9 million	8.9 million	6.8 million	6.4 million	7.7 million

Notes: Numbers may not sum due to rounding.
Source: Kaiser Family Foundation analysis of the CMS Medicare Current Beneficiary Survey Access to Care file, 2008.

benefits to program participants. The plans charge beneficiaries varying premiums and co-payments.

Part D, Medicare's prescription drug benefit, is financed through an annual deductible, monthly premiums, general revenues, and state payments for dual enrollees. As shown in Figure 9, beneficiaries pay an annual deductible, 25% of the cost of drugs up to a set amount ($2,840 in 2011), 100% of the cost of drugs above that amount to a catastrophic threshold ($6,448 in 2011), and 5% of the cost above the catastrophic threshold. The gap in Medicare coverage where the beneficiary pays 100% of the cost of drugs is commonly referred to as the "doughnut hole." In 2007, approximately one-quarter of Part D users purchased drugs in the doughnut hole in 2010 and most plans do not offer coverage in this gap. Under Part D, deductibles, premiums, benefit limits, and catastrophic thresholds are not fixed, but indexed to increase with the growth in per capita Medicare spending for Part D. To offset these charges, the MMA included provisions to assist low-income beneficiaries by reducing or eliminating cost-sharing requirements and the doughnut hole. There are three low-income assistance tiers for beneficiaries who earn up to 150% FPL.[2(p8)]

The ACA included provisions to close the doughnut hole such that beneficiaries will only pay 25% cost-sharing in that range of drug spending by 2020. Beneficiaries received a $250 rebate for purchases made in the doughnut hole in 2010. To close the coverage gap, beneficiaries will receive a phased-in discount for generic and brand name drugs purchased in the doughnut hole going forward. In addition, the amount of out-of-pocket spending needed to reach the catastrophic level was reduced from 2014–2019, but will revert back to its original level in 2020 without further congressional action.[2(p8)]

The MMA also requires that dual enrollees receive their prescription drug benefit through Medicare, not Medicaid. Under the MMA, states are now required to help fund Medicare's prescription drug benefit for dual enrollees through a maintenance-of-effort or "clawback" provision. This provision requires states to pay the federal government a share of expenditures the states would have made to provide prescription drug coverage to dual enrollees. The state share begins at 90% in 2006 and tapers down to 75% in 2015 and beyond. Many states are resisting these requirements and some are threatening not to pay their share. To the extent states adhere to the clawback provision, it represents the first time that states are assisting with Medicare financing. If states choose to provide dual enrollees with prescription drug coverage through Medicaid, states must use 100% of their own dollars to finance the coverage, even if the beneficiary does not enroll in Part D.

Table 6 provides a summary of Medicare financing provisions. Because Part C is financed by parts A and B and is an alternative to A and B, it is not included in the table. Whether beneficiaries have cost-sharing and other

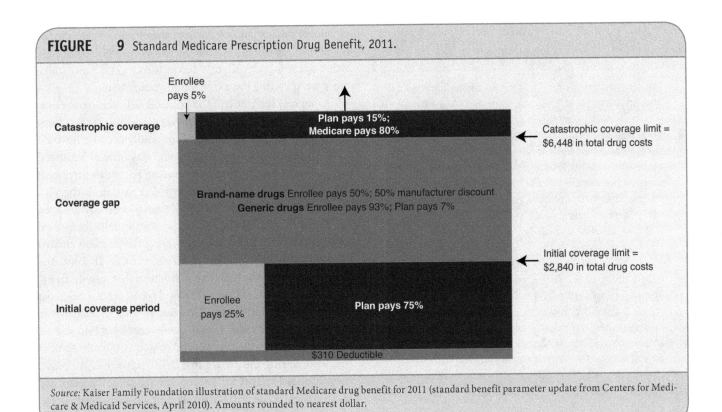

FIGURE 9 Standard Medicare Prescription Drug Benefit, 2011.

Enrollee pays 5%

Catastrophic coverage

Plan pays 15%;
Medicare pays 80%

Catastrophic coverage limit = $6,448 in total drug costs

Coverage gap

Brand-name drugs Enrollee pays 50%; 50% manufacturer discount
Generic drugs Enrollee pays 93%; Plan pays 7%

Initial coverage limit = $2,840 in total drug costs

Initial coverage period

Enrollee pays 25%

Plan pays 75%

$310 Deductible

Source: Kaiser Family Foundation illustration of standard Medicare drug benefit for 2011 (standard benefit parameter update from Centers for Medicare & Medicaid Services, April 2010). Amounts rounded to nearest dollar.

requirements under Part C depends on the specifics of each managed care plan.

Medicare Provider Reimbursement

Medicare's reimbursement rules vary by provider type and by whether care is provided through a fee-for-service arrangement or a Medicare Advantage (i.e., managed care) plan. This section reviews physician and hospital reimbursement methodologies under both payment systems.

Physician Reimbursement

Physicians who are paid by a managed care plan to provide Medicare services to beneficiaries follow the same general rules for managed care reimbursement. However, physicians

TABLE 6 Medicare Financing by Part

Medicare Part	Government Financing Scheme	Beneficiary Payment Requirements		
		Annual Deductible	**Monthly Premium**	**Cost-Sharing**
A	Trust Fund through mandated employer and employee payroll taxes	Yes	No, if Social Security work requirements are met	Yes
B	General federal tax revenue	Yes	Yes	Yes
D	General federal tax revenue and state "clawback" payments for dual enrollees	Yes—except some low-income beneficiaries	Yes—except some low-income beneficiaries	Yes—except some low-income beneficiaries

providing care on a fee-for-service basis are paid according to the Medicare fee schedule, although the ACA includes a 10% bonus payment from 2011–2015 for primary care providers who operate in Health Professional Shortage Areas. The fee schedule assigns a relative weight to every service to reflect the resources needed to provide the service. These weights are adjusted for geographic differences in costs and multiplied by a conversion factor (a way to convert the relative value that defines all medical services on the fee schedule into a dollar amount) to determine the final payment amount. Payment rates are changed through upward or downward shifts in the conversion factor. Although the ratio of Medicare physician fees to private insurance varies considerably by location, overall, Medicare physician fees are about 81% less than those provided by private insurers,[57(p90)] but about 28% higher than reimbursement rates provided by Medicaid.[58]

The formula for reimbursing physicians, referred to as the Sustainable Growth Rate (SGR), has been a focal point of debate. Congress established the SGR in 1997 as a way to control spending for physician services. The formula sets an overall target amount for spending on physician services (and related services such as laboratory tests) in Part B. Payment rates are adjusted to reflect actual spending as compared to the target level—if actual spending is higher than the target level,

payment rates are cut, but if actual spending is lower than the target level, payment rates are raised. From 1997–2001, physician spending was slightly below the target.[59] Since 2003, however, spending has exceeded the target level.

Congress has not had the political will to impose reimbursement cuts called for by the formula. Since 2003, Congress has suspended the formula annually because it would have resulted in rate reductions, and has instead legislated rate increases for physicians. Deferring reimbursement cuts year after year has led to an untenable situation. If the SGR formula were followed in 2010, physician fees would have been cut 21% that year and an additional 5% annually for several more years.[59(p112)] Unfortunately, fixing the problem created by deferred reimbursement is very expensive. In 2008, the Congressional Budget Office estimated that simply freezing physician rates at their 2009 level for 10 years would cost $318 billion. Replacing the SGR with another index (such as the Medicare Economic Index) would cost $439 billion over 10 years.[59(p113)] While Congress discussed options to address this issue during the debate that led to passage of the ACA, they ultimately left it for another day because the price tag was too high. Some critics complain that it is disingenuous to argue that the ACA reduces the deficit when this multi-billion problem was not addressed in the law.

Hospital Reimbursement

Hospitals are paid for acute inpatient services on a prospective basis using "diagnostic related groups" (DRGs). Diagnostic related groups sort patients into more than 500 groups based on their diagnoses. Various diagnoses are grouped together if they have similar clinical profiles and costs. Each DRG is assigned a relative weight based on charges for cases in that group as compared to the national average for all groups. In addition, the part of the DRG covering hospitals' cost of labor is adjusted by a wage index to account for different geographic costs.[60(p43)] Hospitals may also receive additional payments for providing high-cost outlier cases; incurring costs associated with use of new technology; incurring indirect medical education costs; serving a high proportion of low-income patients; or being a qualified sole community provider, a rural referral center, a small Medicare-dependent hospital, a rural hospital treating fewer than 200 admissions, or a critical access hospital (a qualified rural hospital that provides critical care services).[60(pp43–44)]

For outpatient care, hospitals are reimbursed by Medicare using a different prospective system. Each outpatient service is assigned to one of about 800 ambulatory payment classification (APC) groups. Ambulatory payment classifications have a relative weight based on the median cost of the service as compared to the national average. Again, a conversion factor is used to calculate the specific dollar amount per APC and the labor cost portion is adjusted based on a hospital wage index to account for geographic cost differences. Ambulatory payment classification payments may be adjusted when hospitals use new technologies or biologics, and when they treat unusually high-cost patients.[60(p44)]

The ACA included a number of provisions that reduced reimbursement for hospitals and other Medicare providers, including skilled nursing facilities and hospices. These rate reductions include "market basket" updates, which set the prices for a mix of goods and services, and a lowering of Disproportionate Share Hospital payments, which are given to hospitals that provide services to a relatively high proportion of low-income patients. In addition, hospitals will receive reduced payments for services connected to preventable readmissions and hospital-acquired conditions.

Medicare Advantage Reimbursement

Medicare Advantage plans are paid a capitated rate by the federal government to provide Parts A, B, and D benefits to each enrollee in their plan. Plans submit a bid to the federal government that estimates their cost per enrollee and these bids are compared to benchmarks established by statute and that vary by county. The benchmark is the maximum Medicare will pay for Part A and B services in that county.[61] Once a bid is accepted, a contract between plans and the federal government details the services the plan will provide and the premiums, deductibles, and cost sharing it will charge beneficiaries.

The ACA includes significant reductions in Medicare Advantage payments. On average, Medicare Advantage plans had become 9% to 13% more expensive than fee-for-service providers for comparable services.[61] The ACA phases in reduced payments that bring Medicare Advantage plans closer to the benchmark payment for traditional Medicare services in their county. Additional reductions will occur due to changes in the risk-adjustment formula. On the other hand, plans that provide high-quality care may be eligible for additional payments under the new law.[52]

CONCLUSION

This chapter provided you with an overview of the three main public programs that provide health insurance coverage to millions of people in the United States, and raised a series of policy questions for your consideration. Based on the size of the programs, their costs to the federal and state governments, and their importance to millions of (often low-income) individuals, the role and structure of Medicaid, CHIP, and Medicare are constantly being debated. Some people would like to see coverage expanded to ensure that everyone has adequate access to health insurance, others would like to dismantle the programs in the interest of eliminating government-funded entitlements, and still others suggest incremental changes to the programs. The debate continues even with the passage of the ACA. Some want to repeal the law, while others are discussing cuts to entitlement programs as a way to reduce the federal deficit. Each of these decisions, and many others, reflect the recurring themes that have been discussed throughout this chapter: choosing between state flexibility and national uniformity; determining the appropriate role for government, the private sector, and individuals in healthcare financing and delivery; defining a primary decision-making goal (fiscal restraint, equity/social justice, improved health outcomes, uniformity, etc.); and settling on the appropriate scope of coverage to offer beneficiaries. Given these programs' expected increase in beneficiaries and the complementary increase in their cost, it is likely that the debates over Medicaid, CHIP, and Medicare will continue vigorously in the foreseeable future.

REFERENCES

1. Kaiser Family Foundation. *Health coverage of children: The role of Medicaid and CHIP*. 2011. Available at http://www.kff.org/uninsured/7698.cfm. Accessed July 7, 2011; Kaiser Family Foundation. *Medicaid enrollment: June 2010 Snapshot*. Available at http://www.kff.org/medicaid/enrollmentreports.cfm. Accessed July 7, 2011; Kaiser Family Foundation. *Medicare chartbook*. 2010. Available at http://www.kff.org/medicare/8103.cfm. Accessed July 7, 2011.

2. Kaiser Family Foundation. *Medicare: A primer.* 2010. Available at http://www.kff.org/medicare/upload/7615-03.pdf. Accessed July 7, 2011.

3. Social Security Act §§ 1108(f), (g) & 1905(b), 42 U.S.C. §§ 1308 & 1396d(b).

4. Title XIX of the Social Security Act, §§ 1901–1935; 42 U.S.C. §§ 13961396v.

5. 42 C.F.R. Parts 430–498.

6. Centers for Medicaid and Medicare Services. *The state Medicaid manual.* Available at http://www.cms.gov/Manuals/PBM/itemdetail.asp?itemID=CMS021927. Accessed July 8, 2011.

7. Centers for Medicare and Medicaid Services. *State Medicaid director letters.* Available at https://www.cms.gov/SMDL/SMD/. Accessed July 7, 2011.

8. Kaiser Family Foundation. *The Medicaid program at a glance.* 2010. Available at http://www.kff.org/medicaid/upload/7334-04.pdf. Accessed July 7, 2011.

9. Kaiser Family Foundation. *Dual eligibles: Medicaid's role for low-income Medicare beneficiaries,* Kaiser Family Foundation; 2010. Available at http://www.kff.org/medicaid/upload/4091-07.pdf. Accessed March 10, 2011.

10. Kaiser Family Foundation. *Distribution of the nonelderly with Medicaid by Federal Poverty Level (FPL), states (2008–2009), U.S. (2009). State Health Facts.* Available at http://www.statehealthfacts.org/comparebar.jsp?typ=2&ind=156&cat=3&sub=42&cha=1808&o=a. Accessed March 14, 2011.

11. Kaiser Family Foundation. *Health insurance coverage of low income adults 19–64 (under 200% FPL), states (2008–2009), U.S. (2009).* Available at http://www.statehealthfacts.org/comparetable.jsp?typ=1&ind=878&cat=3&sub=177. Accessed March 14, 2011.

12. Kaiser Family Foundation. *Health reform source—frequently asked questions.* Available at http://healthreform.kff.org/faq/who-will-be-eligible-for-medicaid.aspx. Accessed April 4, 2011.

13. Kaiser Family Foundation. *Medicaid financial eligibility: Primary pathways for the elderly and people with disabilities.* 2010. Available at http://www.kff.org/medicaid/8048.cfm. Accessed March 14, 2011.

14. Pub L No. 104-193.

15. Children's Health Insurance Program Reauthorization Act of 2009. Pub L No. 111-3.

16. Fremstad S, Cox L. Covering new Americans: *A review of federal and state policies related to immigrants' eligibility and access to publicly funded health insurance.* Kaiser Family Foundation. 2004. Available at http://www.kff.org/medicaid/7214.cfm. Accessed July 8, 2011.

17. Passell JS. *Unauthorized migrants: Numbers and characteristics.* Pew Hispanic Center. 2005. Available at http://pewhispanic.org/reports/report.php?ReportID=46. Accessed July 8, 2011.

18. Families USA. *Expanding coverage for recent immigrants: CHIPRA gives states new options.* Available at http://www.policyarchive.org/handle/10207/bitstreams/96110.pdf. Accessed April 4, 2011.

19. 42 U.S.C. § 1396d(a)(13); 42 C.F.R. § 440.130.

20. Pub L No. 109-362.

21. 42 U.S.C. § 1937.

22. 42 U.S.C. § 1937(a).

23. 42 U.S.C. § 1937(a)2.

24. Kaiser Family Foundation. *Medicaid enrollment declines for the first time in nearly a decade, but 42 states are planning to expand coverage for uninsured.* Oct. 10, 2007. http://www.kff.org/medicaid/kcmu101007nr.cfm. Accessed July 8, 2011.

25. Kenny GM, Pelletier JE. *Medicaid policy changes in Idaho under the Deficit Reduction Act of 2005: Implementation issues and remaining challenges.* State Health Access Reform Evaluation. June 2010. Available at http://www.shadac.org/files/shadac/publications/IdahoMedicaidDRACaseStudy.pdf. Accessed April 5, 2010.

26. Rosenbaum S. Health policy report: Medicaid. *N Engl J Med.* 2002;346:635–640.

27. Kaiser Family Foundation. *Urban Institute estimates based on data from CMS (form 64).* Available at http://facts.kff.org/chart.aspx?ch=472. Accessed June 29, 2011.

28. Kaiser Family Foundation. *Federal and state share of Medicaid spending, FY 2009.* Available at http://www.statehealthfacts.org/comparemaptable.jsp?typ=2&ind=636&cat=4&sub=47. Accessed March 18, 2011.

29. Kaiser Family Foundation. *Medicaid primer. 2010.* Available at http://www.kff.org/medicaid/upload/7334-04.pdf. Accessed July 8, 2011.

30. Kaiser Family Foundation. *Total Medicaid spending, FY 2009.* Available at http://www.statehealthfacts.org/:comparemaptable.jsp?typ=7&ind=177&cat=4&sub=47. Accessed July 8, 2011.

31. 42 C.F.R. 447.50-.59.

32. 42 U.S.C. § 1916A.

33. Kaiser Family Foundation. *Medicaid and Children's Health Insurance Program provisions in the new health reform law.* April, 2010. Available at http://www.kff.org/healthreform/upload/7952-03.pdf. Accessed June 30, 2011.

34. 42 U.S.C. 1396a(a)(30)(A).

35. Boukus ER, Cassil A, O'Malley AS. *A snapshot of U.S. physicians: Key findings from the 2008 Health Tracking Study Physician Survey.* 2009. Center for Studying Health System Change. Available at http://www.hschange.com/CONTENT/1078/. Accessed July 8, 2011.

36. 42 U.S.C. § 1916A.

37. Centers for Medicare and Medicaid Services. *Medicaid Managed Care Enrollment as of June 30, 2009.* Available at https://www.cms.gov/MedicaidDataSourcesGenInfo/downloads/09June30f.pdf. Accessed July 8, 2011.

38. 42 U.S.C. § 1936u-2.

39. 42 U.S.C. § 1396b(m)(2)(iii); 42 C.F.R. 438.

40. Kaiser Family Foundation. *Five key questions and answers about Section 1115 waivers.* June 2011. Available at http://www.kff.org/medicaid/upload/8196.pdf. Accessed July 8, 2011.

41. 42 U.S.C. §§ 1397aa-1397jj.

42. Kaiser Family Foundation. *Children's health insurance program reauthorization act of 2009.* 2009. Available at http://www.kff.org/medicaid/upload/7863.pdf. Accessed July 6, 2011.

43. Centers for Medicare and Medicaid Services. *CHIP ever enrolled year graph.* 2011. Available at http://www.cms.gov/NationalCHIPPolicy/downloads/CHIPEverEnrolledYearGraph.pdf. Accessed July 8, 2011.

44. Kaiser Commission on Medicaid and the Uninsured. *Health coverage of children: The role of Medicaid and CHIP.* 2010. Available at http://www.kff.org/uninsured/upload/7698-04.pdf. Accessed July 8, 2011.

45. Kaiser Family Foundation. *CHIP Program Name and Type, 2010.* Available at http://www.statehealthfacts.org/comparetable.jsp?cat=4&ind=238. Accessed July 8, 2011.

46. Kaiser Family Foundation. *Enhanced Federal Medical Assistance Percentage (FMAP) for the Children's Health Insurance Program (CHIP).* Health Facts. Available at http://www.statehealthfacts.org/comparetable.jsp?ind=239&cat=4. Accessed July 8, 2011.

47. Ryan K. *The Children's Health Insurance Program: The fundamentals.* National Health Policy Forum. 2009. Available at http://www.nhpf.org/library/details.cfm/2735. Accessed July 6, 2011.

48. Kaiser Family Foundation. *State adoption of coverage and enrollment options in the Children's Health Insurance Reauthorization Act of 2009.* 2011. Available at http://www.kff.org/medicaid/upload/8146.pdf. Accessed July 6, 2011.

49. 42 U.S.C. § 1397cc.

50. Title XXI, § 2102(a); 42 U.S.C. § 1397bb(a).

51. Alliance for Health Reform. *The future of children's health insurance coverage.* Available at http://www.allhealth.org/publications/Child_health_insurance/The_Future_of_Childrens_Health_Coverage_98.pdf. Accessed July 6, 2011.

52. Kaiser Family Foundation. *Summary of key changes to Medicare in the 2010 health reform law.* 2010. Available at http://www.kff.org/healthreform/upload/7948-02.pdf. Accessed July 8, 2011.

53. Kaiser Family Foundation, "Medicare Enrollment 1966–2010," *Medicare Chartbook, Fourth Edition 2010.* Available at http://facts.kff.org/chart.aspx?cb=58&sctn=162&ch=1714. Accessed July 8, 2011.

54. Pub L No. 108-173.

55. Centers for Medicare and Medicaid Services. *National health expenditure projections 2009–2019.* Available at https://www.cms.gov/NationalHealthExpendData/downloads/NHEProjections2009to2019.pdf. Accessed January 25, 2011.

56. Kaiser Family Foundation. *Medicare Fact Sheet: Medicare Spending and Financing.* 2008. Available at http://www.kff.org/medicare/upload/7305_03.pdf. Accessed July 9, 2011.

57. MedPAC. *Report to the Congress: Medicare payment policy.* 2008. Available at http://www.medpac.gov/documents/Mar08_EntireReport.pdf. Accessed July 9, 2011.

58. Zuckerman S, Williams AF, Stockley KE. Trends in Medicaid physician fees, 2003–2008. *Health Aff.* 2009;28(3/4):W511.

59. Congressional Budget Office. *Budget Options: Volume 1—Health Care.* Washington, DC: Congressional Budget Office. 2008. Publication 3185. Available at http://www.cbo.gov/ftpdocs/99xx/doc9925/12-18-HealthOptions.pdf. Accessed July 7, 2011.

60. Medicare Payment Advisory Committee. *Report to Congress: Medicare Payment Policy.* Washington, D.C.: Medicare Payment Advisory Committee; 2005.

61. Kaiser Family Foundation. *Explaining health reform: key changes in the Medicare Advantage program.* 2010. Available at http://www.kff.org/healthreform/upload/8071.pdf. Accessed July 7, 2011.

ENDNOTES

a. Puerto Rico, the U.S. Virgin Islands, Guam, Northern Mariana Islands, and American Samoa participate in Medicaid. However, financing rules are different in these territories than in the 50 states. Federal spending is capped and appropriated by Congress annually.

b. A special 5% adjustment allowed by law effectively brings the eligibility rate to 138% FPL.

c. Community health centers have their own per-visit prospective payment system for reimbursement under Medicaid.

d. Although federal law does not elaborate on the specifics of section 1115 waivers, other federal guidance does. In 1994, HHS prepared a nonbinding notice, "Demonstration Proposal Pursuant to Section 1115(a) of the Social Security Act," 59 Fed. Reg. 49249 (1994), and then the Health Care Financing Administration (now CMS) published a "Review Guide for Section 1115 Research and Demonstration Waiver Proposals for State Health Care Reform." The *State Medicaid Manual* also contains information relating to Section 1115 waivers.

e. Since New Jersey and New York had already expanded coverage to children beyond 300% FPL prior to CHIPRA, those states are allowed to use their enhanced CHIP match up to their capped allotment.

f. Private fee-for-service plans, usually offered at the county level, provide the standard Medicare coverage, but beneficiaries may see only physicians who participate in the plan and must pay premiums and co-payments or co-insurance to the private plan instead of to individual providers. In return, the private plan may offer additional services not covered by Medicare.

GLOSSARY

Abandonment: Unilateral severance by the physician of the professional relationship between himself or herself and the patient without reasonable notice at a time when the patient still needs continuing care.

Abortion: Premature termination of pregnancy at a time when the fetus is incapable of sustaining life independent of the mother.

Ad litem: A Latin term meaning "for the suit." A *guardian ad litem* is a person appointed by a court to defend a legal action on the part of a child or incapacitated person. A *guardian ad litem* is specifically appointed for the purposes of a suit.

Admissibility (of evidence): Refers to the issue of whether a court, applying the rules of evidence, is bound to receive or permit introduction of a particular piece of evidence.

Advance directives: Written instructions expressing one's health care wishes in the event that he or she becomes incapacitated and is unable to make such decisions.

Adverse drug reaction: An unusual or unexpected response to a normal dose of a medication; an injury caused by the use of a drug in the usual, acceptable fashion.

Affidavit: A voluntary statement of facts, or a voluntary declaration in writing of facts, that a person swears to be true before an official authorized to administer an oath.

Agent: An individual who has been designated by a legal document to make decisions on behalf of another individual; a substitute decision maker.

Americans with Disabilities Act (ADA): Federal act that bars employers from discriminating against disabled persons in hiring, promotion, or other provisions of employment.

Appellant: Party who appeals the decision of a lower court to a court of higher jurisdiction.

Appellee: Party against whom an appeal to a higher court is taken.

Artificial nutrition and hydration: Providing food and liquids, such as intravenous feedings, when a patient is unable to eat or drink.

Assault: Intentional act that is designed to make the victim fearful and produces reasonable apprehension of harm.

Attestation: Act of witnessing a document in writing.

Autonomy: Right of an individual to make his or her own independent decisions.

Battery: Intentional touching of one person by another without the consent of the person being touched.

Beneficence: Describes the principle of doing good, demonstrating kindness, and helping others.

Best evidence rule: Legal doctrine requiring that primary evidence of a fact (such as an original document) be introduced or that an acceptable explanation be given before a copy can be introduced or testimony given concerning the fact.

Borrowed servant doctrine: Refers to a situation in which an employee is temporarily placed under the control of someone other than his or her primary employer. It may involve a situation in which an employee is carrying out the specific instructions of a physician. The traditional example is that of a nurse employed by a hospital who is "borrowed" and under the control of the attending surgeon during a procedure in the operating room. The temporary employer of the borrowed servant can be held responsible for the negligent acts of the borrowed servant under the doctrine of *respondeat superior*. This rule is not easily applied, especially if the acts of the employee are for the furtherance of the objectives of the employer. The courts apply a narrow application if the employee is fulfilling the requirement of his or her position.

Captain-of-the-ship doctrine: A doctrine making the physician responsible for the negligent acts of other professionals because he or she had the right to control and oversee the totality of care provided to the patient.

Cardiopulmonary resuscitation: A lifesaving method used by caregivers to restore heartbeat and breathing.

Case citation: Describes where a court's opinion in a particular case can be located. It identifies the parties in the case, the text in which the case can be found, the court writing the opinion, and the year in which the case was decided. For example, the citation *Bouvia v. Superior Court (Glenchur)*, 225 Cal. Rptr. 297 (Ct. App. 1986), is described as follows:

- *Bouvia v. Superior Court (Glenchur)* identifies the basic parties involved in the lawsuit.
- 225 Cal. Rptr. 297 identifies the case as being reported in volume 225 of the California Reporter at page 297.
- Ct. App. 1986 identifies the case as being in the California Court of Appeals in 1986.

Case law: Aggregate of reported cases on a particular legal subject as formed by the decisions of those cases.

Certiorari: Writ that commands a lower court to certify proceedings for review by a higher court. This is the common method of obtaining review by the U.S. Supreme Court.

Charitable immunity: Legal doctrine that developed out of the English court system that held charitable institutions blameless for their negligent acts.

Civil law: Body of law that describes the private rights and responsibilities of individuals. The part of law that does not deal with crimes, it involves actions filed by one individual against another (e.g., actions in tort and contract).

Clinical privileges: On qualification, the diagnostic and therapeutic procedures that an institution allows a physician to perform on a specified patient population. Qualification includes a review of a physician's credentials, such as medical school diploma, state licensure, and residency training.

Closed-shop contract: Labor–management agreement that provides that only members of a particular union may be hired.

Common law: Body of principles that has evolved and continues to evolve and expand from court decisions. Many of the legal principles and rules applied by courts in the United States had their origins in English common law.

Comorbidities: Two or more coexisting medical conditions or disease processes that are additional to an initial diagnosis. [http://medical-dictionary.thefreedictionary.com/Comorbidities].

Complaint: The first pleading, in an alleged negligence action, filed in a court by the plaintiff's attorney. It is the first statement of a case by the plaintiff against the defendant and states a cause of action, notifying the defendant as to the basis for the suit.

Congressional Record: Document in which the proceedings of Congress are published. It is the first record of debate officially reported, printed, and published directly by the federal government. Publication of the *Congressional Record* began March 4, 1873.

Consent: *See Informed consent.*

Consequentialism: A moral theory that determines good or bad, right or wrong, based on good outcomes or consequences.

Contextualism: An ethical doctrine that considers the rightness or wrongness of an action, such as lying, to be based on the particular circumstances of a given situation. The implication is that lying is acceptable in one situation but not in another, even though the situation may be similar. In other words, it depends on the context within which something occurs.

Criminal negligence: Reckless disregard for the safety of others. It is the willful indifference to an injury that could follow an act.

Decision capacity: Having the mental capacity to make one's own decisions. Mental capacity refers to the ability to understand the risks, benefits, alternatives, and consequences of one's actions. Inferred in this interpretation is knowing the decision maker can reasonably distinguish right from wrong and good from bad.

Defamation: Injury of a person's reputation or character caused by the false statements of another made to a third person. Defamation includes both libel and slander.

Defendant: In a criminal case, the person accused of committing a crime. In a civil suit, the party against whom the suit is brought, demanding that he or she pay the other party legal relief.

Demurrer: Formal objection by one of the parties to a lawsuit that the evidence presented by the other party is insufficient to sustain an issue or case.

Deontological ethics: An ethical approach that focuses on duty rather than on the consequences, when determining the right conduct to be followed.

Deposition: A method of pretrial discovery that consists of statements of fact taken by a witness under oath in a question-and-answer format as it would be in a court of law with opportunity given to the adversary to be present for cross-examination. Such statements may be admitted into evidence if it is impossible for a witness to attend a trial in person.

Determinism: The view that nothing happens without a cause.

Directed verdict: When a trial judge decides that the evidence and/or law is clearly in favor of one party, the judge may direct the jury to return a verdict for the appropriate party. The conclusion of the judge must be so clear and obvious that reasonable minds could not arrive at a different conclusion.

Discharge summary: That part of a medical record that summarizes a patient's initial complaints, course of treatment, final diagnosis, and instructions for follow-up care.

Discovery: To ascertain that which was previously unknown through a pretrial investigation; it includes testimony and documents that may be under the exclusive control of the other party.

Dogmatic: The stubborn refusal to consider challenges to your own ethical point of view.

Do not resuscitate (DNR): Directive of a physician to withhold cardiopulmonary resuscitation in the event that a patient experiences cardiac arrest.

Durable power of attorney: Legal instrument enabling an individual to act on another's behalf. In the health care setting, a *durable power of attorney for health care* is the authority to make medical decisions for another.

Ethical conduct: Conducting oneself in a manner consistent with acceptable principles of right and wrong. Such conduct may relate to one's community, country, profession, and so on.

Ethical dilemma: A situation that forces a person to make a decision that involves breaking some ethical norm or contradicting some ethical value. It involves making a decision between two or more possible actions where any one of the actions can be justified as being the right decision, but, whatever action is taken, there always remains some doubt as to whether the correct course of action was chosen. The effect of an action may put others at risk, harm others, or violate the rights of others.

Ethicist: One who specializes in ethics.

Ethics: A set of principles of right and wrong conduct; a theory or system of moral values, of what is right and what is wrong. Ethics is a system of values that guides behavior in relationships among people in accordance with certain social roles.

Ethics committee: A committee created to deal with ethical problems and dilemmas in the delivery of patient care.

Euthanasia: A Greek word meaning "the good death." It is an act conducted for the purpose of causing the merciful death of a person who is suffering from an incurable condition, such as providing a patient with medications to hasten his or her death.

Evidence: Proof of a fact, which is legally presented in a manner prescribed by law, at trial.

Expert witness: Person who has special training, experience, skill, and knowledge in a relevant area and who is allowed to offer an opinion as testimony in court.

Futility: Having no useful result. Futility of treatment, as it relates to medical care, occurs when the physician recognizes that the effect of treatment will be of no benefit to the patient. Morally, the physician has a duty to inform the patient when there is little likelihood of success.

Good Samaritan laws: Laws designed to protect those who stop to render aid in an emergency. These laws generally provide immunity for specified persons from a civil suit arising out of care rendered at the scene of an emergency, provided that the one rendering assistance has not done so in a grossly negligent manner.

Grand jury: Jury called to determine whether there is sufficient evidence that a crime has been committed to justify bringing a case to trial.

Grievance: The process undertaken to resolve a labor–management dispute when there is an allegation by a union member that management has failed in some way to meet the terms of a labor agreement.

Guardian: Person appointed by a court to protect the interests of and make decisions for a person who is incapable of making his or her own decisions.

Health: According to the World Health Organization, "[a] state of complete physical, mental, and social well-being and not merely the absence of disease or infirmity."

Health Care Financing Administration (HCFA): Federal agency that coordinates the federal government's participation in the Medicare and Medicaid programs.

Health care proxy: Document that delegates the authority to make one's own health care decisions to another, known as the health care agent, when one has become incapacitated or is unable to make his or her own decisions.

Hearsay rule: Rule of evidence restricting the admissibility of evidence that is not the personal knowledge of the witness.

Holographic will: A will handwritten by the testator.

Home health agency: An agency that provides home health services. Home health care involves an array of services provided to patients in their homes or foster homes because of acute illness, exacerbation of chronic illness, and disability. Such services are therapeutic and/or preventative.

Home health care: Home health care is an alternative for those who fear leaving the secure environment of their home. Such care is available through home health agencies. These agencies provide a variety of services for the elderly living at home. Such services include part-time or intermittent nursing care; physical, occupational, and speech therapy; medical social services, home health aide services, and nutritional guidance; medical supplies other than drugs and biologicals prescribed by a physician; and the use of medical appliances.

Hospice care: Care provided for terminally ill persons, provided in a setting more economical than that of a hospital or nursing facility. Hospice care is often sought after a decision has been made to discontinue aggressive efforts to prolong life. A hospice program includes such characteristics as support services by training individuals, family involvement, and control of pain and discomfort.

Hydration: Intravenous addition of fluids to the circulatory system.

Immoral: Behavior that is in opposition to accepted societal, religious, cultural, and/or professional standards.

Incapacity: An individual's lack of ability to make decisions for himself or herself.

Incompetent: Individual determined by a court to be incapable of making rational decisions on his or her own behalf.

Independent contractor: One who agrees to undertake work without being under the direct control or direction of an employer.

Indictment: Formal written accusation presented by a grand jury charging a person therein named with criminal conduct.

Informed consent: Legal concept that provides that a patient has the right to know the potential risks, benefits, and alternatives of a proposed procedure prior to undergoing a particular course of treatment. Informed consent implies that a patient understands a particular procedure or treatment, including the risks, benefits, and alternatives; is capable of making a decision; and gives consent voluntarily.

Injunction: Court order either requiring a person to perform a certain act or prohibiting the person from performing a particular act.

In loco parentis: Legal doctrine that permits the courts to assign a person to stand in the place of parents and possess their legal rights, duties, and responsibilities toward a child.

Interrogatories: List of questions sent from one party in a lawsuit to the other party to be answered under oath.

Joint Commission: See *The Joint Commission.*

Judicial notice: An act by which a court, in conducting a trial or forming a decision, will, of its own motion and without evidence, recognize the existence and truth of certain facts bearing on the controversy at bar (e.g., serious falls require X-rays).

Jurisdiction: Right of a court to administer justice by hearing and deciding controversies.

Jurisprudence: Philosophy or science of law on which a particular legal system is built.

Justice: The obligation to be fair in the distribution of benefits and risks.

Kennedy Institute of Ethics: The world's oldest and most comprehensive bioethics center. The institute was established at Georgetown University in 1971 by a grant from the Joseph P. Kennedy, Jr. Foundation.

Larceny: Taking another person's property without consent with the intent to permanently deprive the owner of its use and ownership.

Legal wrong: Invasion of a protected right.

Liability: As it relates to damages, an obligation one has incurred or might incur through a negligent act.

Libel: False or malicious writing that is intended to defame or dishonor another person and is published so that someone other than the one defamed will observe it.

Life support: Medical intervention(s) designed to prolong life (e.g., respirator, kidney dialysis machine, tube feedings).

Living will: A document in which an individual expresses in advance his or her wishes regarding the application of life-sustaining treatment in the event that he or she is incapable of doing so at some future time. A living will describes in advance the kind of care one wants to receive or does not wish to receive in the event that he or she is unable to make decisions for himself or herself. A living will takes effect when a person is in a terminal condition or permanent state of unconsciousness.

Malfeasance: Execution of an unlawful or improper act.

Malpractice: Professional misconduct, improper discharge of professional duties, or failure to meet the standard of care of a professional that results in harm to another; the negligence or carelessness of a professional person such as a nurse, pharmacist, physician, or accountant.

Mandamus: Action brought in a court of competent jurisdiction to compel a lower court or administrative agency to perform—or not to perform—a specific act.

Medicaid: Medical assistance provided in Title XIX of the Social Security Act. Medicaid is a state-administered program for the medically indigent.

Medicare: Medical assistance provided in Title XVIII of the Social Security Act. Medicare is a health insurance program administered by the Social Security Administration for persons aged 65 years and older and for disabled persons who are eligible for benefits. Medicare Part A benefits provide coverage for inpatient hospital care, skilled nursing facility care, home health care, and hospice care. Medicare Part B benefits provide coverage for physician services, outpatient hospital services, diagnostic tests, various therapies, durable medical equipment, medical supplies, and prosthetic devices.

Metaethics: The study of ethical concepts.

Misdemeanor: Unlawful act of a less serious nature than a felony, usually punishable by a jail sentence for a term of less than 1 year and/or a fine.

Misfeasance: Improper performance of an act.

Monotheism: The worship of one God, who is immortal, omniscient, omnipotent, and omnipresent.

Nasogastric tube, insertion of: Involves placing a tube through the patient's nose, down the back of the throat into the esophagus, and then into the stomach. Its purpose is to suction out the contents of the stomach.

Negligence: Omission or commission of an act that a reasonably prudent person would or would not do under given circumstances. It is a form of heedlessness or carelessness that constitutes a departure from the standard of care generally imposed on members of society.

Neiswanger Institute for Bioethics and Health Policy: Dedicated to the threefold mission of research, education, and service, the institute serves the students and faculty of the Stritch School of Medicine, health care professionals and patients of Loyola University Health System, and professionals from the regional community and across the nation.

Non compos mentis: "Not of sound mind"; suffering from some form of mental defect.

Nonfeasance: Failure to act, when there is a duty to act, as a reasonably prudent person would in similar circumstances.

Normative ethics: The study of what is right and wrong.

Norms: Accepted rules and ways of doing things. Without norms, society would be chaotic and unpredictable.

Nuncupative will: An oral statement intended as a last will made in anticipation of death.

Obamacare: An appellation ascribed to the Patient Protection and Affordable Care Act (ACA).

Objectivism: The belief that morality is based on some universal, external, and unchangeable fact. For example, murder is always wrong.

Ombudsman: Person who is designated to speak and act on behalf of a patient/resident, especially in regard to his or her daily needs.

Opined: To give or express as an opinion.

Paternalism: A doctrine that literally means "rule by the father." In health care, it is the concept of physicians making decisions for their patients, whereas the more acceptable approach is autonomy, whereby the physician informs the patient as to the risks, benefits, and alternatives to care and treatment, and then the patient makes the final choice as to what is best.

Patient Protection Affordable Care Act: A federal act passed by Congress, signed into law by President Obama in March 2010, upheld as constitutional by the Supreme Court in 2012, designed to provide better health security by enacting comprehensive health insurance reforms that hold insurance companies accountable, lower health care costs, guarantee more choice, and enhance the quality of care for all Americans.

Perjury: Willful act of giving false testimony under oath.

Plaintiff: Party who brings a civil suit seeking damages or other legal relief.

Polytheism: Belief and worship in many gods.

Privileged communication: Statement made to an attorney, physician, spouse, or anyone else in a position of trust. Because of the confidential nature of such information, the law protects it from being revealed even in court. The term is applied in two distinct situations. First, the communications between certain persons, such as physician and patient, cannot be divulged without the consent of the patient. Second, in some situations, the law provides an exemption from liability for disclosing information for which there is a higher duty to speak, such as statutory reporting requirements.

Probate: A judicial proceeding that determines the existence and validity of a will.

Probate court: A court with jurisdiction over wills. Its powers range from deciding the validity of a will to distributing property.

Process: A series of related actions to achieve a defined outcome.

Prognosis: Informed judgment regarding the likely course and probable outcome of a disease.

Proximate cause: In immediate relation with something else. In negligence cases, the careless act must be the proximate cause of injury.

Rational: Having the capacity to think logically.

Real evidence: Evidence furnished by tangible things (e.g., medical records and equipment).

Rebuttal: Giving of evidence to contradict the effect of evidence introduced by the opposing party.

Relativism: The belief that morality is relative to each individual culture. What is right in one culture may be wrong in another culture. In ethics, it is a theory that conceptions of truth and moral values are not absolute but are relative to the persons or groups holding them.

Relativist: A person who is a proponent of relativism.

Release: Statement signed by one person relinquishing a right or claim against another.

Remand: Referral of a case by an appeals court back to the original court, out of which it came for the purpose of having some action taken there.

Res gestae: "The thing done"; all the surrounding events that become part of an incident. If statements are made as part of the incident, they are admissible in court as res gestae despite the hearsay rule.

Respirator: A machine used to assist in keeping a patient breathing.

Res ipsa loquitur: "The thing speaks for itself"; a doctrine of law applicable to cases in which the defendant had exclusive control over the thing that caused the harm and where the harm ordinarily could not have occurred without negligent conduct.

Res judicata: "The thing is decided"; that which has been acted on or decided by the courts.

Respondeat superior: "Let the master answer"; an aphorism meaning that the employer is responsible for the legal consequences of the acts of the servant or employee who is acting within the scope of his or her employment.

Restraint: Can be either "physical" or "chemical" (medication). Physical restraint involves a device (e.g., safety belts, safety bars, geriatric chairs, bed rails) restricts or limits voluntary movement and which cannot be removed by the patient.

Slander: False oral statement, made in the presence of a third person, that injures the character or reputation of another.

Standard of care: Description of the conduct that is expected of an individual in a given situation. It is a measure against which a defendant's conduct is compared.

Stare decisis: "Let the decision stand"; the legal doctrine that prescribes adherence to those precedents set forth in cases that have been decided.

Statute of limitations: Legal limit on the time allowed for filing suit in civil matters, usually measured from the time of the wrong or from the time when a reasonable person would have discovered the wrong.

Statutory law: Law that is prescribed by legislative enactments.

Stipulation: Agreement, usually in writing, by attorneys on opposite sides of an issue as to any matter pertaining to the proceedings. A stipulation is not binding unless agreed on by the parties involved in the issue.

Subjectivism: A doctrine that says moral judgments are based on personal preferences.

Subpoena ad testificandum: Court order requiring one to appear in court to give testimony.

Subpoena duces tecum: Court order that commands a person to come to court and to produce whatever documents are named in the order.

Subrogation: Substitution of one person for another in reference to a lawful claim or right.

Substituted judgment: In the health care setting, a surrogate decision maker's decisions are accepted as a substitute for the patient in the event the patient becomes incapacitated and unable to make decisions. Decisions are made on the basis of the patient's known health care preferences. Such preferences are generally described in the document appointing the surrogate and/or other documents such as a "living will" or "durable power of attorney for health care."

Summary judgment: Generally, an immediate decision by a judge, without jury deliberation.

Summons: Court order directed to the sheriff or other appropriate official to notify the defendant in a civil suit that a suit has been filed and when and where to appear.

Surrogate decision maker: Individual who has been designated to make decisions on behalf of an individual determined incapable of making his or her own decisions.

Teleological ethics: A theory of morality that derives duty or obligation from what is good or desirable as an end to be achieved.

Terminal condition: A medical condition that is incurable and because of which death will occur.

Testimony: Oral statement of a witness given under oath at trial.

The Joint Commission: A not-for-profit independent organization dedicated to improving the quality of health care in organized health care settings. The major functions of The Joint Commission include developing organizational standards, awarding accreditation decisions, and providing education and consultation to health care organizations.

Theodicy: A vindication of God's goodness and justice in the face of the existence of evil. We often wonder why God allows bad things to happen to good people. The answer often given is that what God allows to happen in the lives of good people is often mysterious to us. We often have difficulty understanding this, and it often provokes anger in us.

Tort: A civil wrong committed by one individual against another. Torts may be classified as either intentional or unintentional. When a tort is classified as a criminal wrong (e.g., assault, battery, false imprisonment), the wrongdoer can be held liable in a criminal and/or civil action.

Tort-feasor: Person who commits a tort.

Trial court: Court where evidence is presented to a judge or jury for decision.

Unethical behavior: Character that describes behavior contrary to admirable traits or a code of conduct that has been endorsed by one's society, community, or profession.

Union-shop contract: Labor–management agreement making continued employment contingent on joining the union.

Utilitarianism: A moral theory that treats pleasure and happiness as the only absolute moral good. Acts that bring about happiness and pleasure are good, and acts that bring about pain and suffering are morally bad.

Value: Worth or usefulness. "Intrinsic values" are those goods that are valuable in their own right. "Instrumental values" are those goods that help us achieve another good.

Value judgment: A judgment that assigns a value to an action.

Venue: Geographic district in which an action is or may be brought.

Verdict: Formal declaration of a jury's findings of fact, signed by the jury foreperson and presented to the court.

Virtue: A moral trade that refers to excellence and righteousness.

Waiver: Intentional giving up of a right, such as allowing another person to testify to information that ordinarily would be protected as a privileged communication.

Will: Legal declaration of the intentions that a person wishes to have carried out after death concerning property, children, or estate. A will designates a person or persons to serve as the executor(s) responsible for carrying out the instructions of the will.

Witness: Person who is called to give testimony in a court of law.

Writ: Written order that is issued to a person or persons requiring the performance of some specified act or giving authority to have it done.

Wrongful birth: Applies to the cause of action of the parents who claim that the negligent advice or treatment deprived them of the choice of aborting conception or of terminating the pregnancy.

Wrongful life: Refers to a cause of action brought by or on behalf of a defective child who claims that but for the defendant (e.g., a laboratory's negligent testing procedures or a physician's negligent advice or treatment of the child's parents), the child would not have been born.

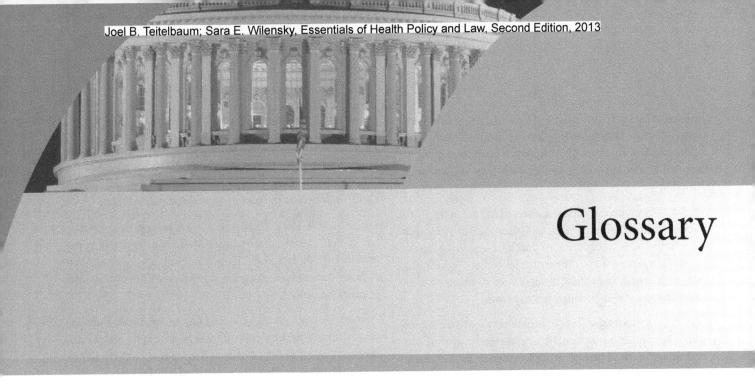

Glossary

Accountable Care Organization (ACO): A group of healthcare providers that is collectively reimbursed for a single patient's care. This arrangement is meant to give providers an incentive to deliver high quality, cost-effective care.

Accreditation: A process applied to healthcare institutions to ensure that all necessary and required processes, standards, competencies, ethics, etc. are up to par.

Administrative Law: The body of law produced by executive (i.e., administrative) agencies of federal, state, and local governments.

Administrative Procedures Act: A federal law that governs the way in which administrative agencies of the federal government may propose and establish regulations.

Adverse Selection: Refers to the idea that individuals with a higher-than-average risk of needing health care are more likely to seek health insurance coverage.

Annual Aggregate Limit: A cap imposed by health insurance companies on the amount a policy will pay during a single year.

Bioterrorism: The threat or use of a biological agent, typically by a non-state actor, to cause death or harm to humans, animals, or plants and specifically targeting civilian populations or resources.

Block Grant: A large sum of money granted by the national government to a regional government with only general provisions as to the way the money is to be spent.

Bundling: Instead of compensating healthcare providers separately for every service performed, "bundling" is an arrangement by which providers are paid a predetermined amount for all services related to treating a specific condition. This arrangement is meant to give providers an incentive to deliver cost-effective care.

"Cadillac" Healthcare Plans: Refers to health insurance plans and other products whose value exceeds a stated annual dollar threshold.

Cafeteria Plans: Employer-sponsored health benefit plans under which employees may set aside wages to be used for medical expenses not otherwise covered by their basic health insurance. Also called Flexible Spending Accounts (FSAs).

Capitation: A method of payment for health services in which a fixed amount is paid for each person served without regard to the actual number or nature of services provided.

Catastrophic Coverage: A health insurance coverage option with limited benefits and a high deductible, intended to protect against medical bankruptcy due to an unforeseen illness or injury.

Centers for Disease Control and Prevention (CDC): The federal agency within the Department of Health and Human Services charged with disease prevention, education, and public health activities.

Centers for Medicare and Medicaid Services (CMS): The federal agency within the Department of Health and Human Services that administers the Medicare and Medicaid programs.

Children's Health Insurance Program (CHIP): A health insurance program targeted to low-income children, established in 1997 and reauthorized in 2009, which is administered by states and funded through a combination of federal and state payments.

COBRA: The nickname for a law, enacted as part of the Consolidated Omnibus Budget Reconciliation Act of 1985, that allows individuals to continue to purchase employee health benefits for a period of 18 to 36 months following a "qualifying event" such as unemployment, death of a wage earner, divorce, or termination of minor dependent coverage.

Coinsurance: Refers to a form of beneficiary cost-sharing for covered health insurance benefits and services, expressed as a percentage of the approved payment amount for the benefit or service (e.g., 20% of the payable amount).

Community Health Centers: A type of community clinic that provides a broad range of healthcare services and that charges on a sliding-scale fee basis. See also *Federally Qualified Health Center.*

Community Rating: Requires health insurance providers to offer health insurance policies within a given territory at the same price to all persons without medical underwriting, regardless of individual health status.

Comparative Effectiveness Research (CER): A type of health services research that compares different approaches to treating medical conditions in order to determine which methods are most likely to produce the best outcomes.

Coordination of Benefits: A process by which health services are paid for by more than one health insurance plan. For example, if a child is insured through both parents, one insurer is generally considered the primary policy, and the secondary policy reimburses for services not covered under the primary policy.

Copayments: Refers to a form of beneficiary cost-sharing for covered health insurance benefits and services, expressed as a flat dollar payment (e.g., $5.00 for a prescription drug).

Cost-sharing: A requirement that insured patients pay a portion of their medical costs, either as coinsurance or as a fixed copayment.

Culturally and Linguistically Appropriate Care: Refers to a federal standard designed to eliminate ethnic and racial disparities in health care.

Deductible: The amount patients must pay out of their own pocket before their health insurance policy begins contributing to the cost of their care.

Department of Health and Human Services: A federal agency that administers federal health and welfare programs and activities.

Dependent Coverage: Health insurance coverage of a spouse, child, or domestic partner of an insured individual.

Diagnostic Related Group (DRG): A system used to classify patients (particularly under Medicare) for the purpose of reimbursing hospitals. Hospitals are paid a fixed fee for each case in a given category, regardless of the actual costs of providing care.

Department of Defense (DoD): A federal agency that, among other things, administers healthcare programs for active military and their dependents through a publicly funded and privately administered health program called TriCare.

Department of Labor (DoL): A federal agency responsible for administration and enforcement of ERISA, a federal law that sets requirements for employer-provided health benefits that are not offered through state-licensed health insurance plans.

Discrimination in Health Care: Failure by providers to treat patients equitably for any of a number of reasons including race, gender, age, ability to pay for care, or severity of illness. Can also be used to describe the insurance company practice of medical underwriting and rating.

Doughnut Hole: A gap in prescription drug coverage under Medicare Part D, for which beneficiaries pay 100% of their prescription drug costs after their total drug spending exceeds an initial coverage limit until they qualify for catastrophic coverage. The coverage gap will be gradually phased out under the Affordable Care Act by 2020.

Electronic Medical Record (EMR): An individual medical record that is stored electronically.

Employee Retirement Income Security Act (ERISA): A 1974 federal law that establishes standards governing both pension plans and "welfare benefit plans" (such as health benefits, dependent care benefits, and other types of benefits and services) and applicable to non-federal employers, multi-employer arrangements, and union plans.

Employer Responsibility: Refers to a requirement that employers assist in covering workers and their dependents, either through the provision of a health plan or through a contribution toward coverage which may be expressed as payment of a flat dollar charge (e.g., $500 per worker), a percentage of payroll, a percentage of an annual insurance premium, or some other amount. Also referred to as an "employer mandate."

Employer-Sponsored Insurance (ESI): A health benefit plan offered by an employer to its employees (and often to employee dependents). Some employers purchase plans from a traditional insurance company, while other (primarily large) employers may choose to directly insure its employees through its own plan.

Entitlement Programs: Refers to a guarantee of access to benefits or services based on established rights or by legislation (e.g., the Medicaid program).

Epidemic: Refers to when new cases of a certain disease, in a given human population during a given period, substantially exceed what is expected based on recent experience.

Epidemiology: The study of patterns of health and illness and associated factors at the population level.

Essential Benefits: A list of core benefits established under the Affordable Care Act that must be included under any health insurance plan in order to meet minimum coverage requirements.

Exchange Eligible Employer: An employer that is permitted to enroll in a health insurance exchange in order to offer health benefits to its employees.

Exchange Eligible Individual: An individual who is permitted to obtain coverage through a health insurance exchange.

Exchange-participating Health Benefit Plans: Health insurance plans offered to individuals and small employers through health insurance exchanges. They must meet federal insurance market and benefit requirements.

Excise Tax: A tax on health insurance and health benefit plans whose annual dollar value exceeds a specified limit, as well as on the sale of specified healthcare items and services such as medical devices and equipment.

Exclusion: The practice by which an insurer or health benefit plan classifies certain otherwise-covered items and treatments as ineligible for coverage. Common exclusions include "experimental," "educational," and "cosmetic" treatments and services.

Executive Order: A presidential directive, with the authority of a law, that directs and governs actions by executive officials and agencies.

Fair Marketing: A term used to encompass a range of health insurance market reforms to protect consumers from medical underwriting and other practices designed to limit the amount an insurer pays for medical claims.

Federal Emergency Management Agency (FEMA): A federal agency responsible for responding to national emergencies, including natural disasters.

Federalism: Refers to a system of government in which sovereignty is constitutionally divided between a central governing authority and constituent political units (e.g., states), and in which the power to govern is shared between the national and state governments.

Federally Qualified Health Center (FQHC): A community health center that either receives funding under Section 440 of the Public Health Service Act, or a center that has been certified as meeting the same criteria.

Fee-for-Service: A method of paying for medical services under which doctors are paid for each service provided. Bills are paid by the patient, who then submits them to the insurance company for reimbursement.

Fraud and Abuse: Refers to a range of wasteful healthcare activities, including billing for services not performed, billing for more expensive services than performed ("up-coding"), and performing inappropriate or unnecessary care.

Gainsharing: A system in which the government passes on savings from providing more-efficient care to insurers and providers.

Guaranteed Issue and Renewal: A rule that bars health insurers from denying or dropping an individual's coverage for any reason other than fraud or nonpayment of health insurance premiums. This is especially important to prevent insurance companies from denying coverage based on individuals' health status.

Healthcare/Public Health Workforce: A term used to define a range of health professionals in private and public practice who provide medical care and public health services such as primary care, disease diagnosis, and public education.

Health Information Privacy and Security: Standards or procedures to ensure that personal health information is not compromised or disclosed in processing healthcare transactions.

Health Information Technology (HIT): Technology that allows the comprehensive management of health information and enables its exchange among health professionals, healthcare providers, healthcare payers, and public health agencies.

Health Insurance Exchange Subsidies: Federal subsidies made available on an income-related basis to exchange-eligible individuals for the purchase of health insurance coverage through health insurance exchanges.

Health Insurance Exchanges: Regulated marketplaces for the sale and purchase of health insurance established under federal law and operated in accordance with federal requirements.

Health Insurance Issuers: Entities that sell health insurance in the individual and employer-sponsored group markets.

Health Insurance Portability and Accountability Act (HIPAA): A federal law that regulates health insurers and health benefit plans in the group market, and provides privacy protections for health information.

Health Maintenance Organization (HMO): A type of health insurance plan that provides a coordinated array of preventive and treatment services for a fixed payment per month. Enrollees receive medically necessary services regardless of whether the cost of those services exceeds the premium paid on the enrollees' behalf.

Health Status: All aspects of physical and mental health and their manifestations in daily living, including impairment, disability, and handicap.

Health Threat: In the context of national or global security, an environmental, biological, chemical, radiological, or physical risk to public or community health.

High-risk Insurance Pool: Refers to an insurance option for patients with existing medical conditions that make them expensive to insure.

Homeland Defense: The protection of U.S. territory, populations, and infrastructure against external threats or aggression.

Incidence: The number of new cases of illness or disease during a specific period of time in a specific population.

Indian Health Care Improvement Act: A federal law creating programs to strengthen healthcare options in Native American communities.

Indian Health Service: A federal health program to provide health care to Native Americans and Alaska natives.

Individual Market: The insurance market for individuals who are purchasing insurance for themselves and their families and are not part of a group plan, such as one offered by an employer. Also known as the "non-group market."

Individual Responsibility: The requirement that all individuals must carry health insurance or pay a penalty. Also referred to as an "individual mandate."

Insurance Pool: A group of individuals whose premiums are used to pay all covered medical costs of its members. Insurance companies may charge higher premiums to a pool whose members are older or less-healthy than other pools in order to cover the risk that its members may submit more medical claims.

Interest Group: An organization that uses various forms of advocacy to influence public opinion and/or policy. Groups vary considerably in size, influence, and purpose. Also referred to as special interest groups, advocacy groups, or lobby groups.

International Health Regulations: A 2005 international treaty obligating all Member States of the World Health Organization to detect, report, and respond to potential public health emergencies of international concern. Aimed at improving global health security through international collaboration and communication.

Large Group Market: The market for health insurance or health benefit plans among employers whose employee numbers exceed a specified threshold size (e.g., 100 full-time workers).

Lifetime Aggregate Limits: Provisions included in health insurance contracts designed to limit the total amount the policy will pay out in claims and benefits over the lifetime of the policy.

Long-term Care: A set of healthcare, personal care, and social services provided to persons who have lost, or never acquired, some degree of functional capacity (e.g., the chronically ill, aged, or disabled) in an institution or at home, on a long-term basis.

Managed Care: Health insurance arrangements that integrate the financing and delivery of services to covered individuals.

Market Failure: Refers to a concept within economic theory in which the allocation of goods and services by a free market is not efficient.

Medicaid: A program established in 1965 to provide health insurance to low-income families and individuals with certain disabilities. It is administered by the states, and funded jointly with the federal government.

Medical Home: A clinic focused on primary care and preventative services that offers a range of coordinated treatment services.

Medical Underwriting: The insurance industry practice of assessing the medical condition of individuals at the time that insurance enrollment is sought in order to identify existing physical or mental health conditions that may affect an individual's or group's eligibility for enrollment, the application of pre-existing condition exclusions or waiting periods, or the price to be charged for coverage.

Medicare: A federal program enacted in 1965 that provides government-sponsored health insurance to individuals ages 65 and older and certain individuals under age 65 with disabilities that meet federal requirements.

Medicare Advantage: Optional private insurance plans in which Medicare beneficiaries may enroll to receive their federal benefits.

Medigap Coverage: Supplemental health insurance designed to cover all or most of the charges that are not covered by Medicare, including the 20% co-payment required for many outpatient services.

National Health Service Corps: A commissioned corps of public health professionals employed by the federal Department of Health and Human Services. Members are assigned to settings that include clinics in underserved areas, state and local health departments, and federal agencies such as the Centers for Disease Control and Prevention.

National Institutes of Health: A federal agency within the Department of Health and Human Services that is primarily responsible for conducting and supporting medical research.

Notifiable Disease: A disease that, once diagnosed, must be reported under the law to a public health authority.

Office of the Inspector General (OIG): Located within the federal Department of Health and Human Services, this office is charged with protecting the integrity of programs administered by the Department, protecting the health and welfare of program beneficiaries, and reporting problems to the Department Secretary and to Congress.

Pandemic: An infectious disease that spreads through human populations across a large region, over multiple continents.

Parity: A term generally used to require that large group insurers or plans pay equivalent benefits for different kinds of services. For example, federal law requires "mental health parity," which means that for health plans that include mental health benefits as well as medical ones, the services must be covered with the same financial requirements and treatment limitations.

Patient Protection and Affordable Care Act: Also known as the Affordable Care Act or ACA, a major federal health reform law enacted in March 2010.

Patient Protections: Laws establishing protections for patients, such as the right to health information, to choice of providers, to access to care, to file a grievance, or to appeal a denied health benefit claim.

Pay-for-Performance (P4P): A healthcare payment system in which providers receive incentives for meeting quality and cost benchmarks (or, in some cases, penalties for not meeting established benchmarks).

Performance Measurement: A set of recommendations, requirements, or data used to determine whether plans, providers, or programs meet or exceed a standard of care.

Policy Analysis: An analysis that provides informed advice to a client that relates to a public policy decision, includes a recommended course of action/inaction, and is framed by the client's powers and values.

Population Health: Health outcomes of a group of individuals, including the distribution of such outcomes within the group.

Pre-existing Conditions: Health conditions that exist prior to or at the time of enrollment into a health insurance or health benefit plan.

Preferred Provider Organization (PPO): A health insurance plan in which providers agree to provide care to covered individuals at a negotiated price. Covered individuals receive all medically necessary services regardless of whether the cost of the services exceeds the premium paid, although members do have cost-sharing obligations.

Premium: The amount a business or individual pays regularly to maintain health insurance coverage.

Premium Rating: An insurance industry practice determining health insurance premiums based on factors including age, health status, gender, industry, geography, or other factors.

Prevalence: The total number of cases of a disease or illness in the population at a given time.

Preventive Services: Measures taken to prevent the development of disease or to treat illnesses early so that they do not become more acute and expensive to treat. Examples include vaccination, weight loss programs, and mammograms.

Primary Care Providers (PCPs): Healthcare providers, such as physicians engaged in the practice of internal medicine, pediatric, or geriatric care, or nurse practitioners, who provide general medical care and coordinate treatment.

Public Health Emergency: An acute event capable of causing large-scale morbidity and mortality, either immediately or over time. These events have the ability to overwhelm normal public health and medical care capabilities.

Public Health Insurance: A health insurance plan that is administered by the government either directly or through the use of private contractors. Medicare, Medicaid, and CHIP all are considered forms of public health insurance.

Public Health Preparedness: The actions and policies associated with preventing, protecting against, responding to, and recovering from a major public health event.

Quarantine: The separation and restriction of movement of people or animals that may have been exposed to an infectious agent.

Reinsurance: Refers to the fact that when health insurers predict how much they will pay out each year in medical claims, they may underestimate and choose to protect themselves against losses by purchasing "reinsurance" from a separate company.

Rescission: A process by which an insurance company seeks to recover the amount paid out for covered services after discovering that information on a beneficiary's initial enrollment form was incomplete or incorrect.

Retiree Health Benefits: Health benefits provided by an employer to its retirees.

Risk Adjustment: A tool for evaluating the relative risk of enrollees within insurance plans and providing for a financial transfer from plans with low-risk enrollees to plans with higher risk enrollees.

Safety Net: The collection of healthcare providers who serve patients regardless of patients' ability to pay for care. Providers include community health centers, public hospitals, local health departments, school- and church-based health clinics, and private physicians and non-profit hospitals committed to serving uninsured and low-income, vulnerable patients.

Skimming: The insurance plan practice of enrolling predominantly healthy individuals in order to reduce the costs to the plan.

Small Group Market: The health insurance market for employers whose size is smaller than a specified threshold (e.g., 100 full-time workers).

Stare Decisis: A Latin term that refers to the legal principle that prior case law decisions should be accorded great deference and should not be frequently overturned.

Surge Capacity: The ability of clinical care facilities and laboratories to accommodate a sharp increase in patients and samples during a public health emergency.

Telehealth: Refers to the use of electronic information and telecommunications technologies to support long-distance clinical health care, patient and professional health-related education, public health, and health administration. Technologies may include videoconferencing, the Internet, store-and-forward imaging, streaming media, and terrestrial and wireless communications.

Uncompensated Care: Services provided by physicians and hospitals for which no payment is received from the patient or from third-party payers.

Underinsured: Those with insurance policies that do not cover all necessary healthcare services, resulting in out-of-pocket expenses that exceed the ability to pay.

Uninsured: Refers to individuals who lack public or private health insurance.

Universal Coverage: The provision of at least basic or medically necessary health insurance for an entire population.

Utilization Review: The examination, usually by an insurer or third-party-administrator (TPA), of the necessity and/or appropriateness of healthcare services provided to a patient.

Weapons of Mass Destruction (WMD): Weapons that cause large-scale destruction, generally including nuclear, radiological, chemical, or biological weapons.

Wellness Programs: Special services and benefits offered by employers to employees in addition to health benefit plans, including nutrition classes, smoking-cessation programs, or gym memberships.

World Health Organization (WHO): The directing and coordinating authority for health within the United Nations system.

The following sources were used, in part, in the compilation of this Glossary:

Health Reform GPS, "Health Reform Glossary," at http://www.healthreformgps.org/glossary/ accessed August 16, 2011.

The Health Policy Institute of Ohio, "Glossary of Health Policy Terms," at http://www.hpio.net/resources/other-resources/glossary.php accessed August 16, 2011.

Health insurance exchanges
    defined, 420
Health Insurance Marketplace, 249
Health Maintenance Organization Act, 393
Health maintenance organizations (HMOs)
    Health Maintenance Organization Act, 393
    Medicare and, 393
Health policy and law, 365, 367-370, 399, 406
    conceptualizing, 365
    introduction, 406
    role of, 365, 369-370
health reform, 367, 408-421, 423-424, 426, 429-430,
    432, 458-459, 475-476
Health reform
    employer mandate, 413, 423-424
    financing, 367, 409, 413, 416, 429, 432, 459
    individual mandate, 417, 419-421, 424, 430
    premium and cost-sharing subsidies, 421
    public health programs, 412
    state health insurance exchanges, 421, 424, 430
    states and, 409
Health reimbursement arrangements (HRAs), 396
health savings accounts (HSAs), 396
Health Security Act, 411, 414, 419
Health status
    defined, 396
    uncertainty, 395-396
Health threat, 474
Healthcare/public health workforce, 473
Heritage Foundation, 389-390
Heterologous artificial insemination, 95
High deductible health plan (HDHP), 396
High-risk insurance pool, 396, 474
Hinduism, 54
Hippocratic Oath, 299-303
HIV/AIDS
    autonomy and, 113
    global situation and trends, 108
    right to treatment, 113
    spread of, 109
HIV/AIDS Services, 431
Holocaust, 68
home care fraud, 213
homeland defense, 474
homologous artificial insemination, 116
honesty, 28, 99, 258
hopefulness, 30
hospital-acquired infections (HAIs), 320
House of Representatives Committee on Ethics, 238
human genetics, 66
Hyde Amendment, 82

I
immigrants, 419-420, 435-437, 458
Immigrants
    Medicaid and, 435, 437, 458
    Medicaid eligibility, 436-437
implied corporate authority, 256-257
income, 369, 376, 379, 388-389, 393, 396, 399-400,
    406-407, 408-410, 412-414, 417, 419,
    421-426, 429, 431, 433-437, 443-448, 450,
    453-454, 457-458, 472-474, 476
Income
Incompetent persons
    consent for, 71, 334
independent contractors, 264
Indian Health Care Improvement Act, 474
indictment, 204, 271, 356
Individual mandate
    tax credits and, 421
individual practice associations (IPAs), 403
Individual responsibility, 474
infliction of mental distress, 202
Informed consent
    reasonable man standard, 70
Insurance pool, 396, 419, 474
Insured, 367, 391-392, 394, 400, 403, 411, 414, 416,
    429, 434-435, 437, 444, 449, 472
intentional torts, 191
interest groups, 369, 372, 381, 388-389, 409-411, 416,
    474
Interest groups
    defined, 372
    policymaking and, 369, 372
Internal Revenue Service, 392
International Health Regulations, 474
Intolerance, 47

intrinsic value, 29
invasion of privacy, 201
involuntary euthanasia, 126
involuntary manslaughter, 214
Islam, 56

J
job lock, 399
Joint Commission (JC)
    compliance with, 125, 278-279
    hospital accreditation, 261
Judaism, 54
judicial branch of government, 181
Justice
    age and, 26
justice
    distributive, 23
Justice
    economic, 27, 179
    physicians and, 23, 77, 210, 290

K
Kennedy Institute of Ethics, 70
Kidney donation, 78
kindness, 1, 106

L
Law
    administrative law, 175
    common law, 14, 66, 126, 175, 325
    contracts, 96, 217, 244, 292
    criminal law, 174, 191
law
    sources of, 95, 173
Law
    statutory law, 126, 175, 200
law
    tort law, 93, 190-191
Leadership
    in Congress, 375, 380, 382, 415-416
legal rights, 369-370
libel, 201
licenses, 368
Lifetime aggregate limits, 474
local government, 388, 404
Local public health agencies (LPHA), 388

M
macroethics, 3
malfeasance, 192
Managed care
    defined, 394, 400, 414, 444-445
    future of, 452, 458
    HMOs, 393-394, 401, 403, 406, 452
    structures, 400, 403
    utilization control tools, 401
Managed care organizations (MCOs)
    defined, 400, 444
Mandatory spending, 379
manslaughter, 213-214
market failure, 474
markets, 368, 403, 424, 474
Markets
    market failure, 474
Massachusetts
    assisted suicide in, 133
Media and confidentiality, 113
Medicaid
    administering, 433
    agency powers, 384
    authorizing legislation, 379
    benefits, 369, 371, 379, 384, 407, 411, 413, 422,
        424, 430, 432-433, 435, 437-440, 442,
        445, 447-450, 452-454, 457, 471,
        473-474, 476
    costs of, 435, 438, 474
    creating, 368, 376, 417, 449, 474
    defined, 384, 432-433, 444-445, 447
    eligibility for, 435-436, 444, 448-449
    financing, 368-369, 388, 409, 413, 416, 425, 429,
        431-433, 438, 443, 445, 447, 449,
        453-455, 457, 459, 474
    future of, 449, 452, 458
    historical perspectives, 369
    oversight of, 184
    provider reimbursement, 425, 444, 447
    rights under, 369
    waivers, 445, 449, 458-459

medical home, 474
Medical integrity, 45
Medical malpractice, 20, 148, 194, 246, 259, 301-302,
    330
medical paternalism, 17
medical records
    falsification of, 60, 308, 358
Medical records
    maintenance of, 27, 262
    nurses and, 212, 280
medical underwriting, 399, 472-474
Medical underwriting
    health insurance, 399, 472-474
Medically necessary, 394, 400-401, 403, 432, 438,
    474-476
Medicare
    benefits, 369, 384, 407, 411, 413-414, 424, 430,
        432-433, 437, 442, 449-454, 457,
        471-472, 475-476
    costs of, 472
    cost-sharing, 414, 424-425, 436, 449-451, 453-455,
        472, 475
    creation of, 426
    defined, 384, 414, 432-433, 444
    dual enrollee, 433
    eligibility, 369, 432-433, 436-437, 442, 444,
        449-450, 453, 458-459, 475
    financing, 368-369, 409, 413, 416, 425, 431-433,
        449, 453-455, 457, 459
    overview, 409, 457
    provider reimbursement, 425, 444
Medicare Part A (Hospital Insurance), 425
    financing, 425
Medicare Payment Advisory Commission, 377
Medications. See also Pharmacies and pharmacists
    forcible administration of, 358
    generics, 186
Medigap coverage, 475
Meditation, 55, 283, 304
mental disability, 438
mental distress, 110, 202
metaethics, 62
microethics, 3
Military Tribunal for War Crimes, 68
Minors. See also Child abuse
    consent by, 87, 333
    emancipated, 332-333
    parental consent for, 82
misdemeanors, 204
misdiagnosis, 41, 311
misfeasance, 192
Moral compass, 60-61
moral dilemmas, 6, 117, 168
Moral integrity, 35, 266
moral judgments, 1
morality
    of abortion, 88
    morning-after pill, 77
Mortality rates
    uninsured, 409
murder, 3, 75, 132-133, 204-205, 354

N
Napoleonic Code, 176
National Health Conference, 412
National Health Insurance Standards Act, 413
National Health Service Corps, 475
National Quality Improvement Strategy, 426
Neanderthal burial sites, 67
negative tolerance, 47
Negligence
    breach of duty, 91, 192, 251, 308
    commission of an act, 191
negligence
    corporate, 249, 255-257, 360
Negligence
    cursory exams, 198
    duty to care, 191-193, 250-251
    of physicians, 271
    omission of an act, 190-192
Negligent sterilization, 90-91
Netherlands, 419
Network HMO, 405
News media and confidentiality, 113
Noncompetition agreements, 219
nonconsequential ethics, 12
nonfeasance, 192
Normative ethics, 7
Notifiable disease, 475

479

CPSIA information can be obtained
at www.ICGtesting.com
Printed in the USA
FSHW021135051019
62638FS